The Complete Guide to ECGs

James H. O'Keefe, Jr., MD
Cardiologist, Mid-America Heart Institute
St. Lukes Hospital, Kansas City, Missouri

Stephen C. Hammill, MD
Director, Electrocardiography and Electrophysiology Laboratories
Mayo Clinic, Rochester, Minnesota

Mark Freed, MD
Cardiologist, William Beaumont Hospital
Royal Oak, Michigan

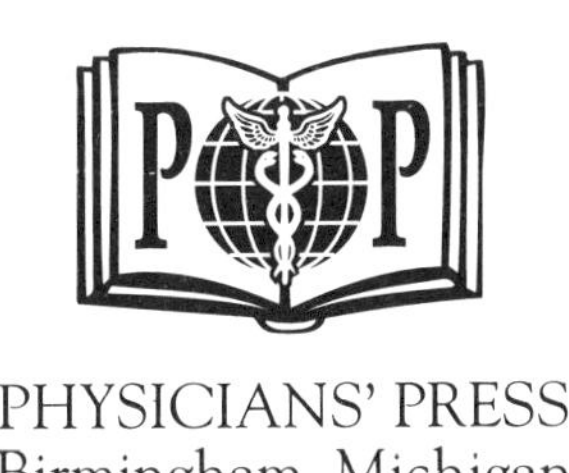

PHYSICIANS' PRESS
Birmingham, Michigan

— About Physicians' Press —

Physicians' Press is a unique entry into the medical publishing industry. Owned and operated by physicians, Physicians' Press specializes in innovative and user-friendly manuals, textbooks, and newsletters in the fields of Clinical Cardiology, Interventional Cardiology, and Internal Medicine. Physicians' Press stands apart from all other medical publishers in being able to produce completely current publications, with literature references ***less than 2 weeks old*** at the time of book release, compared to 18 months old for most other texts! We frequently receive comments such as, "I am astounded at how current your information is...the only books I bother reading are yours, the rest are outdated." Physicians' Press is committed to providing its readers with the most current, practical, and user-friendly information, as we continue to distinguish ourselves as the new gold-standard in medical publishing.

If you are looking for a publisher, or have comments or suggestions you'd like to share, please contact us at:

Physicians' Press
555 South Woodward Ave., Suite 1409
Birmingham, Michigan 48009
Tel: (248) 645-6443
Fax: (248) 642-4949
http://www.physicianspress.com

Printed in the United States of America ISBN: 1-890114-00-6

— Dedication —

To Joan, Jimmy, Evan, and Kathleen; the joys of my life.

James O'Keefe, Jr

To my wife Karen and sons Noel, Eric, Steve, and Danny — thanks for y
and support.

Stephen Hammill

— "Success wasn't meant to be easy, just worth it."

To those who sacrifice in the pursuit of excellence, and to my dear lo
who make the coldest darkest days seem warm and sunny.

Mark Freed

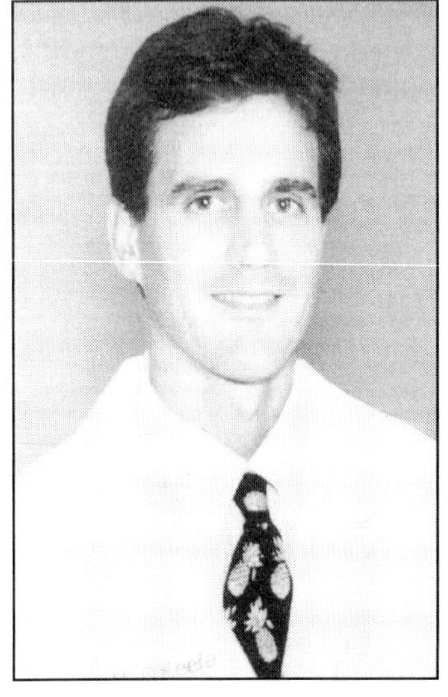

James H. O'Keefe, Jr., MD

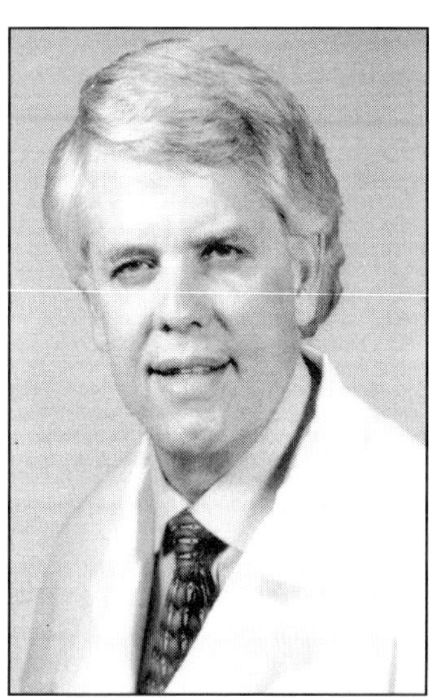

Stephen C. Hammill, MD

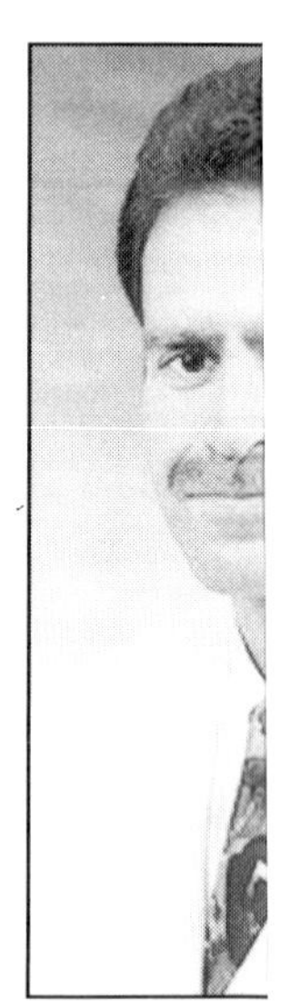

Mark

— Preface —

The Complete Guide to ECGs has been developed as a practical means for clinicians, fellows, residents, interns, medical students, and other medical professionals to improve their ECG interpretation skills. The highly interactive format and comprehensive scope of information are also ideally suited for physicians preparing for the American Board of Internal Medicine Cardiodiovascular Disease or Internal Medicine Board Exams, the American College of Cardiology ECG proficiency test, and other exams requiring ECG interpretation.

This unique reference contains 103 ECGs and more than 1000 questions and answers about specific ECG criteria and interpretive pearls and pitfalls.

We recommend using the answer sheet on many other ECGs in addition to the sample tracings provided. Study groups and regular educational conferences are ideal settings for the presentation of new unknown ECGs and discussion of their correct interpretation. A set of 35 mm slides of each of the ECGs is also available (see ad pages in back of book). Be sure to visit us on the world wide web (www.physicianspress.com), where you'll find an ECG-of-the-week, complete with questions, answers and explanations.

We hope you enjoy reading **The Complete Guide to ECGs** and find it of great practical value.

James O'Keefe, Jr., MD

Stephen Hammill, MD

Mark Freed, MD

— Instructions —

Read each ECG in a thorough and systematic fashion, using the score sheet to record your findings. Be organized. Be compulsive. Be strict in your application of the ECG criteria. And take your time — even the most experienced electrocardiographers miss important ECG diagnoses when hurrying through an interpretation. Be sure to analyze the following 15 features on each ECG:

1. Heart rate
2. P wave morphology and amplitude
3. Origin of the rhythm
4. PR interval
5. QRS width
6. QT interval
7. QRS axis
8. QRS voltage
9. R wave progression in the precordial leads
10. Abnormal Q waves
11. ST segment
12. T wave
13. U wave
14. Baseline
15. Electronic pacemaker

Once these features have been identified, ask yourself the following questions:

1. Is an arrhythmia and/or conduction disturbance present?
2. Is chamber enlargement and/or hypertrophy present?
3. Is ischemia, injury, and/or infarction present?
4. Are any of the clinical disorders (item 14) likely to be present?

It is important to consider each ECG in the context of the clinical history. For example, diffuse ST segment elevation in an asymptomatic patient is likely to represent early repolarization abnormality, whereas the same finding in a patient with chest pain and a friction rub is likely to represent acute pericarditis.

After coding the ECG on the accompanying score sheet, study the correct interpretation and codes on the following page. If ECG diagnoses were missed or improperly selected, turn to the final section of the book and review the appropriate criteria. The ECG criteria expressed in this book represent a consensus among the authors based on previously published literature and their own experience and viewpoints.

Answer the multiple choice, true/false, and fill-in-the-blank questions corresponding to each ECG. Place a check mark next to the questions that were answered incorrectly; at the end of each reading session and at the start of each new reading session, return to these questions and be sure they can be answered correctly. When all the ECGs have been read and all the questions answered, they should be reviewed again until they are mastered.

Common Dilemmas in ECG Interpretation

Questions frequently arise regarding "optimal coding" of ECG tracings, since many specific ECG criteria remain controversial and no single ECG reference standard exists. The following recommendations to some common dilemmas in ECG interpretation represent a consensus among the authors based on previously published literature and their experience and viewpoints.

Problem 1:

Q waves are present in leads V_1 and V_2 only. Should a myocardial infarction be coded?

Recommendation: No. It is important to follow strict coding criteria when interpreting ECGs. To code an anteroseptal myocardial infarction, Q waves must be present in leads V_1, V_2 *and* V_3. In day-to-day clinical medicine, Q waves in V_1 and V_2 are often referred to as "possible" anteroseptal MI or low anterior forces. While this designation is acceptable in clinical cardiology, it is neither acceptable (nor even an option) in standardized testing formats, and an infarct should not be coded.

Problem 2:

The ECG shows an acute myocardial infarction. Should any other ECG diagnoses be coded?

Recommendation: Yes. It is also important to code 12e (ST and/or T abnormalities suggesting myocardial injury) and 14r (coronary artery disease) when acute myocardial infarction is present. Remember to code 12e when ST segment depression is present in leadsV_1 and V_2 in the setting of posterior MI.

Problem 3:

Left bundle branch block is present. Should acute myocardial infarction ever be coded?

Recommendation: No (controversial). Most electrocardiographers are reluctant to diagnosis acute myocardial infarction in the setting of LBBB. However, three criteria have independent value for diagnosing acute myocardial injury (item 7e):

- ST elevation $\geq$ 1 mm concordant to (same direction as) the major deflection of the QRS
- ST depression $\geq$ 1 mm in V_1, V_2, or V_3
- ST elevation $\geq$ 5mm discordant with (opposite direction to) the major deflection of the QRS.

Problem 4:

Acute myocardial infarction is present with ST elevation in one portion of the tracing and ST segment depression in another. Is it necessary to code both ST-T changes suggesting myocardial injury and ST-T changes suggesting myocardial ischemia?

Recommendation: Yes. Many acute myocardial infarctions have significant ST segment elevation in some leads and significant ST segment depression in others. The ST segment depression is usually a manifestation of ischemia adjacent to or remote from the infarct zone. Thus, correct coding for this situation should include item 12d (ST-T abnormalities suggesting myocardial ischemia) and item 12e (ST-T abnormalities suggesting myocardial injury).

Problem 5:

Ischemic-looking ST segment elevation is present without pathological Q waves in a patient with chest pain. Should acute myocardial infarction be coded?

Recommendation: No. Convex upward ST segment elevation without pathological Q waves should be coded as 12e (ST and/or T abnormalities suggesting myocardial injury). Clinically, this usually represents the early stages of acute infarction or transient coronary spasm or occlusion. Nevertheless, in the absence of pathological Q waves (or pathological R waves in the case of posterior infarction), acute myocardial infarction should not be coded. Ischemic ST elevation alone, however, should prompt coding of 14r (coronary artery disease).

Problem 6:

With so many different criteria for the diagnosis of LVH, which should be used as the "gold-standard?"

Recommendation: The Cornell criteria (R wave in aVL + S wave in V_3 > than 24 mm in males and > 20 mm in females) is probably the most accurate of the voltage criteria. However, many ECGs meet voltage criteria in one area of the tracing but not in the others. Therefore, the best policy is know most or all of the various criteria used for the diagnosis of LVH. Remember to code item 10b (LVH with ST-T abnormalities) *and* item 12g (ST-T abnormalities secondary to IVCD or hypertrophy) when LVH with a "strain" pattern is present.

Problem 7:

What are the most important criteria for diagnosing RVH?

Recommendation: RVH, like LVH, is difficult to diagnosis due to the numerous different criteria that have been proposed. No single finding is diagnostic of RVH. Essential elements include right axis deviation, and a dominant R wave with secondary ST-T changes in leads V_1 and V_2. Right atrial abnormality is also commonly seen.

Problem 8:

Mobitz Type I second-degree AV block is present. Should first-degree AV block also be coded if the PR interval exceeds 0.20 seconds?

Recommendation: Not necessarily. Mobitz Type I second-degree AV block (Wenckebach) can occur with or without first-degree AV block. If the ***shortest*** PR interval — usually the first PR interval after a nonconducted P wave — exceeds 0.20 seconds, first-degree AV block (item 6a) should be coded.

Problem 9:

A dominant junctional or ventricular rhythm is present. Is it necessary to code the underlying atrial rhythm if one is present?

Recommendation: Yes. If in addition to the presence of a dominant junctional or ventricular rhythm, an atrial rhythm is also apparent, the atrial rhythm should also be coded (e.g., ventricular tachycardia and sinus rhythm). This applies to significant AV block as well (e.g., sinus tachycardia with third-degree AV block).

Problem 10:

Should left axis deviation be coded when left anterior fascicular block is present? Similarly, should right axis deviation be coded when left posterior fascicular block is present?

Recommendation: Yes. The QRS axis is merely a descriptor of the major QRS vector. If left anterior fascicular block or left posterior fascicular block is present, the axis should also be coded.

Problem 11:

Wolff-Parkinson-White pattern is present. How should the associated ST-T abnormalities be coded? When should myocardial infarction be coded?

Recommendation: The ECG pattern noted in WPW is usually associated with ST-T abnormalities, which are most appropriately coded as item 12g (ST-T abnormalities secondary to IVCD or hypertrophy). WPW results in abnormal interventricular conduction due to the coalescence of two electrical wavefronts entering the ventricle from different locations. Therefore, fusion complexes (item 5a) should also be coded. Acute MI should not be diagnosed in the presence of WPW; negative delta waves are frequently mistaken for Q waves ("pseudoinfarction" pattern).

Problem 12:

Atrial fibrillation is present with intermittent episodes of atrial flutter. Should atrial fibrillation or atrial flutter be coded?

Recommendation: Atrial fibrillation. Atrial fibrillation often manifests as "fib/flutter;" however, on formal testing, you must choose one or the other. The best strategy in this setting is to code atrial fibrillation; atrial flutter should be reserved for tracings that show continuous atrial flutter without interspersed episodes of fibrillation.

— Acknowledgments —

We would like to express our deep and sincere gratitude to David M. Steinhaus, MD, and Robert C. Canby, MD, clinical electrophysiologists at the Mid-America Heart Institute, St. Lukes Hospital, Kansas City, Missouri, for their thoughtful comments and suggestions, and their careful review of the manuscript. We also wish to acknowledge Lori Maher, Dianna Frye, and Monica Crowder for their outstanding work in typing and formatting this guide, and Norm Lyle of The Lyle Group for the cover art, cartoons and ad pages. Finally, we wish to acknowledge Dickinson Press, particularly Mike DeFoe, for their printing expertise and for ensuring high-quality reproduction of the ECG tracings. We are indebted to these individuals, and hope their efforts are well-received.

James O'Keefe, Jr., MD
Stephen Hammill, MD
Mark Freed, MD

— Notice —

The ECG interpretations and criteria expressed in this book represent a consensus among the authors based on previously published literature and their own experience and viewpoints. The authors and publisher disclaim responsibility for adverse effects resulting from omissions or undetected errors or adverse results obtained from the use of such information. Readers are encouraged to review other references on ECG interpretation to further expand their knowlege and interpretation skills.

— Abbreviations —

APC	*Atrial premature contraction*	**RVH**	*Right ventricular hypertrophy*
AV	*Atrioventricular*	**SA**	*Sinoatrial*
COPD	*Chronic obstructive pulmonary*	**SVT**	*Supraventricular tachycardia*
LAFB	*Left anterior fascicular block*	**VA**	*Ventriculoatrial*
LBBB	*Left bundle branch block*	**VF**	*Ventricular fibrillation*
LPFB	*Left posterior fascicular block*	**VPC**	*Ventricular premature contraction*
LVH	*Left ventricular hypertrophy*	**VT**	*Ventricular tachycardia*
MI	*Myocardial infarction*	**WPW**	*Wolff-Parkinson-White*
RBBB	*Right bundle branch block*		

— Nomenclature —

The relative amplitudes of the component waves of the QRS complex are described using small (lower case) and large (upper case) letters. For example: an "rS complex" describes a QRS with a small R wave and a large S wave; a "qRs complex" describes a QRS with a small Q wave, a large R wave, and a small S wave; and an "RSR' complex" describes a QRS with a large R wave, a large S wave, and a large secondary R wave (R'). When the QRS complex consists solely of a Q wave, a "QS" designation is used.

— Section I —

So You Think You Know ECGs...

ECG 1. 46-year-old male in the emergency room with chest discomfort:

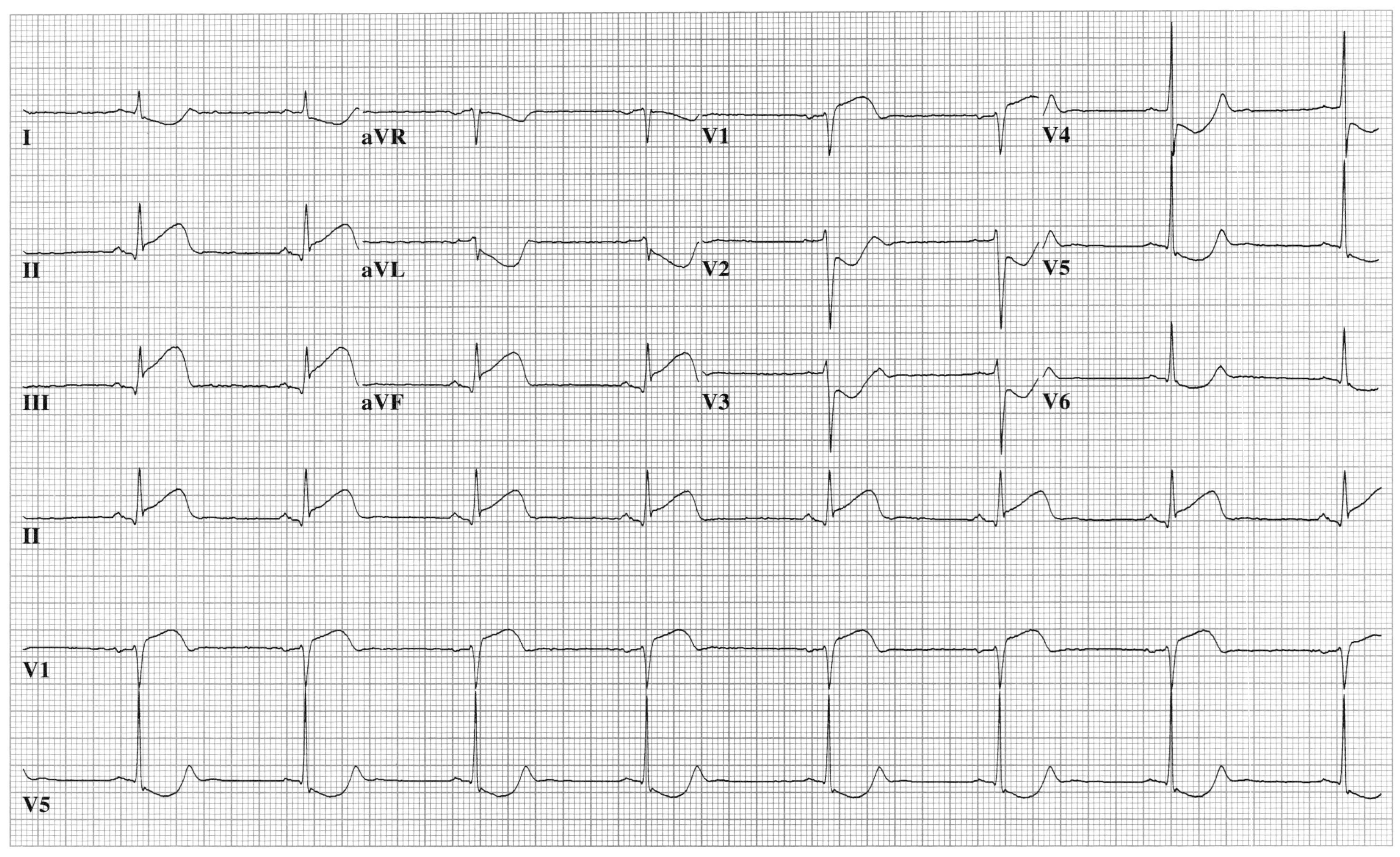

1. GENERAL FEATURES
- ☐ a. Normal ECG
- ☐ b. Borderline normal ECG or normal variant
- ☐ c. Incorrect electrode placement
- ☐ d. Artifact due to tremor

2. ATRIAL RHYTHMS
- ☐ a. Sinus rhythm
- ☐ b. Sinus arrhythmia
- ☐ c. Sinus bradycardia (< 60)
- ☐ d. Sinus tachycardia (> 100)
- ☐ e. Sinus pause or arrest
- ☐ f. Sinoatrial exit block
- ☐ g. Ecoptic atrial rhythm
- ☐ h. Wandering atrial pacemaker
- ☐ i. Atrial premature complexes, normally conducted
- ☐ j. Atrial premature complexes, nonconducted
- ☐ k. Atrial premature complexes with aberrant intraventricular conduction
- ☐ l. Atrial tachycardia (regular, sustained, 1:1 conduction)
- ☐ m. Atrial tachycardia, repetitive (short paroxysms)
- ☐ n. Atrial tachycardia, multifocal
- ☐ o. Atrial tachycardia with AV block
- ☐ p. Supraventricular tachycardia, unspecific
- ☐ q. Supraventricular tachycardia, paroxysmal
- ☐ r. Atrial flutter
- ☐ s. Atrial fibrillation
- ☐ t. Retrograde atrial activation

3. AV JUNCTIONAL RHYTHMS
- ☐ a. AV junctional premature complexes
- ☐ b. AV junctional escape complexes
- ☐ c. AV junctional rhythm, accelerated
- ☐ d. AV junctional rhythm

4. VENTRICULAR RHYTHMS
- ☐ a. Ventricular premature complex(es), uniform, fixed coupling
- ☐ b. Ventricular premature complex(es), uniform, nonfixed coupling
- ☐ c. Ventricular premature complexes(es), multiform
- ☐ d. Ventricular premature complexes, in pairs
- ☐ e. Ventricular parasystole
- ☐ f. Ventricular tachycardia (≥ 3 consecutive complexes)
- ☐ g. Accelerated idioventricular rhythm
- ☐ h. Ventricular escape complexes or rhythm
- ☐ i. Ventricular fibrillation

5. ATRIAL-VENTRICULAR INTERACTIONS IN ARRHYTHMIAS
- ☐ a. Fusion complexes
- ☐ b. Reciprocal (echo) complexes
- ☐ c. Ventricular capture complexes
- ☐ d. AV dissociation
- ☐ e. Ventriculophasic sinus arrhythmia

6. AV CONDUCTION ABNORMALITIES
- ☐ a. AV block, 1°
- ☐ b. AV block, 2° - Mobitz type I (Wenckebach)
- ☐ c. AV block, 2° - Mobitz type II
- ☐ d. AV block, 2:1
- ☐ e. AV block, 3°
- ☐ f. AV block, variable
- ☐ g. Short PR interval (with sinus rhythm and normal QRS duration)
- ☐ h. Wolff-Parkinson-White pattern

7. INTRAVENTRICULAR CONDUCTION DISTURBANCES
- ☐ a. RBBB, incomplete
- ☐ b. RBBB, complete
- ☐ c. Left anterior fascicular block
- ☐ d. Left posterior fascicular block
- ☐ e. LBBB, with ST-T wave suggestive of acute myocardial injury or infarction
- ☐ f. LBBB, complete
- ☐ g. LBBB, intermittent
- ☐ h. Intraventricular conduction disturbance, nonspecific
- ☐ i. Aberrant intraventricular conduction with supraventricular arrhythmia

8. P WAVE ABNORMALITIES
- ☐ a. Right atrial abnormality
- ☐ b. Left atrial abnormalities
- ☐ c. Nonspecific atrial abnormality

9. ABNORMALITIES OF QRS VOLTAGE OR AXIS
- ☐ a. Low voltage, limb leads only
- ☐ b. Low voltage, limb and precordial leads
- ☐ c. Left axis deviation (> - 30%)
- ☐ d. Right axis deviation (> + 100)
- ☐ e. Electrical alternans

10. VENTRICULAR HYPERTROPHY
- ☐ a. LVH by voltage only
- ☐ b. LVH by voltage and ST-T segment abnormalities
- ☐ c. RVH
- ☐ d. Combined ventricular hypertrophy

11. Q WAVE MYOCARDIAL INFARCTION

	Probably Acute or Recent	Probably Old or Age Indeterminate
Anterolateral	☐ a.	☐ g.
Anterior	☐ b.	☐ h
Anteroseptal	☐ c.	☐ i.
Lateral/High lateral	☐ d.	☐ j.
Inferior	☐ e.	☐ k
Posterior	☐ f.	☐ l.

- ☐ m. Probably ventricular aneurysm

12. ST, T, U, WAVE ABNORMALITIES
- ☐ a. Normal variant, early repolarization
- ☐ b. Normal variant, juvenile T waves
- ☐ c. Nonspecific ST and/or T wave abnormalities
- ☐ d. ST and/or T wave abnormalities suggesting myocardial ischemia
- ☐ e. ST and/or T wave abnormalities suggesting myocardial injury
- ☐ f. ST and/or T wave abnormalities suggesting acute pericarditis
- ☐ g. ST-T segment abnormalities secondary to intraventricular conduction disturbance or hypertrophy
- ☐ h. Post-extrasystolic T wave abnormality
- ☐ i. Isolated J point depression
- ☐ j. Peaked T waves
- ☐ k. Prolonged QT interval
- ☐ l. Prominent U waves

13. PACEMAKER FUNCTION AND RHYTHM
- ☐ a. Atrial or coronary sinus pacing
- ☐ b. Ventricular demand pacing
- ☐ c. AV sequential pacing
- ☐ d. Ventricular pacing, complete control
- ☐ e. Dual chamber, atrial sensing pacemaker
- ☐ f. Pacemaker malfunction, not constantly capturing (atrium or ventricle)
- ☐ g. Pacemaker malfunction, not constantly sensing (atrium or ventricle)
- ☐ h. Pacemaker malfunction, not firing
- ☐ i. Pacemaker malfunction, slowing

14. SUGGESTED OR PROBABLE CLINICAL DISORDERS
- ☐ a. Digitalis effect
- ☐ b. Digitalis toxicity
- ☐ c. Antiarrhythmic drug effect
- ☐ d. Antiarrhythmic drug toxicity
- ☐ e. Hyperkalemia
- ☐ f. Hypokalemia
- ☐ g. Hypercalcemia
- ☐ h. Hypocalcemia
- ☐ i. Atrial septal defect, secundum
- ☐ j. Atrial septal defect, primum
- ☐ k. Dextrocardia, mirror image
- ☐ l. Mitral valve disease
- ☐ m. Chronic lung disease
- ☐ n. Acute cor pulmonale, including pulmonary embolus
- ☐ o. Pericardial effusion
- ☐ p. Acute pericarditis
- ☐ q. Hypertrophic cardiomyopathy
- ☐ r. Coronary artery disease
- ☐ s. Central nervous system disorder
- ☐ t. Myxedema
- ☐ u. Hypothermia
- ☐ v. Sick sinus syndrome

ECG 1 was obtained in a 46-year-old male who is being evaluated in the emergency department with chest discomfort. The ECG shows sinus bradycardia at 47 beats/minute with findings compatible with an acute posterior and inferior myocardial infarction with evolving Q waves. ST segment changes suggesting injury and coronary artery disease are also present. The Q waves inferiorly (arrows) and the R wave in V_1 (arrowhead) do not yet meet criteria for inferoposterior myocardial infarction (although they probably would within an hour or two after this tracing). Thus, criteria are not yet met for acute infarction. Of interest, the ST elevation in V_1 is likely due to right ventricular infarction.

Codes:

2c	Sinus bradycardia
12e	ST and/or T wave abnormalities suggesting myocardial injury
14r	Coronary artery disease

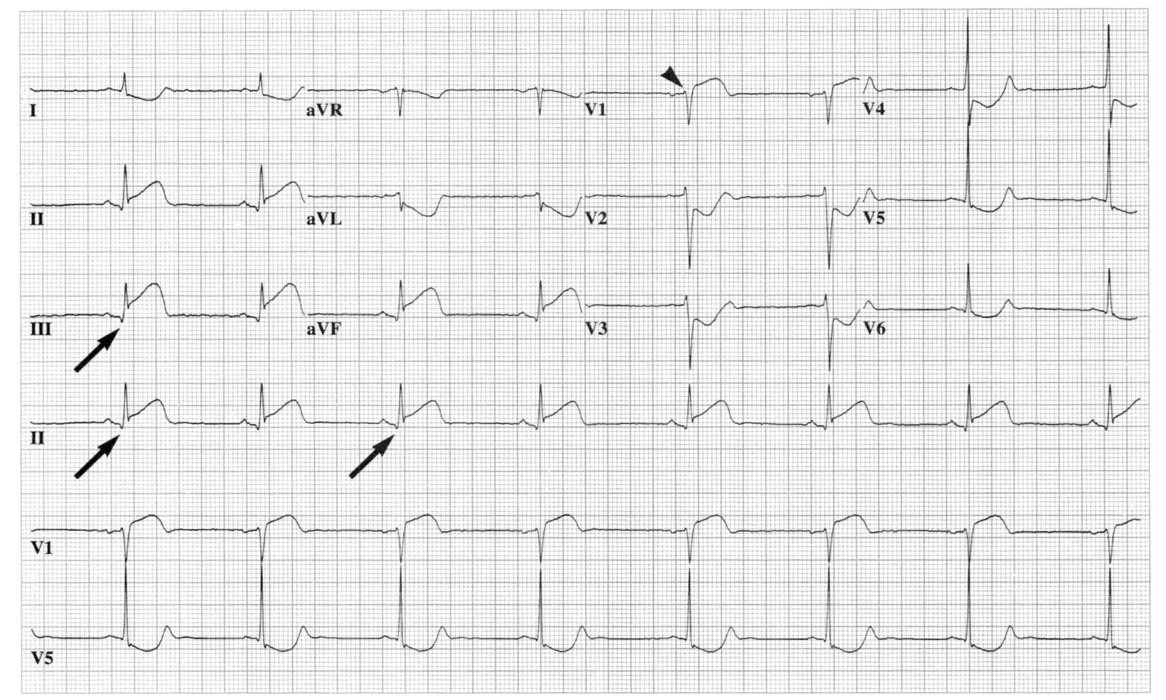

Questions: ECG 1

1. Isoelectric ST segments and deep T wave inversion associated with Q waves are suggestive of:

   a. Recent MI
   b. Acute MI
   c. Old MI

2. Upwardly concave ST elevation is typically seen in the setting of:

   a. Acute MI
   b. Pericarditis
   c. Normal variant
   d. Coronary spasm

Answers: ECG 1

1. The repolarization abnormalities associated with acute myocardial infarction typically evolve in a relatively predictable fashion. Usually, the earliest finding is marked peaking of the T waves ("hyperacute T waves") in the region of the infarct; these are often missed since they occur very early in the course of the acute event and are transient. If transmural ischemia persists for more than a few minutes, the peaked T waves evolve into ST segment elevation, which should be $\geq$1 mm in height to be considered significant. The ST segment elevation of myocardial infarction is usually upwardly ***convex***, in contrast to acute pericarditis or normal variant early repolarization, in which the ST elevation is usually upwardly ***concave***. As the acute infarction continues to evolve, the ST segment elevation decreases and the T waves begin to invert. The T waves usually become progressively deeper as the ST segment elevation subsides. An isoelectric ST segment with upward convexity and deeply inverted T waves is often associated with subacute or recent myocardial infarction; however, sometimes these changes persist for weeks or months. (Answer: a)

2. Upwardly concave ST segment elevation is typically seen in the setting of pericarditis or normal variant early repolarization abnormality. In contrast, the ST segment elevation of transmural ischemia or acute myocardial infarction is typically upwardly convex (although the ST segment may still be somewhat concave

in configuration in the early stages of acute infarction). Other clues to help distinguish pericarditis or normal variant findings from acute infarction include: (1) the diffuseness of ST elevation (generally in a few leads — acute infarction; in all or almost all leads except aVR — pericarditis; in V_2 - V_5 and the inferior leads — early repolarization); (2) the presence of reciprocal ST depression (often present in acute MI but not pericarditis or early repolarization); and (3) the presence of PR depression (often present in acute pericarditis, sometimes in early repolarization, and rarely in early acute MI). (Answer: b, c)

— Quick Review 1 —

Sinus bradycardia	
• Rate < ____ per minute	60
• If sinus rate is < 40 per minute, think of 2:1 ____	sinoatrial exit block
ST and/or T wave changes suggesting myocardial injury	
• Acute ST segment (elevation/depression) with upward (convexity/concavity) in the leads representing the area of infarction	elevation convexity
• T waves invert (before/after) ST segments return to baseline	before
• Associated ST (elevation/depression) in the noninfarct leads is common	depression
• Acute ____ wall injury often has horizontal or downsloping ST segment depression with upright T waves in V_1-V_3, with or without a prominent R wave in these same leads	posterior

— POP QUIZ —

Make The Diagnosis

<u>Instructions</u>: Determine the clinical disorder that best corresponds to the ECG features listed below (see item 14 of score sheet for options)

ECG Features	Answer
• "Classic changes" usually occur in the precordial leads ‣ Large upright or deeply inverted T waves ‣ Prolonged QT interval (often marked) ‣ Prominent U waves • Other changes: ‣ ST segment changes: • Can mimic acute pericarditis or acute injury_ • ST depression may also occur ‣ Abnormal Q waves mimicking MI ‣ Almost any rhythm abnormality including sinus tachycardia or bradycardia, junctional rhythm, VPCs, ventricular tachycardia, etc.	CNS disorder
• Low QRS voltage in all leads • Sinus bradycardia • T wave flattened or inverted • PR interval may be prolonged • Frequently associated with pericardial effusion • Electrical alternans may occur	Myxedema
• Sinus bradycardia • PR, QRS, and QT prolonged) • Osborne ("J") wave: late upright terminal deflection of QRS complex • Atrial fibrillation in 50-60%	Hypothermia

ECG 2. 48-year-old man with a history of aortic valve disease:

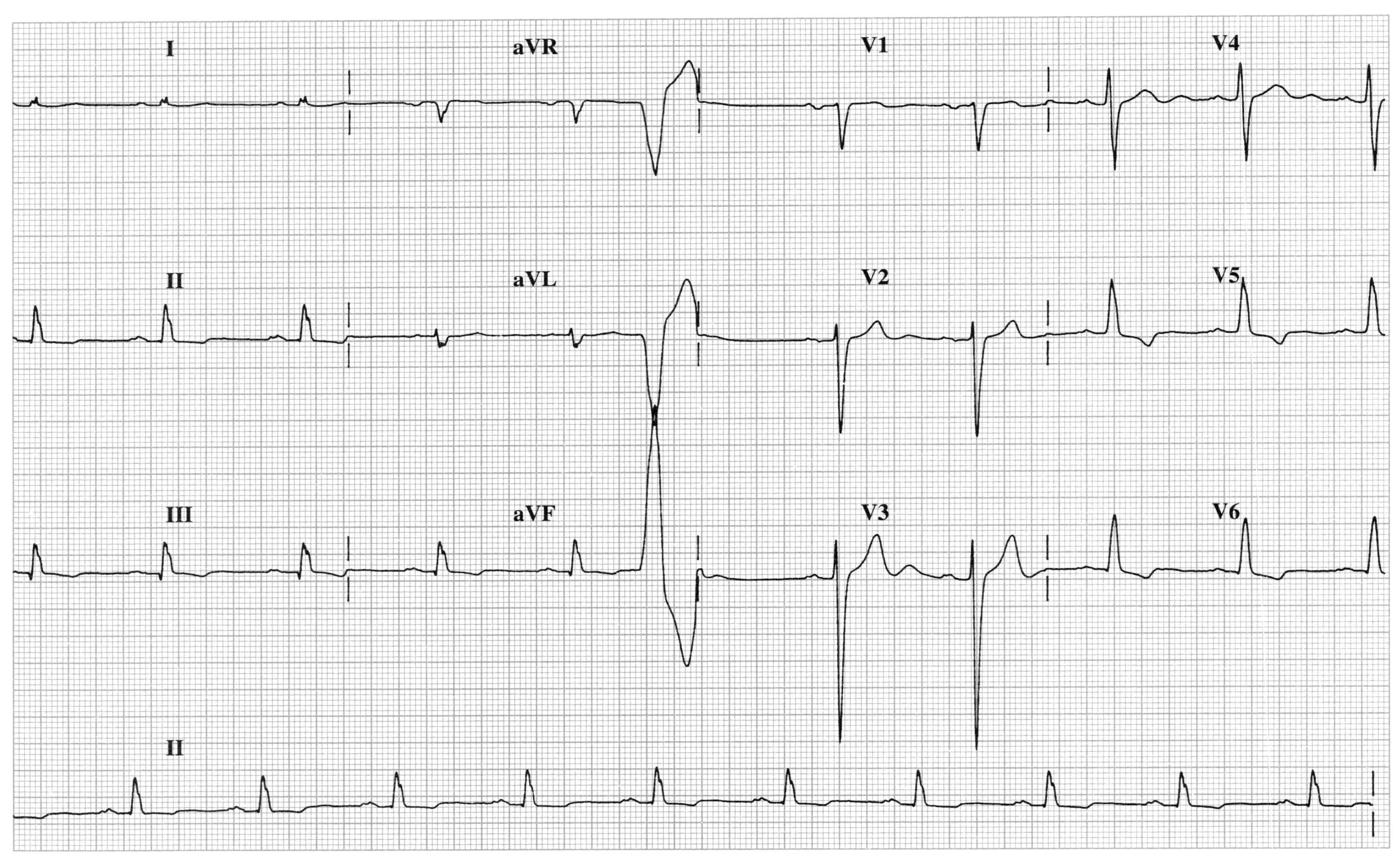

1. GENERAL FEATURES

☐ a. Normal ECG
☐ b. Borderline normal ECG or normal variant
☐ c. Incorrect electrode placement
☐ d. Artifact due to tremor

2. ATRIAL RHYTHMS

☐ a. Sinus rhythm
☐ b. Sinus arrhythmia
☐ c. Sinus bradycardia (< 60)
☐ d. Sinus tachycardia (> 100)
☐ e. Sinus pause or arrest
☐ f. Sinoatrial exit block
☐ g. Ecoptic atrial rhythm
☐ h. Wandering atrial pacemaker
☐ i. Atrial premature complexes, normally conducted
☐ j. Atrial premature complexes, nonconducted
☐ k. Atrial premature complexes with aberrant intraventricular conduction
☐ l. Atrial tachycardia (regular, sustained, 1:1 conduction)
☐ m. Atrial tachycardia, repetitive (short paroxysms)
☐ n. Atrial tachycardia, multifocal
☐ o. Atrial tachycardia with AV block
☐ p. Supraventricular tachycardia, unspecific
☐ q. Supraventricular tachycardia, paroxysmal
☐ r. Atrial flutter
☐ s. Atrial fibrillation
☐ t. Retrograde atrial activation

3. AV JUNCTIONAL RHYTHMS

☐ a. AV junctional premature complexes
☐ b. AV junctional escape complexes
☐ c. AV junctional rhythm, accelerated
☐ d. AV junctional rhythm

4. VENTRICULAR RHYTHMS

☐ a. Ventricular premature complex(es), uniform, fixed coupling
☐ b. Ventricular premature complex(es), uniform, nonfixed coupling
☐ c. Ventricular premature complexes(es), multiform
☐ d. Ventricular premature complexes, in pairs
☐ e. Ventricular parasystole
☐ f. Ventricular tachycardia (≥ 3 consecutive complexes)
☐ g. Accelerated idioventricular rhythm
☐ h. Ventricular escape complexes or rhythm
☐ i. Ventricular fibrillation

5. ATRIAL-VENTRICULAR INTERACTIONS IN ARRHYTHMIAS

☐ a. Fusion complexes
☐ b. Reciprocal (echo) complexes
☐ c. Ventricular capture complexes
☐ d. AV dissociation

☐ e. Ventriculophasic sinus arrhythmia

6. AV CONDUCTION ABNORMALITIES

☐ a. AV block, 1°
☐ b. AV block, 2° - Mobitz type I (Wenckebach)
☐ c. AV block, 2° - Mobitz type II
☐ d. AV block, 2:1
☐ e. AV block, 3°
☐ f. AV block, variable
☐ g. Short PR interval (with sinus rhythm and normal QRS duration)
☐ h. Wolff-Parkinson-White pattern

7. INTRAVENTRICULAR CONDUCTION DISTURBANCES

☐ a. RBBB, incomplete
☐ b. RBBB, complete
☐ c. Left anterior fascicular block
☐ d. Left posterior fascicular block
☐ e. LBBB, with ST-T wave suggestive of acute myocardial injury or infarction
☐ f. LBBB, complete
☐ g. LBBB, intermittent
☐ h. Intraventricular conduction disturbance, nonspecific
☐ i. Aberrant intraventricular conduction with supraventricular arrhythmia

8. P WAVE ABNORMALITIES

☐ a. Right atrial abnormality
☐ b. Left atrial abnormalities
☐ c. Nonspecific atrial abnormality

9. ABNORMALITIES OF QRS VOLTAGE OR AXIS

☐ a. Low voltage, limb leads only
☐ b. Low voltage, limb and precordial leads
☐ c. Left axis deviation (> - 30%)
☐ d. Right axis deviation (> + 100)
☐ e. Electrical alternans

10. VENTRICULAR HYPERTROPHY

☐ a. LVH by voltage only
☐ b. LVH by voltage and ST-T segment abnormalities
☐ c. RVH
☐ d. Combined ventricular hypertrophy

11. Q WAVE MYOCARDIAL INFARCTION

	Probably Acute or Recent	Probably Old or Age Indeterminate
Anterolateral	☐ a.	☐ g.
Anterior	☐ b.	☐ h.
Anteroseptal	☐ c.	☐ i.
Lateral/High lateral	☐ d.	☐ j.
Inferior	☐ e.	☐ k.
Posterior	☐ f.	☐ l.

☐ m. Probably ventricular aneurysm

12. ST, T, U, WAVE ABNORMALITIES

☐ a. Normal variant, early repolarization
☐ b. Normal variant, juvenile T waves
☐ c. Nonspecific ST and/or T wave abnormalities
☐ d. ST and/or T wave abnormalities suggesting myocardial ischemia
☐ e. ST and/or T wave abnormalities suggesting myocardial injury
☐ f. ST and/or T wave abnormalities suggesting acute pericarditis
☐ g. ST-T segment abnormalities secondary to intraventricular conduction disturbance or hypertrophy
☐ h. Post-extrasystolic T wave abnormality
☐ i. Isolated J point depression
☐ j. Peaked T waves
☐ k. Prolonged QT interval
☐ l. Prominent U waves

13. PACEMAKER FUNCTION AND RHYTHM

☐ a. Atrial or coronary sinus pacing
☐ b. Ventricular demand pacing
☐ c. AV sequential pacing
☐ d. Ventricular pacing, complete control
☐ e. Dual chamber, atrial sensing pacemaker
☐ f. Pacemaker malfunction, not constantly capturing (atrium or ventricle)
☐ g. Pacemaker malfunction, not constantly sensing (atrium or ventricle)
☐ h. Pacemaker malfunction, not firing
☐ i. Pacemaker malfunction, slowing

14. SUGGESTED OR PROBABLE CLINICAL DISORDERS

☐ a. Digitalis effect
☐ b. Digitalis toxicity
☐ c. Antiarrhythmic drug effect
☐ d. Antiarrhythmic drug toxicity
☐ e. Hyperkalemia
☐ f. Hypokalemia
☐ g. Hypercalcemia
☐ h. Hypocalcemia
☐ i. Atrial septal defect, secundum
☐ j. Atrial septal defect, primum
☐ k. Dextrocardia, mirror image
☐ l. Mitral valve disease
☐ m. Chronic lung disease
☐ n. Acute cor pulmonale, including pulmonary embolus
☐ o. Pericardial effusion
☐ p. Acute pericarditis
☐ q. Hypertrophic cardiomyopathy
☐ r. Coronary artery disease
☐ s. Central nervous system disorder
☐ t. Myxedema
☐ u. Hypothermia
☐ v. Sick sinus syndrome

ECG 2 was obtained in a 48-year-old male with a history of aortic valve disease. The ECG shows a sinus rhythm with a single ventricular premature complex. LVH is apparent with an R wave in aVL + S wave in $V_3 > 24$ mm (Cornell criteria). Repolarization abnormalities (downsloping ST depression and asymmetrical T wave inversion) secondary to LVH are present (arrows) as well as prominent U waves (arrowhead), a common finding in LVH.

Codes:

2a	Sinus rhythm
4a	Ventricular premature complex(es), uniform, fixed coupling
10b	LVH by both voltage and ST-T segment abnormalities
12g	ST-T segment abnormalities secondary to IVCD or hypertrophy
12l	Prominent U waves

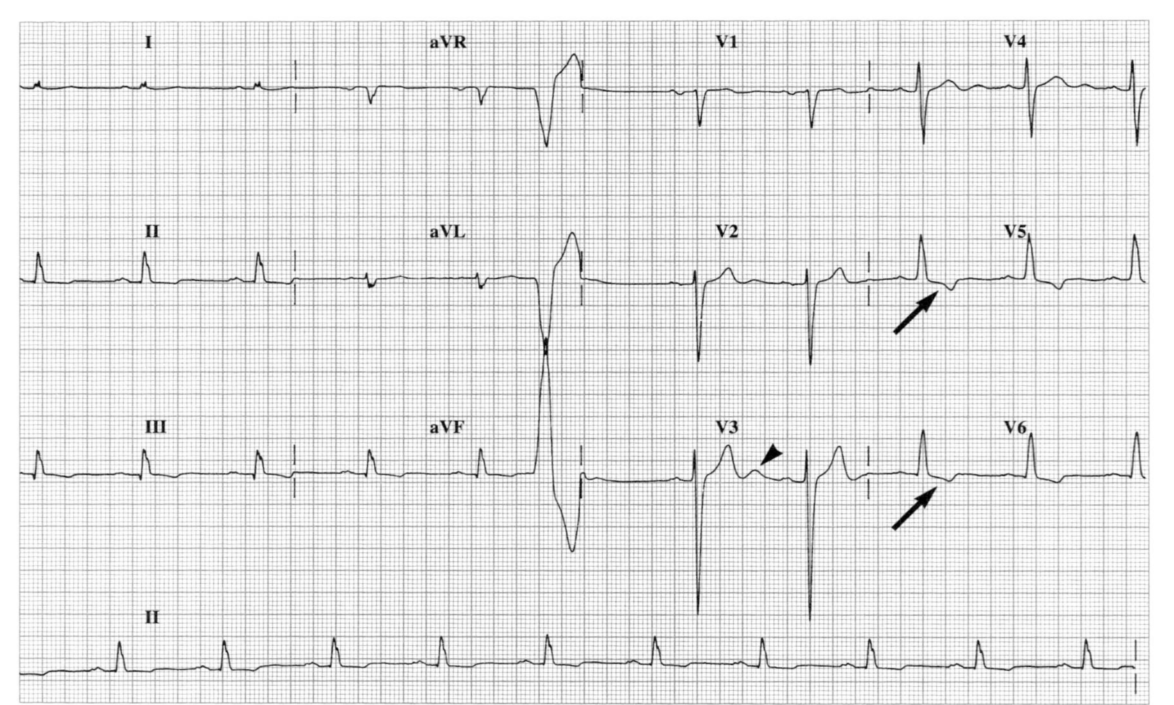

Questions: ECG 2

1. Findings in this ECG that can be attributed to LVH include:

   a. Left atrial abnormality
   b. Prominent U wave
   c. ST segment depression and T wave inversion
   d. Intraventricular conduction delay
   e. Poor R wave progression
   f. Absent Q wave in V_5
   g. ST elevation in V_3

2. The differential diagnosis for prominent U waves includes:

   a. Hypokalemia
   b. Hyperkalemia
   c. Digitalis
   d. Quinidine
   e. Amiodarone
   f. Central nervous system disorders
   g. LVH

3. Anatomical LVH is more likely to be present when repolarization (ST and T wave) changes exist in addition to voltage criteria:

   a. True
   b. False

4. Which of the following ECG criteria is most specific (i.e., fewest false-positives) for the diagnosis of LVH?

   a. R in V_5 or V_6 + S in V_1 > 35 mm
   b. R in aVL > 12 mm
   c. Any R + S in the precordial leads > 45 mm
   d. R in aVL + S in V_3 > 24 mm (20 mm in females)

5. Which of the following ECG criteria is the most sensitive (i.e., fewest false-negatives) for the diagnosis of LVH?

   a. R in V_5 or V_6 + S in V_1 > 35 mm
   b. R in aVL > 12 mm
   c. Any R + S in the precordial leads > 45 mm
   d. Left axis deviation > -30°
   e. R in aVL + S in V_3 > 24 mm (> 20 mm in females)

6. Factors/conditions reducing the sensitivity for the diagnosis of LVH by voltage criteria include:

   a. Obesity
   b. Thin body habitus
   c. Severe COPD
   d. Pericardial or plural effusion
   e. Coronary artery disease
   f. Pneumothorax

g. Sarcoidosis or amyloidosis of the heart
h. Severe right ventricular hypertrophy
i. Left bundle branch block
j. Left anterior fascicular block

7. Patients with LVH on ECG have higher 5-10 year mortality rates than those without LVH:

   a. True
   b. False

Answers: ECG 2

1. The ECG diagnosis of left ventricular hypertrophy (LVH) is based primarily on the presence of large amplitude QRS complexes generated from the hypertrophic left ventricle. LVH also frequently results in non-voltage based changes, some of which are evident in this ECG tracing. ***Left atrial abnormality***, while not a direct manifestation of LVH, increases the probability that LVH is present, and is given 3 points in the point score system for LVH by Romhilt and Estes (Table 1). A ***prominent U wave*** is often seen in the right precordial leads (V_2, V_3) but is neither sensitive nor specific for the diagnosis of LVH. ***ST and T wave changes*** are very common in advanced stages of LVH; when present, the ECG specificity for the diagnosis of anatomical LVH is increased: In the left precordial leads (V_4 - V_6), these changes typically consist of downsloping ST segment depression with a slight upward concavity, and asymmetrical T wave inversion, with more gentle sloping of the descending limb compared to the ascending limb. In the right precordial leads (V_1 - V_3), reciprocal ST segment elevation and tall T waves are often seen, which, in conjunction with ***poor R wave progression*** (or even Q waves or QS complexes) may mimic anteroseptal or anterior MI. In the limb leads, ST and T wave changes appear in a direction opposite from the main QRS forces (i.e., in leads with largely positive QRS complexes, ST depression and T wave inversion are present; in leads with largely negative QRS complexes, ST elevation and tall T waves are present). Other changes in this ECG consistent with LVH include ***delayed onset of intrinsicoid deflection*** (onset of QRS to peak R wave $\geq$ 0.05 seconds; due to a delay in intraventricular conduction), and ***inferior Q waves***, the mechanism of which is unknown. Findings not present in this tracing but often evident in LVH include ***notching of the QRS complex*** and ***left axis deviation***. (Answer: All)

2. Mild hyperkalemia (5.5 - 6.5 mEq/L) can result in T waves that are tall, peaked, and symmetrical, and shortening of the QT interval. Moderate hyperkalemia (6.5 - 8.0 mEq/L) can result in a decrease in P wave and R wave amplitudes, lengthening of the PR interval and QRS duration, and depression or elevation of the ST segment; ventricular premature complexes may also be seen. In severe hyperkalemia, the P wave may be undetectable and the QRS complex markedly widened, giving the appearance of a sine wave. Rhythms may include sinoventricular rhythm (no P waves apparent), idioventricular rhythm, accelerated idioventricular

rhythm, ventricular tachycardia, ventricular fibrillation, and asystole. U waves, however, are not typically seen. (Answer: All except b)

3. As shown in Table 1, the sensitivity and specificity for the ECG diagnosis of anatomical LVH depend on the ECG criteria. Although ST and T wave changes "typical" for LVH may be caused by other conditions (e.g., myocardial ischemia), their presence increases the specificity for the diagnosis of LVH by voltage criteria. (Answer: a)

4. As shown in Table 1, an R wave in aVL ≥ 12 mm in the absence of left anterior fascicular block is highly specific for the diagnosis of LVH. However, only 11% of individuals with LVH. meet this criteria (i.e., poor sensitivity). **CAVEAT:** Since the presence of left anterior fascicular block results in large leftward forces (R waves) in leads I and aVL, voltage criteria using these leads (i.e., R wave in aVL > 12 mm; R wave in lead I + S wave in lead III > 25 mm; R wave in aVL + S wave in V_3 > 24 mm [Cornell criteria]) will overestimate the diagnosis of LVH. (Answer: b)

5. As shown in Table 1, an R wave in V_5 or V_6 + S wave in V_1 > 35 mm, or any R + S wave in the precordial leads > 45 mm has equally high sensitivity (~ 45%) for the diagnosis of LVH. (Answer: a, c)

6. The amplitude of the QRS as recorded by the surface electrocardiogram (and the sensitivity for the diagnosis of LVH by voltage criteria) is often decreased by conditions that increase the amount of body tissue (obesity), air (COPD, pneumothorax), fluid (pericardial or plural effusion), or fibrous tissue (coronary artery disease, sarcoid or amyloid of the heart) between the myocardium and ECG electrodes. Severe RVH can also underestimate the ECG diagnosis of LVH by cancelling prominent QRS forces from the thickened LV. Left bundle branch block may also reduce QRS amplitude as well. In contrast, thin body habitus and the presence of left anterior fascicular block may increase QRS amplitude in the absence of LVH, thus decreasing the specificity of the voltage criteria. (Answer: All except b and j)

Table 1. Sensitivity & Specificity for Selected Criteria for LVH

Criterion	Sensitivity (%)	Specificity (%) (false-positives)
S in V_1 + R in V_5 or V_6 > 35 mm	43	5
Any R + S > 45 mm	45	7
R in aVL + S in V_3 > 24 mm (> 20 mm in females)	20	2
R in I + S in III > 25 mm	11	0
S in aVR > 14 mm	7	0
R in aVL > 11 mm	11	0
R in aVF > 20 mm	1	1

Adapted from Romhilt et al. Circulation 1969;40:185.

7. Answer: True

— Quick Review 2 —

LVH by both voltage and ST-T segment abnormalities	
• Voltage criteria for LVH and one or more ST-T abnormalities:	
▸ ST segment and T wave deviation in (same/opposite) direction to the major deflection of QRS	opposite
▸ ST segment (elevation/depression) in leads I, aVL, III, aVF, and/or V_4-V_6	depression
▸ Subtle (< 1-2 mm) ST (elevation/depression) in leads V_1-V_3	elevation
▸ Inverted ____ waves in leads I, aVL, V_4-V_6	T
▸ (Absent/prominent) U waves	prominent

— POP QUIZ —

Find The Mistake

<u>Instructions</u>: Identify the incorrect ECG feature(s) for each of the ECG diagnoses listed below

ECG Features	Answer
Pericarditis • Classic evolutionary ST-T pattern consists of 4 stages: 1) Diffuse upwardly concave ST elevation; 2) T waves invert; 3) ST junction returns to baseline & T wave amplitude decreases; 4) ECG returns to normal • Other clues include sinus tachycardia, PR depression late, and low voltage QRS	ST junction returns to baseline before (not after) the T waves invert; PR depression occurs early (not late)
Digitalis effect • Sagging ST segment depression with upward convexity • T wave flat, inverted, or biphasic • QT interval shortened • U wave amplitude increased • PR interval lengthened	ST segments have upward concavity (not convexity)
Digitalis toxicity • Typical abnormalities include paroxysmal atrial tachycardia with block, atrial fibrillation with complete heart block, second- or third-degree AV block, complete heart block with accelerated junctional or idioventricular rhythm, and bundle branch block	Isolated bundle branch block is not a manifestation of digitalis toxicity
Antiarrhythmic drug effect • Prominent U waves (one of the earliest findings) • Prolonged QT interval • Nonspecific ST and/or T wave changes • Widening of the QRS complex and QT interval • Various degrees of AV block	Widening of the QRS complex & QT interval, and AV block are consistent with drug toxicity (not drug effect)

ECG 3. 71-year-old male with previous episodes of tachycardia:

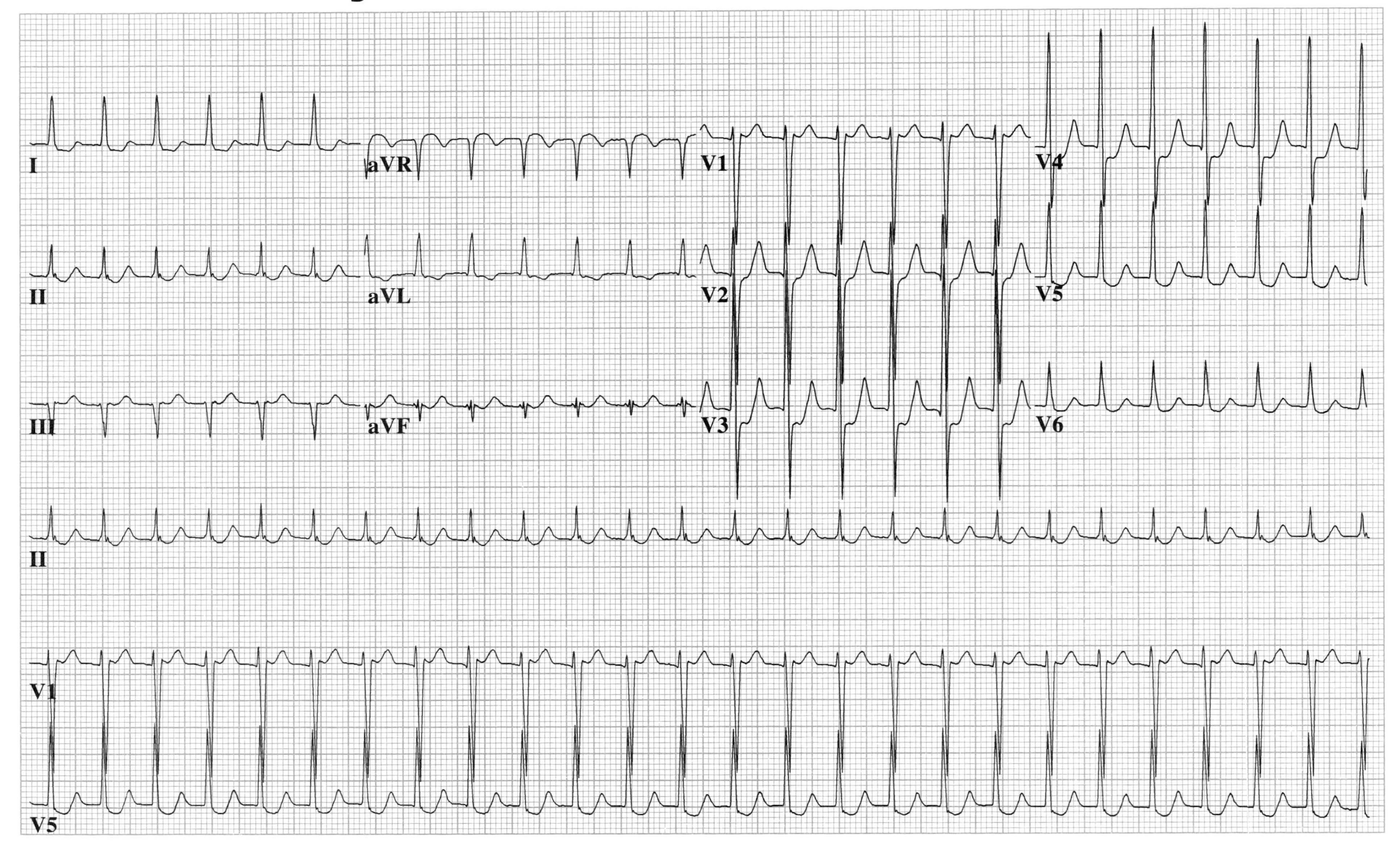

1. GENERAL FEATURES
- ☐ a. Normal ECG
- ☐ b. Borderline normal ECG or normal variant
- ☐ c. Incorrect electrode placement
- ☐ d. Artifact due to tremor

2. ATRIAL RHYTHMS
- ☐ a. Sinus rhythm
- ☐ b. Sinus arrhythmia
- ☐ c. Sinus bradycardia (< 60)
- ☐ d. Sinus tachycardia (> 100)
- ☐ e. Sinus pause or arrest
- ☐ f. Sinoatrial exit block
- ☐ g. Ecoptic atrial rhythm
- ☐ h. Wandering atrial pacemaker
- ☐ i. Atrial premature complexes, normally conducted
- ☐ j. Atrial premature complexes, nonconducted
- ☐ k. Atrial premature complexes with aberrant intraventricular conduction
- ☐ l. Atrial tachycardia (regular, sustained, 1:1 conduction)
- ☐ m. Atrial tachycardia, repetitive (short paroxysms)
- ☐ n. Atrial tachycardia, multifocal
- ☐ o. Atrial tachycardia with AV block
- ☐ p. Supraventricular tachycardia, unspecific
- ☐ q. Supraventricular tachycardia, paroxysmal
- ☐ r. Atrial flutter
- ☐ s. Atrial fibrillation
- ☐ t. Retrograde atrial activation

3. AV JUNCTIONAL RHYTHMS
- ☐ a. AV junctional premature complexes
- ☐ b. AV junctional escape complexes
- ☐ c. AV junctional rhythm, accelerated
- ☐ d. AV junctional rhythm

4. VENTRICULAR RHYTHMS
- ☐ a. Ventricular premature complex(es), uniform, fixed coupling
- ☐ b. Ventricular premature complex(es), uniform, nonfixed coupling
- ☐ c. Ventricular premature complexes(es), multiform
- ☐ d. Ventricular premature complexes, in pairs
- ☐ e. Ventricular parasystole
- ☐ f. Ventricular tachycardia (≥ 3 consecutive complexes)
- ☐ g. Accelerated idioventricular rhythm
- ☐ h. Ventricular escape complexes or rhythm
- ☐ i. Ventricular fibrillation

5. ATRIAL-VENTRICULAR INTERACTIONS IN ARRHYTHMIAS
- ☐ a. Fusion complexes
- ☐ b. Reciprocal (echo) complexes
- ☐ c. Ventricular capture complexes
- ☐ d. AV dissociation
- ☐ e. Ventriculophasic sinus arrhythmia

6. AV CONDUCTION ABNORMALITIES
- ☐ a. AV block, 1°
- ☐ b. AV block, 2° - Mobitz type I (Wenckebach)
- ☐ c. AV block, 2° - Mobitz type II
- ☐ d. AV block, 2:1
- ☐ e. AV block, 3°
- ☐ f. AV block, variable
- ☐ g. Short PR interval (with sinus rhythm and normal QRS duration)
- ☐ h. Wolff-Parkinson-White pattern

7. INTRAVENTRICULAR CONDUCTION DISTURBANCES
- ☐ a. RBBB, incomplete
- ☐ b. RBBB, complete
- ☐ c. Left anterior fascicular block
- ☐ d. Left posterior fascicular block
- ☐ e. LBBB, with ST-T wave suggestive of acute myocardial injury or infarction
- ☐ f. LBBB, complete
- ☐ g. LBBB, intermittent
- ☐ h. Intraventricular conduction disturbance, nonspecific
- ☐ i. Aberrant intraventricular conduction with supraventricular arrhythmia

8. P WAVE ABNORMALITIES
- ☐ a. Right atrial abnormality
- ☐ b. Left atrial abnormalities
- ☐ c. Nonspecific atrial abnormality

9. ABNORMALITIES OF QRS VOLTAGE OR AXIS
- ☐ a. Low voltage, limb leads only
- ☐ b. Low voltage, limb and precordial leads
- ☐ c. Left axis deviation (> - 30%)
- ☐ d. Right axis deviation (> + 100)
- ☐ e. Electrical alternans

10. VENTRICULAR HYPERTROPHY
- ☐ a. LVH by voltage only
- ☐ b. LVH by voltage and ST-T segment abnormalities
- ☐ c. RVH
- ☐ d. Combined ventricular hypertrophy

11. Q WAVE MYOCARDIAL INFARCTION

	Probably Acute or Recent	Probably Old or Age Indeterminate
Anterolateral	☐ a.	☐ g.
Anterior	☐ b.	☐ h.
Anteroseptal	☐ c.	☐ i.
Lateral/High lateral	☐ d.	☐ j.
Inferior	☐ e.	☐ k.
Posterior	☐ f.	☐ l.

- ☐ m. Probably ventricular aneurysm

12. ST, T, U, WAVE ABNORMALITIES
- ☐ a. Normal variant, early repolarization
- ☐ b. Normal variant, juvenile T waves
- ☐ c. Nonspecific ST and/or T wave abnormalities
- ☐ d. ST and/or T wave abnormalities suggesting myocardial ischemia
- ☐ e. ST and/or T wave abnormalities suggesting myocardial injury
- ☐ f. ST and/or T wave abnormalities suggesting acute pericarditis
- ☐ g. ST-T segment abnormalities secondary to intraventricular conduction disturbance or hypertrophy
- ☐ h. Post-extrasystolic T wave abnormality
- ☐ i. Isolated J point depression
- ☐ j. Peaked T waves
- ☐ k. Prolonged QT interval
- ☐ l. Prominent U waves

13. PACEMAKER FUNCTION AND RHYTHM
- ☐ a. Atrial or coronary sinus pacing
- ☐ b. Ventricular demand pacing
- ☐ c. AV sequential pacing
- ☐ d. Ventricular pacing, complete control
- ☐ e. Dual chamber, atrial sensing pacemaker
- ☐ f. Pacemaker malfunction, not constantly capturing (atrium or ventricle)
- ☐ g. Pacemaker malfunction, not constantly sensing (atrium or ventricle)
- ☐ h. Pacemaker malfunction, not firing
- ☐ i. Pacemaker malfunction, slowing

14. SUGGESTED OR PROBABLE CLINICAL DISORDERS
- ☐ a. Digitalis effect
- ☐ b. Digitalis toxicity
- ☐ c. Antiarrhythmic drug effect
- ☐ d. Antiarrhythmic drug toxicity
- ☐ e. Hyperkalemia
- ☐ f. Hypokalemia
- ☐ g. Hypercalcemia
- ☐ h. Hypocalcemia
- ☐ i. Atrial septal defect, secundum
- ☐ j. Atrial septal defect, primum
- ☐ k. Dextrocardia, mirror image
- ☐ l. Mitral valve disease
- ☐ m. Chronic lung disease
- ☐ n. Acute cor pulmonale, including pulmonary embolus
- ☐ o. Pericardial effusion
- ☐ p. Acute pericarditis
- ☐ q. Hypertrophic cardiomyopathy
- ☐ r. Coronary artery disease
- ☐ s. Central nervous system disorder
- ☐ t. Myxedema
- ☐ u. Hypothermia
- ☐ v. Sick sinus syndrome

ECG 3 was obtained in a 71-year-old male with previous episodes of tachycardia. The ECG shows a regular narrow complex tachycardia at 153 beats/minute with ST depression in V_3-V_6 suggesting subendocardial ischemia (arrows). Retrograde P waves are most noticeable in lead II, immediately following the QRS complex (arrowhead; also see full-size ECG on previous page). This tracing is most appropriately coded as supraventricular tachycardia, unspecified, with retrograde atrial activation. Electrical alternans is commonly seen in SVT and is present in this tracing (asterisk). Also noted is a prolonged QT interval. At electrophysiologic study, this patient was shown to have AV nodal re-entry tachycardia.

Codes:

2p	Supraventricular tachycardia, unspecified
2t	Retrograde atrial activation
9e	Electrical alternans
12d	ST and/or T wave abnormalities suggesting myocardial ischemia
12k	Prolonged QT interval

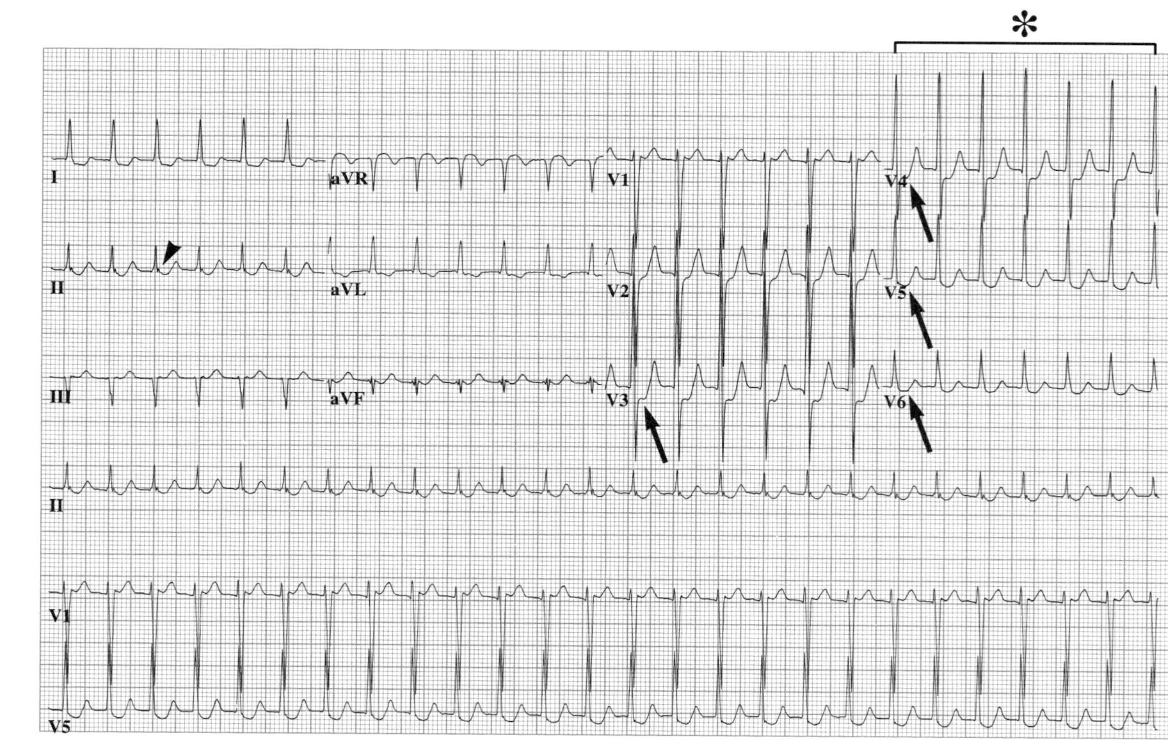

Questions: ECG 3

1. Retrograde P waves are usually inverted in leads II, III, and aVF:

   a. True
   b. False

2. ECG features consistent with a supraventricular origin rather than a ventricular origin for a tachycardia include:

   a. Capture or fusion beats
   b. Narrow QRS width
   c. Left axis deviation
   d. AV dissociation

Answers: ECG 3

1. Retrograde atrial activation results in inverted P waves in leads II, III, and aVF. The retrograde atrial wavefront moves in a superior direction away from the AV node and inferior leads, resulting in inverted P waves in these leads. Retrograde P waves typically occur with junctional beats and AV nodal re-entrant tachycardia, and sometimes with ventricular tachycardia or VPCs (if retrograde AV nodal conduction is present). (Answer: a)

2. The differentiation of a supraventricular from a ventricular rhythm is an important and frequent encountered clinical dilemma.

   A supraventricular origin is favored if:
   - The QRS is narrow
   - QRS morphology is similar to that noted during a sinus rhythm or during an aberrantly conducted atrial premature complex
   - The tachyarrhythmia is initiated by an atrial premature complex

   A ventricular origin is favored if:
   - The QRS is wide ($\geq$0.14 seconds in duration)
   - AV dissociation, capture beats, and/or fusion beats are present
   - The QRS axis is leftward or northwest
   - Ventricular concordance is present
   - The dysrhythmia is initiated by a VPC

(Answer: b)

— Quick Review 3 —

SVT, unspecified	
• (Regular/irregular) rhythm	Regular
• Rate > ____ per minute	100
• P waves (easily/not easily) identified	not easily
• QRS complex is usually (narrow/wide)	narrow
• If rate is 150 per minute, consider ____	atrial flutter with 2:1 block
Retrograde atrial activation	
• Inverted P waves in leads ____	II, III and aVF
Electrical alternans	
• Alteration in the ____ and/or ____ of the P, QRS and/or T waves	amplitude, direction

— POP QUIZ —

Make The Diagnosis

<u>Instructions</u>: Determine the ECG diagnosis that best corresponds to the ECG features listed below (see score sheet for options)

ECG Features	Diagnosis
• Resultant ECG mimics dextrocardia with inversion of the P-QRS-T in leads I and aVL	Incorrect lead placement
• Sinus P wave • Longest and shortest PP intervals vary by > 0.16 seconds or 10%	Sinus arrhythmia
• PP interval > 1.6 - 2.0 seconds • Resumption of sinus rhythm at a PP interval that is not a multiple of the basic sinus PP interval	Sinus pause or arrest
• Sinus P wave • Some sinus impulses fail to reach the atria • " Group beating" with: (1) Shortening of the PP interval prior to absent P wave (2) Constant PR interval (3) PP pause less than twice the normal PP interval	Mobitz Type I, second-degree sinoatrial exit block
• Sinus P wave • Some sinus impulses fail to reach the atria • Constant PP interval followed by a pause that is a multiple (2x, 3x, etc.) of the normal PP interval	Mobitz Type II, second-degree sinoatrial exit block
• Non-sinus P wave • Rate < 100 per minute • PR interval > 0.11 seconds	Ectopic atrial rhythm
• Rate < 100 per minute • P waves with ≥ 3 morphologies • PR, RR, and RP intervals vary	Wandering atrial pacemaker

ECG 4. 79-year-old asymptomatic male with a prior cardiac history:

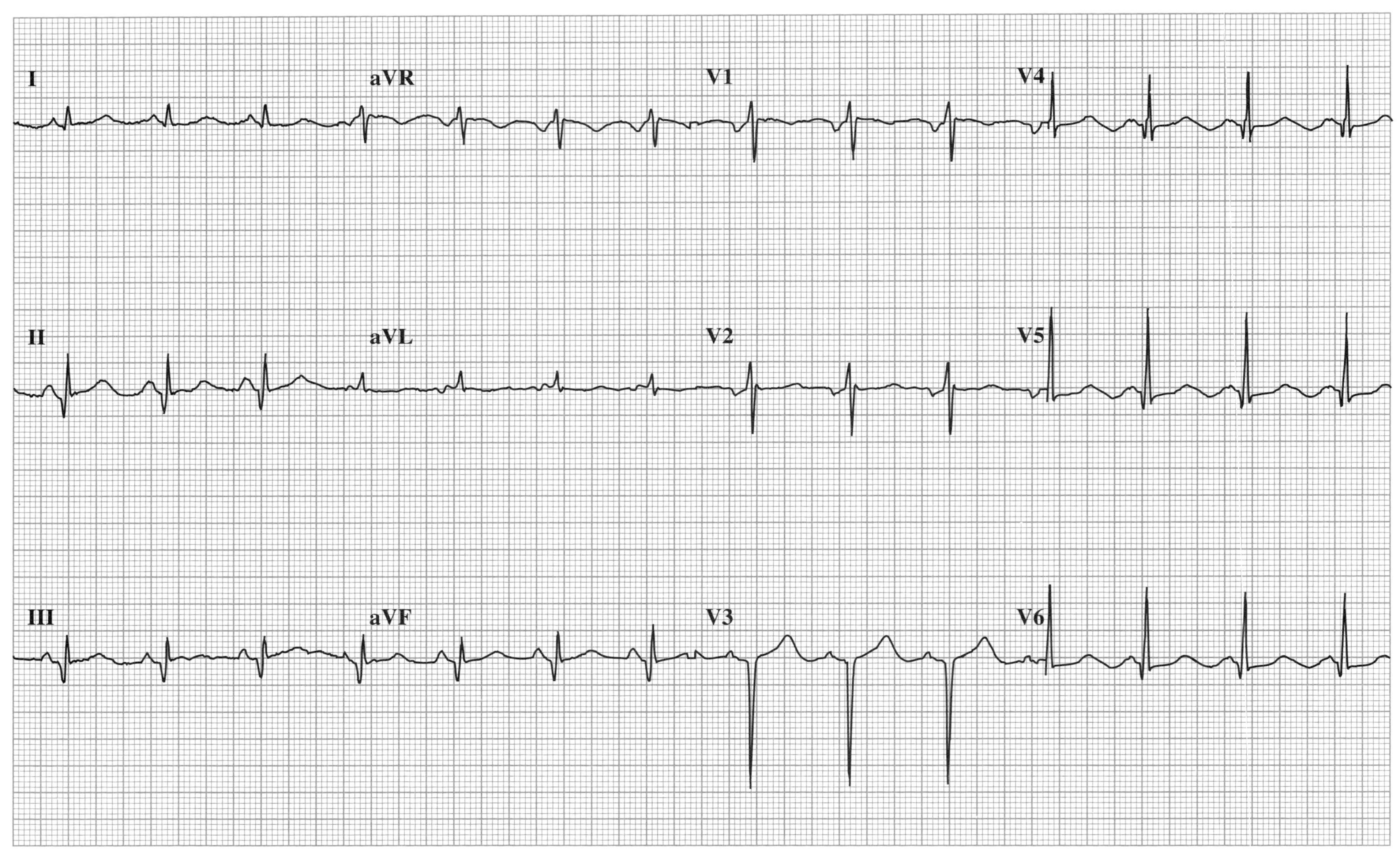

1. GENERAL FEATURES

☐ a. Normal ECG
☐ b. Borderline normal ECG or normal variant
☐ c. Incorrect electrode placement
☐ d. Artifact due to tremor

2. ATRIAL RHYTHMS

☐ a. Sinus rhythm
☐ b. Sinus arrhythmia
☐ c. Sinus bradycardia (< 60)
☐ d. Sinus tachycardia (> 100)
☐ e. Sinus pause or arrest
☐ f. Sinoatrial exit block
☐ g. Ecoptic atrial rhythm
☐ h. Wandering atrial pacemaker
☐ i. Atrial premature complexes, normally conducted
☐ j. Atrial premature complexes, nonconducted
☐ k. Atrial premature complexes with aberrant intraventricular conduction
☐ l. Atrial tachycardia (regular, sustained, 1:1 conduction)
☐ m. Atrial tachycardia, repetitive (short paroxysms)
☐ n. Atrial tachycardia, multifocal
☐ o. Atrial tachycardia with AV block
☐ p. Supraventricular tachycardia, unspecific
☐ q. Supraventricular tachycardia, paroxysmal
☐ r. Atrial flutter
☐ s. Atrial fibrillation
☐ t. Retrograde atrial activation

3. AV JUNCTIONAL RHYTHMS

☐ a. AV junctional premature complexes
☐ b. AV junctional escape complexes
☐ c. AV junctional rhythm, accelerated
☐ d. AV junctional rhythm

4. VENTRICULAR RHYTHMS

☐ a. Ventricular premature complex(es), uniform, fixed coupling
☐ b. Ventricular premature complex(es), uniform, nonfixed coupling
☐ c. Ventricular premature complexes(es), multiform
☐ d. Ventricular premature complexes, in pairs
☐ e. Ventricular parasystole
☐ f. Ventricular tachycardia (≥ 3 consecutive complexes)
☐ g. Accelerated idioventricular rhythm
☐ h. Ventricular escape complexes or rhythm
☐ i. Ventricular fibrillation

5. ATRIAL-VENTRICULAR INTERACTIONS IN ARRHYTHMIAS

☐ a. Fusion complexes
☐ b. Reciprocal (echo) complexes
☐ c. Ventricular capture complexes
☐ d. AV dissociation
☐ e. Ventriculophasic sinus arrhythmia

6. AV CONDUCTION ABNORMALITIES

☐ a. AV block, 1°
☐ b. AV block, 2° - Mobitz type I (Wenckebach)
☐ c. AV block, 2° - Mobitz type II
☐ d. AV block, 2:1
☐ e. AV block, 3°
☐ f. AV block, variable
☐ g. Short PR interval (with sinus rhythm and normal QRS duration)
☐ h. Wolff-Parkinson-White pattern

7. INTRAVENTRICULAR CONDUCTION DISTURBANCES

☐ a. RBBB, incomplete
☐ b. RBBB, complete
☐ c. Left anterior fascicular block
☐ d. Left posterior fascicular block
☐ e. LBBB, with ST-T wave suggestive of acute myocardial injury or infarction
☐ f. LBBB, complete
☐ g. LBBB, intermittent
☐ h. Intraventricular conduction disturbance, nonspecific
☐ i. Aberrant intraventricular conduction with supraventricular arrhythmia

8. P WAVE ABNORMALITIES

☐ a. Right atrial abnormality
☐ b. Left atrial abnormalities
☐ c. Nonspecific atrial abnormality

9. ABNORMALITIES OF QRS VOLTAGE OR AXIS

☐ a. Low voltage, limb leads only
☐ b. Low voltage, limb and precordial leads
☐ c. Left axis deviation (> - 30%)
☐ d. Right axis deviation (> + 100)
☐ e. Electrical alternans

10. VENTRICULAR HYPERTROPHY

☐ a. LVH by voltage only
☐ b. LVH by voltage and ST-T segment abnormalities
☐ c. RVH
☐ d. Combined ventricular hypertrophy

11. Q WAVE MYOCARDIAL INFARCTION

	Probably Acute or Recent	Probably Old or Age Indeterminate
Anterolateral	☐ a.	☐ g.
Anterior	☐ b.	☐ h.
Anteroseptal	☐ c.	☐ i.
Lateral/High lateral	☐ d.	☐ j.
Inferior	☐ e.	☐ k.
Posterior	☐ f.	☐ l

☐ m. Probably ventricular aneurysm

12. ST, T, U, WAVE ABNORMALITIES

☐ a. Normal variant, early repolarization
☐ b. Normal variant, juvenile T waves
☐ c. Nonspecific ST and/or T wave abnormalities
☐ d. ST and/or T wave abnormalities suggesting myocardial ischemia
☐ e. ST and/or T wave abnormalities suggesting myocardial injury
☐ f. ST and/or T wave abnormalities suggesting acute pericarditis
☐ g. ST-T segment abnormalities secondary to intraventricular conduction disturbance or hypertrophy
☐ h. Post-extrasystolic T wave abnormality
☐ i. Isolated J point depression
☐ j. Peaked T waves
☐ k. Prolonged QT interval
☐ l. Prominent U waves

13. PACEMAKER FUNCTION AND RHYTHM

☐ a. Atrial or coronary sinus pacing
☐ b. Ventricular demand pacing
☐ c. AV sequential pacing
☐ d. Ventricular pacing, complete control
☐ e. Dual chamber, atrial sensing pacemaker
☐ f. Pacemaker malfunction, not constantly capturing (atrium or ventricle)
☐ g. Pacemaker malfunction, not constantly sensing (atrium or ventricle)
☐ h. Pacemaker malfunction, not firing
☐ i. Pacemaker malfunction, slowing

14. SUGGESTED OR PROBABLE CLINICAL DISORDERS

☐ a. Digitalis effect
☐ b. Digitalis toxicity
☐ c. Antiarrhythmic drug effect
☐ d. Antiarrhythmic drug toxicity
☐ e. Hyperkalemia
☐ f. Hypokalemia
☐ g. Hypercalcemia
☐ h. Hypocalcemia
☐ i. Atrial septal defect, secundum
☐ j. Atrial septal defect, primum
☐ k. Dextrocardia, mirror image
☐ l. Mitral valve disease
☐ m. Chronic lung disease
☐ n. Acute cor pulmonale, including pulmonary embolus
☐ o. Pericardial effusion
☐ p. Acute pericarditis
☐ q. Hypertrophic cardiomyopathy
☐ r. Coronary artery disease
☐ s. Central nervous system disorder
☐ t. Myxedema
☐ u. Hypothermia
☐ v. Sick sinus syndrome

ECG 4 was obtained from a 79-year-old man with a prior cardiac history who is currently asymptomatic. The ECG shows sinus rhythm, left and right atrial abnormalities(arrows), and Q waves meeting criteria for age indeterminate anterior, anterolateral and inferior infarctions (arrowheads). Nonspecific ST-T abnormalities are present (the subtle ST segment elevation does not meet 1 mm in the inferior leads and thus, is not diagnostic for either aneurysm or acute injury). The prominent R wave in leads V_1 and V_2 is likely a reflection of posterior infarction although this does not meet strict criteria for posterior infarction. The Q waves are consistent with coronary artery disease. The corrected QT is prolonged (486 msec).

Codes:

2a	Sinus rhythm
8a	Right atrial abnormality
8b	Left atrial abnormality
11g	Anterolateral Q wave MI, probably old or age indeterminate
11h	Anterior Q wave MI, probably old or age indeterminate
11k	Inferior Q wave MI, probably old or age indeterminate
12c	Nonspecific ST and/or T wave abnormalities
14r	Coronary artery disease

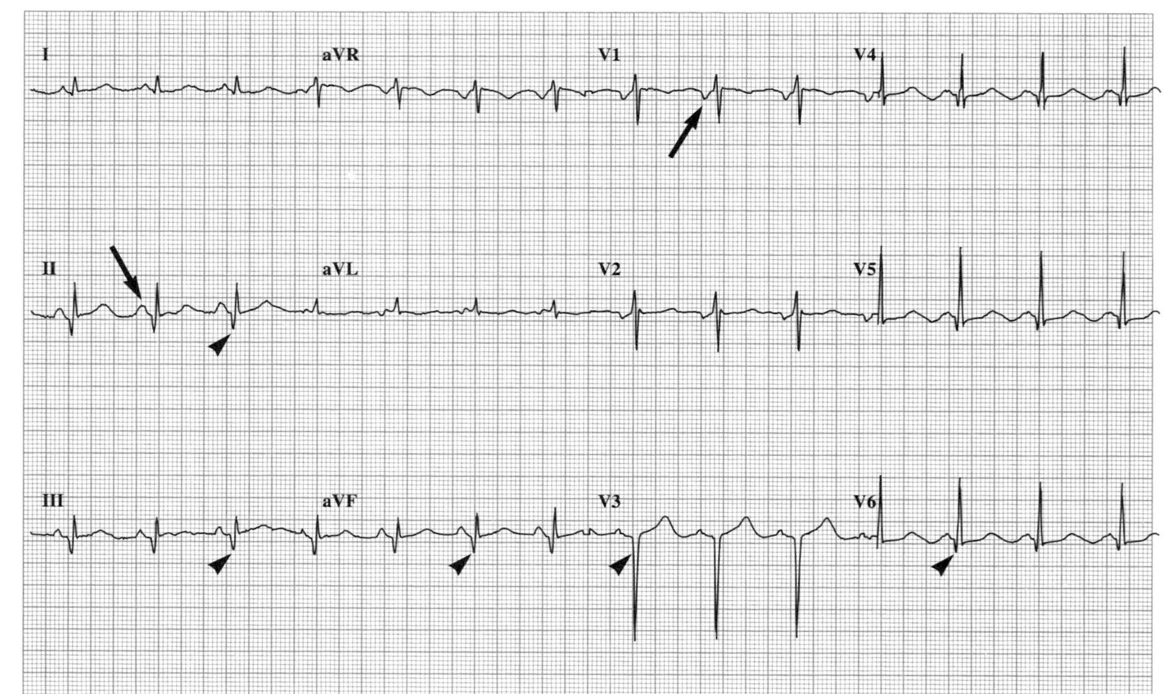

Questions: ECG 4

1. Conditions associated with pathological Q waves that can mimic myocardial infarction include

   a. Wolff-Parkinson-White syndrome
   b. Pericarditis
   c. Left bundle branch block
   d. COPD
   e. Pneumothorax
   f. Severe right ventricular hypertrophy
   g. Cardiomyopathy
   h. Infiltrative diseases of the myocardium (e.g., tumor, sarcoid)
   i. Pulmonary embolism

2. Drugs that can prolong the QT interval include:

   a. Quinidine
   b. Sotalol
   c. Disopyramide
   d. Tricyclic antidepressants
   e. Lithium
   f. Procainamide
   g. Amiodarone
   h. Phenothiazines

3. What is the likely age of this MI?

   a. Minutes to hours
   b. Hours to days
   c. Months to years

4. The presence of a Q wave can be used to distinguish transmural from subendocardial infarction:

   a. True
   b. False

5. The absence of a Q wave can be used to distinguish transmural from subendocardial infarction:

   a. True
   b. False

6. The most likely explanation for the tall R wave in V_1 is:

   a. Posterior myocardial infarction
   b. Right ventricular hypertrophy
   c. Incomplete right bundle branch block

Answers: ECG 4

1. While abnormal Q waves are most commonly associated with myocardial infarction (MI), several other conditions may produce abnormal Q waves on ECG, including WPW syndrome, left bundle branch block (LBBB), COPD, pneumothorax, cardiomyopathy, pulmonary embolism and others. In the WPW syndrome, negative delta-waves can occur in the inferior leads and mimic MI. In left bundle branch block, QS complexes in leads V_1 - V_4, (often accompanied by 1 - 2 mm of ST elevation) can be mistaken for anteroseptal MI. In COPD, Q waves usually occur in the inferior and/or right/mid precordial leads; other findings include poor R wave progression, P pulmonale, low voltage QRS, and $S_1S_2S_3$ pattern. Pneumothorax can cause a loss of R waves in the right precordial leads (QS complex), and along with the presence of symmetrical T wave inversion, can mimic anterior MI. In hypertrophic cardiomyopathy, abnormal Q waves are frequently seen in leads I, aVL, V_4 - V_6 due to septal hypertrophy. Abnormal Q waves may also be seen in infiltrative diseases of the myocardium, where electrically-active tissue may be replaced by fibrous tissue or electrically-inert substances (e.g., amyloid). Finally, Q waves may be seen in lead III and sometimes in aVF in pulmonary embolism, which can be accompanied by ST and T waves changes and confused with acute inferior MI; however, unlike inferior MI, Q waves in lead II are rare. (Answer: All except b, f)

2. Many drugs increase ventricular repolarization to cause prolongation of the QT interval, especially Type IA antiarrhythmics (quinidine, procainamide, disopyramide), sotalol and amiodarone. Significant QT prolongation increases the risk of torsade de pointes, syncope, and sudden cardiac death. (Answer: All)

3. The development of Q waves, and evolutionary changes in the T wave and ST segment can be used to approximate the age of myocardial infarction:

   - **T waves**: The development of large upright T waves is often the earliest manifestations of acute MI, occurring within minutes and lasting for minutes to hours. T wave inversion, which begins while ST segments are still elevated, may last for months to years, persist indefinitely, or regress to nonspecific T wave changes.

   - **ST segment**: ST elevation usually develops in the minutes to hours following acute MI. Resolution may occur within hours, but usually requires a few days for complete return to baseline. Persistence beyond 4 weeks should raise the suspicion of ventricular aneurysm.

   - **Q waves**: Abnormal Q waves usually develop in the first several hours to days following acute infarction. In most patients, they persist indefinitely, but may regress to no longer meet the criteria for abnormal Q waves; in some patients (< 15%), Q waves disappear entirely.

In the ECG in question, the presence of inferior Q waves accompanied by isoelectric ST segments and upright T waves suggest that the infarction is not acute, but rather, months or years in age. (Answer: c)

4. Q waves were once thought to be the hallmark of transmural infarction, but pathological studies have confirmed that Q waves can occur in subendocardial infarction as well. The presence of a Q wave cannot be used to reliably distinguish transmural from subendocardial MI. (Answer: b)

5. Non-Q-wave MI can be seen in both transmural infarction (especially when the culprit vessel is the left circumflex coronary artery) and subendocardial infarction. (Answer: b)

6. Tall R waves in lead V_1 occur in both right ventricular hypertrophy and incomplete RBBB. However, since multiple (inferior, anterior, lateral) infarcts are evident in the present tracing, posterior MI is the most likely diagnosis (even though strict criteria for R > S are not satisfied). (Answer: a)

— Quick Review 4 —

Anterolateral MI, age indeterminate or probably old	
• Abnormal Q waves (with/without) ST segment elevation in leads ____	without V_4-V_6
Anterior MI, age indeterminate or probably old	
• rS in lead ____, *followed by* QS or QR complexes (with/without) ST segment elevation in leads ____, *or* (increasing/decreasing) R wave amplitude from V_2-V_5	V_1 without, V_2-V_4 decreasing
Inferior MI, age indeterminate or probably old	
• Abnormal Q waves (with/without) ST elevation in at least two of leads ____	without II, III, aVF

ECG 5. 78-year-old female with dizziness:

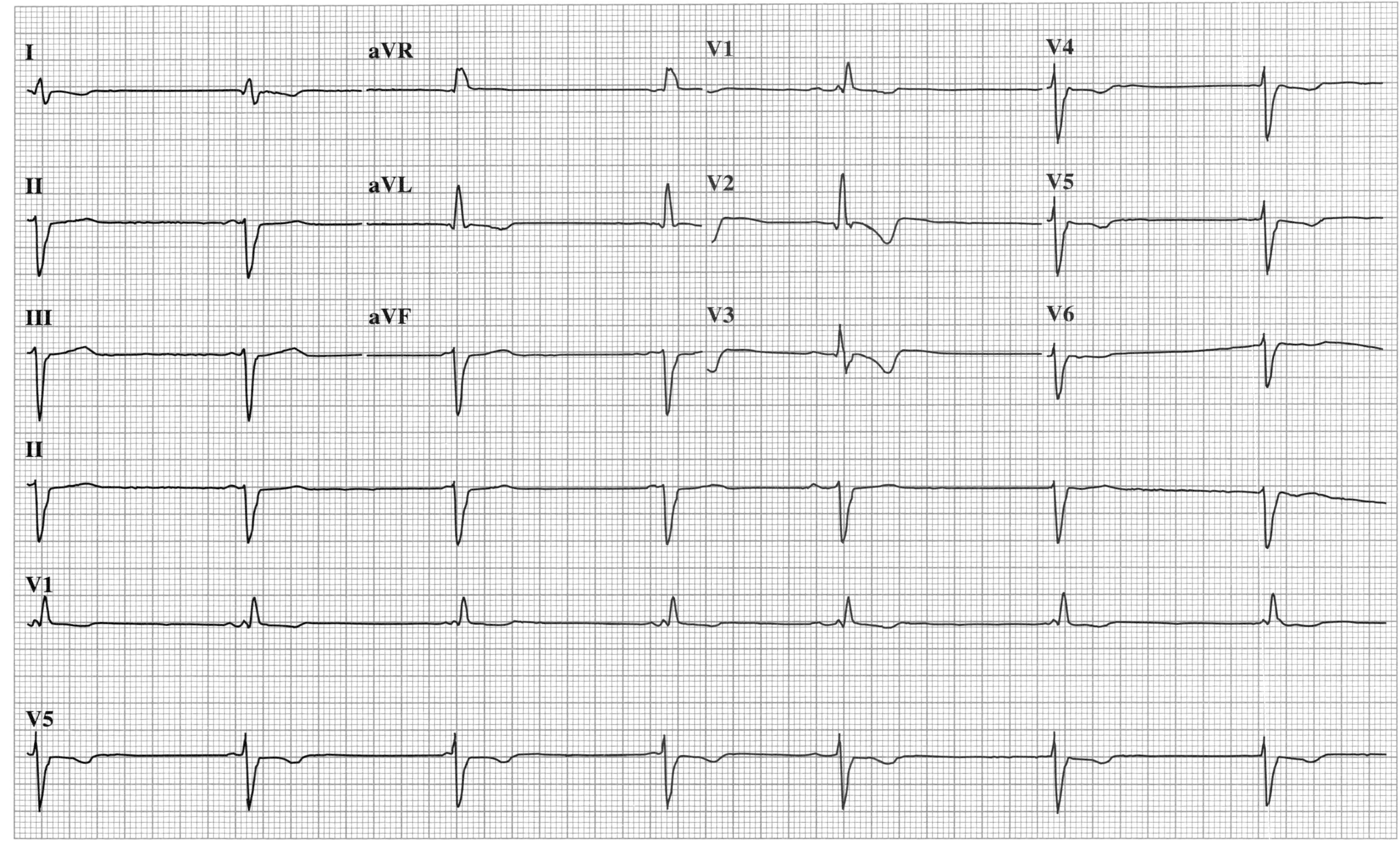

1. GENERAL FEATURES

☐ a. Normal ECG
☐ b. Borderline normal ECG or normal variant
☐ c. Incorrect electrode placement
☐ d. Artifact due to tremor

2. ATRIAL RHYTHMS

☐ a. Sinus rhythm
☐ b. Sinus arrhythmia
☐ c. Sinus bradycardia (< 60)
☐ d. Sinus tachycardia (> 100)
☐ e. Sinus pause or arrest
☐ f. Sinoatrial exit block
☐ g. Ecoptic atrial rhythm
☐ h. Wandering atrial pacemaker
☐ i. Atrial premature complexes, normally conducted
☐ j. Atrial premature complexes, nonconducted
☐ k. Atrial premature complexes with aberrant intraventricular conduction
☐ l. Atrial tachycardia (regular, sustained, 1:1 conduction)
☐ m. Atrial tachycardia, repetitive (short paroxysms)
☐ n. Atrial tachycardia, multifocal
☐ o. Atrial tachycardia with AV block
☐ p. Supraventricular tachycardia, unspecific
☐ q. Supraventricular tachycardia, paroxysmal
☐ r. Atrial flutter
☐ s. Atrial fibrillation
☐ t. Retrograde atrial activation

3. AV JUNCTIONAL RHYTHMS

☐ a. AV junctional premature complexes
☐ b. AV junctional escape complexes
☐ c. AV junctional rhythm, accelerated
☐ d. AV junctional rhythm

4. VENTRICULAR RHYTHMS

☐ a. Ventricular premature complex(es), uniform, fixed coupling
☐ b. Ventricular premature complex(es), uniform, nonfixed coupling
☐ c. Ventricular premature complexes(es), multiform
☐ d. Ventricular premature complexes, in pairs
☐ e. Ventricular parasystole
☐ f. Ventricular tachycardia (≥ 3 consecutive complexes)
☐ g. Accelerated idioventricular rhythm
☐ h. Ventricular escape complexes or rhythm
☐ i. Ventricular fibrillation

5. ATRIAL-VENTRICULAR INTERACTIONS IN ARRHYTHMIAS

☐ a. Fusion complexes
☐ b. Reciprocal (echo) complexes
☐ c. Ventricular capture complexes
☐ d. AV dissociation
☐ e. Ventriculophasic sinus arrhythmia

6. AV CONDUCTION ABNORMALITIES

☐ a. AV block, 1°
☐ b. AV block, 2° - Mobitz type I (Wenckebach)
☐ c. AV block, 2° - Mobitz type II
☐ d. AV block, 2:1
☐ e. AV block, 3°
☐ f. AV block, variable
☐ g. Short PR interval (with sinus rhythm and normal QRS duration)
☐ h. Wolff-Parkinson-White pattern

7. INTRAVENTRICULAR CONDUCTION DISTURBANCES

☐ a. RBBB, incomplete
☐ b. RBBB, complete
☐ c. Left anterior fascicular block
☐ d. Left posterior fascicular block
☐ e. LBBB, with ST-T wave suggestive of acute myocardial injury or infarction
☐ f. LBBB, complete
☐ g. LBBB, intermittent
☐ h. Intraventricular conduction disturbance, nonspecific
☐ i. Aberrant intraventricular conduction with supraventricular arrhythmia

8. P WAVE ABNORMALITIES

☐ a. Right atrial abnormality
☐ b. Left atrial abnormalities
☐ c. Nonspecific atrial abnormality

9. ABNORMALITIES OF QRS VOLTAGE OR AXIS

☐ a. Low voltage, limb leads only
☐ b. Low voltage, limb and precordial leads
☐ c. Left axis deviation (> - 30%)
☐ d. Right axis deviation (> + 100)
☐ e. Electrical alternans

10. VENTRICULAR HYPERTROPHY

☐ a. LVH by voltage only
☐ b. LVH by voltage and ST-T segment abnormalities
☐ c. RVH
☐ d. Combined ventricular hypertrophy

11. Q WAVE MYOCARDIAL INFARCTION

	Probably Acute or Recent	Probably Old or Age Indeterminate
Anterolateral	☐ a.	☐ g.
Anterior	☐ b.	☐ h.
Anteroseptal	☐ c.	☐ i.
Lateral/High lateral	☐ d.	☐ j.
Inferior	☐ e.	☐ k.
Posterior	☐ f.	☐ l.

☐ m. Probably ventricular aneurysm

12. ST, T, U, WAVE ABNORMALITIES

☐ a. Normal variant, early repolarization
☐ b. Normal variant, juvenile T waves
☐ c. Nonspecific ST and/or T wave abnormalities
☐ d. ST and/or T wave abnormalities suggesting myocardial ischemia
☐ e. ST and/or T wave abnormalities suggesting myocardial injury
☐ f. ST and/or T wave abnormalities suggesting acute pericarditis
☐ g. ST-T segment abnormalities secondary to intraventricular conduction disturbance or hypertrophy
☐ h. Post-extrasystolic T wave abnormality
☐ i. Isolated J point depression
☐ j. Peaked T waves
☐ k. Prolonged QT interval
☐ l. Prominent U waves

13. PACEMAKER FUNCTION AND RHYTHM

☐ a. Atrial or coronary sinus pacing
☐ b. Ventricular demand pacing
☐ c. AV sequential pacing
☐ d. Ventricular pacing, complete control
☐ e. Dual chamber, atrial sensing pacemaker
☐ f. Pacemaker malfunction, not constantly capturing (atrium or ventricle)
☐ g. Pacemaker malfunction, not constantly sensing (atrium or ventricle)
☐ h. Pacemaker malfunction, not firing
☐ i. Pacemaker malfunction, slowing

14. SUGGESTED OR PROBABLE CLINICAL DISORDERS

☐ a. Digitalis effect
☐ b. Digitalis toxicity
☐ c. Antiarrhythmic drug effect
☐ d. Antiarrhythmic drug toxicity
☐ e. Hyperkalemia
☐ f. Hypokalemia
☐ g. Hypercalcemia
☐ h. Hypocalcemia
☐ i. Atrial septal defect, secundum
☐ j. Atrial septal defect, primum
☐ k. Dextrocardia, mirror image
☐ l. Mitral valve disease
☐ m. Chronic lung disease
☐ n. Acute cor pulmonale, including pulmonary embolus
☐ o. Pericardial effusion
☐ p. Acute pericarditis
☐ q. Hypertrophic cardiomyopathy
☐ r. Coronary artery disease
☐ s. Central nervous system disorder
☐ t. Myxedema
☐ u. Hypothermia
☐ v. Sick sinus syndrome

ECG 5 was obtained in a 78-year-old female complaining of dizziness. The ECG shows a profound sinus bradycardia at 40 BPM (arrows mark sinus P waves) competing with a junctional rhythm (arrowheads mark junctional QRS complexes) and resulting in AV dissociation. Also present are sinus arrhythmia, RBBB with secondary ST-T changes, and left axis deviation (due to left anterior fascicular block). The fifth complex on the tracing shows a normally conducted P wave resulting in a ventricular capture complex (which is premature compared to the junctional complexes)(asterisk). These findings are consistent with sick sinus syndrome.

Codes:

2b	Sinus arrhythmia
2c	Sinus bradycardia < 60
3d	AV junctional rhythm
5c	Ventricular capture complexes
5d	AV dissociation
7b	RBBB, complete
7c	Left anterior fascicular block
9c	Left axis deviation (>-30°)
12g	ST-T segment abnormalities secondary to IVCD or hypertrophy
14v	Sick sinus syndrome

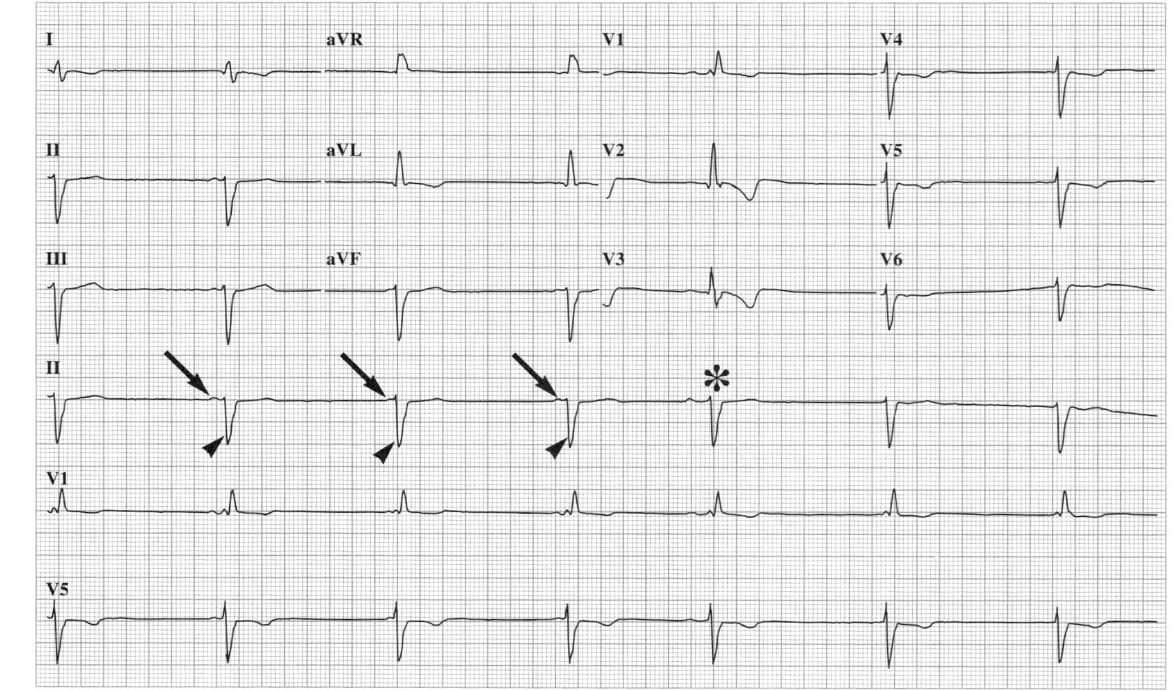

Questions: ECG 5

1. Left anterior fascicular block requires an axis leftward of:

   a. - 45°
   b. - 30°
   c. 0°
   d. - 90°

2. Which of the following statements about junctional escape rhythms are true:

   a. The usual heart rate is 60-80 BPM
   b. Retrograde atrial activation is always evident
   c. AV dissociation is common
   d. The P wave may proceed the QRS

3. Incomplete RBBB and complete RBBB requires a QRS duration of ____ and ____ seconds, respectively:

   a. 0.09-0.12 and ≥ 0.12
   b. 0.09-0.11 and ≥ 0.11
   c. 0.09 to < 0.12, and ≥ 0.12
   d. 0.11 and 0.14

Answers: ECG 5

1. Left anterior fascicular block (LAFB) requires a QRS axis between - 45° and -90°, and is typically associated with a normal to slightly prolonged QRS duration (0.08-0.10 seconds). Since LAFB is a diagnosis of exclusion, be sure to exclude other causes of left axis deviation (e.g., LVH, inferior infarction LBBB, emphysema) before coding LAFB. (Answer: a)

2. The usual heart rate noted with a junctional escape rhythm is between 40-60 BPM. Junctional rhythms are often associated with isorhythmic AV dissociation (P waves and QRS complexes appear to bear a close relationship to each other but actually represent independent atrial and ventricular activation) or retrograde atrial activation (inverted P waves in leads II, III, and aVF). The P wave inscribed by a junctional pacemaker may proceed (by ≤ 0.11), be superimposed upon, or follow the QRS complex. (Answer: c, d)

3. Complete RBBB requires a QRS duration of ≥ 0.12 seconds (whereas incomplete RBBB requires a QRS duration between 0.09 and < 0.12 seconds). Lead V_1 is usually the most helpful lead for diagnosing RBBB, and typically displays an rSr' pattern. RBBB is not usually associated with extensive and diffuse ST-T wave (repolarization) abnormalities, although T wave inversions are often present in leads V_1 - V_3. (Answer: c)

— Quick Review 5 —

AV dissociation	
• Atrial and ventricular rhythms are ____ of each other	independent
• Ventricular rate is (</≥) than the atrial rate	≥
RBBB, complete	
• QRS duration ≥ ____ seconds	0.12
• Secondary R wave (R') in lead ____ is usually	V_1
(shorter/taller) than the initial R wave	taller
• Onset of intrinsicoid deflection in leads V_1 and V_2 > ____ seconds	0.05
• ST segment ____ and T wave	depression
____ in V_1, V_2	inversion
• Wide slurred S wave in leads ____	I, aVL, V_5, V_6
• QRS axis is usually (normal/leftward/rightward)	normal
• RBBB (does/does not) interfere with the ECG diagnosis of ventricular hypertrophy or Q wave MI	does not
Left anterior fascicular block	
• ____ axis deviation with a mean QRS axis between	left
____ and ____ degrees	-45, -90
• (qR/rS) complex in leads I and aVL	qR
• (qR/rS) complex in lead III	rS
• Normal or slightly prolonged QRS duration (true/false)	true
• No other cause for left axis deviation should be present (true/false)	true
• Poor R wave progression is (common/uncommon)	common

— POP QUIZ —

2:1 AV Block: Mobitz Type I or II

Instructions: Decide if the ECG features listed below favor Mobitz Type I (Wenkebach) or Mobitz Type II second-degree AV block

ECG Feature	Mobitz Type I or II
Wide QRS complex	II
AV block improves in response to maneuvers that increase heart rate & AV conduction (e.g., atropine, exercise)	I
AV block improves in response to maneuvers that reduce heart rate & AV conduction (e.g., carotid sinus massage)	II
2:1 block develops during anterior MI	II
Type I on another part of ECG	I
History of syncope	II

ECG 6. 66-year-old female complaining of rapid, irregular heart beating:

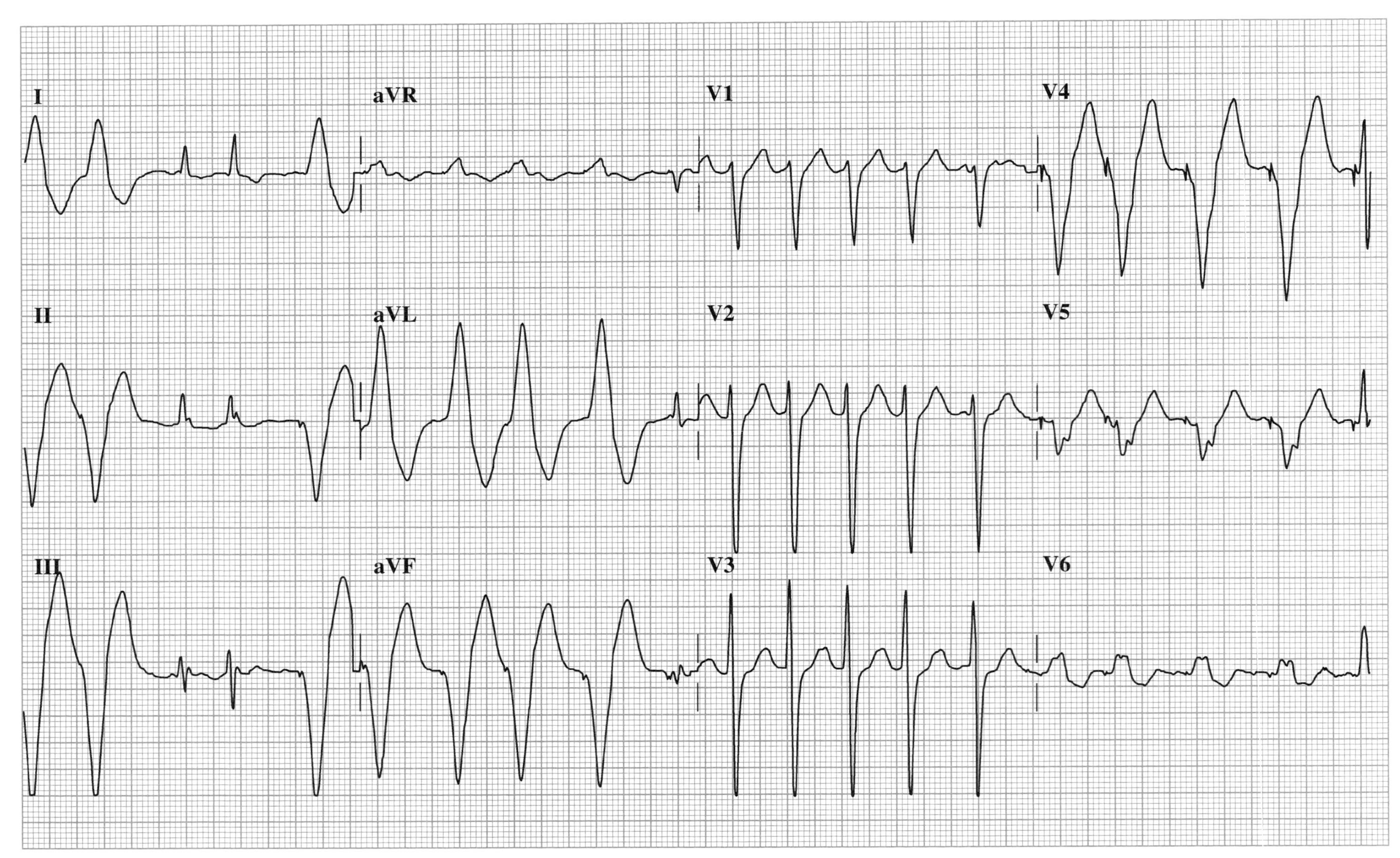

1. GENERAL FEATURES
☐ a. Normal ECG
☐ b. Borderline normal ECG or normal variant
☐ c. Incorrect electrode placement
☐ d. Artifact due to tremor

2. ATRIAL RHYTHMS
☐ a. Sinus rhythm
☐ b. Sinus arrhythmia
☐ c. Sinus bradycardia (< 60)
☐ d. Sinus tachycardia (> 100)
☐ e. Sinus pause or arrest
☐ f. Sinoatrial exit block
☐ g. Ecoptic atrial rhythm
☐ h. Wandering atrial pacemaker
☐ i. Atrial premature complexes, normally conducted
☐ j. Atrial premature complexes, nonconducted
☐ k. Atrial premature complexes with aberrant intraventricular conduction
☐ l. Atrial tachycardia (regular, sustained, 1:1 conduction)
☐ m. Atrial tachycardia, repetitive (short paroxysms)
☐ n. Atrial tachycardia, multifocal
☐ o. Atrial tachycardia with AV block
☐ p. Supraventricular tachycardia, unspecific
☐ q. Supraventricular tachycardia, paroxysmal
☐ r. Atrial flutter
☐ s. Atrial fibrillation
☐ t. Retrograde atrial activation

3. AV JUNCTIONAL RHYTHMS
☐ a. AV junctional premature complexes
☐ b. AV junctional escape complexes
☐ c. AV junctional rhythm, accelerated
☐ d. AV junctional rhythm

4. VENTRICULAR RHYTHMS
☐ a. Ventricular premature complex(es), uniform, fixed coupling
☐ b. Ventricular premature complex(es), uniform, nonfixed coupling
☐ c. Ventricular premature complexes(es), multiform
☐ d. Ventricular premature complexes, in pairs
☐ e. Ventricular parasystole
☐ f. Ventricular tachycardia (≥ 3 consecutive complexes)
☐ g. Accelerated idioventricular rhythm
☐ h. Ventricular escape complexes or rhythm
☐ i. Ventricular fibrillation

5. ATRIAL-VENTRICULAR INTERACTIONS IN ARRHYTHMIAS
☐ a. Fusion complexes
☐ b. Reciprocal (echo) complexes
☐ c. Ventricular capture complexes
☐ d. AV dissociation

☐ e. Ventriculophasic sinus arrhythmia

6. AV CONDUCTION ABNORMALITIES
☐ a. AV block, 1°
☐ b. AV block, 2° - Mobitz type I (Wenckebach)
☐ c. AV block, 2° - Mobitz type II
☐ d. AV block, 2:1
☐ e. AV block, 3°
☐ f. AV block, variable
☐ g. Short PR interval (with sinus rhythm and normal QRS duration)
☐ h. Wolff-Parkinson-White pattern

7. INTRAVENTRICULAR CONDUCTION DISTURBANCES
☐ a. RBBB, incomplete
☐ b. RBBB, complete
☐ c. Left anterior fascicular block
☐ d. Left posterior fascicular block
☐ e. LBBB, with ST-T wave suggestive of acute myocardial injury or infarction
☐ f. LBBB, complete
☐ g. LBBB, intermittent
☐ h. Intraventricular conduction disturbance, nonspecific
☐ i. Aberrant intraventricular conduction with supraventricular arrhythmia

8. P WAVE ABNORMALITIES
☐ a. Right atrial abnormality
☐ b. Left atrial abnormalities
☐ c. Nonspecific atrial abnormality

9. ABNORMALITIES OF QRS VOLTAGE OR AXIS
☐ a. Low voltage, limb leads only
☐ b. Low voltage, limb and precordial leads
☐ c. Left axis deviation (> - 30%)
☐ d. Right axis deviation (> + 100)
☐ e. Electrical alternans

10. VENTRICULAR HYPERTROPHY
☐ a. LVH by voltage only
☐ b. LVH by voltage and ST-T segment abnormalities
☐ c. RVH
☐ d. Combined ventricular hypertrophy

11. Q WAVE MYOCARDIAL INFARCTION

	Probably Acute or Recent	Probably Old or Age Indeterminate
Anterolateral	☐ a.	☐ g.
Anterior	☐ b.	☐ h.
Anteroseptal	☐ c.	☐ i.
Lateral/High lateral	☐ d.	☐ j.
Inferior	☐ e.	☐ k.
Posterior	☐ f.	☐ l.

☐ m. Probably ventricular aneurysm

12. ST, T, U, WAVE ABNORMALITIES
☐ a. Normal variant, early repolarization
☐ b. Normal variant, juvenile T waves
☐ c. Nonspecific ST and/or T wave abnormalities
☐ d. ST and/or T wave abnormalities suggesting myocardial ischemia
☐ e. ST and/or T wave abnormalities suggesting myocardial injury
☐ f. ST and/or T wave abnormalities suggesting acute pericarditis
☐ g. ST-T segment abnormalities secondary to intraventricular conduction disturbance or hypertrophy
☐ h. Post-extrasystolic T wave abnormality
☐ i. Isolated J point depression
☐ j. Peaked T waves
☐ k. Prolonged QT interval
☐ l. Prominent U waves

13. PACEMAKER FUNCTION AND RHYTHM
☐ a. Atrial or coronary sinus pacing
☐ b. Ventricular demand pacing
☐ c. AV sequential pacing
☐ d. Ventricular pacing, complete control
☐ e. Dual chamber, atrial sensing pacemaker
☐ f. Pacemaker malfunction, not constantly capturing (atrium or ventricle)
☐ g. Pacemaker malfunction, not constantly sensing (atrium or ventricle)
☐ h. Pacemaker malfunction, not firing
☐ i. Pacemaker malfunction, slowing

14. SUGGESTED OR PROBABLE CLINICAL DISORDERS
☐ a. Digitalis effect
☐ b. Digitalis toxicity
☐ c. Antiarrhythmic drug effect
☐ d. Antiarrhythmic drug toxicity
☐ e. Hyperkalemia
☐ f. Hypokalemia
☐ g. Hypercalcemia
☐ h. Hypocalcemia
☐ i. Atrial septal defect, secundum
☐ j. Atrial septal defect, primum
☐ k. Dextrocardia, mirror image
☐ l. Mitral valve disease
☐ m. Chronic lung disease
☐ n. Acute cor pulmonale, including pulmonary embolus
☐ o. Pericardial effusion
☐ p. Acute pericarditis
☐ q. Hypertrophic cardiomyopathy
☐ r. Coronary artery disease
☐ s. Central nervous system disorder
☐ t. Myxedema
☐ u. Hypothermia
☐ v. Sick sinus syndrome

ECG 6 was obtained from a 66-year-old female complaining of rapid, irregular heart beating. The ECG shows atrial fibrillation with a rapid ventricular response, sometimes resulting in aberrant conduction as seen in the 4th beat on the tracing (arrow). Intermittent irregular ventricular pacing is present (arrowheads). This is the result of sensed atrial fibrillation/flutter waves with subsequent ventricular pacing (normal DDD pacemaker function). The 10th beat in the tracing is a fusion complex (asterisk), which results from simultaneous ventricular pacing and normal conduction through the AV node. The native QRS complexes show a nonspecific intraventricular conduction defect.

Codes:

2s	Atrial fibrillation
5a	Fusion complexes
7h	IVCD, nonspecific type
7i	Aberrant intraventricular conduction with supraventricular arrhythmia
12g	ST-T segment abnormalities secondary to IVCD or hypertrophy
13e	Dual chamber, atrial sensing pacemaker

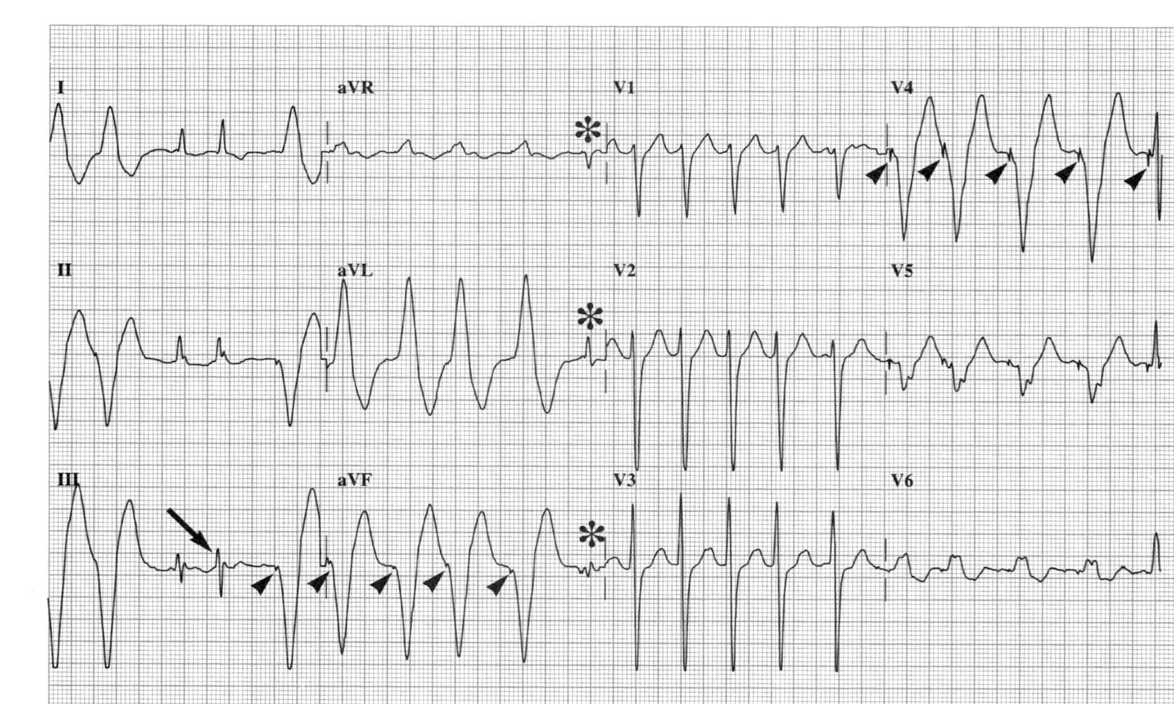

Questions: ECG 6

1. A DDD pacemaker senses:

   a. The ventricle only
   b. The atrium only
   c. The atrium and the ventricle
   d. Neither the atrium nor the ventricle

2. Which of the following statements about the effects of atrial fibrillation on DDD pacemakers are true:

   a. Rapid irregular pacing may occur
   b. Complete inhibition of pacemaker activity may occur
   c. Upper rate pacing occurs when the fibrillation waves are large and sensed

Answers: ECG 6

1. DDD pacemakers sense and pace both the right atrium and the right ventricle, resulting in inhibition or triggering of pulse generator impulses on either the atrial or ventricular channels. (Answer: c)

2. In atrial fibrillation, atrial sensing of the rapid irregular fibrillation/flutter waves can result in rapid irregular pacing of the ventricle. On the other hand, if the ventricular response rate (to native AV nodal conduction) is in excess of the upper rate limit of the pacemaker, the pacemaker will be inhibited without any pacemaker activity apparent on the 12-lead ECG. If the atrial fibrillation/flutter waves are large, and for the most part entirely sensed, the pacemaker response will be upper rate limit ventricular pacing with some irregularity. Some of the newer pacemaker models have programmed adaptive features to respond specifically to the development of atrial fibrillation or supraventricular tachycardia. One of these algorithms involves "automatic mode switching" — when the atrium senses atrial fibrillation, the pacemaker is automatically reprogrammed to a VVI mode (to avoid tracking the rapid irregular fibrillation and/or flutter waves). (Answer: All)

— Quick Review 6 —

Atrial fibrillation	
• ____ waves are absent	P
• Atrial activity is totally ____ and represented by fibrillatory (f) waves of varying amplitudes, duration and morphology	irregular
• Atrial activity is best seen in the ____ and ____ leads	right precordial, inferior
• Ventricular rhythm is (regularly/irregularly) irregular	irregularly
• ____ toxicity may result in regularization of the RR interval due to complete heart block with junctional tachycardia	Digitalis
• Ventricular rate is usually ____ per minute in the absence of drugs	100-180
▸ Think ____ if the ventricular rate is > 200 per minute and the QRS is > 0.12 seconds	Wolff-Parkinson-White
Fusion complexes	
• Due to simultaneous activation of the ventricle from ____ sources, resulting in a QRS complex that is ____ in morphology between each source	2 intermediate
Dual chamber, atrial-sensing pacemaker	
• For atrial sensing, need to demonstrate inhibition of (atrial/ventricular) output and/or triggering of the (atrial/ventricular) stimulus in response to intrinsic atrial depolarization	atrial ventricular
• Includes ____ and possibly VAT or VDD pacemakers	DDD

Common Dilemmas in ECG Interpretation

Problem:

The ECG shows an acute myocardial infarction. Should any other ECG diagnoses be coded?

Recommendation

Yes. It is also important to code 12e (ST and/or T abnormalities suggesting myocardial injury) and 14r (coronary artery disease) when acute myocardial infarction is present. Remember to code 12e when ST segment depression is present in leads V_1 and V_2 in the setting of posterior MI.

ECG 7. 58-year-old male with recent epigastric discomfort:

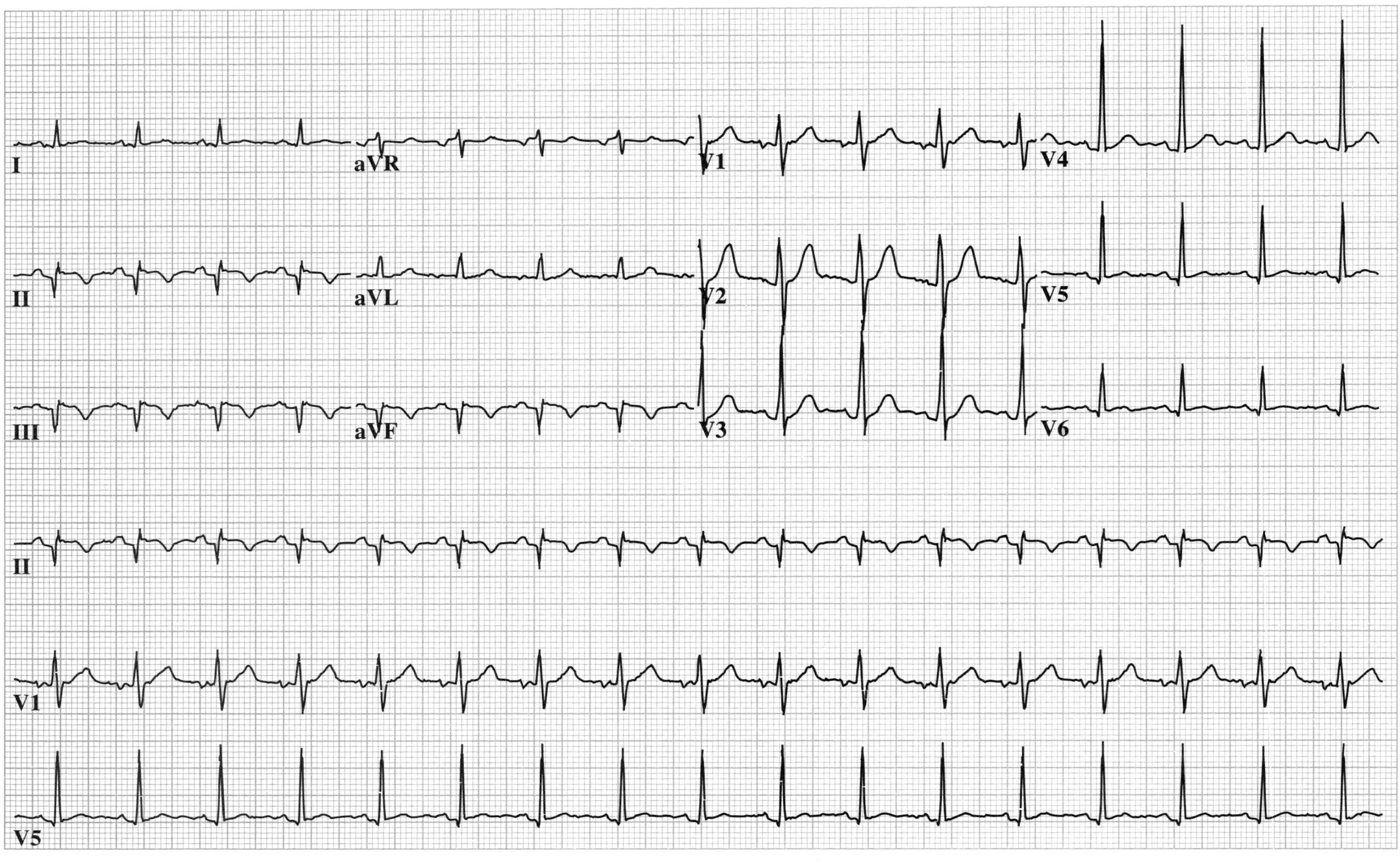

1. GENERAL FEATURES

☐ a. Normal ECG
☐ b. Borderline normal ECG or normal variant
☐ c. Incorrect electrode placement
☐ d. Artifact due to tremor

2. ATRIAL RHYTHMS

☐ a. Sinus rhythm
☐ b. Sinus arrhythmia
☐ c. Sinus bradycardia (< 60)
☐ d. Sinus tachycardia (> 100)
☐ e. Sinus pause or arrest
☐ f. Sinoatrial exit block
☐ g. Ecoptic atrial rhythm
☐ h. Wandering atrial pacemaker
☐ i. Atrial premature complexes, normally conducted
☐ j. Atrial premature complexes, nonconducted
☐ k. Atrial premature complexes with aberrant intraventricular conduction
☐ l. Atrial tachycardia (regular, sustained, 1:1 conduction)
☐ m. Atrial tachycardia, repetitive (short paroxysms)
☐ n. Atrial tachycardia, multifocal
☐ o. Atrial tachycardia with AV block
☐ p. Supraventricular tachycardia, unspecific
☐ q. Supraventricular tachycardia, paroxysmal
☐ r. Atrial flutter
☐ s. Atrial fibrillation
☐ t. Retrograde atrial activation

3. AV JUNCTIONAL RHYTHMS

☐ a. AV junctional premature complexes
☐ b. AV junctional escape complexes
☐ c. AV junctional rhythm, accelerated
☐ d. AV junctional rhythm

4. VENTRICULAR RHYTHMS

☐ a. Ventricular premature complex(es), uniform, fixed coupling
☐ b. Ventricular premature complex(es), uniform, nonfixed coupling
☐ c. Ventricular premature complexes(es), multiform
☐ d. Ventricular premature complexes, in pairs
☐ e. Ventricular parasystole
☐ f. Ventricular tachycardia (≥ 3 consecutive complexes)
☐ g. Accelerated idioventricular rhythm
☐ h. Ventricular escape complexes or rhythm
☐ i. Ventricular fibrillation

5. ATRIAL-VENTRICULAR INTERACTIONS IN ARRHYTHMIAS

☐ a. Fusion complexes
☐ b. Reciprocal (echo) complexes
☐ c. Ventricular capture complexes
☐ d. AV dissociation
☐ e. Ventriculophasic sinus arrhythmia

6. AV CONDUCTION ABNORMALITIES

☐ a. AV block, 1°
☐ b. AV block, 2° - Mobitz type I (Wenckebach)
☐ c. AV block, 2° - Mobitz type II
☐ d. AV block, 2:1
☐ e. AV block, 3°
☐ f. AV block, variable
☐ g. Short PR interval (with sinus rhythm and normal QRS duration)
☐ h. Wolff-Parkinson-White pattern

7. INTRAVENTRICULAR CONDUCTION DISTURBANCES

☐ a. RBBB, incomplete
☐ b. RBBB, complete
☐ c. Left anterior fascicular block
☐ d. Left posterior fascicular block
☐ e. LBBB, with ST-T wave suggestive of acute myocardial injury or infarction
☐ f. LBBB, complete
☐ g. LBBB, intermittent
☐ h. Intraventricular conduction disturbance, nonspecific
☐ i. Aberrant intraventricular conduction with supraventricular arrhythmia

8. P WAVE ABNORMALITIES

☐ a. Right atrial abnormality
☐ b. Left atrial abnormalities
☐ c. Nonspecific atrial abnormality

9. ABNORMALITIES OF QRS VOLTAGE OR AXIS

☐ a. Low voltage, limb leads only
☐ b. Low voltage, limb and precordial leads
☐ c. Left axis deviation (> - 30%)
☐ d. Right axis deviation (> + 100)
☐ e. Electrical alternans

10. VENTRICULAR HYPERTROPHY

☐ a. LVH by voltage only
☐ b. LVH by voltage and ST-T segment abnormalities
☐ c. RVH
☐ d. Combined ventricular hypertrophy

11. Q WAVE MYOCARDIAL INFARCTION

	Probably Acute or Recent	Probably Old or Age Indeterminate
Anterolateral	☐ a.	☐ g.
Anterior	☐ b.	☐ h.
Anteroseptal	☐ c.	☐ i.
Lateral/High lateral	☐ d.	☐ j.
Inferior	☐ e.	☐ k.
Posterior	☐ f.	☐ l.

☐ m. Probably ventricular aneurysm

12. ST, T, U, WAVE ABNORMALITIES

☐ a. Normal variant, early repolarization
☐ b. Normal variant, juvenile T waves
☐ c. Nonspecific ST and/or T wave abnormalities
☐ d. ST and/or T wave abnormalities suggesting myocardial ischemia
☐ e. ST and/or T wave abnormalities suggesting myocardial injury
☐ f. ST and/or T wave abnormalities suggesting acute pericarditis
☐ g. ST-T segment abnormalities secondary to intraventricular conduction disturbance or hypertrophy
☐ h. Post-extrasystolic T wave abnormality
☐ i. Isolated J point depression
☐ j. Peaked T waves
☐ k. Prolonged QT interval
☐ l. Prominent U waves

13. PACEMAKER FUNCTION AND RHYTHM

☐ a. Atrial or coronary sinus pacing
☐ b. Ventricular demand pacing
☐ c. AV sequential pacing
☐ d. Ventricular pacing, complete control
☐ e. Dual chamber, atrial sensing pacemaker
☐ f. Pacemaker malfunction, not constantly capturing (atrium or ventricle)
☐ g. Pacemaker malfunction, not constantly sensing (atrium or ventricle)
☐ h. Pacemaker malfunction, not firing
☐ i. Pacemaker malfunction, slowing

14. SUGGESTED OR PROBABLE CLINICAL DISORDERS

☐ a. Digitalis effect
☐ b. Digitalis toxicity
☐ c. Antiarrhythmic drug effect
☐ d. Antiarrhythmic drug toxicity
☐ e. Hyperkalemia
☐ f. Hypokalemia
☐ g. Hypercalcemia
☐ h. Hypocalcemia
☐ i. Atrial septal defect, secundum
☐ j. Atrial septal defect, primum
☐ k. Dextrocardia, mirror image
☐ l. Mitral valve disease
☐ m. Chronic lung disease
☐ n. Acute cor pulmonale, including pulmonary embolus
☐ o. Pericardial effusion
☐ p. Acute pericarditis
☐ q. Hypertrophic cardiomyopathy
☐ r. Coronary artery disease
☐ s. Central nervous system disorder
☐ t. Myxedema
☐ u. Hypothermia
☐ v. Sick sinus syndrome

ECG 7 was obtained in a 58-year-old male with recent epigastric discomfort. The tracing shows a sinus tachycardia at 102 beats/minute. ST segment elevation is present in leads II, III and aVF (arrowheads) consistent with an injury pattern and an acute or recent inferior myocardial infarction. The prominent R wave in lead V_1 (arrow) is consistent with acute or recent posterior myocardial infarction. Left axis deviation is present, probably due to the inferior wall MI. Coronary artery disease should also be coded.

Codes:

2d	Sinus tachycardia
9c	Left axis deviation (>-30°)
11e	Inferior Q wave MI, probably acute or recent
11f	Posterior MI, probably acute or recent
12e	ST and/or T wave abnormalities suggesting myocardial injury
14r	Coronary artery disease

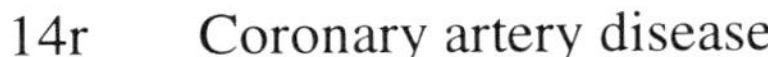

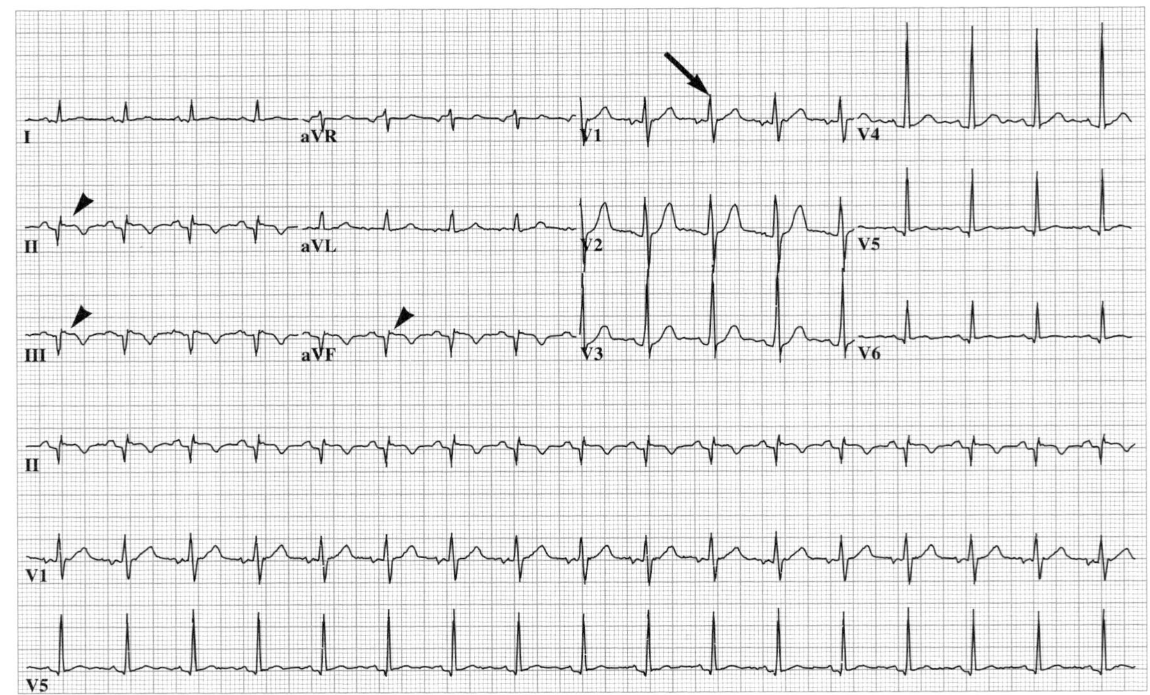

Questions: ECG 7

1. Sinus tachycardia requires a:

   a. Normal P wave axis
   b. Normal PR interval
   c. Rate > 100 BPM
   d. Normal QRS axis

2. Upwardly convex ST elevation is typically due to myocardial infarction/injury:

   a. True
   b. False

3. ECG findings consistent with coronary artery disease include:

   a. Abnormal Q waves
   b. Convex ST segment elevation
   c. Nonspecific ST and/or T wave changes

Answers: ECG 7

1. Sinus tachycardia requires a normal P wave axis and a rate greater than 100 BPM. The PR interval may be short, normal, or prolonged, and the QRS axis may be normal, leftward, or rightward; they are generally not helpful in determining whether the atrial rhythm originates in the sinus node. (Answer: a, c)

2. Upwardly convex ST segment elevation is typically due to myocardial injury or infarction. In the setting of acute MI, Q waves generally develop in leads with ST elevation. Prompt and complete resolution of ST segment elevation is usually good evidence of adequate reperfusion during primary angioplasty or thrombolytic therapy. (Answer: a)

3. The diagnosis of coronary artery disease (14r) is one of the most frequently coded criteria on the ECG section of the Cardiovascular Disease board examination. To make this diagnosis, there should be very strong evidence of coronary disease such as pathological Q waves and/or ischemic ST segment elevation. Neither nonspecific ST-T changes nor isolated ST depression is sufficient to diagnose coronary disease. However, if ST depression in V_1 - V_3 is associated with a tall R wave in $V_1 \geq 0.04$ seconds in a patient with chest pain, acute posterior myocardial infarction and coronary disease should be coded. (Answer: a, b)

— Quick Review 7 —

Sinus tachycardia (>100)	
• Rate > ____ per minute	100
• P wave amplitude often (increases/decreases) and PR interval often (increases/decreases) with increasing heart rate	increases decreases
Inferior MI, recent or probably acute	
• Abnormal Q waves and ST elevation in at least two of leads ____	II, III, aVF
• Associated ST depression is usually evident in leads I, aVL, V_1-V_3 (true/false)	true
Posterior MI, recent or probably acute	
• Initial R wave ≥ ____ seconds in leads ____ and ____ with:	0.04, V_1 V_2
▸ R wave amplitude (greater than/less than) S wave amplitude, *and* ST segment (elevation/depression) with (upright/inverted) T waves	greater than depression, upright
• Posterior MI is usually seen in the setting of acute inferior MI (true/false)	true
• RVH, WPW and RBBB (do/do not) interfere with the ECG diagnosis of posterior MI	do

Don't Get Confused!

Atrial Fibrillation

P waves are absent; atrial activity is totally irregular and represented by fibrillatory (f) waves of varying amplitudes, duration and morphology, causing random oscillation of the baseline; ventricular rhythm is irregularly irregular (unless third-degree AV block is present).

May be confused with:

Multifocal atrial tachycardia

Atrial rate is >100 per minute; P waves have 3 or more different morphologies; and PR, RR and RP intervals vary.

Paroxysmal atrial tachycardia with block

P wave axis or morphology is different from the sinus node; atrial rate is 150-240 per minute; isoelectric intervals are seen between P waves in all leads; second- or third-degree AV block is present; and the rhythm is regular.

Atrial flutter

Rapid regular atrial undulations (flutter or "F" waves) occur at a rate of 240-340 per minute; QRS complex may be normal or aberrant; rate and regularity of QRS complexes depend on the AV conduction sequence; and a distinct isoelectric baseline is absent (except possibly in lead V_1).

ECG 8. 97-year-old female with confusion and weakness:

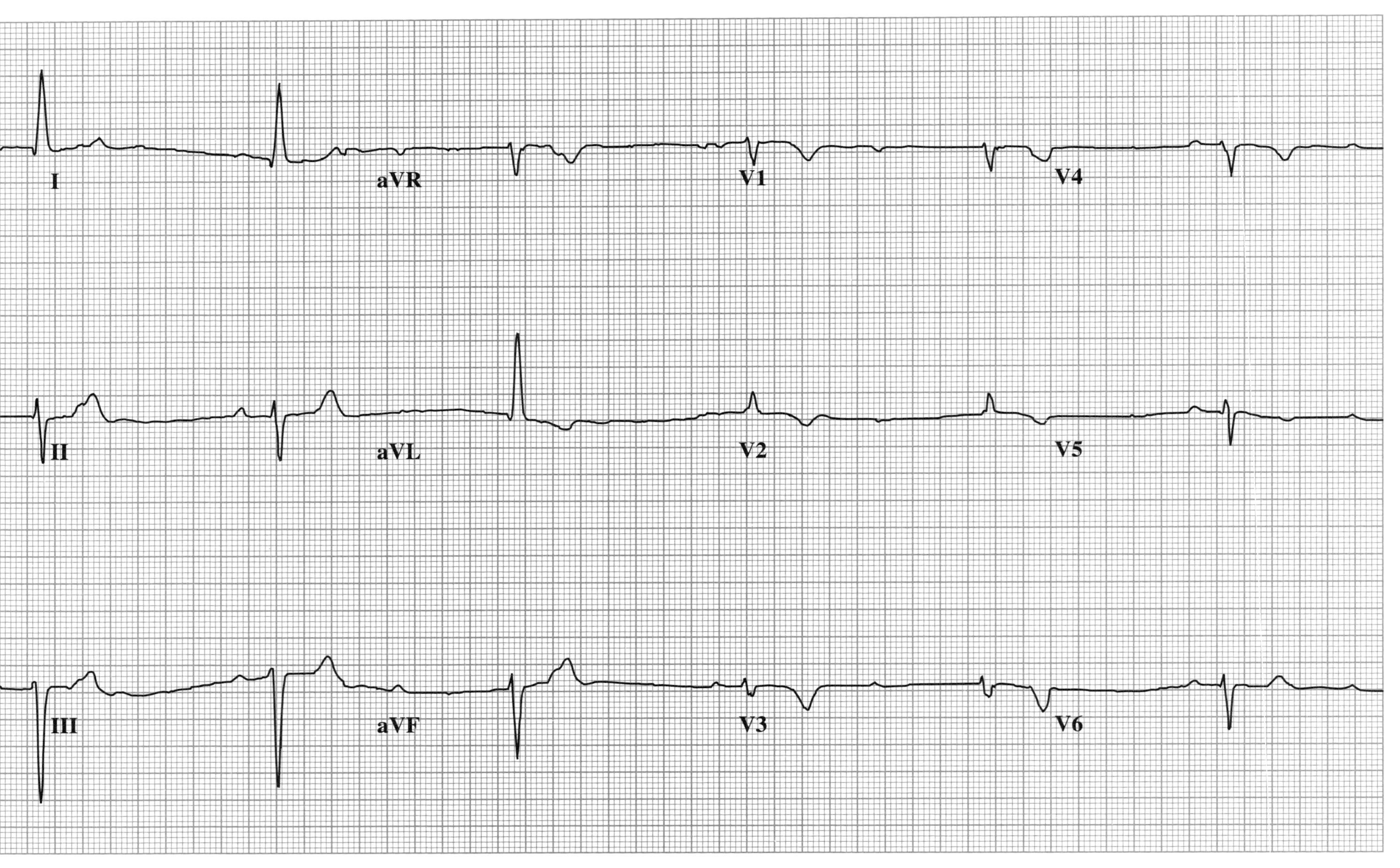

1. GENERAL FEATURES

☐ a. Normal ECG
☐ b. Borderline normal ECG or normal variant
☐ c. Incorrect electrode placement
☐ d. Artifact due to tremor

2. ATRIAL RHYTHMS

☐ a. Sinus rhythm
☐ b. Sinus arrhythmia
☐ c. Sinus bradycardia (< 60)
☐ d. Sinus tachycardia (> 100)
☐ e. Sinus pause or arrest
☐ f. Sinoatrial exit block
☐ g. Ecoptic atrial rhythm
☐ h. Wandering atrial pacemaker
☐ i. Atrial premature complexes, normally conducted
☐ j. Atrial premature complexes, nonconducted
☐ k. Atrial premature complexes with aberrant intraventricular conduction
☐ l. Atrial tachycardia (regular, sustained, 1:1 conduction)
☐ m. Atrial tachycardia, repetitive (short paroxysms)
☐ n. Atrial tachycardia, multifocal
☐ o. Atrial tachycardia with AV block
☐ p. Supraventricular tachycardia, unspecific
☐ q. Supraventricular tachycardia, paroxysmal
☐ r. Atrial flutter
☐ s. Atrial fibrillation
☐ t. Retrograde atrial activation

3. AV JUNCTIONAL RHYTHMS

☐ a. AV junctional premature complexes
☐ b. AV junctional escape complexes
☐ c. AV junctional rhythm, accelerated
☐ d. AV junctional rhythm

4. VENTRICULAR RHYTHMS

☐ a. Ventricular premature complex(es), uniform, fixed coupling
☐ b. Ventricular premature complex(es), uniform, nonfixed coupling
☐ c. Ventricular premature complexes(es), multiform
☐ d. Ventricular premature complexes, in pairs
☐ e. Ventricular parasystole
☐ f. Ventricular tachycardia (≥ 3 consecutive complexes)
☐ g. Accelerated idioventricular rhythm
☐ h. Ventricular escape complexes or rhythm
☐ i. Ventricular fibrillation

5. ATRIAL-VENTRICULAR INTERACTIONS IN ARRHYTHMIAS

☐ a. Fusion complexes
☐ b. Reciprocal (echo) complexes
☐ c. Ventricular capture complexes
☐ d. AV dissociation
☐ e. Ventriculophasic sinus arrhythmia

6. AV CONDUCTION ABNORMALITIES

☐ a. AV block, 1°
☐ b. AV block, 2° - Mobitz type I (Wenckebach)
☐ c. AV block, 2° - Mobitz type II
☐ d. AV block, 2:1
☐ e. AV block, 3°
☐ f. AV block, variable
☐ g. Short PR interval (with sinus rhythm and normal QRS duration)
☐ h. Wolff-Parkinson-White pattern

7. INTRAVENTRICULAR CONDUCTION DISTURBANCES

☐ a. RBBB, incomplete
☐ b. RBBB, complete
☐ c. Left anterior fascicular block
☐ d. Left posterior fascicular block
☐ e. LBBB, with ST-T wave suggestive of acute myocardial injury or infarction
☐ f. LBBB, complete
☐ g. LBBB, intermittent
☐ h. Intraventricular conduction disturbance, nonspecific
☐ i. Aberrant intraventricular conduction with supraventricular arrhythmia

8. P WAVE ABNORMALITIES

☐ a. Right atrial abnormality
☐ b. Left atrial abnormalities
☐ c. Nonspecific atrial abnormality

9. ABNORMALITIES OF QRS VOLTAGE OR AXIS

☐ a. Low voltage, limb leads only
☐ b. Low voltage, limb and precordial leads
☐ c. Left axis deviation (> - 30%)
☐ d. Right axis deviation (> + 100)
☐ e. Electrical alternans

10. VENTRICULAR HYPERTROPHY

☐ a. LVH by voltage only
☐ b. LVH by voltage and ST-T segment abnormalities
☐ c. RVH
☐ d. Combined ventricular hypertrophy

11. Q WAVE MYOCARDIAL INFARCTION

	Probably Acute or Recent	Probably Old or Age Indeterminate
Anterolateral	☐ a.	☐ g.
Anterior	☐ b.	☐ h.
Anteroseptal	☐ c.	☐ i.
Lateral/High lateral	☐ d.	☐ j.
Inferior	☐ e.	☐ k.
Posterior	☐ f.	☐ l.

☐ m. Probably ventricular aneurysm

12. ST, T, U, WAVE ABNORMALITIES

☐ a. Normal variant, early repolarization
☐ b. Normal variant, juvenile T waves
☐ c. Nonspecific ST and/or T wave abnormalities
☐ d. ST and/or T wave abnormalities suggesting myocardial ischemia
☐ e. ST and/or T wave abnormalities suggesting myocardial injury
☐ f. ST and/or T wave abnormalities suggesting acute pericarditis
☐ g. ST-T segment abnormalities secondary to intraventricular conduction disturbance or hypertrophy
☐ h. Post-extrasystolic T wave abnormality
☐ i. Isolated J point depression
☐ j. Peaked T waves
☐ k. Prolonged QT interval
☐ l. Prominent U waves

13. PACEMAKER FUNCTION AND RHYTHM

☐ a. Atrial or coronary sinus pacing
☐ b. Ventricular demand pacing
☐ c. AV sequential pacing
☐ d. Ventricular pacing, complete control
☐ e. Dual chamber, atrial sensing pacemaker
☐ f. Pacemaker malfunction, not constantly capturing (atrium or ventricle)
☐ g. Pacemaker malfunction, not constantly sensing (atrium or ventricle)
☐ h. Pacemaker malfunction, not firing
☐ i. Pacemaker malfunction, slowing

14. SUGGESTED OR PROBABLE CLINICAL DISORDERS

☐ a. Digitalis effect
☐ b. Digitalis toxicity
☐ c. Antiarrhythmic drug effect
☐ d. Antiarrhythmic drug toxicity
☐ e. Hyperkalemia
☐ f. Hypokalemia
☐ g. Hypercalcemia
☐ h. Hypocalcemia
☐ i. Atrial septal defect, secundum
☐ j. Atrial septal defect, primum
☐ k. Dextrocardia, mirror image
☐ l. Mitral valve disease
☐ m. Chronic lung disease
☐ n. Acute cor pulmonale, including pulmonary embolus
☐ o. Pericardial effusion
☐ p. Acute pericarditis
☐ q. Hypertrophic cardiomyopathy
☐ r. Coronary artery disease
☐ s. Central nervous system disorder
☐ t. Myxedema
☐ u. Hypothermia
☐ v. Sick sinus syndrome

ECG 8 was obtained from a 97-year-old female who presents with confusion and weakness. The ECG shows a sinus bradycardia with complete heart block and a junctional escape rhythm at 35 BPM (arrows mark P waves; arrowheads mark junctional escape complexes). The junctional escape complexes show evidence for LVH (R wave in I ≥ 14 mm; R wave in aVL ≥ 12 mm; R wave in aVL + S wave in III > 20 mm) with associated ST-T changes, nonspecific IVCD, and left axis deviation. The sinus bradycardia, complete heart block, and junctional escape are all consistent with the diagnosis of sick sinus syndrome.

Codes:

2c	Sinus bradycardia
3b	AV junctional escape complexes
6e	AV block, 3°
9c	Left axis deviation (> -30°)
10b	LVH by both voltage and ST-T segment abnormalities
12g	ST-T segment abnormalities secondary to IVCD or hypertrophy
14v	Sick sinus syndrome

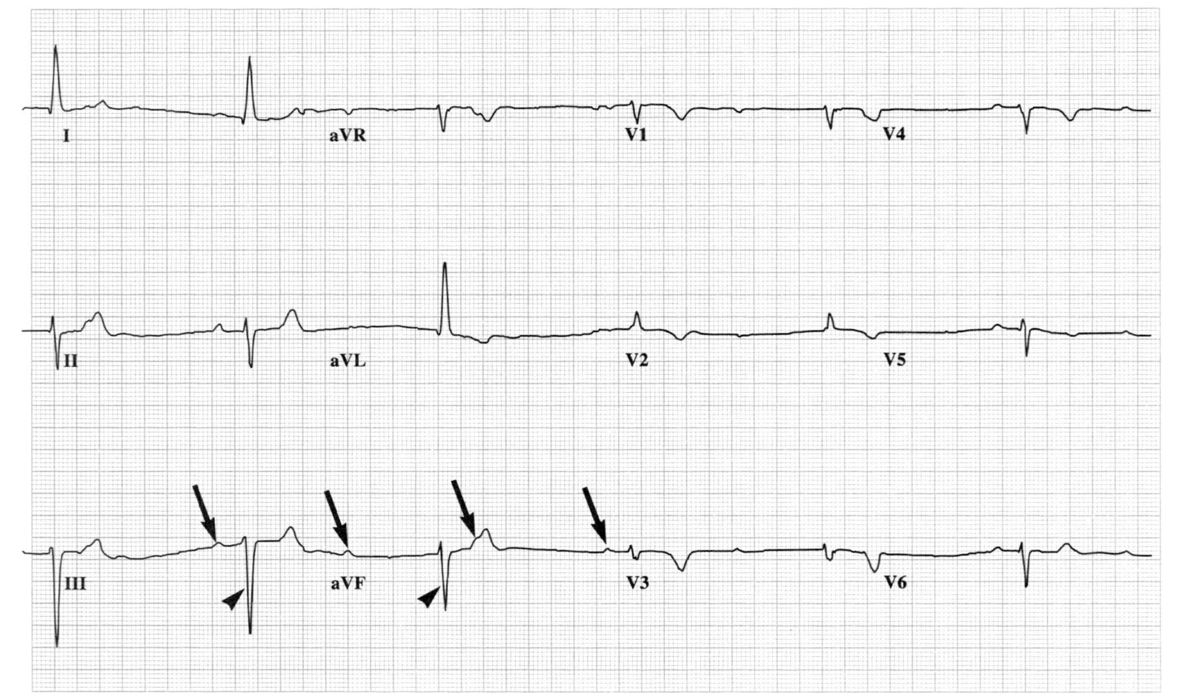

Questions: ECG 8

1. The distorted T wave best seen in the first beat in leads II, III, and aVF is due to:

   a. Repolarization abnormality
   b. Artifact
   c. Superimposed P wave

2. Is ventriculophasic sinus arrhythmia present?

   a. Yes
   b. No

3. Can the diagnosis of left anterior fascicular block be made with certainty on this tracing?

   a. Yes
   b. No

4. Which leads (or combination of leads) in this tracing manifest voltage criteria for LVH?

   a. R wave in lead I
   b. R wave in lead aVL + S wave in lead III
   c. R wave in lead V_1 + S wave in lead V_6
   d. R wave in lead aVL
   e. S wave in lead aVR

5. Complete AV block can be diagnosed when the ventricular rate is faster than the atrial rate:

   a. True
   b. False

6. Causes of complete heart block include:

   a. Hyperkalemia
   b. Hypokalemia
   c. Endocarditis
   d. Acute MI
   e. Digitalis toxicity
   f. Lyme disease

7. In patients with complete congenital heart block, the site of block is typically the:

   a. AV node
   b. Bundle of His
   c. His-Purinkje system

Answers: ECG 8

1. Complete heart block occurs when atrial impulses consistently fail to reach the ventricles (i.e., atria and ventricles beat independently of each other). On ECG, the PP and RR intervals are constant, but the PR interval varies (since the P wave bares no constant relationship to the QRS complex). The P wave may precede, be buried within (and not visualized), or follow the QRS to deform the ST segment or T wave, as seen in several beats in the present tracing. The presence of bifid T waves in the first but not the second beats in leads II and III speaks against repolarization abnormality, which, if present in one beat, should be present in all beats in that lead. Artifact may deform the T wave, but this diagnosis is unlikely since the positive deflection appears in the early portion of the T wave and nowhere else on the ECG. (Answer: c)

2. Ventriculophasic sinus arrhythmia occurs in approximately 30% of cases of complete heart block, and is said to be present when the PP interval containing a QRS complex is shorter than the PP interval not containing a QRS complex. In the present tracing, the PP intervals are regular, so ventriculophasic sinus arrhythmia is not present. (Answer: b)

3. Left anterior fascicular block (LAFB) is a diagnosis of exclusion, and can only be made with certainty when other conditions causing left axis deviation are absent, such as left ventricular hypertrophy (which is present on this tracing), inferior myocardial infarction, and chronic lung disease. (Answer: b)

4. Voltage criteria satisfied in this tracing include an R wave in lead I $\geq$ 14 mm, and an R wave in lead aVL $\geq$ 12 mm. (Answer: a, d)

5. The diagnosis of complete heart block requires that atrial and ventricular activity are independent of each other, <u>and</u> that the atrial rate is *faster* than the ventricular rate. When the ventricular rate exceeds the atrial rate, *AV dissociation* (as opposed to AV block) is said to be present; in this situation, the rapidly beating ventricles may be refractory to incoming atrial impulses, even though AV conduction is intact. (Answer: b)

6. Complete heart block may occur in advanced hyperkalemia, although death is usually from ventricular tachyarrhythmias. In endocarditis, inflammation and edema of the septum and peri-AV nodal tissues may cause conduction failure and complete heart block; PR prolongation usually precedes this event. Five to fifteen percent of acute myocardial infarctions are complicated by complete heart block: In inferior MI, complete heart block is usually preceded by first-degree AV block or Type I second-degree AV block, usually occurs at the level of the AV node, is typically transient (< 1 week), and is usually associated with a stable junctional escape rhythm (narrow QRS; rate $\geq$ 40 BPM). In anterior MI, complete heart block occurs as a result of extensive damage to the left ventricle, is typically preceded by Type II second-degree AV block or bifascicular block, and is associated with mortality rates as high as 70% due to pump failure rather than heart block per se. Digitalis toxicity is one of

the most common causes of reversible complete AV block, and is usually associated with a junctional escape rhythm (narrow QRS), which is often accelerated. Lyme disease, which is caused by a tick-borne spirochete (Borrelia burgdorferi), can also cause complete heart block. This disorder begins with a characteristic skin rash (erythema chronicum migrans), and may be followed in subsequent weeks to months by joint, cardiac and neurological involvement. Cardiac involvement includes AV block, which may be partial or complete, usually occurs at the level of the AV node, and may be accompanied by syncope. Other causes of complete heart block include infiltrative diseases of the myocardium (amyloid, sarcoid), myocardial contusion, acute rheumatic fever, aortic valve disease, degenerative diseases of the conduction system (Lev's disease, Lenegre's disease), and others. (Answer: All except b)

7. Complete congenital heart block usually occurs at the level of the AV node, and is typically associated with a stable junctional escape. Many very young patients have escape heart rates > 55 BPM and do not require permanent pacing until age 25-30. (Answer: a)

— Quick Review 8 —

AV junctional escape complexes	
• QRS complex occurs as a ____ phenomenon in response to decreased sinus impulse formation or conduction, or high-degree AV block	secondary
• Rate is typically ____ per minute	40-60
• Atrial mechanism may be sinus rhythm, paroxysmal atrial tachycardia, atrial flutter, or atrial fibrillation (true/false)	true
• QRS morphology is (similar to/different from) the sinus or supraventricular impulse	similar to
AV block, 3°	
• Atrial and ventricular rhythms are ____ of each other	independent
• Atrial rate is (faster/slower) than the ventricular rate	faster
Sick sinus syndrome	
• Marked sinus ____	bradycardia
• ____ arrest or ____ exit block	Sinus, sinoatrial
• Bradycardia alternating with ____	tachycardia
• Atrial fibrillation with ____ ventricular response preceded or followed by sinus bradycardia, sinus arrest, or sinoatrial exit block	slow
• Prolonged sinus node ____ time after atrial premature complex or atrial tachyarrhythmias	recovery
• AV junctional ____ rhythm	escape
• Additional conduction system disease is often present, including AV block, IVCD, and/or bundle branch block (true/false)	true

ECG 9. 63-year-old female with high blood pressure:

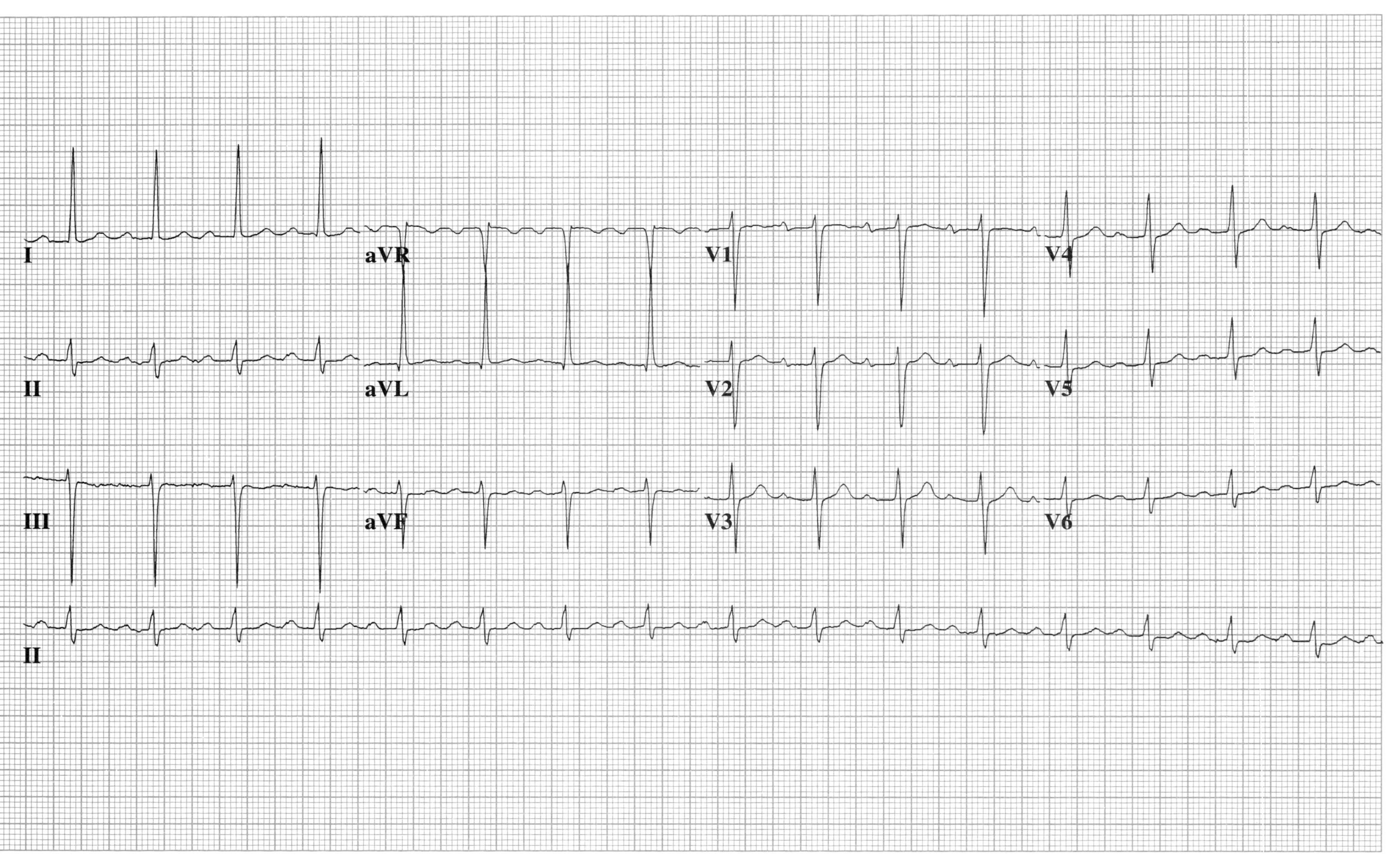

1. GENERAL FEATURES

- ☐ a. Normal ECG
- ☐ b. Borderline normal ECG or normal variant
- ☐ c. Incorrect electrode placement
- ☐ d. Artifact due to tremor

2. ATRIAL RHYTHMS

- ☐ a. Sinus rhythm
- ☐ b. Sinus arrhythmia
- ☐ c. Sinus bradycardia (< 60)
- ☐ d. Sinus tachycardia (> 100)
- ☐ e. Sinus pause or arrest
- ☐ f. Sinoatrial exit block
- ☐ g. Ecoptic atrial rhythm
- ☐ h. Wandering atrial pacemaker
- ☐ i. Atrial premature complexes, normally conducted
- ☐ j. Atrial premature complexes, nonconducted
- ☐ k. Atrial premature complexes with aberrant intraventricular conduction
- ☐ l. Atrial tachycardia (regular, sustained, 1:1 conduction)
- ☐ m. Atrial tachycardia, repetitive (short paroxysms)
- ☐ n. Atrial tachycardia, multifocal
- ☐ o. Atrial tachycardia with AV block
- ☐ p. Supraventricular tachycardia, unspecific
- ☐ q. Supraventricular tachycardia, paroxysmal
- ☐ r. Atrial flutter
- ☐ s. Atrial fibrillation
- ☐ t. Retrograde atrial activation

3. AV JUNCTIONAL RHYTHMS

- ☐ a. AV junctional premature complexes
- ☐ b. AV junctional escape complexes
- ☐ c. AV junctional rhythm, accelerated
- ☐ d. AV junctional rhythm

4. VENTRICULAR RHYTHMS

- ☐ a. Ventricular premature complex(es), uniform, fixed coupling
- ☐ b. Ventricular premature complex(es), uniform, nonfixed coupling
- ☐ c. Ventricular premature complexes(es), multiform
- ☐ d. Ventricular premature complexes, in pairs
- ☐ e. Ventricular parasystole
- ☐ f. Ventricular tachycardia (≥ 3 consecutive complexes)
- ☐ g. Accelerated idioventricular rhythm
- ☐ h. Ventricular escape complexes or rhythm
- ☐ i. Ventricular fibrillation

5. ATRIAL-VENTRICULAR INTERACTIONS IN ARRHYTHMIAS

- ☐ a. Fusion complexes
- ☐ b. Reciprocal (echo) complexes
- ☐ c. Ventricular capture complexes
- ☐ d. AV dissociation
- ☐ e. Ventriculophasic sinus arrhythmia

6. AV CONDUCTION ABNORMALITIES

- ☐ a. AV block, 1°
- ☐ b. AV block, 2° - Mobitz type I (Wenckebach)
- ☐ c. AV block, 2° - Mobitz type II
- ☐ d. AV block, 2:1
- ☐ e. AV block, 3°
- ☐ f. AV block, variable
- ☐ g. Short PR interval (with sinus rhythm and normal QRS duration)
- ☐ h. Wolff-Parkinson-White pattern

7. INTRAVENTRICULAR CONDUCTION DISTURBANCES

- ☐ a. RBBB, incomplete
- ☐ b. RBBB, complete
- ☐ c. Left anterior fascicular block
- ☐ d. Left posterior fascicular block
- ☐ e. LBBB, with ST-T wave suggestive of acute myocardial injury or infarction
- ☐ f. LBBB, complete
- ☐ g. LBBB, intermittent
- ☐ h. Intraventricular conduction disturbance, nonspecific
- ☐ i. Aberrant intraventricular conduction with supraventricular arrhythmia

8. P WAVE ABNORMALITIES

- ☐ a. Right atrial abnormality
- ☐ b. Left atrial abnormalities
- ☐ c. Nonspecific atrial abnormality

9. ABNORMALITIES OF QRS VOLTAGE OR AXIS

- ☐ a. Low voltage, limb leads only
- ☐ b. Low voltage, limb and precordial leads
- ☐ c. Left axis deviation (> - 30%)
- ☐ d. Right axis deviation (> + 100)
- ☐ e. Electrical alternans

10. VENTRICULAR HYPERTROPHY

- ☐ a. LVH by voltage only
- ☐ b. LVH by voltage and ST-T segment abnormalities
- ☐ c. RVH
- ☐ d. Combined ventricular hypertrophy

11. Q WAVE MYOCARDIAL INFARCTION

	Probably Acute or Recent	Probably Old or Age Indeterminate
Anterolateral	☐ a.	☐ g.
Anterior	☐ b.	☐ h.
Anteroseptal	☐ c.	☐ i.
Lateral/High lateral	☐ d.	☐ j.
Inferior	☐ e.	☐ k.
Posterior	☐ f.	☐ l.

☐ m. Probably ventricular aneurysm

12. ST, T, U, WAVE ABNORMALITIES

- ☐ a. Normal variant, early repolarization
- ☐ b. Normal variant, juvenile T waves
- ☐ c. Nonspecific ST and/or T wave abnormalities
- ☐ d. ST and/or T wave abnormalities suggesting myocardial ischemia
- ☐ e. ST and/or T wave abnormalities suggesting myocardial injury
- ☐ f. ST and/or T wave abnormalities suggesting acute pericarditis
- ☐ g. ST-T segment abnormalities secondary to intraventricular conduction disturbance or hypertrophy
- ☐ h. Post-extrasystolic T wave abnormality
- ☐ i. Isolated J point depression
- ☐ j. Peaked T waves
- ☐ k. Prolonged QT interval
- ☐ l. Prominent U waves

13. PACEMAKER FUNCTION AND RHYTHM

- ☐ a. Atrial or coronary sinus pacing
- ☐ b. Ventricular demand pacing
- ☐ c. AV sequential pacing
- ☐ d. Ventricular pacing, complete control
- ☐ e. Dual chamber, atrial sensing pacemaker
- ☐ f. Pacemaker malfunction, not constantly capturing (atrium or ventricle)
- ☐ g. Pacemaker malfunction, not constantly sensing (atrium or ventricle)
- ☐ h. Pacemaker malfunction, not firing
- ☐ i. Pacemaker malfunction, slowing

14. SUGGESTED OR PROBABLE CLINICAL DISORDERS

- ☐ a. Digitalis effect
- ☐ b. Digitalis toxicity
- ☐ c. Antiarrhythmic drug effect
- ☐ d. Antiarrhythmic drug toxicity
- ☐ e. Hyperkalemia
- ☐ f. Hypokalemia
- ☐ g. Hypercalcemia
- ☐ h. Hypocalcemia
- ☐ i. Atrial septal defect, secundum
- ☐ j. Atrial septal defect, primum
- ☐ k. Dextrocardia, mirror image
- ☐ l. Mitral valve disease
- ☐ m. Chronic lung disease
- ☐ n. Acute cor pulmonale, including pulmonary embolus
- ☐ o. Pericardial effusion
- ☐ p. Acute pericarditis
- ☐ q. Hypertrophic cardiomyopathy
- ☐ r. Coronary artery disease
- ☐ s. Central nervous system disorder
- ☐ t. Myxedema
- ☐ u. Hypothermia
- ☐ v. Sick sinus syndrome

ECG 9 was obtained in a 63-year-old female with high blood pressure. The ECG shows a sinus rhythm at 98 BPM with first-degree AV block and LVH by voltage criteria (R wave in I ≥ 14 mm; R wave in aVL + S wave in V_3 > 20 mm; R wave in aVL ≥ 12 mm).

Codes:

2a	Sinus rhythm
6a	AV block, 1°
10a	Left ventricular hypertrophy by voltage only

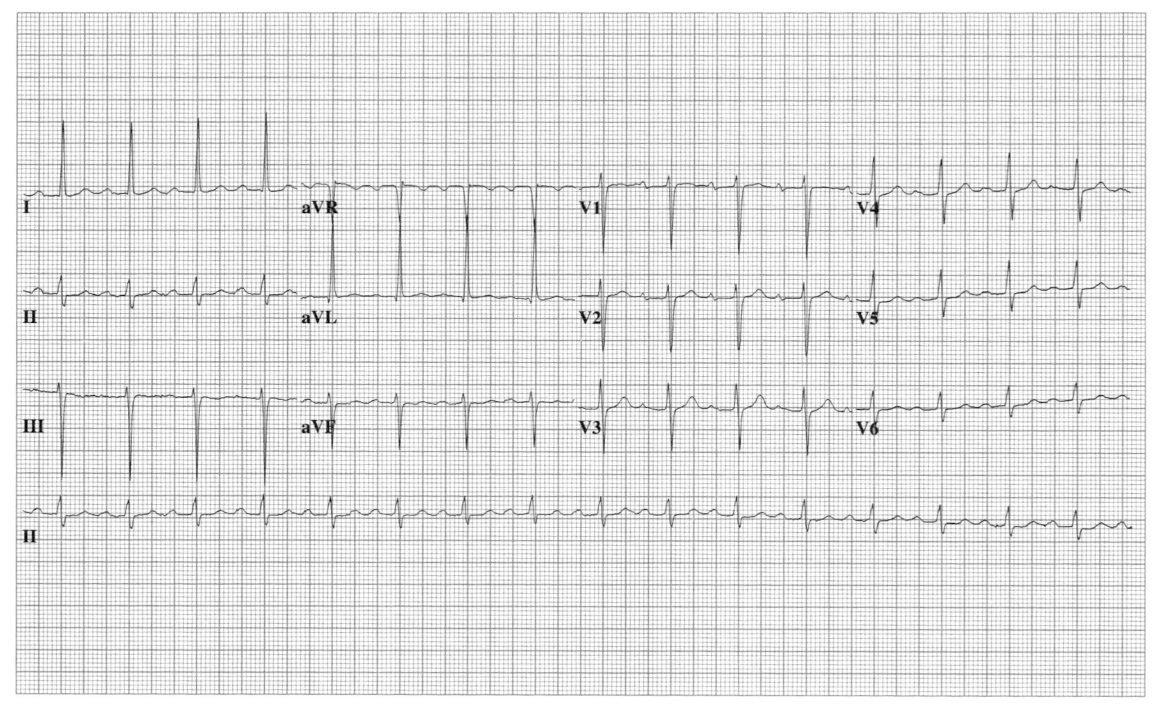

Questions: ECG 9

1. Characteristic repolarization changes associated with LVH include ST segment and T wave deviation in a direction opposite to the major deflection of the QRS:

   a. True
   b. False

2. A prolonged PR interval may result from delay in the:

   a. Sinoatrial node
   b. AV node
   c. His bundle
   d. Bundle branches

3. An R wave in lead aVL ≥ ___ mm is consistent with LVH:

   a. 10 mm
   b. 15 mm
   c. 12 mm
   d. 14 mm

Answers: ECG 9

1. Typical repolarization abnormalities associated with left ventricular hypertrophy include ST segment and T wave deviation opposite to the major QRS vector. This usually manifests as ST segment depression and T wave inversion in leads with dominant R waves (V_4 - V_6), and subtle ST segment elevation and tall T waves in leads with a dominant S wave (V_1 - V_3). ST segment changes in the limb leads are generally directed away from the main QRS forces. The repolarization abnormalities associated with LVH are often mistaken for lateral myocardial ischemia (due to the presence of lateral ST depression and T wave inversions) or anterior/inferior myocardial infarction (due to the presence of Q waves in II, III, aVF, V_1-V_2 and ST elevation in V_1 - V_2). LVH is probably the most common cause for false positive exercise treadmill ECG tests. Since patients with hypertension are at increased risk for coronary artery disease, when such patients present with chest pain and ECG findings of LVH with a "strain pattern," it is important to pursue further diagnostic testing (e.g., nuclear stress perfusion imaging or stress echocardiography) to rule out ischemic heart disease. (Answer: a)

2. The normal PR interval is defined as 0.12 - 0.20 seconds. A PR interval exceeding 0.20 seconds identifies the presence of first-degree AV block, and a PR interval less than 0.12 seconds identifies the presence of a short PR interval. The PR interval

represents the interval from the onset of atrial depolarization to the onset of ventricular depolarization; it does not, however, represent conduction from the sinoatrial node to the atrium. Prolongation of the PR interval, therefore, may be caused by conduction delay within the atrium, AV node, His bundle or bundle branches, but not the sinoatrial node. When the QRS complex is narrow, conduction delay usually occurs at the level of the AV node. When the QRS complex is wide, conduction delay usually occurs within the bundle branches. (Answer: b, c, d)

3. An R wave in lead aVL ≥ 12 mm is consistent with and highly specific for the diagnosis of LVH. The specificity of this finding is reduced when left anterior fascicular block is present. Despite its high specificity, only 10-15% of patients with proven LVH meet this criteria. (Answer: b, c, d)

— Quick Review 9 —

AV block, 1°	
• PR interval ≥ ____ seconds	0.20
LVH by voltage only	
• **Cornell Criteria** (most accurate): R in aVL + S in V_3 > ____ mm in males or > ____ mm in females	24, 20
• **Other commonly used voltage-based criteria**	
▸ Precordial leads (one or more)	
(1) R wave in V_5 or V_6 + S wave in V_1	
▸ > ____ mm if age > 30 years	35
(2) Maximum R wave + S wave in precordial leads > ____ mm	45
(3) R wave in V_5 > ____ mm	26
(4) R wave in V_6 > ____ mm	20
▸ Limb leads (one or more)	
(1) R wave in I + S in lead II ≥ ____ mm	26
(2) R wave in lead I ≥ ____ mm	14
(3) S wave in aVR ≥ ____ mm	15
(4) R wave in aVL ≥ ____ mm	12
(5) R wave in aVF ≥ ____ mm	21

Don't Forget!

- An S_1 S_2 S_3 pattern (S wave in leads I, II, and III) is present in up to 20% of healthy adults
- Parkinson's tremor (~ 300 per minute) may be mistaken for atrial flutter
- If sinus bradycardia is present at a rate < 40 per minute, think of 2:1 sinoatrial exit block (item 2f)
- P wave amplitude often increases and PR interval often shortens with increasing heart rate (e.g., during exercise)
- The post-extrasystolic pause of normally conducted APCs is usually *noncompensatory* (i.e., PP interval containing the APC is less than two times the normal PP interval)
- In nonconducted (blocked) APCs, the P waves are often hidden in the preceding T wave — when you see an RR pause, look for a deformed T wave immediately preceding the pause to identify the presence of a nonconducted atrial premature beat

ECG 10. 51-year-old female with a history of asthma:

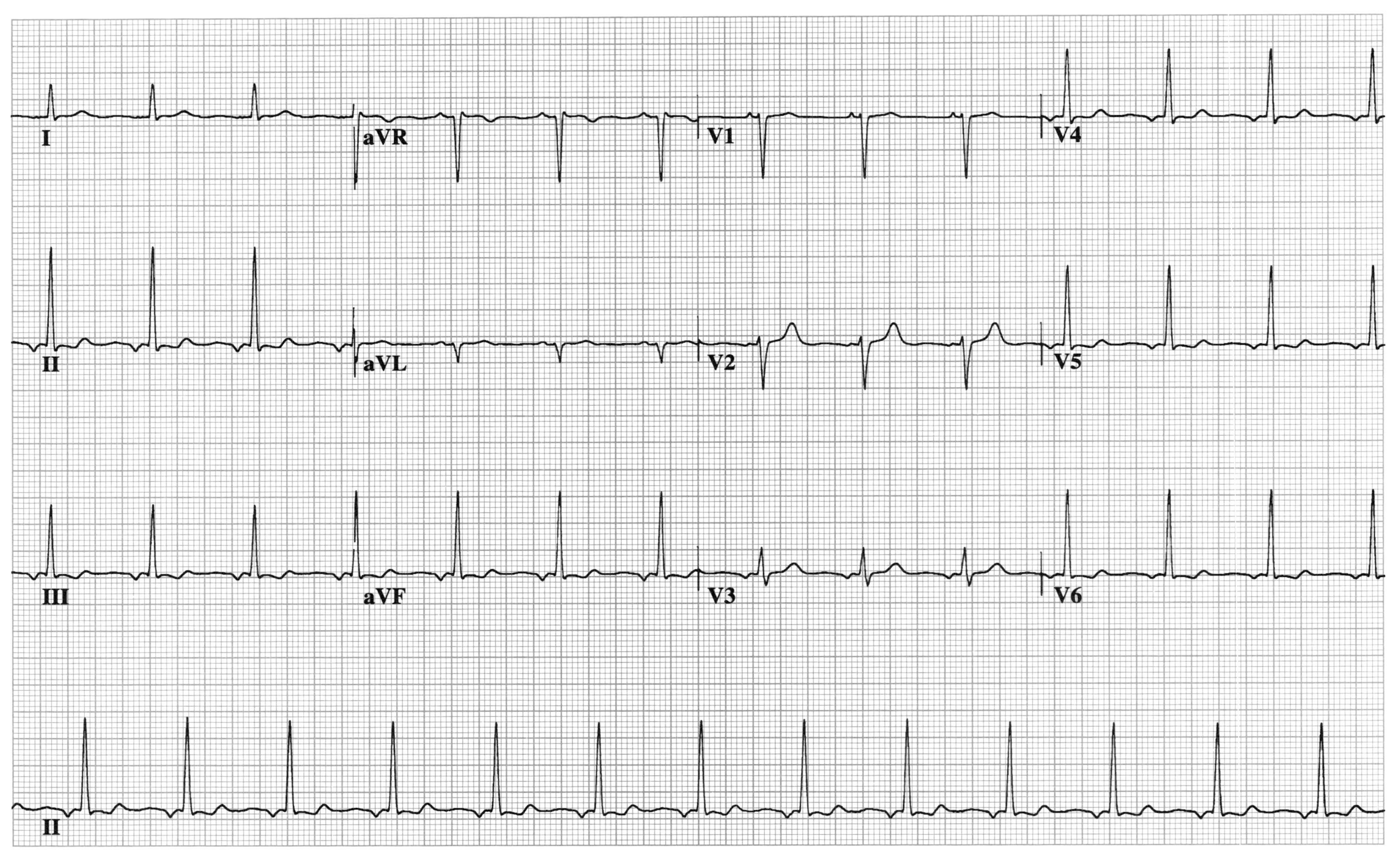

1. GENERAL FEATURES

- ☐ a. Normal ECG
- ☐ b. Borderline normal ECG or normal variant
- ☐ c. Incorrect electrode placement
- ☐ d. Artifact due to tremor

2. ATRIAL RHYTHMS

- ☐ a. Sinus rhythm
- ☐ b. Sinus arrhythmia
- ☐ c. Sinus bradycardia (< 60)
- ☐ d. Sinus tachycardia (> 100)
- ☐ e. Sinus pause or arrest
- ☐ f. Sinoatrial exit block
- ☐ g. Ecoptic atrial rhythm
- ☐ h. Wandering atrial pacemaker
- ☐ i. Atrial premature complexes, normally conducted
- ☐ j. Atrial premature complexes, nonconducted
- ☐ k. Atrial premature complexes with aberrant intraventricular conduction
- ☐ l. Atrial tachycardia (regular, sustained, 1:1 conduction)
- ☐ m. Atrial tachycardia, repetitive (short paroxysms)
- ☐ n. Atrial tachycardia, multifocal
- ☐ o. Atrial tachycardia with AV block
- ☐ p. Supraventricular tachycardia, unspecific
- ☐ q. Supraventricular tachycardia, paroxysmal
- ☐ r. Atrial flutter
- ☐ s. Atrial fibrillation
- ☐ t. Retrograde atrial activation

3. AV JUNCTIONAL RHYTHMS

- ☐ a. AV junctional premature complexes
- ☐ b. AV junctional escape complexes
- ☐ c. AV junctional rhythm, accelerated
- ☐ d. AV junctional rhythm

4. VENTRICULAR RHYTHMS

- ☐ a. Ventricular premature complex(es), uniform, fixed coupling
- ☐ b. Ventricular premature complex(es), uniform, nonfixed coupling
- ☐ c. Ventricular premature complexes(es), multiform
- ☐ d. Ventricular premature complexes, in pairs
- ☐ e. Ventricular parasystole
- ☐ f. Ventricular tachycardia (≥ 3 consecutive complexes)
- ☐ g. Accelerated idioventricular rhythm
- ☐ h. Ventricular escape complexes or rhythm
- ☐ i. Ventricular fibrillation

5. ATRIAL-VENTRICULAR INTERACTIONS IN ARRHYTHMIAS

- ☐ a. Fusion complexes
- ☐ b. Reciprocal (echo) complexes
- ☐ c. Ventricular capture complexes
- ☐ d. AV dissociation
- ☐ e. Ventriculophasic sinus arrhythmia

6. AV CONDUCTION ABNORMALITIES

- ☐ a. AV block, 1°
- ☐ b. AV block, 2° - Mobitz type I (Wenckebach)
- ☐ c. AV block, 2° - Mobitz type II
- ☐ d. AV block, 2:1
- ☐ e. AV block, 3°
- ☐ f. AV block, variable
- ☐ g. Short PR interval (with sinus rhythm and normal QRS duration)
- ☐ h. Wolff-Parkinson-White pattern

7. INTRAVENTRICULAR CONDUCTION DISTURBANCES

- ☐ a. RBBB, incomplete
- ☐ b. RBBB, complete
- ☐ c. Left anterior fascicular block
- ☐ d. Left posterior fascicular block
- ☐ e. LBBB, with ST-T wave suggestive of acute myocardial injury or infarction
- ☐ f. LBBB, complete
- ☐ g. LBBB, intermittent
- ☐ h. Intraventricular conduction disturbance, nonspecific
- ☐ i. Aberrant intraventricular conduction with supraventricular arrhythmia

8. P WAVE ABNORMALITIES

- ☐ a. Right atrial abnormality
- ☐ b. Left atrial abnormalities
- ☐ c. Nonspecific atrial abnormality

9. ABNORMALITIES OF QRS VOLTAGE OR AXIS

- ☐ a. Low voltage, limb leads only
- ☐ b. Low voltage, limb and precordial leads
- ☐ c. Left axis deviation (> - 30%)
- ☐ d. Right axis deviation (> + 100)
- ☐ e. Electrical alternans

10. VENTRICULAR HYPERTROPHY

- ☐ a. LVH by voltage only
- ☐ b. LVH by voltage and ST-T segment abnormalities
- ☐ c. RVH
- ☐ d. Combined ventricular hypertrophy

11. Q WAVE MYOCARDIAL INFARCTION

	Probably Acute or Recent	Probably Old or Age Indeterminate
Anterolateral	☐ a.	☐ g.
Anterior	☐ b.	☐ h.
Anteroseptal	☐ c.	☐ i.
Lateral/High lateral	☐ d.	☐ j.
Inferior	☐ e.	☐ k.
Posterior	☐ f.	☐ l.

- ☐ m. Probably ventricular aneurysm

12. ST, T, U, WAVE ABNORMALITIES

- ☐ a. Normal variant, early repolarization
- ☐ b. Normal variant, juvenile T waves
- ☐ c. Nonspecific ST and/or T wave abnormalities
- ☐ d. ST and/or T wave abnormalities suggesting myocardial ischemia
- ☐ e. ST and/or T wave abnormalities suggesting myocardial injury
- ☐ f. ST and/or T wave abnormalities suggesting acute pericarditis
- ☐ g. ST-T segment abnormalities secondary to intraventricular conduction disturbance or hypertrophy
- ☐ h. Post-extrasystolic T wave abnormality
- ☐ i. Isolated J point depression
- ☐ j. Peaked T waves
- ☐ k. Prolonged QT interval
- ☐ l. Prominent U waves

13. PACEMAKER FUNCTION AND RHYTHM

- ☐ a. Atrial or coronary sinus pacing
- ☐ b. Ventricular demand pacing
- ☐ c. AV sequential pacing
- ☐ d. Ventricular pacing, complete control
- ☐ e. Dual chamber, atrial sensing pacemaker
- ☐ f. Pacemaker malfunction, not constantly capturing (atrium or ventricle)
- ☐ g. Pacemaker malfunction, not constantly sensing (atrium or ventricle)
- ☐ h. Pacemaker malfunction, not firing
- ☐ i. Pacemaker malfunction, slowing

14. SUGGESTED OR PROBABLE CLINICAL DISORDERS

- ☐ a. Digitalis effect
- ☐ b. Digitalis toxicity
- ☐ c. Antiarrhythmic drug effect
- ☐ d. Antiarrhythmic drug toxicity
- ☐ e. Hyperkalemia
- ☐ f. Hypokalemia
- ☐ g. Hypercalcemia
- ☐ h. Hypocalcemia
- ☐ i. Atrial septal defect, secundum
- ☐ j. Atrial septal defect, primum
- ☐ k. Dextrocardia, mirror image
- ☐ l. Mitral valve disease
- ☐ m. Chronic lung disease
- ☐ n. Acute cor pulmonale, including pulmonary embolus
- ☐ o. Pericardial effusion
- ☐ p. Acute pericarditis
- ☐ q. Hypertrophic cardiomyopathy
- ☐ r. Coronary artery disease
- ☐ s. Central nervous system disorder
- ☐ t. Myxedema
- ☐ u. Hypothermia
- ☐ v. Sick sinus syndrome

ECG 10 was obtained in this 51-year-old female with a history of asthma. The tracing shows an ectopic atrial rhythm at 81 beats/minute. The inverted P waves (arrows) are consistent with a rhythm originating in the lower part of the atrium or the AV junction. The PR interval greater than 110 ms (the PR interval on this tracing is approximately 125 msec) is consistent with an ectopic atrial rhythm rather than an accelerated junctional rhythm with retrograde atrial conduction. Nonspecific repolarization abnormalities are present.

Codes:

2g Ectopic atrial rhythm
12c Nonspecific ST and/or T wave abnormalities

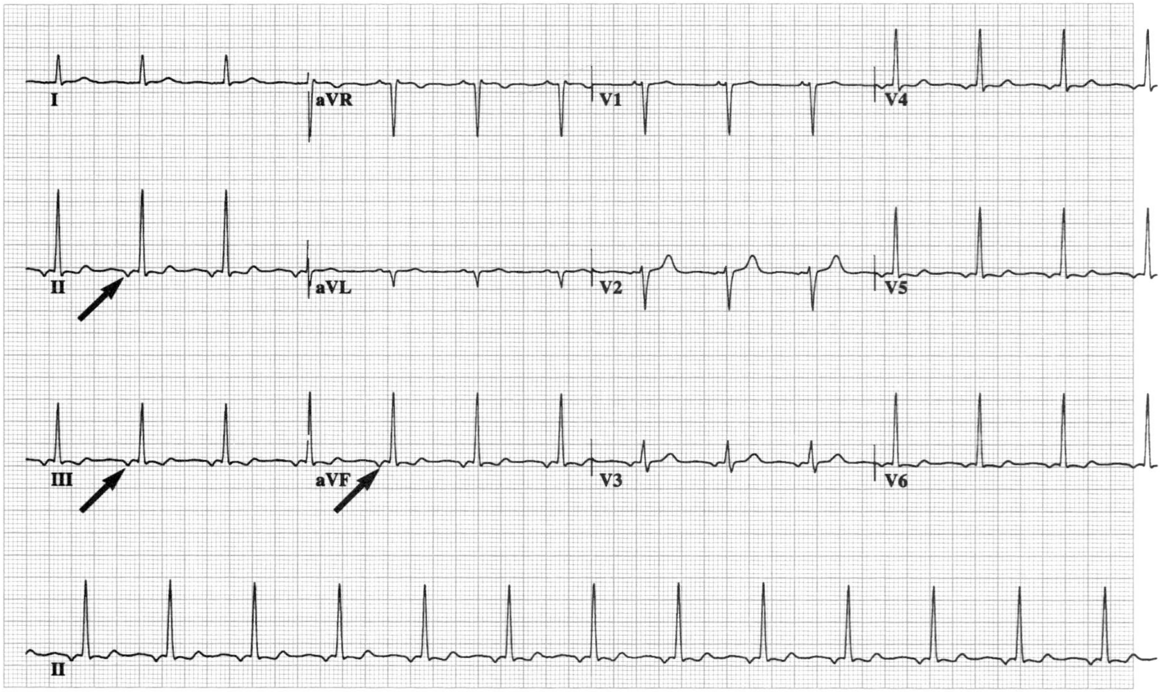

Questions: ECG 10

1. Rhythms consistent with this ECG include:

   a. Sinus rhythm
   b. Sinus tachycardia with 2:1 second-degree sinoatrial exit block
   c. Accelerated junctional rhythm with retrograde atrial activation
   d. Ectopic atrial rhythm
   e Accelerated idioventricular rhythm with retrograde atrial activation

2. Which of the following statements about ectopic atrial rhythm are true?

   a. P wave may be upright or inverted
   b. PR interval may be prolonged, normal, or short
   c. QT interval is usually prolonged

Answers: ECG 10

1. This ECG is consistent with a low atrial rhythm or junctional rhythm with retrograde atrial activation. The inverted P wave in lead II excludes the diagnosis of sinus rhythm or sinus tachycardia with second degree 2:1 sinoatrial exit block, since sinus P waves are always upright in this lead. The narrow QRS complex essentially excludes idioventricular rhythm, although a ventricular rhythm originating high in the septum may produce a relatively narrow QRS complex. (Answer: c, d, e)

2. Ectopic atrial rhythms can have P waves that are upright (when atrial activity originates near the sinus node) or inverted (when the ectopic focus originates in the lower atrium). The PR interval may be prolonged, normal, or short, depending on the proximity of the ectopic atrial impulse to the AV node, and whether delay is present in the AV conduction system. The QT interval, which represents the duration of ventricular depolarization and repolarization, is typically normal in ectopic atrial rhythm. (Answer: a, b)

— Quick Review 10 —

Ectopic atrial rhythm	
• (Sinus/nonsinus) P wave	nonsinus
• Rate < ____ per minute	100
• PR interval > ____ seconds	0.11
• Inverted P waves in II, III, aVF suggest either an AV junctional rhythm with retrograde atrial activation or a low atrial rhythm:	
▸ PR > 0.11 seconds suggests (low atrial/AV junctional) rhythm	low atrial
▸ PR ≤ 0.11 seconds suggests (low atrial/AV junctional) rhythm	AV junctional
Nonspecific ST and/or T wave abnormalities	
• Slight ____ segment depression or elevation	ST
• Slightly inverted or flat ____ wave	T

— Comic Relief —

Good work! Enjoy a break before moving on to the next set of ECGs...

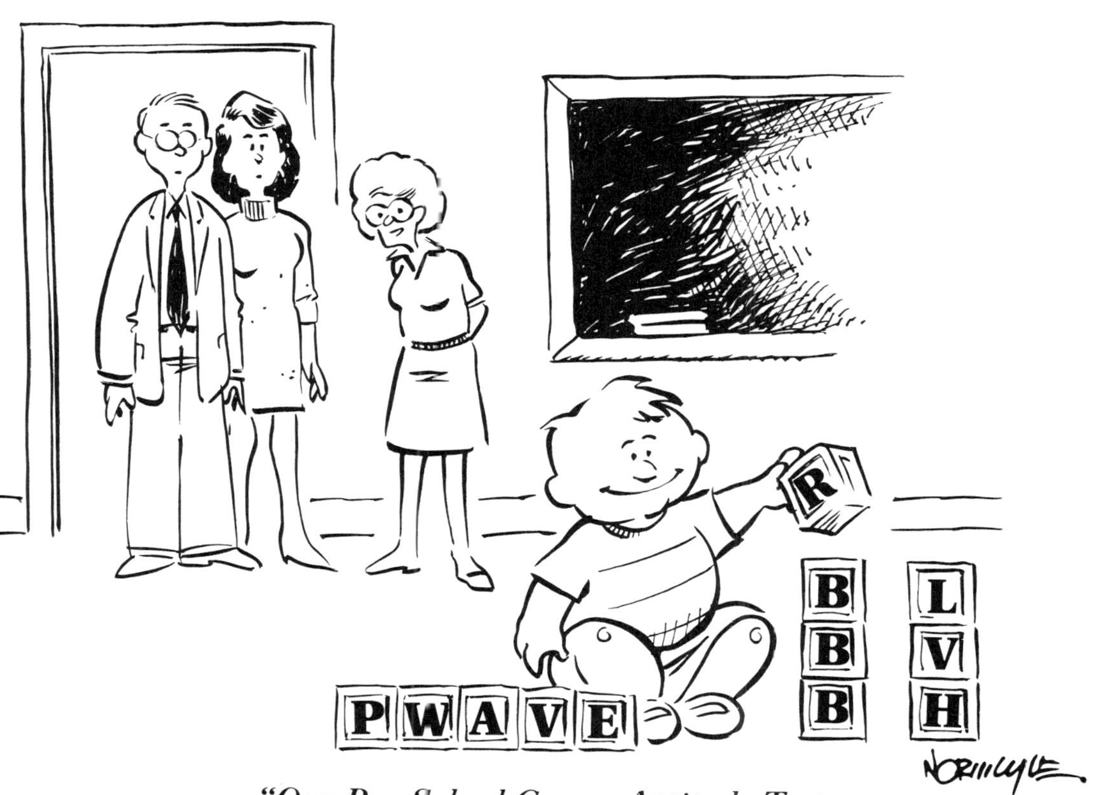

"Our Pre-School Career Aptitude Tests indicate little Mark will make a very fine cardiologist".

ECG 11. 79-year-old male with lightheadedness:

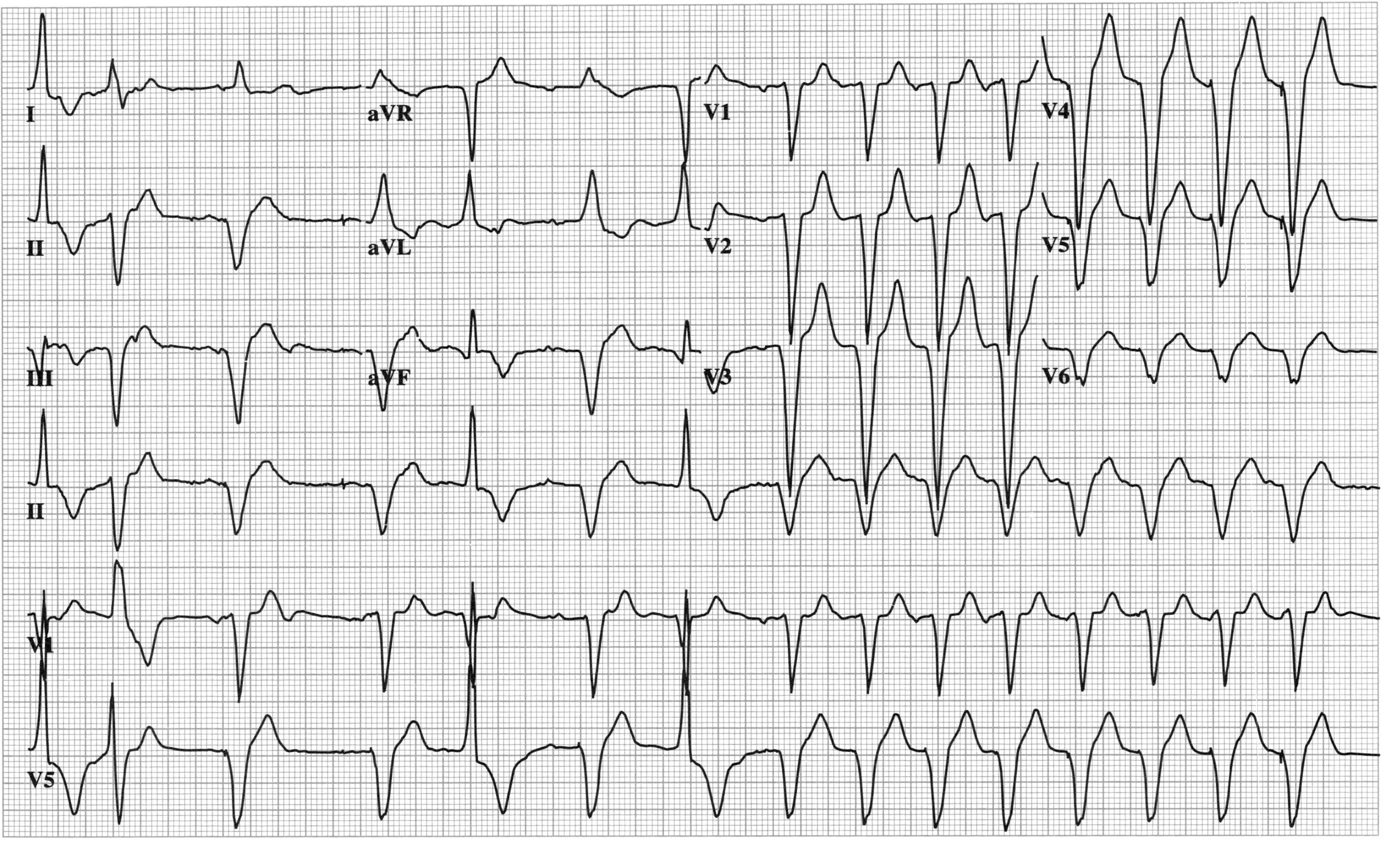

1. GENERAL FEATURES

- ☐ a. Normal ECG
- ☐ b. Borderline normal ECG or normal variant
- ☐ c. Incorrect electrode placement
- ☐ d. Artifact due to tremor

2. ATRIAL RHYTHMS

- ☐ a. Sinus rhythm
- ☐ b. Sinus arrhythmia
- ☐ c. Sinus bradycardia (< 60)
- ☐ d. Sinus tachycardia (> 100)
- ☐ e. Sinus pause or arrest
- ☐ f. Sinoatrial exit block
- ☐ g. Ecoptic atrial rhythm
- ☐ h. Wandering atrial pacemaker
- ☐ i. Atrial premature complexes, normally conducted
- ☐ j. Atrial premature complexes, nonconducted
- ☐ k. Atrial premature complexes with aberrant intraventricular conduction
- ☐ l. Atrial tachycardia (regular, sustained, 1:1 conduction)
- ☐ m. Atrial tachycardia, repetitive (short paroxysms)
- ☐ n. Atrial tachycardia, multifocal
- ☐ o. Atrial tachycardia with AV block
- ☐ p. Supraventricular tachycardia, unspecific
- ☐ q. Supraventricular tachycardia, paroxysmal
- ☐ r. Atrial flutter
- ☐ s. Atrial fibrillation
- ☐ t. Retrograde atrial activation

3. AV JUNCTIONAL RHYTHMS

- ☐ a. AV junctional premature complexes
- ☐ b. AV junctional escape complexes
- ☐ c. AV junctional rhythm, accelerated
- ☐ d. AV junctional rhythm

4. VENTRICULAR RHYTHMS

- ☐ a. Ventricular premature complex(es), uniform, fixed coupling
- ☐ b. Ventricular premature complex(es), uniform, nonfixed coupling
- ☐ c. Ventricular premature complexes(es), multiform
- ☐ d. Ventricular premature complexes, in pairs
- ☐ e. Ventricular parasystole
- ☐ f. Ventricular tachycardia (≥ 3 consecutive complexes)
- ☐ g. Accelerated idioventricular rhythm
- ☐ h. Ventricular escape complexes or rhythm
- ☐ i. Ventricular fibrillation

5. ATRIAL-VENTRICULAR INTERACTIONS IN ARRHYTHMIAS

- ☐ a. Fusion complexes
- ☐ b. Reciprocal (echo) complexes
- ☐ c. Ventricular capture complexes
- ☐ d. AV dissociation
- ☐ e. Ventriculophasic sinus arrhythmia

6. AV CONDUCTION ABNORMALITIES

- ☐ a. AV block, 1°
- ☐ b. AV block, 2° - Mobitz type I (Wenckebach)
- ☐ c. AV block, 2° - Mobitz type II
- ☐ d. AV block, 2:1
- ☐ e. AV block, 3°
- ☐ f. AV block, variable
- ☐ g. Short PR interval (with sinus rhythm and normal QRS duration)
- ☐ h. Wolff-Parkinson-White pattern

7. INTRAVENTRICULAR CONDUCTION DISTURBANCES

- ☐ a. RBBB, incomplete
- ☐ b. RBBB, complete
- ☐ c. Left anterior fascicular block
- ☐ d. Left posterior fascicular block
- ☐ e. LBBB, with ST-T wave suggestive of acute myocardial injury or infarction
- ☐ f. LBBB, complete
- ☐ g. LBBB, intermittent
- ☐ h. Intraventricular conduction disturbance, nonspecific
- ☐ i. Aberrant intraventricular conduction with supraventricular arrhythmia

8. P WAVE ABNORMALITIES

- ☐ a. Right atrial abnormality
- ☐ b. Left atrial abnormalities
- ☐ c. Nonspecific atrial abnormality

9. ABNORMALITIES OF QRS VOLTAGE OR AXIS

- ☐ a. Low voltage, limb leads only
- ☐ b. Low voltage, limb and precordial leads
- ☐ c. Left axis deviation (> - 30%)
- ☐ d. Right axis deviation (> + 100)
- ☐ e. Electrical alternans

10. VENTRICULAR HYPERTROPHY

- ☐ a. LVH by voltage only
- ☐ b. LVH by voltage and ST-T segment abnormalities
- ☐ c. RVH
- ☐ d. Combined ventricular hypertrophy

11. Q WAVE MYOCARDIAL INFARCTION

	Probably Acute or Recent	Probably Old or Age Indeterminate
Anterolateral	☐ a.	☐ g.
Anterior	☐ b.	☐ h.
Anteroseptal	☐ c.	☐ i.
Lateral/High Lateral	☐ d.	☐ j.
Inferior	☐ e.	☐ k.
Posterior	☐ f.	☐ l.

- ☐ m. Probably ventricular aneurysm

12. ST, T, U, WAVE ABNORMALITIES

- ☐ a. Normal variant, early repolarization
- ☐ b. Normal variant, juvenile T waves
- ☐ c. Nonspecific ST and/or T wave abnormalities
- ☐ d. ST and/or T wave abnormalities suggesting myocardial ischemia
- ☐ e. ST and/or T wave abnormalities suggesting myocardial injury
- ☐ f. ST and/or T wave abnormalities suggesting acute pericarditis
- ☐ g. ST-T segment abnormalities secondary to intraventricular conduction disturbance or hypertrophy
- ☐ h. Post-extrasystolic T wave abnormality
- ☐ i. Isolated J point depression
- ☐ j. Peaked T waves
- ☐ k. Prolonged QT interval
- ☐ l. Prominent U waves

13. PACEMAKER FUNCTION AND RHYTHM

- ☐ a. Atrial or coronary sinus pacing
- ☐ b. Ventricular demand pacing
- ☐ c. AV sequential pacing
- ☐ d. Ventricular pacing, complete control
- ☐ e. Dual chamber, atrial sensing pacemaker
- ☐ f. Pacemaker malfunction, not constantly capturing (atrium or ventricle)
- ☐ g. Pacemaker malfunction, not constantly sensing (atrium or ventricle)
- ☐ h. Pacemaker malfunction, not firing
- ☐ i. Pacemaker malfunction, slowing

14. SUGGESTED OR PROBABLE CLINICAL DISORDERS

- ☐ a. Digitalis effect
- ☐ b. Digitalis toxicity
- ☐ c. Antiarrhythmic drug effect
- ☐ d. Antiarrhythmic drug toxicity
- ☐ e. Hyperkalemia
- ☐ f. Hypokalemia
- ☐ g. Hypercalcemia
- ☐ h. Hypocalcemia
- ☐ i. Atrial septal defect, secundum
- ☐ j. Atrial septal defect, primum
- ☐ k. Dextrocardia, mirror image
- ☐ l. Mitral valve disease
- ☐ m. Chronic lung disease
- ☐ n. Acute cor pulmonale, including pulmonary embolus
- ☐ o. Pericardial effusion
- ☐ p. Acute pericarditis
- ☐ q. Hypertrophic cardiomyopathy
- ☐ r. Coronary artery disease
- ☐ s. Central nervous system disorder
- ☐ t. Myxedema
- ☐ u. Hypothermia
- ☐ v. Sick sinus syndrome

ECG 11 was obtained in a 79-year-old male with complaints of lightheadedness. The ECG shows a normally functioning dual chamber atrial sensing (DDD) pacemaker (asterisk). Paroxysmal atrial tachycardia is seen in the latter half of the tracing, with atrial tracking of the SVT resulting in ventricular pacing (arrows mark pacer spikes). Single, multifocal VPCs are most prominent in the rhythm strips (arrowheads). The combination of bradycardia and tachycardia suggests sick sinus syndrome.

Codes:

2m	Atrial tachycardia, repetitive (short paroxysms)
4c	Ventricular premature complex(es), multiform
13e	Dual chamber, atrial sensing pacemaker
14v	Sick sinus syndrome

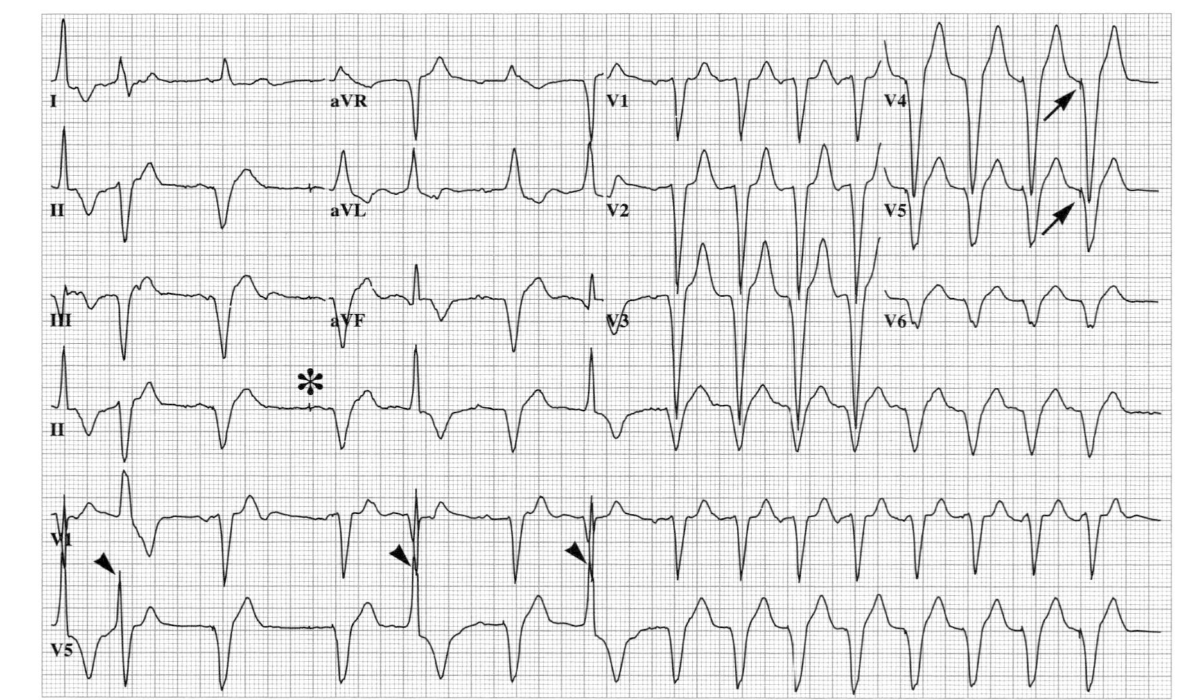

Questions: ECG 11

1. ECG clues to suggest a ventricular premature contraction rather than an atrial premature contraction include:

   a. Initial QRS vector different from sinus beats
   b. QRS duration > 0.12 seconds
   c. Retrograde P waves

2. Arrhythmias and conduction disturbances found in patients with Sick Sinus Syndrome include:

   a. Marked sinus bradycardia
   b. Sinus arrest or sinoatrial exit block
   c. Bradycardia alternating with tachycardia
   d. Atrial fibrillation with slow ventricular response preceded or followed by sinus bradycardia, sinus arrest, or sinoatrial exit block
   e. Prolonged sinus node recovery time after atrial premature complex or atrial tachyarrhythmias
   f. AV junctional escape rhythm

Answers: ECG 11

1. Clues on the electrocardiogram suggestive of a ventricular (rather than atrial) origin of an ectopic beat include an initial QRS vector different from the sinus beats, QRS duration > 0.12 seconds, retrograde P waves (caused by retrograde conduction through the AV node), and the presence of a fully compensatory pause. (Answer: All)

2. In addition to the listed abnormalities, additional conduction system disease is often present, including AV block, IVCD, and bundle branch block. (Answer: All)

— Quick Review 11 —	
Atrial tachycardia, repetitive (short paroxysm)	
• Recurring short runs of atrial tachycardia interrupted by ____	normal sinus rhythm
Dual chamber, atrial-sensing pacemaker	
• For atrial sensing, need to demonstrate inhibition of (atrial/ventricular) output and/or triggering of the (atrial/ventricular) stimulus in response to intrinsic atrial depolarization	atrial ventricular
• Includes____ and VAT or VDD pacemakers	DDD

ECG 12. 25-year-old male with syncope:

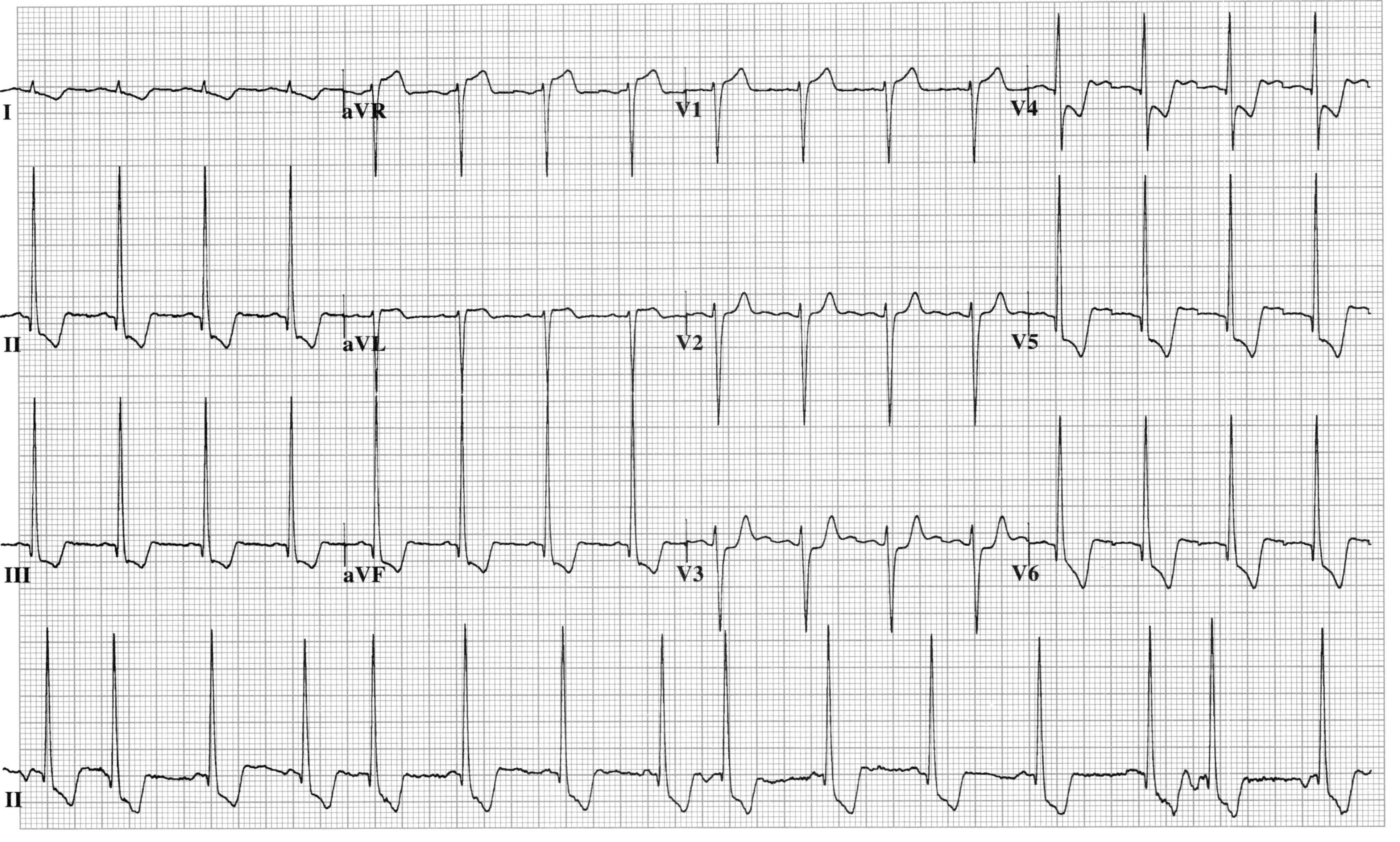

1. GENERAL FEATURES

☐ a. Normal ECG
☐ b. Borderline normal ECG or normal variant
☐ c. Incorrect electrode placement
☐ d. Artifact due to tremor

2. ATRIAL RHYTHMS

☐ a. Sinus rhythm
☐ b. Sinus arrhythmia
☐ c. Sinus bradycardia (< 60)
☐ d. Sinus tachycardia (> 100)
☐ e. Sinus pause or arrest
☐ f. Sinoatrial exit block
☐ g. Ecoptic atrial rhythm
☐ h. Wandering atrial pacemaker
☐ i. Atrial premature complexes, normally conducted
☐ j. Atrial premature complexes, nonconducted
☐ k. Atrial premature complexes with aberrant intraventricular conduction
☐ l. Atrial tachycardia (regular, sustained, 1:1 conduction)
☐ m. Atrial tachycardia, repetitive (short paroxysms)
☐ n. Atrial tachycardia, multifocal
☐ o. Atrial tachycardia with AV block
☐ p. Supraventricular tachycardia, unspecific
☐ q. Supraventricular tachycardia, paroxysmal
☐ r. Atrial flutter
☐ s. Atrial fibrillation
☐ t. Retrograde atrial activation

3. AV JUNCTIONAL RHYTHMS

☐ a. AV junctional premature complexes
☐ b. AV junctional escape complexes
☐ c. AV junctional rhythm, accelerated
☐ d. AV junctional rhythm

4. VENTRICULAR RHYTHMS

☐ a. Ventricular premature complex(es), uniform, fixed coupling
☐ b. Ventricular premature complex(es), uniform, nonfixed coupling
☐ c. Ventricular premature complexes(es), multiform
☐ d. Ventricular premature complexes, in pairs
☐ e. Ventricular parasystole
☐ f. Ventricular tachycardia (≥ 3 consecutive complexes)
☐ g. Accelerated idioventricular rhythm
☐ h. Ventricular escape complexes or rhythm
☐ i. Ventricular fibrillation

5. ATRIAL-VENTRICULAR INTERACTIONS IN ARRHYTHMIAS

☐ a. Fusion complexes
☐ b. Reciprocal (echo) complexes
☐ c. Ventricular capture complexes
☐ d. AV dissociation
☐ e. Ventriculophasic sinus arrhythmia

6. AV CONDUCTION ABNORMALITIES

☐ a. AV block, 1°
☐ b. AV block, 2° - Mobitz type I (Wenckebach)
☐ c. AV block, 2° - Mobitz type II
☐ d. AV block, 2:1
☐ e. AV block, 3°
☐ f. AV block, variable
☐ g. Short PR interval (with sinus rhythm and normal QRS duration)
☐ h. Wolff-Parkinson-White pattern

7. INTRAVENTRICULAR CONDUCTION DISTURBANCES

☐ a. RBBB, incomplete
☐ b. RBBB, complete
☐ c. Left anterior fascicular block
☐ d. Left posterior fascicular block
☐ e. LBBB, with ST-T wave suggestive of acute myocardial injury or infarction
☐ f. LBBB, complete
☐ g. LBBB, intermittent
☐ h. Intraventricular conduction disturbance, nonspecific
☐ i. Aberrant intraventricular conduction with supraventricular arrhythmia

8. P WAVE ABNORMALITIES

☐ a. Right atrial abnormality
☐ b. Left atrial abnormalities
☐ c. Nonspecific atrial abnormality

9. ABNORMALITIES OF QRS VOLTAGE OR AXIS

☐ a. Low voltage, limb leads only
☐ b. Low voltage, limb and precordial leads
☐ c. Left axis deviation (> - 30%)
☐ d. Right axis deviation (> + 100)
☐ e. Electrical alternans

10. VENTRICULAR HYPERTROPHY

☐ a. LVH by voltage only
☐ b. LVH by voltage and ST-T segment abnormalities
☐ c. RVH
☐ d. Combined ventricular hypertrophy

11. Q WAVE MYOCARDIAL INFARCTION

	Probably Acute or Recent	Probably Old or Age Indeterminate
Anterolateral	☐ a.	☐ g.
Anterior	☐ b.	☐ h.
Anteroseptal	☐ c.	☐ i.
Lateral/High lateral	☐ d.	☐ j.
Inferior	☐ e.	☐ k.
Posterior	☐ f.	☐ l.

☐ m. Probably ventricular aneurysm

12. ST, T, U, WAVE ABNORMALITIES

☐ a. Normal variant, early repolarization
☐ b. Normal variant, juvenile T waves
☐ c. Nonspecific ST and/or T wave abnormalities
☐ d. ST and/or T wave abnormalities suggesting myocardial ischemia
☐ e. ST and/or T wave abnormalities suggesting myocardial injury
☐ f. ST and/or T wave abnormalities suggesting acute pericarditis
☐ g. ST-T segment abnormalities secondary to intraventricular conduction disturbance or hypertrophy
☐ h. Post-extrasystolic T wave abnormality
☐ i. Isolated J point depression
☐ j. Peaked T waves
☐ k. Prolonged QT interval
☐ l. Prominent U waves

13. PACEMAKER FUNCTION AND RHYTHM

☐ a. Atrial or coronary sinus pacing
☐ b. Ventricular demand pacing
☐ c. AV sequential pacing
☐ d. Ventricular pacing, complete control
☐ e. Dual chamber, atrial sensing pacemaker
☐ f. Pacemaker malfunction, not constantly capturing (atrium or ventricle)
☐ g. Pacemaker malfunction, not constantly sensing (atrium or ventricle)
☐ h. Pacemaker malfunction, not firing
☐ i. Pacemaker malfunction, slowing

14. SUGGESTED OR PROBABLE CLINICAL DISORDERS

☐ a. Digitalis effect
☐ b. Digitalis toxicity
☐ c. Antiarrhythmic drug effect
☐ d. Antiarrhythmic drug toxicity
☐ e. Hyperkalemia
☐ f. Hypokalemia
☐ g. Hypercalcemia
☐ h. Hypocalcemia
☐ i. Atrial septal defect, secundum
☐ j. Atrial septal defect, primum
☐ k. Dextrocardia, mirror image
☐ l. Mitral valve disease
☐ m. Chronic lung disease
☐ n. Acute cor pulmonale, including pulmonary embolus
☐ o. Pericardial effusion
☐ p. Acute pericarditis
☐ q. Hypertrophic cardiomyopathy
☐ r. Coronary artery disease
☐ s. Central nervous system disorder
☐ t. Myxedema
☐ u. Hypothermia
☐ v. Sick sinus syndrome

ECG 12 was obtained from a 25-year-old male with syncope shows a sinus rhythm with normally conducted APCs (asterisks). LVH (S wave in aVR ≥ 15mm; R wave in aVF ≥ 21mm; R wave in V_5 + S wave in V_1≥ 40mm; R wave in V_6> 20mm) and ST-T abnormalities are noted. The markedly increased QRS voltage and ST-T abnormalities in a young person with syncope suggest the diagnosis of hypertrophic cardiomyopathy (the Q waves inferiorly and anterolaterally are secondary to the hypertrophic cardiomyopathy and not previous infarction).

Codes:

2a	Sinus rhythm
2i	Atrial premature complexes, normally conducted
10b	Left ventricular hypertrophy by both voltage and ST-T segment abnormalities
12g	ST-T segment abnormalities secondary to IVCD or hypertrophy
14q	Hypertrophic cardiomyopathy

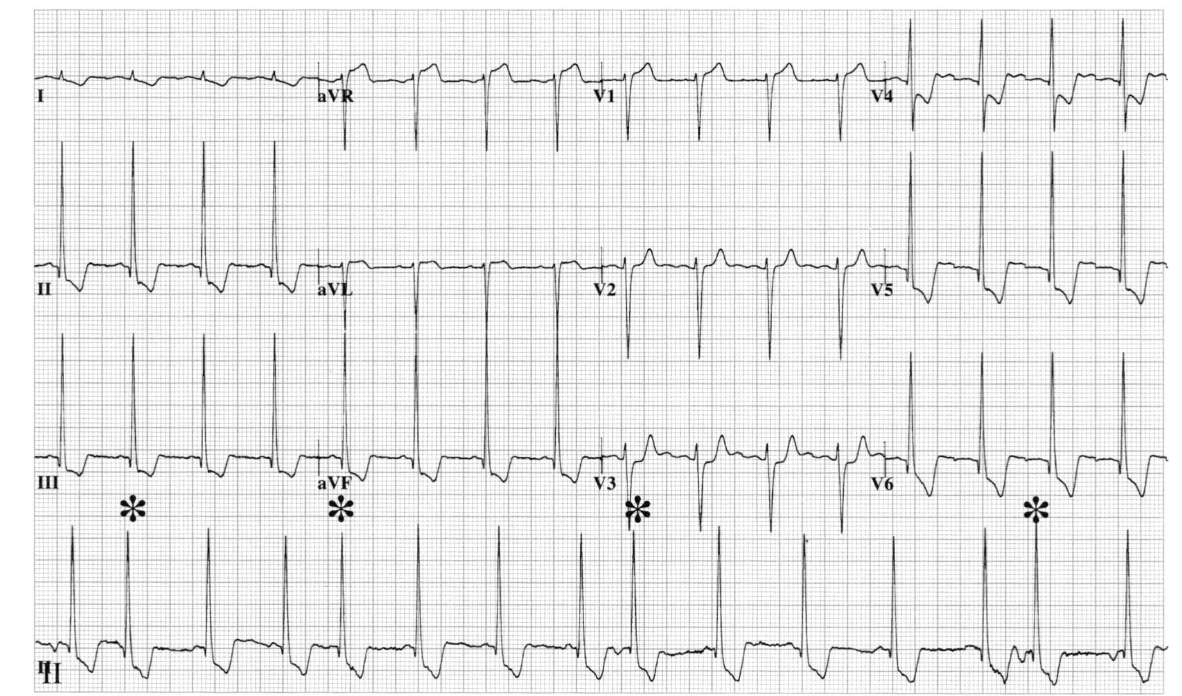

Questions: ECG 12

1. Which of the following statements about hypertrophic obstructive cardiomyopathy are true?

   a. Left atrial abnormality is frequently seen
   b. Right axis deviation occurs in ~ 30% of cases
   c. LVH is present in > 90% of cases
   d. Pathological Q waves occur in 20-30% of cases
   e. ST and T wave changes are the most common finding
   f. Sinus node disease and AV block are common
   g. Non-sustained VT is a risk factor for sudden death

2. Causes of ST segment depression include:

   a. Hypokalemia
   b. Hyperkalemia
   c. Digoxin
   d. Quinidine
   e. Mitral valve prolapse

3. Among the causes of ST segment depression listed in question 2, which is likely to be present given the following additional ECG findings?

   a Atrial fibrillation with a regular ventricular response
   b. Prominent U waves

4. The diagnosis of LVH by voltage criteria is less specific in young patients compared to older patients:

   a True
   b. False

Answers: ECG 12

1. Hypertrophic cardiomyopathy is an uncommon disorder characterized by altered myocyte shape, size and alignment, which along with increased myocardial fibrosis, results in marked ventricular hypertrophy, LV stiffness, and diastolic dysfunction. The vast majority of patients have abnormal ECGs, with LVH in 50-65%, left atrial abnormality in 20-40%, and pathological Q waves (especially leads I, aVL, V_4 - V_5) in 20-30%. ST and T wave changes (repolarization abnormalities secondary to LVH) are the most common ECG findings, while right axis deviation is rare. The most frequent cause of mortality is sudden death, with risk factors including young age and a history of syncope and/or asymptomatic ventricular tachycardia on ambulatory monitoring. Sinus node disease and AV block are uncommon manifestations of this disorder. (Answer: a, d, e, g)

2. ST depression is a common manifestation of hypokalemia, along with decreased T wave amplitude and prominent U waves. Classical digitalis effect produces ST depression that pulls down the first portion of the T wave to create a diphasic T wave, initially negative and then positive. ST depression can also be seen in patients taking quinidine, in conjunction with prolonged QT interval, flat or inverted T waves, and a prominent U wave. Approximately 20-40% of patients with mitral valve prolapse manifest some degree of ST depression and/or T wave inversion, especially in the inferior leads. ST segment depression is not a usual manifestation of hyperkalemia, although ST segment elevation can occur in advanced cases. (Answer: All except b)

3. Atrial fibrillation with a regular ventricular response should raise the suspicion of digitalis toxicity. In this case, regularization of the ventricular response is due to complete heart block and accelerated junctional rhythm. Digitalis toxicity may be exacerbated by hypokalemia, hypomagnesemia, and hypercalcemia. Electrical cardioversion of atrial fibrillation is contraindicated in the setting of digitalis toxicity due to the risk of ventricular fibrillation. (Answer to 3a: c; Answer to 3b: a, c, d, e)

4. Increased QRS voltage is commonly observed in young adults with normal hearts. Many electrocardiographers are reluctant to diagnose LVH by voltage criteria alone in patients under the age of 40, and require other changes to be present (e.g., strain pattern, left axis deviation, delayed onset of intrinsicoid deflection, poor R wave progression). (Answer: a)

— Quick Review 12 —

Hypertrophic cardiomyopathy	
• (Right/left) atrial abnormality is common;	left
(right/left) atrial abnormality on occasion	right
• Majority have abnormal QRS complexes (true/false):	true
▸ (Small/large) amplitude QRS	large
▸ Large abnormal ____ waves (can give pseudoinfarct pattern in inferior, lateral, and anterior precordial leads)	Q
▸ Tall R wave with inverted T wave in V_1 simulating ____	RVH
▸ Nonspecific ST and/or T wave abnormalities are common (true/false)	false
▸ Apical variant of hypertrophic cardiomyopathy has deep T wave inversions in leads ____	V_4-V_6
▸ (Right/left) axis deviation in 20%	left

Differential Diagnosis

Prolonged QT Interval

(i.e., corrected QT interval (QTc) $\geq$ 0.42-0.46 sec)

- Drugs (quinidine, procainamide, disopyramide, amiodarone, sotalol, phenothiazine, tricyclics, lithium) (item 14c, d)
- Hypomagnesemia
- Hypocalcemia (item 14h)
- Marked bradyarrhythmias
- Intracranial hemorrhage (item 14s)
- Myocarditis
- Mitral valve prolapse
- Hypothyroidism (item 14t)
- Hypothermia (item 14u)
- Liquid protein diets
- Romano-Ward syndrome (normal hearing)
- Jervell and Lange-Nielson syndrome (deafness)

ECG 13. 52-year-old female with chest pain:

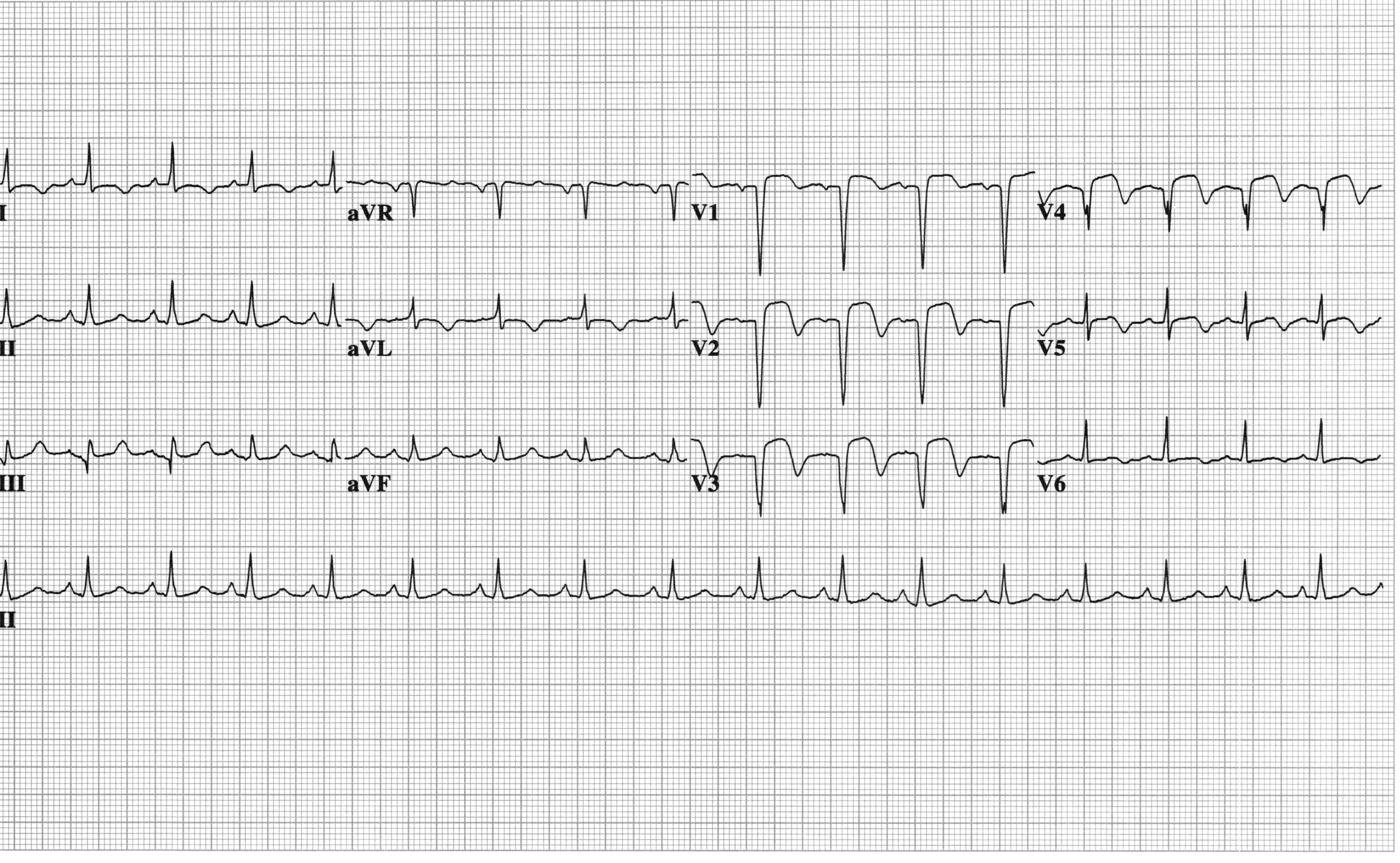

1. GENERAL FEATURES

- ☐ a. Normal ECG
- ☐ b. Borderline normal ECG or normal variant
- ☐ c. Incorrect electrode placement
- ☐ d. Artifact due to tremor

2. ATRIAL RHYTHMS

- ☐ a. Sinus rhythm
- ☐ b. Sinus arrhythmia
- ☐ c. Sinus bradycardia (< 60)
- ☐ d. Sinus tachycardia (> 100)
- ☐ e. Sinus pause or arrest
- ☐ f. Sinoatrial exit block
- ☐ g. Ecoptic atrial rhythm
- ☐ h. Wandering atrial pacemaker
- ☐ i. Atrial premature complexes, normally conducted
- ☐ j. Atrial premature complexes, nonconducted
- ☐ k. Atrial premature complexes with aberrant intraventricular conduction
- ☐ l. Atrial tachycardia (regular, sustained, 1:1 conduction)
- ☐ m. Atrial tachycardia, repetitive (short paroxysms)
- ☐ n. Atrial tachycardia, multifocal
- ☐ o. Atrial tachycardia with AV block
- ☐ p. Supraventricular tachycardia, unspecific
- ☐ q. Supraventricular tachycardia, paroxysmal
- ☐ r. Atrial flutter
- ☐ s. Atrial fibrillation
- ☐ t. Retrograde atrial activation

3. AV JUNCTIONAL RHYTHMS

- ☐ a. AV junctional premature complexes
- ☐ b. AV junctional escape complexes
- ☐ c. AV junctional rhythm, accelerated
- ☐ d. AV junctional rhythm

4. VENTRICULAR RHYTHMS

- ☐ a. Ventricular premature complex(es), uniform, fixed coupling
- ☐ b. Ventricular premature complex(es), uniform, nonfixed coupling
- ☐ c. Ventricular premature complexes(es), multiform
- ☐ d. Ventricular premature complexes, in pairs
- ☐ e. Ventricular parasystole
- ☐ f. Ventricular tachycardia (≥ 3 consecutive complexes)
- ☐ g. Accelerated idioventricular rhythm
- ☐ h. Ventricular escape complexes or rhythm
- ☐ i. Ventricular fibrillation

5. ATRIAL-VENTRICULAR INTERACTIONS IN ARRHYTHMIAS

- ☐ a. Fusion complexes
- ☐ b. Reciprocal (echo) complexes
- ☐ c. Ventricular capture complexes
- ☐ d. AV dissociation
- ☐ e. Ventriculophasic sinus arrhythmia

6. AV CONDUCTION ABNORMALITIES

- ☐ a. AV block, 1°
- ☐ b. AV block, 2° - Mobitz type I (Wenckebach)
- ☐ c. AV block, 2° - Mobitz type II
- ☐ d. AV block, 2:1
- ☐ e. AV block, 3°
- ☐ f. AV block, variable
- ☐ g. Short PR interval (with sinus rhythm and normal QRS duration)
- ☐ h. Wolff-Parkinson-White pattern

7. INTRAVENTRICULAR CONDUCTION DISTURBANCES

- ☐ a. RBBB, incomplete
- ☐ b. RBBB, complete
- ☐ c. Left anterior fascicular block
- ☐ d. Left posterior fascicular block
- ☐ e. LBBB, with ST-T wave suggestive of acute myocardial injury or infarction
- ☐ f. LBBB, complete
- ☐ g. LBBB, intermittent
- ☐ h. Intraventricular conduction disturbance, nonspecific
- ☐ i. Aberrant intraventricular conduction with supraventricular arrhythmia

8. P WAVE ABNORMALITIES

- ☐ a. Right atrial abnormality
- ☐ b. Left atrial abnormalities
- ☐ c. Nonspecific atrial abnormality

9. ABNORMALITIES OF QRS VOLTAGE OR AXIS

- ☐ a. Low voltage, limb leads only
- ☐ b. Low voltage, limb and precordial leads
- ☐ c. Left axis deviation (> - 30%)
- ☐ d. Right axis deviation (> + 100)
- ☐ e. Electrical alternans

10. VENTRICULAR HYPERTROPHY

- ☐ a. LVH by voltage only
- ☐ b. LVH by voltage and ST-T segment abnormalities
- ☐ c. RVH
- ☐ d. Combined ventricular hypertrophy

11. Q WAVE MYOCARDIAL INFARCTION

	Probably Acute or Recent	Probably Old or Age Indeterminate
Anterolateral	☐ a.	☐ g.
Anterior	☐ b.	☐ h.
Anteroseptal	☐ c.	☐ i.
Lateral/High lateral	☐ d.	☐ j.
Inferior	☐ e.	☐ k.
Posterior	☐ f.	☐ l.

☐ m. Probably ventricular aneurysm

12. ST, T, U, WAVE ABNORMALITIES

- ☐ a. Normal variant, early repolarization
- ☐ b. Normal variant, juvenile T waves
- ☐ c. Nonspecific ST and/or T wave abnormalities
- ☐ d. ST and/or T wave abnormalities suggesting myocardial ischemia
- ☐ e. ST and/or T wave abnormalities suggesting myocardial injury
- ☐ f. ST and/or T wave abnormalities suggesting acute pericarditis
- ☐ g. ST-T segment abnormalities secondary to intraventricular conduction disturbance or hypertrophy
- ☐ h. Post-extrasystolic T wave abnormality
- ☐ i. Isolated J point depression
- ☐ j. Peaked T waves
- ☐ k. Prolonged QT interval
- ☐ l. Prominent U waves

13. PACEMAKER FUNCTION AND RHYTHM

- ☐ a. Atrial or coronary sinus pacing
- ☐ b. Ventricular demand pacing
- ☐ c. AV sequential pacing
- ☐ d. Ventricular pacing, complete control
- ☐ e. Dual chamber, atrial sensing pacemaker
- ☐ f. Pacemaker malfunction, not constantly capturing (atrium or ventricle)
- ☐ g. Pacemaker malfunction, not constantly sensing (atrium or ventricle)
- ☐ h. Pacemaker malfunction, not firing
- ☐ i. Pacemaker malfunction, slowing

14. SUGGESTED OR PROBABLE CLINICAL DISORDERS

- ☐ a. Digitalis effect
- ☐ b. Digitalis toxicity
- ☐ c. Antiarrhythmic drug effect
- ☐ d. Antiarrhythmic drug toxicity
- ☐ e. Hyperkalemia
- ☐ f. Hypokalemia
- ☐ g. Hypercalcemia
- ☐ h. Hypocalcemia
- ☐ i. Atrial septal defect, secundum
- ☐ j. Atrial septal defect, primum
- ☐ k. Dextrocardia, mirror image
- ☐ l. Mitral valve disease
- ☐ m. Chronic lung disease
- ☐ n. Acute cor pulmonale, including pulmonary embolus
- ☐ o. Pericardial effusion
- ☐ p. Acute pericarditis
- ☐ q. Hypertrophic cardiomyopathy
- ☐ r. Coronary artery disease
- ☐ s. Central nervous system disorder
- ☐ t. Myxedema
- ☐ u. Hypothermia
- ☐ v. Sick sinus syndrome

ECG 13 was obtained in a 52-year-old female with chest pain. The ECG shows sinus tachycardia and acute anteroseptal myocardial infarction (Q waves and ST segment elevation in V_1-V_4) (asterisks). T wave inversions in leads I and aVL (arrows) suggest high lateral ischemia. Coronary artery disease should also be coded.

Codes:

2d	Sinus tachycardia
11c	Anteroseptal Q wave MI, probably acute or recent
12d	ST and/or T wave abnormalities suggesting myocardial ischemia
12e	ST and/or T wave abnormalities suggest myocardial injury
14r	Coronary artery disease

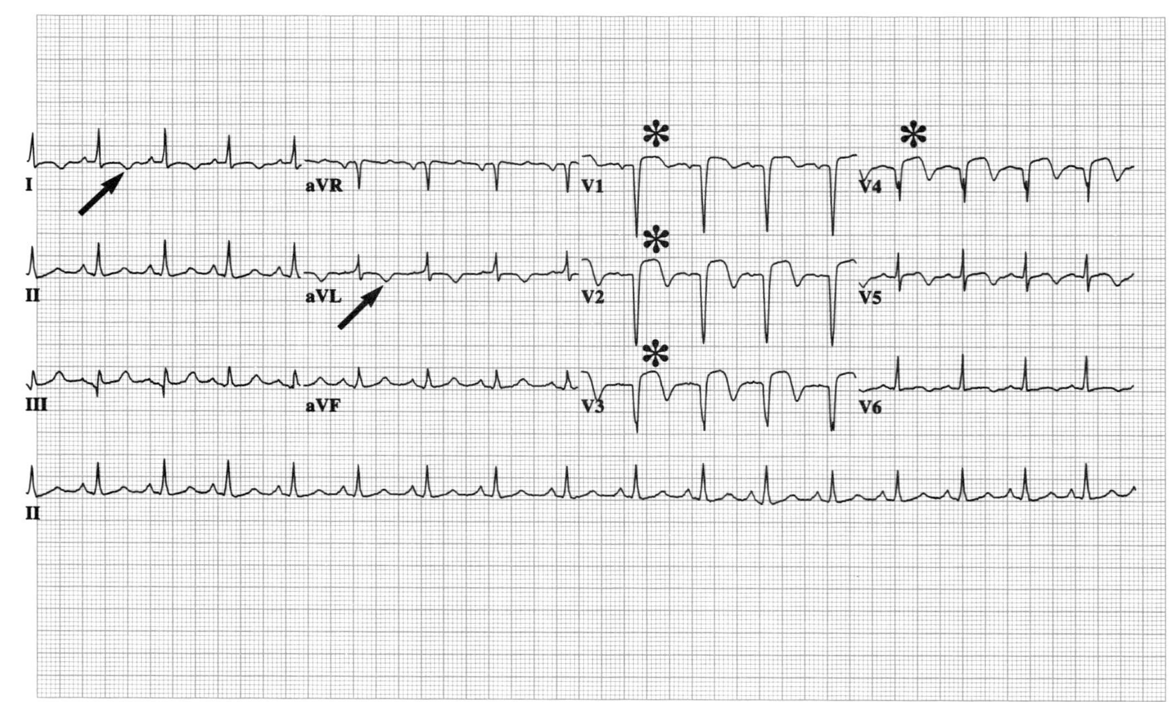

Questions: ECG 13

1. ST elevation that persists for longer than ____ weeks post-MI suggests the presence of left ventricular aneurysm:

   a. 8
   b. 2
   c. 1
   d. 4

2. The ECG diagnosis of anteroseptal myocardial infarction requires the presence of an abnormal Q wave in V_1:

   a. True
   b. False

Answers: ECG 13

1. Extensive transmural myocardial infarction may develop into a ventricular aneurysm, which manifests on the ECG as ST segment elevation persisting longer than 4 weeks in leads demonstrating pathological Q waves. Ventricular aneurysm occurs most commonly in the setting of anteroseptal and anteroapical infarction, as is the case in the present tracing. (Answer: d)

2. The diagnosis of anteroseptal myocardial infarction requires the presence of pathological Q waves in leads V_1-V_3. If pathological Q waves are present in leads V_2-V_4, but not V_1, the infarction should be classified as anterior rather than anteroseptal. (Answer: a)

— Quick Review 13 —	
Sinus tachycardia	
• Rate > ____ per minute	100
• P wave amplitude often (increases/decreases) and PR interval often (increases/decreases) with increasing heart rate	increases shortens
Anteroseptal MI, recent or probably acute	
• Abnormal Q or QS deflection and ST elevation in leads ____ (and sometimes V_4)	V_1-V_3
• The presence of a Q wave in lead ____ distinguishes anteroseptal from anterior infarction	V_1

ECG 14. 68-year-old male with fatigue and dyspnea:

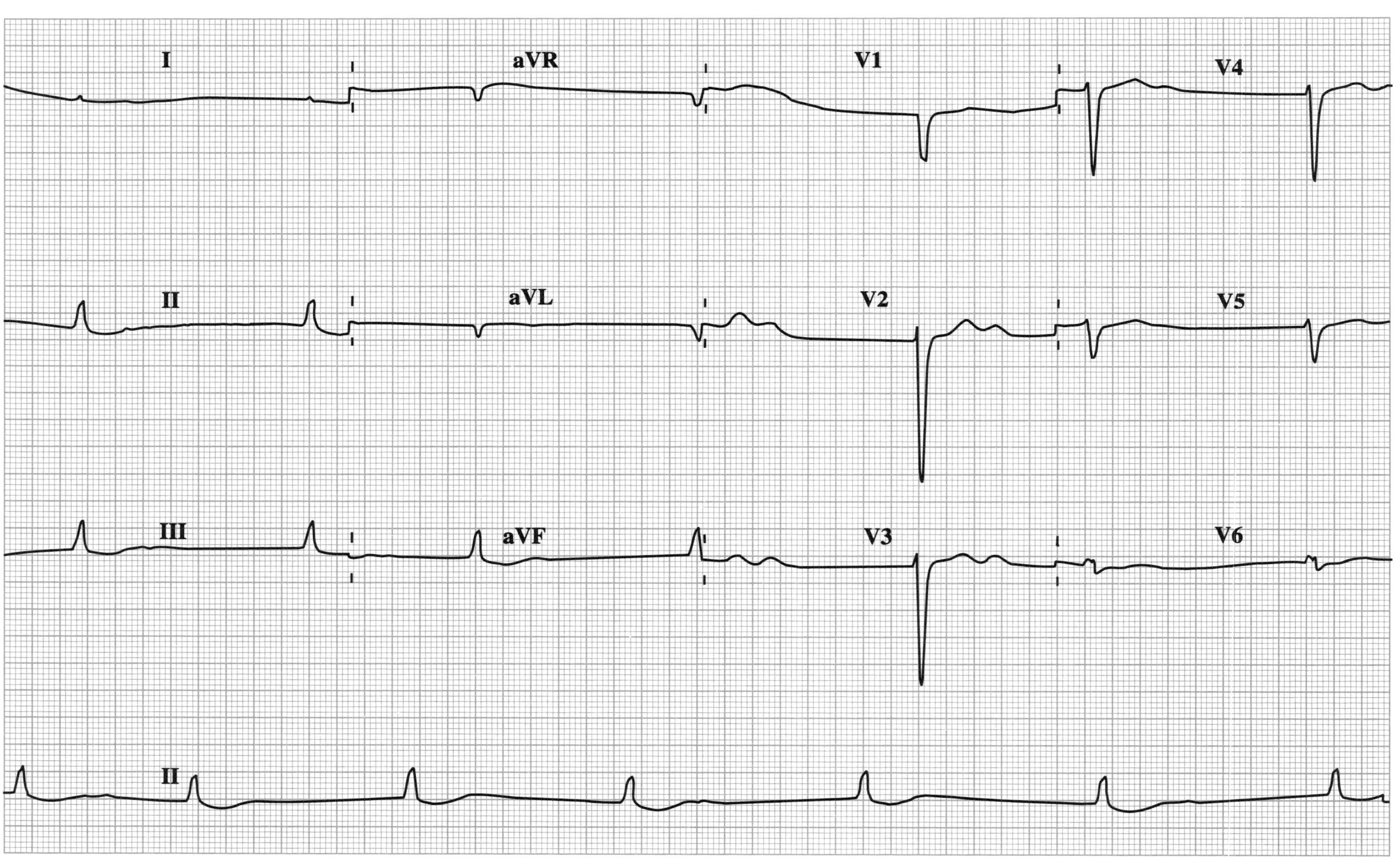

1. GENERAL FEATURES

☐ a. Normal ECG
☐ b. Borderline normal ECG or normal variant
☐ c. Incorrect electrode placement
☐ d. Artifact due to tremor

2. ATRIAL RHYTHMS

☐ a. Sinus rhythm
☐ b. Sinus arrhythmia
☐ c. Sinus bradycardia (< 60)
☐ d. Sinus tachycardia (> 100)
☐ e. Sinus pause or arrest
☐ f. Sinoatrial exit block
☐ g. Ecoptic atrial rhythm
☐ h. Wandering atrial pacemaker
☐ i. Atrial premature complexes, normally conducted
☐ j. Atrial premature complexes, nonconducted
☐ k. Atrial premature complexes with aberrant intraventricular conduction
☐ l. Atrial tachycardia (regular, sustained, 1:1 conduction)
☐ m. Atrial tachycardia, repetitive (short paroxysms)
☐ n. Atrial tachycardia, multifocal
☐ o. Atrial tachycardia with AV block
☐ p. Supraventricular tachycardia, unspecific
☐ q. Supraventricular tachycardia, paroxysmal
☐ r. Atrial flutter
☐ s. Atrial fibrillation
☐ t. Retrograde atrial activation

3. AV JUNCTIONAL RHYTHMS

☐ a. AV junctional premature complexes
☐ b. AV junctional escape complexes
☐ c. AV junctional rhythm, accelerated
☐ d. AV junctional rhythm

4. VENTRICULAR RHYTHMS

☐ a. Ventricular premature complex(es), uniform, fixed coupling
☐ b. Ventricular premature complex(es), uniform, nonfixed coupling
☐ c. Ventricular premature complexes(es), multiform
☐ d. Ventricular premature complexes, in pairs
☐ e. Ventricular parasystole
☐ f. Ventricular tachycardia (≥ 3 consecutive complexes)
☐ g. Accelerated idioventricular rhythm
☐ h. Ventricular escape complexes or rhythm
☐ i. Ventricular fibrillation

5. ATRIAL-VENTRICULAR INTERACTIONS IN ARRHYTHMIAS

☐ a. Fusion complexes
☐ b. Reciprocal (echo) complexes
☐ c. Ventricular capture complexes
☐ d. AV dissociation
☐ e. Ventriculophasic sinus arrhythmia

6. AV CONDUCTION ABNORMALITIES

☐ a. AV block, 1°
☐ b. AV block, 2° - Mobitz type I (Wenckebach)
☐ c. AV block, 2° - Mobitz type II
☐ d. AV block, 2:1
☐ e. AV block, 3°
☐ f. AV block, variable
☐ g. Short PR interval (with sinus rhythm and normal QRS duration)
☐ h. Wolff-Parkinson-White pattern

7. INTRAVENTRICULAR CONDUCTION DISTURBANCES

☐ a. RBBB, incomplete
☐ b. RBBB, complete
☐ c. Left anterior fascicular block
☐ d. Left posterior fascicular block
☐ e. LBBB, with ST-T wave suggestive of acute myocardial injury or infarction
☐ f. LBBB, complete
☐ g. LBBB, intermittent
☐ h. Intraventricular conduction disturbance, nonspecific
☐ i. Aberrant intraventricular conduction with supraventricular arrhythmia

8. P WAVE ABNORMALITIES

☐ a. Right atrial abnormality
☐ b. Left atrial abnormalities
☐ c. Nonspecific atrial abnormality

9. ABNORMALITIES OF QRS VOLTAGE OR AXIS

☐ a. Low voltage, limb leads only
☐ b. Low voltage, limb and precordial leads
☐ c. Left axis deviation (> - 30%)
☐ d. Right axis deviation (> + 100)
☐ e. Electrical alternans

10. VENTRICULAR HYPERTROPHY

☐ a. LVH by voltage only
☐ b. LVH by voltage and ST-T segment abnormalities
☐ c. RVH
☐ d. Combined ventricular hypertrophy

11. Q WAVE MYOCARDIAL INFARCTION

	Probably Acute or Recent	Probably Old or Age Indeterminate
Anterolateral	☐ a.	☐ g.
Anterior	☐ b.	☐ h.
Anteroseptal	☐ c.	☐ i.
Lateral/High lateral	☐ d.	☐ j.
Inferior	☐ e.	☐ k.
Posterior	☐ f.	☐ l.

☐ m. Probably ventricular aneurysm

12. ST, T, U, WAVE ABNORMALITIES

☐ a. Normal variant, early repolarization
☐ b. Normal variant, juvenile T waves
☐ c. Nonspecific ST and/or T wave abnormalities
☐ d. ST and/or T wave abnormalities suggesting myocardial ischemia
☐ e. ST and/or T wave abnormalities suggesting myocardial injury
☐ f. ST and/or T wave abnormalities suggesting acute pericarditis
☐ g. ST-T segment abnormalities secondary to intraventricular conduction disturbance or hypertrophy
☐ h. Post-extrasystolic T wave abnormality
☐ i. Isolated J point depression
☐ j. Peaked T waves
☐ k. Prolonged QT interval
☐ l. Prominent U waves

13. PACEMAKER FUNCTION AND RHYTHM

☐ a. Atrial or coronary sinus pacing
☐ b. Ventricular demand pacing
☐ c. AV sequential pacing
☐ d. Ventricular pacing, complete control
☐ e. Dual chamber, atrial sensing pacemaker
☐ f. Pacemaker malfunction, not constantly capturing (atrium or ventricle)
☐ g. Pacemaker malfunction, not constantly sensing (atrium or ventricle)
☐ h. Pacemaker malfunction, not firing
☐ i. Pacemaker malfunction, slowing

14. SUGGESTED OR PROBABLE CLINICAL DISORDERS

☐ a. Digitalis effect
☐ b. Digitalis toxicity
☐ c. Antiarrhythmic drug effect
☐ d. Antiarrhythmic drug toxicity
☐ e. Hyperkalemia
☐ f. Hypokalemia
☐ g. Hypercalcemia
☐ h. Hypocalcemia
☐ i. Atrial septal defect, secundum
☐ j. Atrial septal defect, primum
☐ k. Dextrocardia, mirror image
☐ l. Mitral valve disease
☐ m. Chronic lung disease
☐ n. Acute cor pulmonale, including pulmonary embolus
☐ o. Pericardial effusion
☐ p. Acute pericarditis
☐ q. Hypertrophic cardiomyopathy
☐ r. Coronary artery disease
☐ s. Central nervous system disorder
☐ t. Myxedema
☐ u. Hypothermia
☐ v. Sick sinus syndrome

ECG 14 was obtained from a 68-year-old male with fatigue and dyspnea shows sinus arrest with a junctional rhythm at approximately 40 beats/minute. The slight irregularity in the early portion of the rhythm strip is due to the presence of an AV junctional premature complex (asterisk). The sagging ST segment depression (arrowheads) is typical for digitalis effect (but could also be as nonspecific ST-T abnormalities). Prominent U waves are present (arrows). This constellation of findings is consistent with digitalis toxicity.

Codes:

2e	Sinus pause or arrest
3a	AV junctional premature complexes
3d	AV junctional rhythm
12l	Prominent U waves
14a	Digitalis effect
14b	Digitalis toxicity

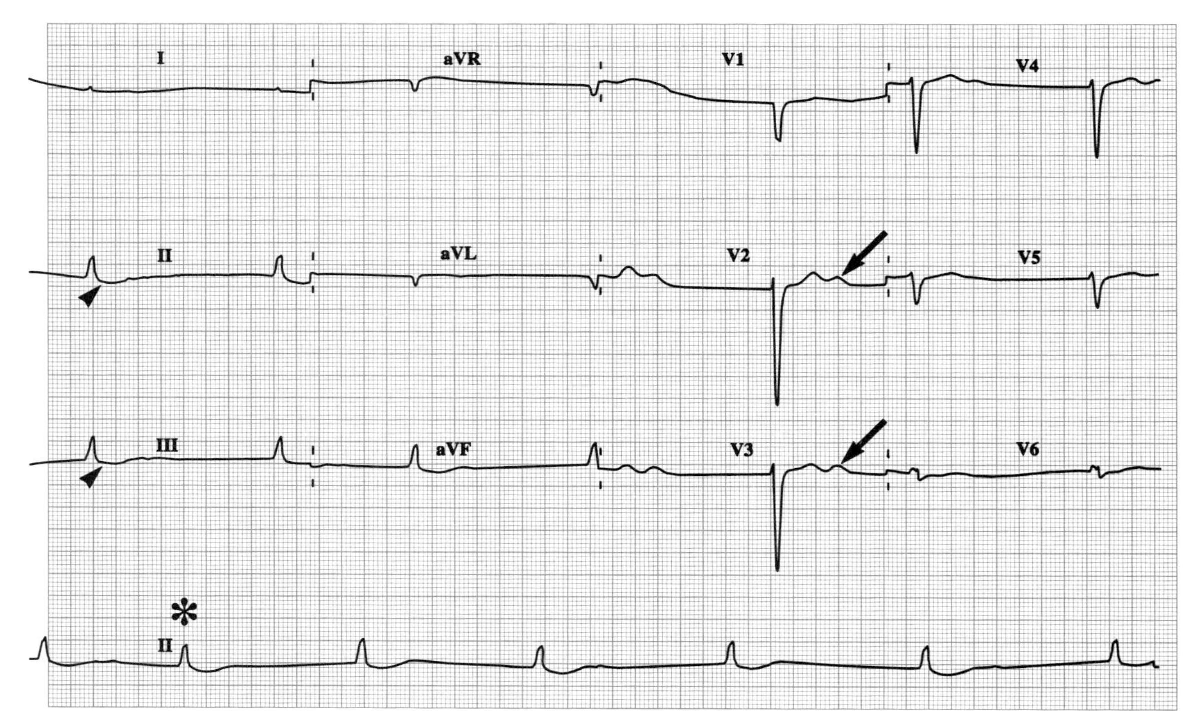

Questions: ECG 14

1. Which of the following ECG findings are due to digitalis effect and which are due to digitalis toxicity?

   a. Sagging ST segment depression
   b. Decreased T wave amplitude
   c. Shortening of the QT interval
   d. U waves
   e. Increased PR interval
   f. Left bundle branch block
   g. Right bundle branch block
   h. Paroxysmal atrial tachycardia with block
   I. Atrial fibrillation with regular ventricular response
   j. Bidirectional ventricular tachycardia
   k. Complete heart block

2. Findings on this ECG that speak against hyperkalemia include:

   a. Absent P waves
   b. Absence of peaked T waves
   c. Intraventricular conduction delay
   d. Prominent U waves

Answers: ECG 14

1. Typical digitalis effects include prolonged PR interval, sagging ST segment depression, decreased T wave amplitude, shortened QT interval, and prominent U waves. Arrhythmias and conduction disturbances associated with digitalis toxicity include paroxysmal atrial tachycardia (PAT) with block, atrial fibrillation with a regular ventricular response, junctional tachycardia, bidirectional ventricular tachycardia, and complete heart block. Digitalis does not produce bundle branch block or atrial flutter. (Answer: Digitalis effect: a - e; Digitalis toxicity: h - k)

2. The lack of P waves and the presence of IVCD are consistent with the diagnosis of hyperkalemia. However, normal T wave amplitude speaks strongly against this diagnosis, especially when hyperkalemia is acute. Prominent U waves are frequently observed in hypokalemia, not hyperkalemia. (Answer: b, d)

— Quick Review 14 —

Sinus pause or arrest	
• PP interval > _____ seconds	1.6-2.0
• Resumption of sinus rhythm at a PP interval that (is/is not) a multiple of the basic sinus PP interval	is not
• If sinus rhythm resumes at a multiple of the basic PP, consider _____	sinoatrial exit block
AV junctional rhythm	
• Rate≤ ____ per minute	60
• QRS complex may be narrow or aberrant (true/false)	true
• Inverted P waves in leads ____ and upright P waves in leads ____ are common	II, III, aVF I, aVL
• RR interval of escape rhythm is usually (constant/variable)	constant
Digitalis toxicity	
• Digitalis toxicity can cause almost any type of cardiac dysrhythmia or conduction disturbance except _____	bundle branch block
• Typical abnormalities include:	
▸ Paroxysmal ____ tachycardia with block	atrial
▸ Atrial fibrillation with ____ heart block	complete
▸ Second or third-degree ____ block	AV
▸ Complete heart block with accelerated ____ or ____ rhythm	junctional idioventricular
▸ Supraventricular tachycardia with ____ bundle branch block	alternating

— POP QUIZ —

Find The Mistake

Instructions: Identify the incorrect ECG feature(s) for each of the ECG diagnoses listed below

ECG Features	Answer
Multifocal atrial tachycardia • Atrial rate > 100 per minute • P waves with ≥ 3 morphologies • PR, RR intervals vary • RP interval is constant	PR, RR, *and* RP intervals vary
Atrial tachycardia with block • Sinus P waves • Atrial rate of 150-240 per minute • Isoelectric intervals between P waves in some but not all leads • Second- or third-degree AV block • Rhythm is regular	Non-sinus (not sinus) P waves are present; isoelectric intervals are present in all leads
Atrial flutter • Rapid regular atrial undulations at 240-340 per minute • Undulations in leads II, III, AVF, and V_1 are typically inverted without an isoelectric baseline	In V_1, flutter waves are typically small positive deflections with a distinct isoelectric baseline
Atrial fibrillation • Totally irregular atrial activity manifests as undulations of varying amplitude, duration and morphology • Ventricular rhythm is irregularly irregular • Atrial activity may regularize with digitalis toxicity	Ventricular activity may regularize with digitalis toxicity, but atrial activity remains irregular

ECG 15. 73-year-old male with dyspnea:

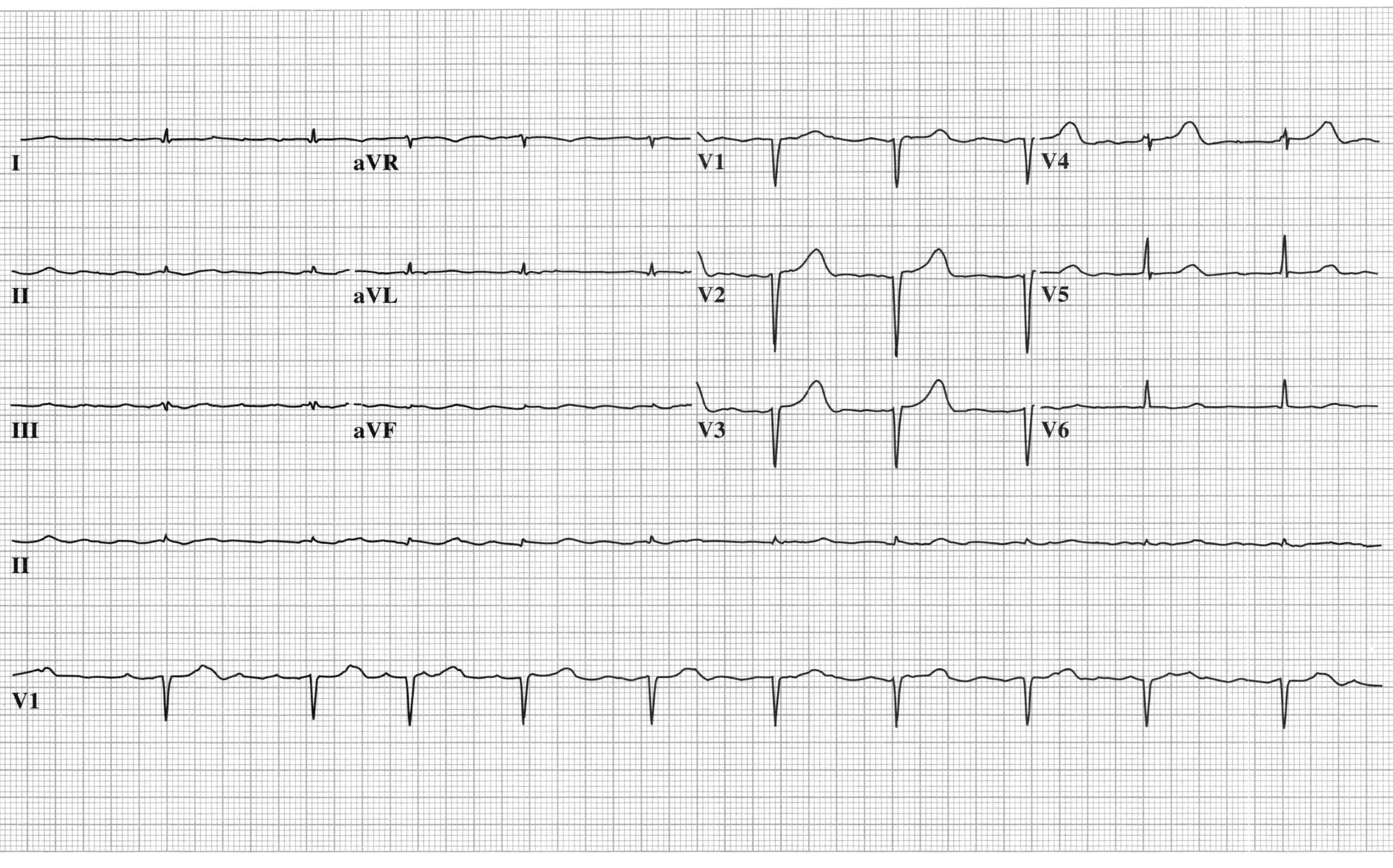

1. GENERAL FEATURES

- ☐ a. Normal ECG
- ☐ b. Borderline normal ECG or normal variant
- ☐ c. Incorrect electrode placement
- ☐ d. Artifact due to tremor

2. ATRIAL RHYTHMS

- ☐ a. Sinus rhythm
- ☐ b. Sinus arrhythmia
- ☐ c. Sinus bradycardia (< 60)
- ☐ d. Sinus tachycardia (> 100)
- ☐ e. Sinus pause or arrest
- ☐ f. Sinoatrial exit block
- ☐ g. Ecoptic atrial rhythm
- ☐ h. Wandering atrial pacemaker
- ☐ i. Atrial premature complexes, normally conducted
- ☐ j. Atrial premature complexes, nonconducted
- ☐ k. Atrial premature complexes with aberrant intraventricular conduction
- ☐ l. Atrial tachycardia (regular, sustained, 1:1 conduction)
- ☐ m. Atrial tachycardia, repetitive (short paroxysms)
- ☐ n. Atrial tachycardia, multifocal
- ☐ o. Atrial tachycardia with AV block
- ☐ p. Supraventricular tachycardia, unspecific
- ☐ q. Supraventricular tachycardia, paroxysmal
- ☐ r. Atrial flutter
- ☐ s. Atrial fibrillation
- ☐ t. Retrograde atrial activation

3. AV JUNCTIONAL RHYTHMS

- ☐ a. AV junctional premature complexes
- ☐ b. AV junctional escape complexes
- ☐ c. AV junctional rhythm, accelerated
- ☐ d. AV junctional rhythm

4. VENTRICULAR RHYTHMS

- ☐ a. Ventricular premature complex(es), uniform, fixed coupling
- ☐ b. Ventricular premature complex(es), uniform, nonfixed coupling
- ☐ c. Ventricular premature complexes(es), multiform
- ☐ d. Ventricular premature complexes, in pairs
- ☐ e. Ventricular parasystole
- ☐ f. Ventricular tachycardia (≥ 3 consecutive complexes)
- ☐ g. Accelerated idioventricular rhythm
- ☐ h. Ventricular escape complexes or rhythm
- ☐ i. Ventricular fibrillation

5. ATRIAL-VENTRICULAR INTERACTIONS IN ARRHYTHMIAS

- ☐ a. Fusion complexes
- ☐ b. Reciprocal (echo) complexes
- ☐ c. Ventricular capture complexes
- ☐ d. AV dissociation
- ☐ e. Ventriculophasic sinus arrhythmia

6. AV CONDUCTION ABNORMALITIES

- ☐ a. AV block, 1°
- ☐ b. AV block, 2° - Mobitz type I (Wenckebach)
- ☐ c. AV block, 2° - Mobitz type II
- ☐ d. AV block, 2:1
- ☐ e. AV block, 3°
- ☐ f. AV block, variable
- ☐ g. Short PR interval (with sinus rhythm and normal QRS duration)
- ☐ h. Wolff-Parkinson-White pattern

7. INTRAVENTRICULAR CONDUCTION DISTURBANCES

- ☐ a. RBBB, incomplete
- ☐ b. RBBB, complete
- ☐ c. Left anterior fascicular block
- ☐ d. Left posterior fascicular block
- ☐ e. LBBB, with ST-T wave suggestive of acute myocardial injury or infarction
- ☐ f. LBBB, complete
- ☐ g. LBBB, intermittent
- ☐ h. Intraventricular conduction disturbance, nonspecific
- ☐ i. Aberrant intraventricular conduction with supraventricular arrhythmia

8. P WAVE ABNORMALITIES

- ☐ a. Right atrial abnormality
- ☐ b. Left atrial abnormalities
- ☐ c. Nonspecific atrial abnormality

9. ABNORMALITIES OF QRS VOLTAGE OR AXIS

- ☐ a. Low voltage, limb leads only
- ☐ b. Low voltage, limb and precordial leads
- ☐ c. Left axis deviation (> - 30%)
- ☐ d. Right axis deviation (> + 100)
- ☐ e. Electrical alternans

10. VENTRICULAR HYPERTROPHY

- ☐ a. LVH by voltage only
- ☐ b. LVH by voltage and ST-T segment abnormalities
- ☐ c. RVH
- ☐ d. Combined ventricular hypertrophy

11. Q WAVE MYOCARDIAL INFARCTION

	Probably Acute or Recent	Probably Old or Age Indeterminate
Anterolateral	☐ a.	☐ g.
Anterior	☐ b.	☐ h.
Anteroseptal	☐ c.	☐ i.
Lateral/High Lateral	☐ d.	☐ j.
Inferior	☐ e.	☐ k.
Posterior	☐ f.	☐ l.

☐ m. Probably ventricular aneurysm

12. ST, T, U, WAVE ABNORMALITIES

- ☐ a. Normal variant, early repolarization
- ☐ b. Normal variant, juvenile T waves
- ☐ c. Nonspecific ST and/or T wave abnormalities
- ☐ d. ST and/or T wave abnormalities suggesting myocardial ischemia
- ☐ e. ST and/or T wave abnormalities suggesting myocardial injury
- ☐ f. ST and/or T wave abnormalities suggesting acute pericarditis
- ☐ g. ST-T segment abnormalities secondary to intraventricular conduction disturbance or hypertrophy
- ☐ h. Post-extrasystolic T wave abnormality
- ☐ i. Isolated J point depression
- ☐ j. Peaked T waves
- ☐ k. Prolonged QT interval
- ☐ l. Prominent U waves

13. PACEMAKER FUNCTION AND RHYTHM

- ☐ a. Atrial or coronary sinus pacing
- ☐ b. Ventricular demand pacing
- ☐ c. AV sequential pacing
- ☐ d. Ventricular pacing, complete control
- ☐ e. Dual chamber, atrial sensing pacemaker
- ☐ f. Pacemaker malfunction, not constantly capturing (atrium or ventricle)
- ☐ g. Pacemaker malfunction, not constantly sensing (atrium or ventricle)
- ☐ h. Pacemaker malfunction, not firing
- ☐ i. Pacemaker malfunction, slowing

14. SUGGESTED OR PROBABLE CLINICAL DISORDERS

- ☐ a. Digitalis effect
- ☐ b. Digitalis toxicity
- ☐ c. Antiarrhythmic drug effect
- ☐ d. Antiarrhythmic drug toxicity
- ☐ e. Hyperkalemia
- ☐ f. Hypokalemia
- ☐ g. Hypercalcemia
- ☐ h. Hypocalcemia
- ☐ i. Atrial septal defect, secundum
- ☐ j. Atrial septal defect, primum
- ☐ k. Dextrocardia, mirror image
- ☐ l. Mitral valve disease
- ☐ m. Chronic lung disease
- ☐ n. Acute cor pulmonale, including pulmonary embolus
- ☐ o. Pericardial effusion
- ☐ p. Acute pericarditis
- ☐ q. Hypertrophic cardiomyopathy
- ☐ r. Coronary artery disease
- ☐ s. Central nervous system disorder
- ☐ t. Myxedema
- ☐ u. Hypothermia
- ☐ v. Sick sinus syndrome

ECG 15 was obtained in a 73-year-old male with dyspnea. The ECG shows atrial fibrillation/flutter with a ventricular rate of 66 beats/minute. Low voltage in the limb leads and nonspecific ST-T abnormalities are also evident. This patient was subsequently diagnosed with amyloid heart disease, which was undoubtedly the reason for the very low anterior R wave forces in leads V_1-V_3 (asterisks).

Codes:		
	2s	Atrial fibrillation
	9a	Low voltage, limb leads only
	12c	Nonspecific ST and/or T wave abnormalities

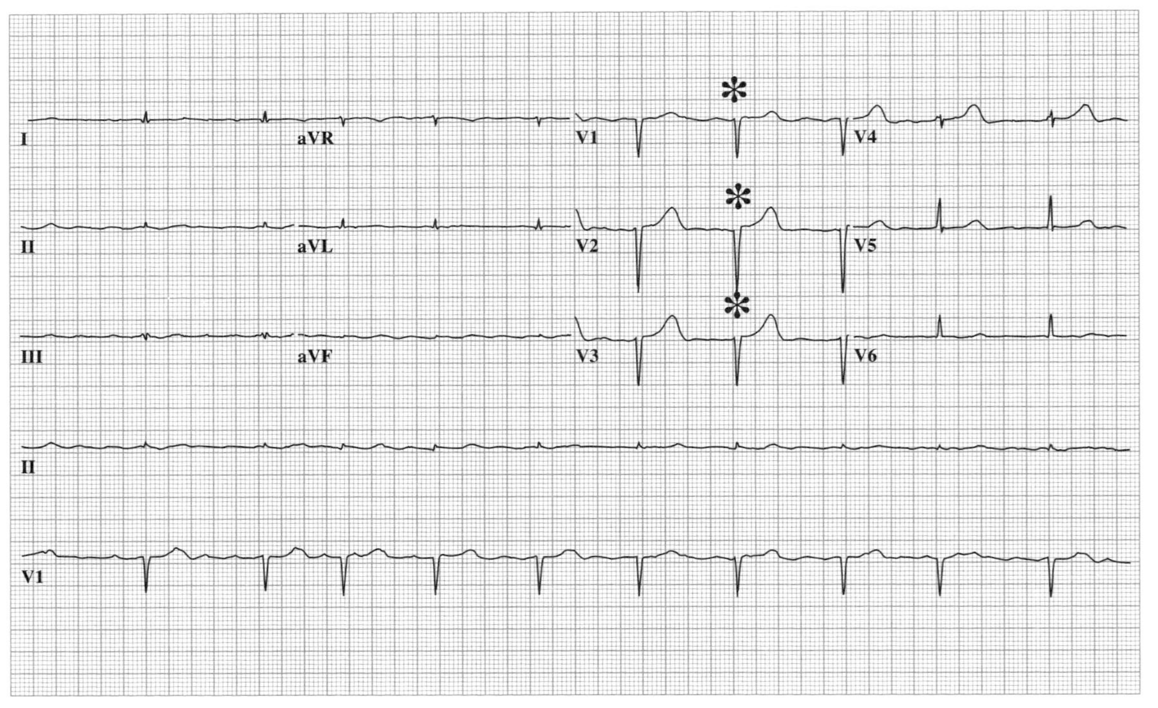

Questions: ECG 15

1. The definition of low voltage requires a total of QRS amplitude (R + S wave) < ___ mm in each limb lead and < ___ mm in each precordial lead:

   a. 5 and 10
   b. 10 and 5
   c. 5 and 15
   d. 10 and 20

2. ECG manifestations of hypothyroidism include all of the following except:

   a. Atrial fibrillation
   b. Low voltage
   c. T wave flattening
   d. Sinus bradycardia
   e. First-degree AV block
   f. Sinus tachycardia
   g. Osborne waves

Answers: ECG 15

1. The definition of low QRS voltage requires an R + S wave < 5 mm in the limb leads and < 10 mm in the precordial leads. The low QRS voltage and very low R wave anterior forces present in this tracing are characteristic of amyloid heart disease, which was diagnosed in this patient. (Answer: a)

2. ECG manifestations of hypothyroidism include low voltage QRS, T wave flattening, sinus bradycardia, and first-degree AV block. Sinus tachycardia and atrial fibrillation are associated with hyperthyroidism, not hypothyroidism. Osborne waves are extra positive deflections in the terminal portion of the QRS and are seen in hypothermia. (Answer: a, f)

— Quick Review 15 —	
Low voltage, limb leads only • Amplitude of the entire QRS complex (R+S) < ____ mm in each limb leads	5
Nonspecific ST-T abnormalities • ST depression or elevation < ____ mm • T wave flat or slightly ____	 1 inverted

ECG 16. 62-year-old female with a history of tachycardia:

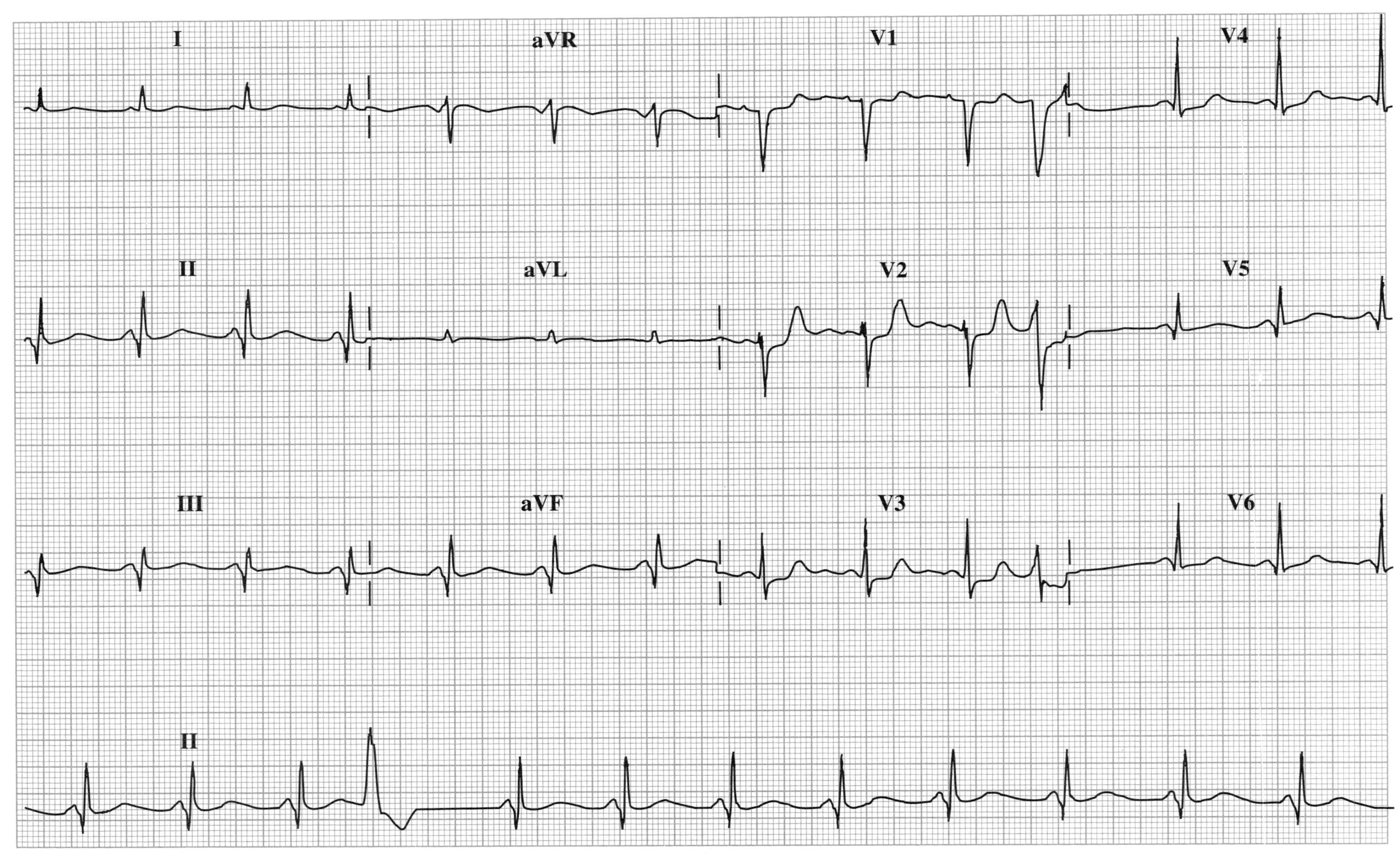

1. GENERAL FEATURES

☐ a. Normal ECG
☐ b. Borderline normal ECG or normal variant
☐ c. Incorrect electrode placement
☐ d. Artifact due to tremor

2. ATRIAL RHYTHMS

☐ a. Sinus rhythm
☐ b. Sinus arrhythmia
☐ c. Sinus bradycardia (< 60)
☐ d. Sinus tachycardia (> 100)
☐ e. Sinus pause or arrest
☐ f. Sinoatrial exit block
☐ g. Ecoptic atrial rhythm
☐ h. Wandering atrial pacemaker
☐ i. Atrial premature complexes, normally conducted
☐ j. Atrial premature complexes, nonconducted
☐ k. Atrial premature complexes with aberrant intraventricular conduction
☐ l. Atrial tachycardia (regular, sustained, 1:1 conduction)
☐ m. Atrial tachycardia, repetitive (short paroxysms)
☐ n. Atrial tachycardia, multifocal
☐ o. Atrial tachycardia with AV block
☐ p. Supraventricular tachycardia, unspecific
☐ q. Supraventricular tachycardia, paroxysmal
☐ r. Atrial flutter
☐ s. Atrial fibrillation
☐ t. Retrograde atrial activation

3. AV JUNCTIONAL RHYTHMS

☐ a. AV junctional premature complexes
☐ b. AV junctional escape complexes
☐ c. AV junctional rhythm, accelerated
☐ d. AV junctional rhythm

4. VENTRICULAR RHYTHMS

☐ a. Ventricular premature complex(es), uniform, fixed coupling
☐ b. Ventricular premature complex(es), uniform, nonfixed coupling
☐ c. Ventricular premature complexes(es), multiform
☐ d. Ventricular premature complexes, in pairs
☐ e. Ventricular parasystole
☐ f. Ventricular tachycardia (≥ 3 consecutive complexes)
☐ g. Accelerated idioventricular rhythm
☐ h. Ventricular escape complexes or rhythm
☐ i. Ventricular fibrillation

5. ATRIAL-VENTRICULAR INTERACTIONS IN ARRHYTHMIAS

☐ a. Fusion complexes
☐ b. Reciprocal (echo) complexes
☐ c. Ventricular capture complexes
☐ d. AV dissociation

☐ e. Ventriculophasic sinus arrhythmia

6. AV CONDUCTION ABNORMALITIES

☐ a. AV block, 1°
☐ b. AV block, 2° - Mobitz type I (Wenckebach)
☐ c. AV block, 2° - Mobitz type II
☐ d. AV block, 2:1
☐ e. AV block, 3°
☐ f. AV block, variable
☐ g. Short PR interval (with sinus rhythm and normal QRS duration)
☐ h. Wolff-Parkinson-White pattern

7. INTRAVENTRICULAR CONDUCTION DISTURBANCES

☐ a. RBBB, incomplete
☐ b. RBBB, complete
☐ c. Left anterior fascicular block
☐ d. Left posterior fascicular block
☐ e. LBBB, with ST-T wave suggestive of acute myocardial injury or infarction
☐ f. LBBB, complete
☐ g. LBBB, intermittent
☐ h. Intraventricular conduction disturbance, nonspecific
☐ i. Aberrant intraventricular conduction with supraventricular arrhythmia

8. P WAVE ABNORMALITIES

☐ a. Right atrial abnormality
☐ b. Left atrial abnormalities
☐ c. Nonspecific atrial abnormality

9. ABNORMALITIES OF QRS VOLTAGE OR AXIS

☐ a. Low voltage, limb leads only
☐ b. Low voltage, limb and precordial leads
☐ c. Left axis deviation (> - 30%)
☐ d. Right axis deviation (> + 100)
☐ e. Electrical alternans

10. VENTRICULAR HYPERTROPHY

☐ a. LVH by voltage only
☐ b. LVH by voltage and ST-T segment abnormalities
☐ c. RVH
☐ d. Combined ventricular hypertrophy

11. Q WAVE MYOCARDIAL INFARCTION

	Probably Acute or Recent	Probably Old or Age Indeterminate
Anterolateral	☐ a.	☐ g.
Anterior	☐ b.	☐ h.
Anteroseptal	☐ c.	☐ i.
Lateral/High lateral	☐ d.	☐ j.
Inferior	☐ e.	☐ k.
Posterior	☐ f.	☐ l.

☐ m. Probably ventricular aneurysm

12. ST, T, U, WAVE ABNORMALITIES

☐ a. Normal variant, early repolarization
☐ b. Normal variant, juvenile T waves
☐ c. Nonspecific ST and/or T wave abnormalities
☐ d. ST and/or T wave abnormalities suggesting myocardial ischemia
☐ e. ST and/or T wave abnormalities suggesting myocardial injury
☐ f. ST and/or T wave abnormalities suggesting acute pericarditis
☐ g. ST-T segment abnormalities secondary to intraventricular conduction disturbance or hypertrophy
☐ h. Post-extrasystolic T wave abnormality
☐ i. Isolated J point depression
☐ j. Peaked T waves
☐ k. Prolonged QT interval
☐ l. Prominent U waves

13. PACEMAKER FUNCTION AND RHYTHM

☐ a. Atrial or coronary sinus pacing
☐ b. Ventricular demand pacing
☐ c. AV sequential pacing
☐ d. Ventricular pacing, complete control
☐ e. Dual chamber, atrial sensing pacemaker
☐ f. Pacemaker malfunction, not constantly capturing (atrium or ventricle)
☐ g. Pacemaker malfunction, not constantly sensing (atrium or ventricle)
☐ h. Pacemaker malfunction, not firing
☐ i. Pacemaker malfunction, slowing

14. SUGGESTED OR PROBABLE CLINICAL DISORDERS

☐ a. Digitalis effect
☐ b. Digitalis toxicity
☐ c. Antiarrhythmic drug effect
☐ d. Antiarrhythmic drug toxicity
☐ e. Hyperkalemia
☐ f. Hypokalemia
☐ g. Hypercalcemia
☐ h. Hypocalcemia
☐ i. Atrial septal defect, secundum
☐ j. Atrial septal defect, primum
☐ k. Dextrocardia, mirror image
☐ l. Mitral valve disease
☐ m. Chronic lung disease
☐ n. Acute cor pulmonale, including pulmonary embolus
☐ o. Pericardial effusion
☐ p. Acute pericarditis
☐ q. Hypertrophic cardiomyopathy
☐ r. Coronary artery disease
☐ s. Central nervous system disorder
☐ t. Myxedema
☐ u. Hypothermia
☐ v. Sick sinus syndrome

ECG 16 was obtained from a 62-year-old female with a past history of tachycardia. Normal sinus rhythm is present. The PR interval is just over 120 msec in leads V_1 and V_6 and thus is within normal limits (always look for the longest PR interval on the ECG). Abnormal Q waves (arrows) are noted in the inferior leads suggesting previous inferior infarction (and a past history of coronary artery disease). Nonspecific ST-T abnormalities are present. Abnormal notching of the QRS complex in lead V_2 could be coded as nonspecific IVCD (arrowhead; also see full-size ECG on previous page for closer inspection).

Codes:

2a	Sinus rhythm
4a	Ventricular premature complex(es), uniform, fixed coupling
6g	Short PR interval (with sinus rhythm and normal QRS duration)
7h	IVCD, nonspecific type
11k	Inferior Q wave MI, probably old or age indeterminate
12c	Nonspecific ST and/or T wave abnormalities
14r	Coronary artery disease

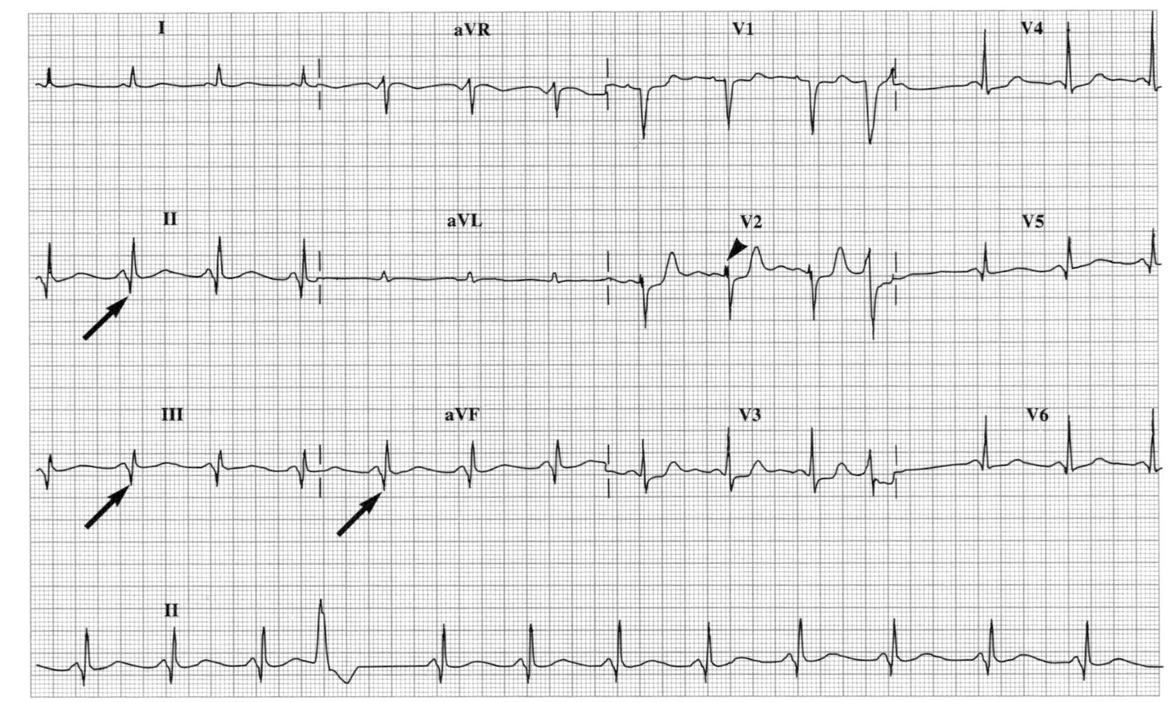

Questions: ECG 16

1. Is a compensatory pause present?

   a. Yes
   b. No

2. Conditions associated with a short PR interval include:

   a. AV junctional rhythm
   b. Wolff-Parkinson-White syndrome
   c. Lown-Ganong-Levine syndrome
   d. Normal variant
   e. Pericarditis

3. The Q waves in leads II, III, and AVF are most consistent with the diagnosis of:

   a. Ischemic heart disease
   b. Wolff-Parkinson-White syndrome
   c. Mitral valve prolapse
   d. Hypertrophic cardiomyopathy

4. In a patient with a short PR interval, delta waves and a prolonged QRS are needed for the diagnosis of WPW?

   a. True
   b. False

5. Is the QT interval prolonged?

   a. Yes
   b. No

Answers: ECG 16

1. Ventricular premature complexes (VPC) may be associated with complete or incomplete compensatory pauses, or no pause at all (i.e., interpolated VPC). The VPC in the present tracing shows a compensatory pause (i.e., the RR interval containing the VPC is equal to 2 times the normal RR interval). VPCs must be distinguished from supraventricular beats with aberration; features favoring the presence of a VPC include the lack of a preceding P wave, a left bundle branch block pattern in V_1, a compensatory pause, and an RP interval $\geq$ 0.20 seconds when retrograde atrial activation is present. (Answer: a)

2. The PR interval represents the time from the onset of atrial depolarization to the onset of ventricular depolarization (i.e., conduction from the atria → AV node → bundle of His → Purkinje fibers → ventricle). AV junctional rhythms can result in a short PR interval when retrograde atrial activation occurs before the antegrade impulse reaches the ventricles. In the WPW syndrome, the presence of an accessory AV pathway (bundle of Kent), which connects the atria directly to the ventricles and bypasses the normal conduction delay in the AV node, prematurely activates the ventricles to result in a short PR. In the Lown-Ganong-Levine (LGL) syndrome, many experts believe that the short PR interval is due to "enhanced AV node conduction" from an immature AV node — not, as was once thought, from conduction down distinct atrioHisian fibers. In LGL syndrome, the QRS is normal in duration and configuration, unlike the WPW syndrome, in which more than 2/3 of cases show initial slurring of the QRS (delta wave) with a QRS duration ≥ 0.11 seconds. A short PR interval may also occur as a normal variant, although it is much more common in the pediatric population (as opposed to adults) and at faster (as compared to slower) heart rates. Pericarditis is associated with PR segment depression, but a short PR interval is not a characteristic finding. (Answer: All except e)

3. Ischemic heart disease is the most likely diagnosis based on the prevalence of coronary artery disease in the aged population. In the WPW syndrome, negative delta waves may occur in the inferior leads and resemble Q waves, but lack of initial slurring of the QRS in the present tracing rules against this diagnosis. In mitral valve prolapse, inferior Q waves (leads II, aVF) can be seen but are uncommon. Finally, in hypertrophic cardiomyopathy, large septal Q waves (from hypertrophy of the septum) are present in approximately 25% of cases and are usually seen in leads I, aVL, and V_4 - V_6. (Answer: a)

4. In approximately 1/3 of patients with WPW syndrome, the QRS duration is ≤ 0.10 seconds. In these cases, the ventricles are depolarized almost entirely by the sinus impulse (via the normal AV conduction system), with minimal contribution from antegrade conduction along the accessory pathway. (Answer: b)

5. At first glance, leads III and aVF appear to show QT prolongation. However, closer inspection of this ECG demonstrates that this "pseudo" QT prolongation is caused by superimposition of the U wave on the preceding T wave. (U waves are best seen in leads V_2 and V_3.) (Answer: b)

— Quick Review 16 —

Ventricular premature complex(es), uniform, fixed coupling	
• A wide, notched or slurred ____ complex that is premature relative to the normal RR interval and is not preceded by a ____ wave	QRS P
• QRS duration is almost always > ____ seconds	0.12
• Initial direction of the QRS is often (similar to/different from) the QRS during sinus rhythm	different from
• Secondary ST & T wave changes in the (same/opposite) direction as the major deflection of the QRS (i.e., ST depression & T wave inversion in leads with a dominant _____wave; ST elevation and upright T wave in leads with a dominant _____ wave or ____ complex)	opposite R S QS
• Coupling interval is constant or varies by < ____ seconds	0.08
• Morphology of VPCs in any given lead is (the same/different)	the same
• Retrograde capture of atria may occur (true/false)	true
• A full ____ pause (PP interval containing the VPC is twice the normal PP interval) is usually evident	compensatory
Intraventricular conduction disturbance, nonspecific type	
• QRS ≥ ____ seconds in duration but morphology does not meet criteria for LBBB or RBBB, *or* abnormal ____ without widening of the QRS complex	0.11 notching

ECG 17. 87-year-old male hospitalized with chest tightness and dyspnea:

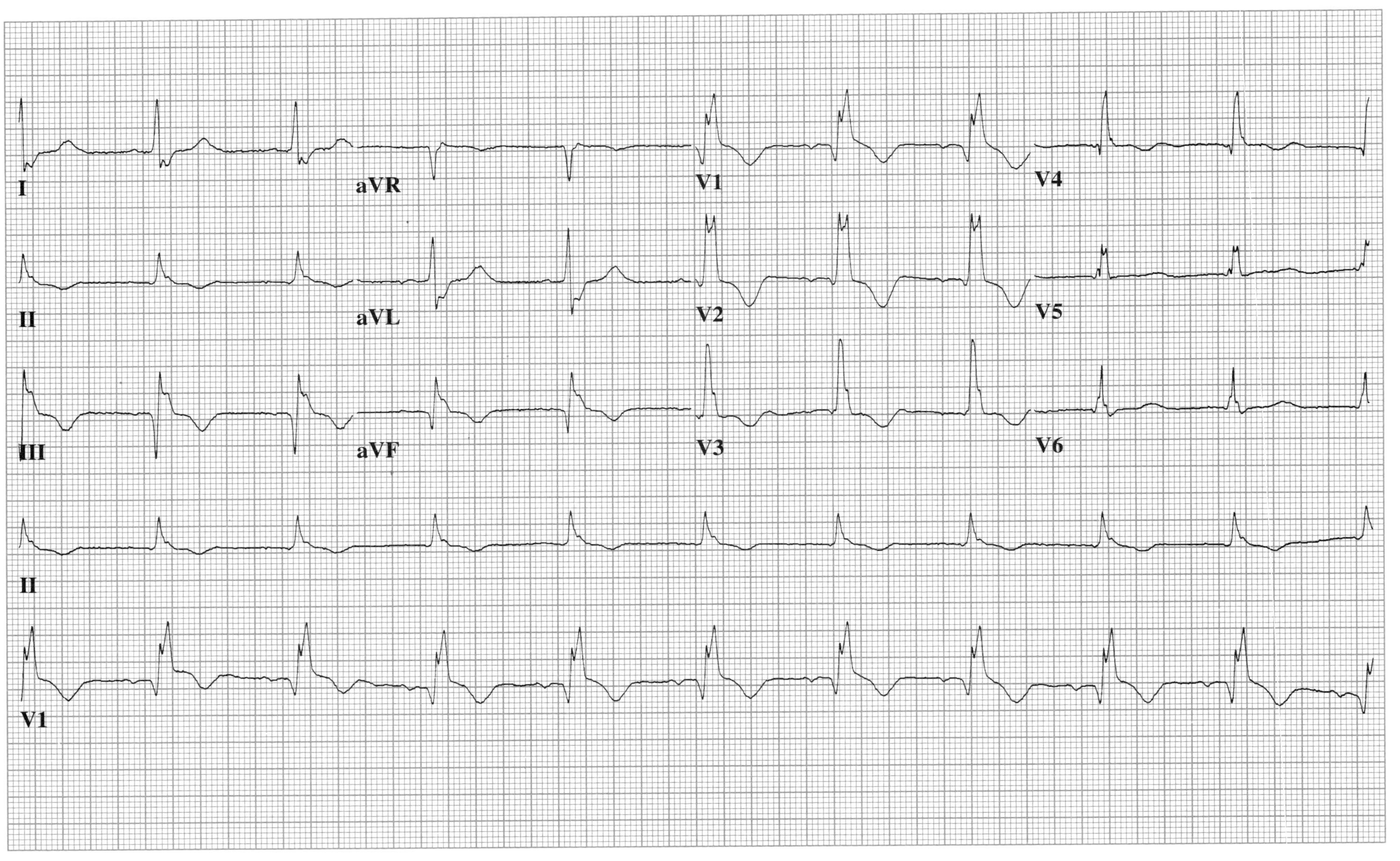

1. GENERAL FEATURES

- ☐ a. Normal ECG
- ☐ b. Borderline normal ECG or normal variant
- ☐ c. Incorrect electrode placement
- ☐ d. Artifact due to tremor

2. ATRIAL RHYTHMS

- ☐ a. Sinus rhythm
- ☐ b. Sinus arrhythmia
- ☐ c. Sinus bradycardia (< 60)
- ☐ d. Sinus tachycardia (> 100)
- ☐ e. Sinus pause or arrest
- ☐ f. Sinoatrial exit block
- ☐ g. Ecoptic atrial rhythm
- ☐ h. Wandering atrial pacemaker
- ☐ i. Atrial premature complexes, normally conducted
- ☐ j. Atrial premature complexes, nonconducted
- ☐ k. Atrial premature complexes with aberrant intraventricular conduction
- ☐ l. Atrial tachycardia (regular, sustained, 1:1 conduction)
- ☐ m. Atrial tachycardia, repetitive (short paroxysms)
- ☐ n. Atrial tachycardia, multifocal
- ☐ o. Atrial tachycardia with AV block
- ☐ p. Supraventricular tachycardia, unspecific
- ☐ q. Supraventricular tachycardia, paroxysmal
- ☐ r. Atrial flutter
- ☐ s. Atrial fibrillation
- ☐ t. Retrograde atrial activation

3. AV JUNCTIONAL RHYTHMS

- ☐ a. AV junctional premature complexes
- ☐ b. AV junctional escape complexes
- ☐ c. AV junctional rhythm, accelerated
- ☐ d. AV junctional rhythm

4. VENTRICULAR RHYTHMS

- ☐ a. Ventricular premature complex(es), uniform, fixed coupling
- ☐ b. Ventricular premature complex(es), uniform, nonfixed coupling
- ☐ c. Ventricular premature complexes(es), multiform
- ☐ d. Ventricular premature complexes, in pairs
- ☐ e. Ventricular parasystole
- ☐ f. Ventricular tachycardia (≥ 3 consecutive complexes)
- ☐ g. Accelerated idioventricular rhythm
- ☐ h. Ventricular escape complexes or rhythm
- ☐ i. Ventricular fibrillation

5. ATRIAL-VENTRICULAR INTERACTIONS IN ARRHYTHMIAS

- ☐ a. Fusion complexes
- ☐ b. Reciprocal (echo) complexes
- ☐ c. Ventricular capture complexes
- ☐ d. AV dissociation
- ☐ e. Ventriculophasic sinus arrhythmia

6. AV CONDUCTION ABNORMALITIES

- ☐ a. AV block, 1°
- ☐ b. AV block, 2° - Mobitz type I (Wenckebach)
- ☐ c. AV block, 2° - Mobitz type II
- ☐ d. AV block, 2:1
- ☐ e. AV block, 3°
- ☐ f. AV block, variable
- ☐ g. Short PR interval (with sinus rhythm and normal QRS duration)
- ☐ h. Wolff-Parkinson-White pattern

7. INTRAVENTRICULAR CONDUCTION DISTURBANCES

- ☐ a. RBBB, incomplete
- ☐ b. RBBB, complete
- ☐ c. Left anterior fascicular block
- ☐ d. Left posterior fascicular block
- ☐ e. LBBB, with ST-T wave suggestive of acute myocardial injury or infarction
- ☐ f. LBBB, complete
- ☐ g. LBBB, intermittent
- ☐ h. Intraventricular conduction disturbance, nonspecific
- ☐ i. Aberrant intraventricular conduction with supraventricular arrhythmia

8. P WAVE ABNORMALITIES

- ☐ a. Right atrial abnormality
- ☐ b. Left atrial abnormalities
- ☐ c. Nonspecific atrial abnormality

9. ABNORMALITIES OF QRS VOLTAGE OR AXIS

- ☐ a. Low voltage, limb leads only
- ☐ b. Low voltage, limb and precordial leads
- ☐ c. Left axis deviation (> - 30%)
- ☐ d. Right axis deviation (> + 100)
- ☐ e. Electrical alternans

10. VENTRICULAR HYPERTROPHY

- ☐ a. LVH by voltage only
- ☐ b. LVH by voltage and ST-T segment abnormalities
- ☐ c. RVH
- ☐ d. Combined ventricular hypertrophy

11. Q WAVE MYOCARDIAL INFARCTION

	Probably Acute or Recent	Probably Old or Age Indeterminate
Anterolateral	☐ a.	☐ g.
Anterior	☐ b.	☐ h.
Anteroseptal	☐ c.	☐ i.
Lateral/High lateral	☐ d.	☐ j.
Inferior	☐ e.	☐ k.
Posterior	☐ f.	☐ l.

☐ m. Probably ventricular aneurysm

12. ST, T, U, WAVE ABNORMALITIES

- ☐ a. Normal variant, early repolarization
- ☐ b. Normal variant, juvenile T waves
- ☐ c. Nonspecific ST and/or T wave abnormalities
- ☐ d. ST and/or T wave abnormalities suggesting myocardial ischemia
- ☐ e. ST and/or T wave abnormalities suggesting myocardial injury
- ☐ f. ST and/or T wave abnormalities suggesting acute pericarditis
- ☐ g. ST-T segment abnormalities secondary to intraventricular conduction disturbance or hypertrophy
- ☐ h. Post-extrasystolic T wave abnormality
- ☐ i. Isolated J point depression
- ☐ j. Peaked T waves
- ☐ k. Prolonged QT interval
- ☐ l. Prominent U waves

13. PACEMAKER FUNCTION AND RHYTHM

- ☐ a. Atrial or coronary sinus pacing
- ☐ b. Ventricular demand pacing
- ☐ c. AV sequential pacing
- ☐ d. Ventricular pacing, complete control
- ☐ e. Dual chamber, atrial sensing pacemaker
- ☐ f. Pacemaker malfunction, not constantly capturing (atrium or ventricle)
- ☐ g. Pacemaker malfunction, not constantly sensing (atrium or ventricle)
- ☐ h. Pacemaker malfunction, not firing
- ☐ i. Pacemaker malfunction, slowing

14. SUGGESTED OR PROBABLE CLINICAL DISORDERS

- ☐ a. Digitalis effect
- ☐ b. Digitalis toxicity
- ☐ c. Antiarrhythmic drug effect
- ☐ d. Antiarrhythmic drug toxicity
- ☐ e. Hyperkalemia
- ☐ f. Hypokalemia
- ☐ g. Hypercalcemia
- ☐ h. Hypocalcemia
- ☐ i. Atrial septal defect, secundum
- ☐ j. Atrial septal defect, primum
- ☐ k. Dextrocardia, mirror image
- ☐ l. Mitral valve disease
- ☐ m. Chronic lung disease
- ☐ n. Acute cor pulmonale, including pulmonary embolus
- ☐ o. Pericardial effusion
- ☐ p. Acute pericarditis
- ☐ q. Hypertrophic cardiomyopathy
- ☐ r. Coronary artery disease
- ☐ s. Central nervous system disorder
- ☐ t. Myxedema
- ☐ u. Hypothermia
- ☐ v. Sick sinus syndrome

ECG 17 was obtained in an 87-year-old male hospitalized with chest tightness and dyspnea. The ECG shows a sinus rhythm at 61 BPM, first-degree AV block, and RBBB. Q waves and ST-T changes in leads III and aVF (asterisks) are consistent with the diagnosis of recent inferior MI. An age indeterminate anteroseptal myocardial infarction is also present (arrows).

Codes:

2a	Sinus rhythm
6a	AV block, 1°
7b	RBBB, complete
11e	Inferior Q wave MI, probably acute or recent
11i	Anteroseptal Q wave MI, probably old or age indeterminate
12d	ST and/or T wave abnormalities suggesting myocardial injury
14r	Coronary artery disease

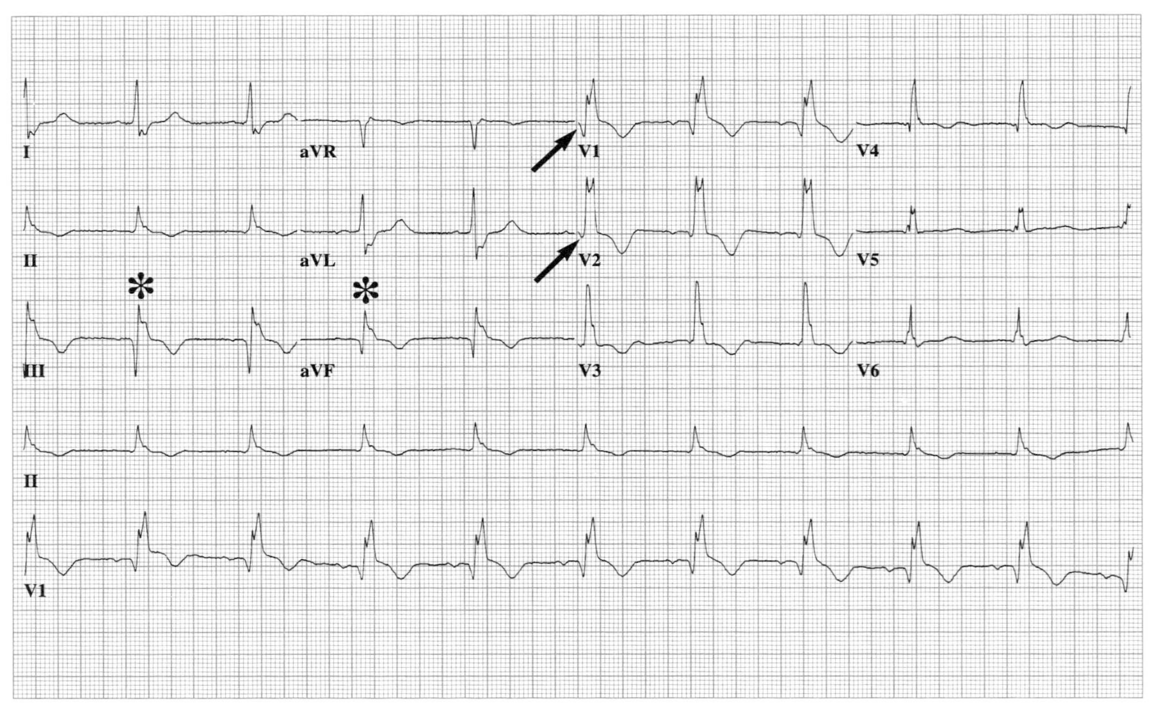

Questions: ECG 17

1. Pathologic Q waves in leads V_2-V_6 must be at least _____ seconds in duration:

   a. 0.02
   b. 0.03
   c. 0.04
   d. 0.06

2. An isolated Q wave in lead III is enough to make the diagnosis of inferior myocardial infarction:

   a. True
   b. False

Answers: ECG 17

1. Leads I, II, and V_2-V_6 require a Q wave duration ≥ 0.03 seconds to be considered pathological, and must be ≥ 0.04 seconds in leads III, aVL, aVF, and V_1. (Answer: b)

2. The diagnosis of inferior myocardial infarction requires the presence of pathological Q waves in 2 or more of leads II, III, and aVF. (Answer: b)

— Quick Review 17 —

AV block, 1°	
• PR interval ≥ ____ seconds	0.20
RBBB, complete	
• QRS duration ≥ ____ seconds	0.12
• Secondary R wave (R') in lead ____ is usually	V_1
(shorter/taller) than the initial R wave	taller
• Onset of intrinsicoid deflection in leads V_1 and V_2 > ____ seconds	0.05
• ST segment (depression/elevation) and	depression
(upright/inverted) T waves in V_1, V_2	inverted
• Wide slurred S wave in leads ____	I, aVL, V_5, V_6
• QRS axis is usually (normal/leftward/rightward)	normal
• RBBB (does/does not) interfere with the ECG diagnosis of ventricular hypertrophy or Q wave MI	does not
Inferior MI, recent or probably acute	
• Abnormal Q waves and ST elevation in at least two of leads ____	II, III, aVF
• Associated ST depression is usually evident in leads I, aVL, V_1-V_3 (true/false)	true

ECG 18. 46-year-old male four years status-post cardiac transplantation:

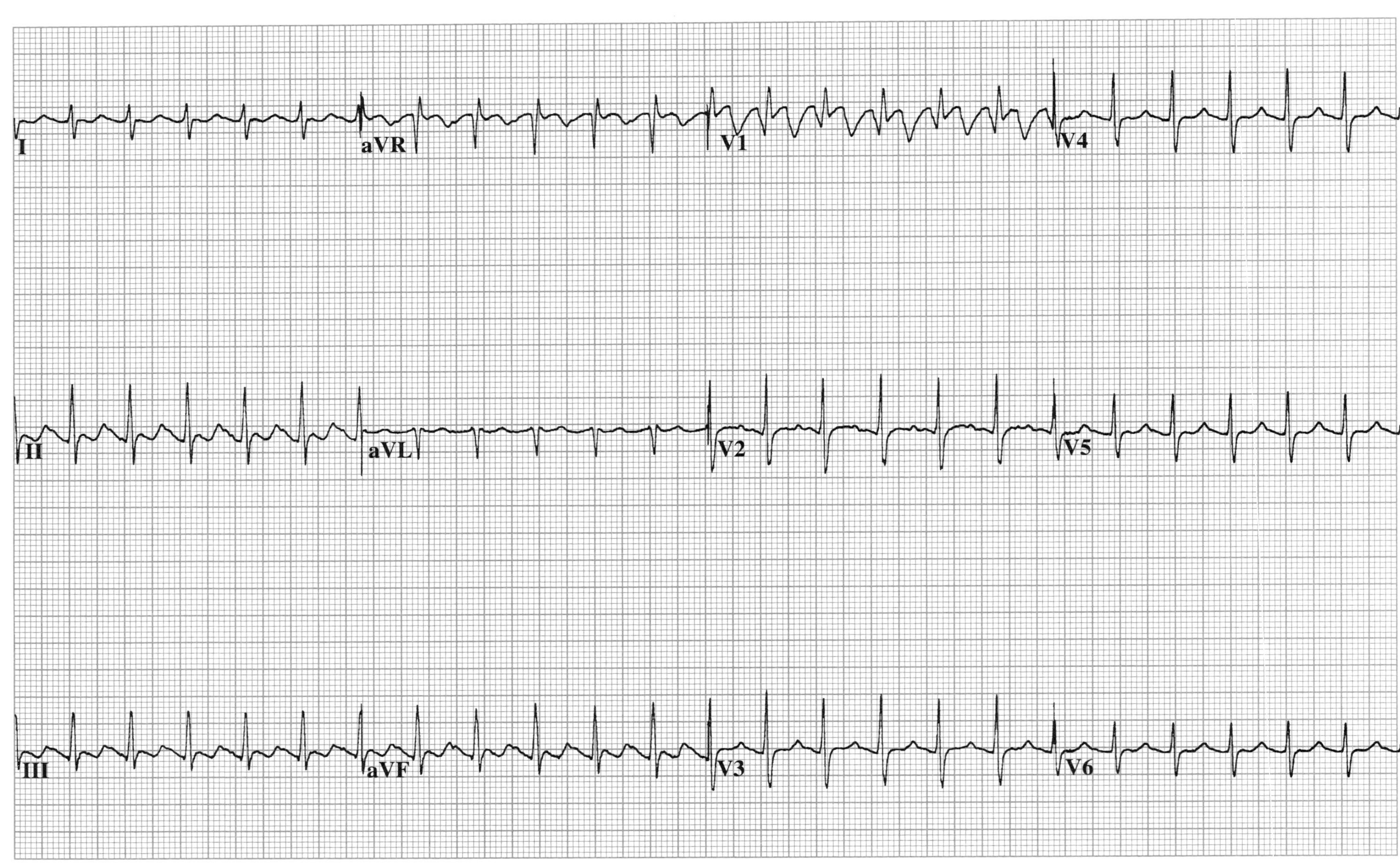

1. GENERAL FEATURES
- ☐ a. Normal ECG
- ☐ b. Borderline normal ECG or normal variant
- ☐ c. Incorrect electrode placement
- ☐ d. Artifact due to tremor

2. ATRIAL RHYTHMS
- ☐ a. Sinus rhythm
- ☐ b. Sinus arrhythmia
- ☐ c. Sinus bradycardia (< 60)
- ☐ d. Sinus tachycardia (> 100)
- ☐ e. Sinus pause or arrest
- ☐ f. Sinoatrial exit block
- ☐ g. Ecoptic atrial rhythm
- ☐ h. Wandering atrial pacemaker
- ☐ i. Atrial premature complexes, normally conducted
- ☐ j. Atrial premature complexes, nonconducted
- ☐ k. Atrial premature complexes with aberrant intraventricular conduction
- ☐ l. Atrial tachycardia (regular, sustained, 1:1 conduction)
- ☐ m. Atrial tachycardia, repetitive (short paroxysms)
- ☐ n. Atrial tachycardia, multifocal
- ☐ o. Atrial tachycardia with AV block
- ☐ p. Supraventricular tachycardia, unspecific
- ☐ q. Supraventricular tachycardia, paroxysmal
- ☐ r. Atrial flutter
- ☐ s. Atrial fibrillation
- ☐ t. Retrograde atrial activation

3. AV JUNCTIONAL RHYTHMS
- ☐ a. AV junctional premature complexes
- ☐ b. AV junctional escape complexes
- ☐ c. AV junctional rhythm, accelerated
- ☐ d. AV junctional rhythm

4. VENTRICULAR RHYTHMS
- ☐ a. Ventricular premature complex(es), uniform, fixed coupling
- ☐ b. Ventricular premature complex(es), uniform, nonfixed coupling
- ☐ c. Ventricular premature complexes(es), multiform
- ☐ d. Ventricular premature complexes, in pairs
- ☐ e. Ventricular parasystole
- ☐ f. Ventricular tachycardia (≥ 3 consecutive complexes)
- ☐ g. Accelerated idioventricular rhythm
- ☐ h. Ventricular escape complexes or rhythm
- ☐ i. Ventricular fibrillation

5. ATRIAL-VENTRICULAR INTERACTIONS IN ARRHYTHMIAS
- ☐ a. Fusion complexes
- ☐ b. Reciprocal (echo) complexes
- ☐ c. Ventricular capture complexes
- ☐ d. AV dissociation
- ☐ e. Ventriculophasic sinus arrhythmia

6. AV CONDUCTION ABNORMALITIES
- ☐ a. AV block, 1°
- ☐ b. AV block, 2° - Mobitz type I (Wenckebach)
- ☐ c. AV block, 2° - Mobitz type II
- ☐ d. AV block, 2:1
- ☐ e. AV block, 3°
- ☐ f. AV block, variable
- ☐ g. Short PR interval (with sinus rhythm and normal QRS duration)
- ☐ h. Wolff-Parkinson-White pattern

7. INTRAVENTRICULAR CONDUCTION DISTURBANCES
- ☐ a. RBBB, incomplete
- ☐ b. RBBB, complete
- ☐ c. Left anterior fascicular block
- ☐ d. Left posterior fascicular block
- ☐ e. LBBB, with ST-T wave suggestive of acute myocardial injury or infarction
- ☐ f. LBBB, complete
- ☐ g. LBBB, intermittent
- ☐ h. Intraventricular conduction disturbance, nonspecific
- ☐ i. Aberrant intraventricular conduction with supraventricular arrhythmia

8. P WAVE ABNORMALITIES
- ☐ a. Right atrial abnormality
- ☐ b. Left atrial abnormalities
- ☐ c. Nonspecific atrial abnormality

9. ABNORMALITIES OF QRS VOLTAGE OR AXIS
- ☐ a. Low voltage, limb leads only
- ☐ b. Low voltage, limb and precordial leads
- ☐ c. Left axis deviation (> - 30%)
- ☐ d. Right axis deviation (> + 100)
- ☐ e. Electrical alternans

10. VENTRICULAR HYPERTROPHY
- ☐ a. LVH by voltage only
- ☐ b. LVH by voltage and ST-T segment abnormalities
- ☐ c. RVH
- ☐ d. Combined ventricular hypertrophy

11. Q WAVE MYOCARDIAL INFARCTION

	Probably Acute or Recent	Probably Old or Age Indeterminate
Anterolateral	☐ a.	☐ g.
Anterior	☐ b.	☐ h.
Anteroseptal	☐ c.	☐ i.
Lateral/High lateral	☐ d.	☐ j.
Inferior	☐ e.	☐ k.
Posterior	☐ f.	☐ l.

- ☐ m. Probably ventricular aneurysm

12. ST, T, U, WAVE ABNORMALITIES
- ☐ a. Normal variant, early repolarization
- ☐ b. Normal variant, juvenile T waves
- ☐ c. Nonspecific ST and/or T wave abnormalities
- ☐ d. ST and/or T wave abnormalities suggesting myocardial ischemia
- ☐ e. ST and/or T wave abnormalities suggesting myocardial injury
- ☐ f. ST and/or T wave abnormalities suggesting acute pericarditis
- ☐ g. ST-T segment abnormalities secondary to intraventricular conduction disturbance or hypertrophy
- ☐ h. Post-extrasystolic T wave abnormality
- ☐ i. Isolated J point depression
- ☐ j. Peaked T waves
- ☐ k. Prolonged QT interval
- ☐ l. Prominent U waves

13. PACEMAKER FUNCTION AND RHYTHM
- ☐ a. Atrial or coronary sinus pacing
- ☐ b. Ventricular demand pacing
- ☐ c. AV sequential pacing
- ☐ d. Ventricular pacing, complete control
- ☐ e. Dual chamber, atrial sensing pacemaker
- ☐ f. Pacemaker malfunction, not constantly capturing (atrium or ventricle)
- ☐ g. Pacemaker malfunction, not constantly sensing (atrium or ventricle)
- ☐ h. Pacemaker malfunction, not firing
- ☐ i. Pacemaker malfunction, slowing

14. SUGGESTED OR PROBABLE CLINICAL DISORDERS
- ☐ a. Digitalis effect
- ☐ b. Digitalis toxicity
- ☐ c. Antiarrhythmic drug effect
- ☐ d. Antiarrhythmic drug toxicity
- ☐ e. Hyperkalemia
- ☐ f. Hypokalemia
- ☐ g. Hypercalcemia
- ☐ h. Hypocalcemia
- ☐ i. Atrial septal defect, secundum
- ☐ j. Atrial septal defect, primum
- ☐ k. Dextrocardia, mirror image
- ☐ l. Mitral valve disease
- ☐ m. Chronic lung disease
- ☐ n. Acute cor pulmonale, including pulmonary embolus
- ☐ o. Pericardial effusion
- ☐ p. Acute pericarditis
- ☐ q. Hypertrophic cardiomyopathy
- ☐ r. Coronary artery disease
- ☐ s. Central nervous system disorder
- ☐ t. Myxedema
- ☐ u. Hypothermia
- ☐ v. Sick sinus syndrome

ECG 18 was obtained from a 46-year-old male who is four years status-post cardiac transplantation. The tracing shows a narrow complex tachycardia. Atrial flutter waves (arrowheads) are apparent in the inferior leads and lead V_1. Two-to-one AV block and right axis deviation are noted.

Codes:

2r	Atrial flutter
6d	AV block, 2:1
9d	Right axis deviation (> +100°)

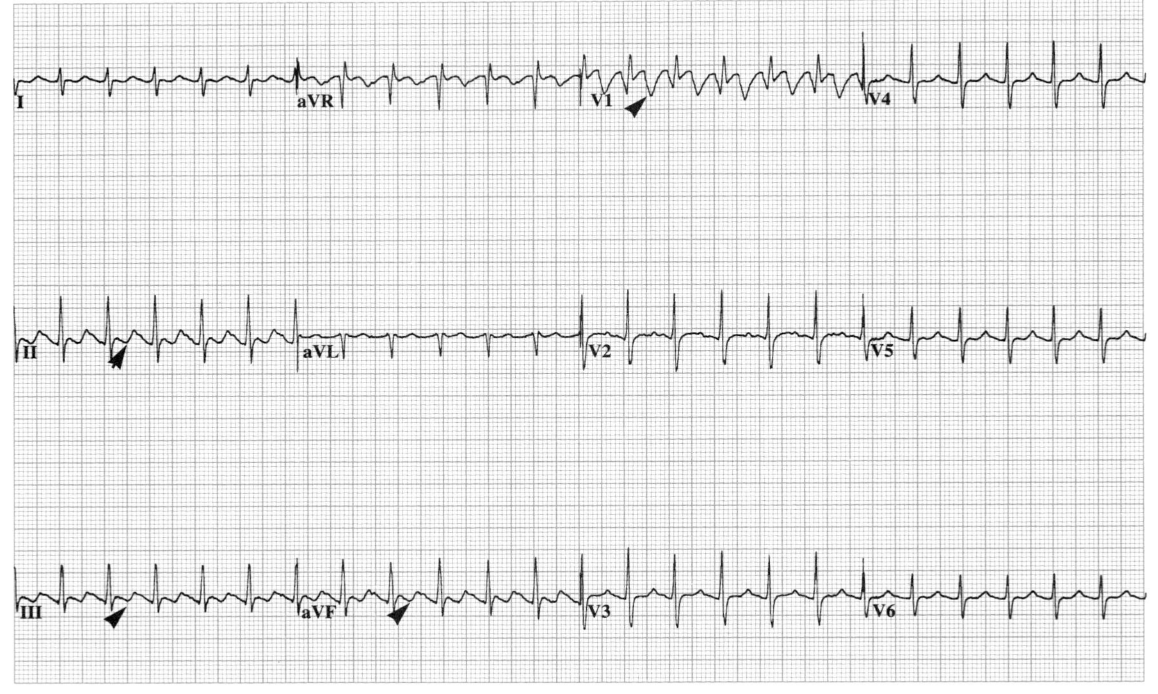

Questions: ECG 18

1. Right axis deviation is associated with all of the following conditions except:

   a. COPD
   b. Right ventricular hypertrophy
   c. Right bundle branch block
   d. Anterior MI
   e. Lateral MI
   f. Left anterior fascicular block
   g. Left posterior fascicular block
   h. Dextrocardia
   i. Lead reversal
   j. WPW syndrome

2. The typical response of atrial flutter to carotid sinus massage is:

   a. No effect
   b. Slowing of flutter rate; no change in ventricular response
   c. No change in flutter rate; transient increase in AV block
   d. Conversion to normal sinus rhythm

Answers: ECG 18

1. (Answer: c, d, f)

2. In patients with atrial flutter, carotid sinus massage typically causes a transient increase in AV block and slowing of the ventricular response, without a change in the atrial flutter rate; less commonly, no effect is seen. When 2:1 AV block is present and atrial flutter is suspected, carotid sinus massage may unmask flutter waves and help confirm the diagnosis. Upon discontinuation of carotid sinus massage, the usual response is return to the original ventricular rate. (Answer: c)

— Quick Review 18 —

Atrial flutter	
• Rapid (regular/irregular) atrial undulations ("F" waves) at a rate of ____ per minute	regular 240-340
• Flutter rate may (increase/decrease) in the presence of Types IA, IC or III antiarrhythmic drugs	decrease
• Flutter waves in leads II, III, AVF are typically (inverted/upright) (with/without) an isoelectric baseline	inverted,without
• Flutter waves in lead V_1 are typically small (positive/negative) deflections (with/without) a distinct isoelectric baseline	positive, with
• QRS complex may be normal or aberrant (true/false)	true
• AV conduction ratio (ratio of flutter waves to QRS complexes) is usually (fixed/variable)	fixed
▸ Conduction ratios of 1:1 and 3:1 are (common/uncommon)	uncommon
▸ In untreated patients, AV block ≥ ____ suggests the coexistence of AV conduction disease	4:1
Right axis deviation	
• Mean QRS axis between ____ and ____ degrees	101, 254

Common Dilemmas in ECG Interpretation

Problem

Left bundle branch block is present. Should acute myocardial infarction ever be coded?

Recommendation

No (controversial). Most electrocardiographers are reluctant to diagnosis acute myocardial infarction in the setting of LBBB. However, three criteria have independent value for diagnosing acute myocardial injury (item 7e):

- ST elevation $\geq$ 1 mm concordant to (same direction as) the major deflection of the QRS
- ST depression $\geq$ 1 mm in V_1, V_2, or V_3
- ST elevation $\geq$ 5mm discordant with (opposite direction to) the major deflection of the QRS

ECG 19. 24-year-old female with post-partum cardiomyopathy and palpitations:

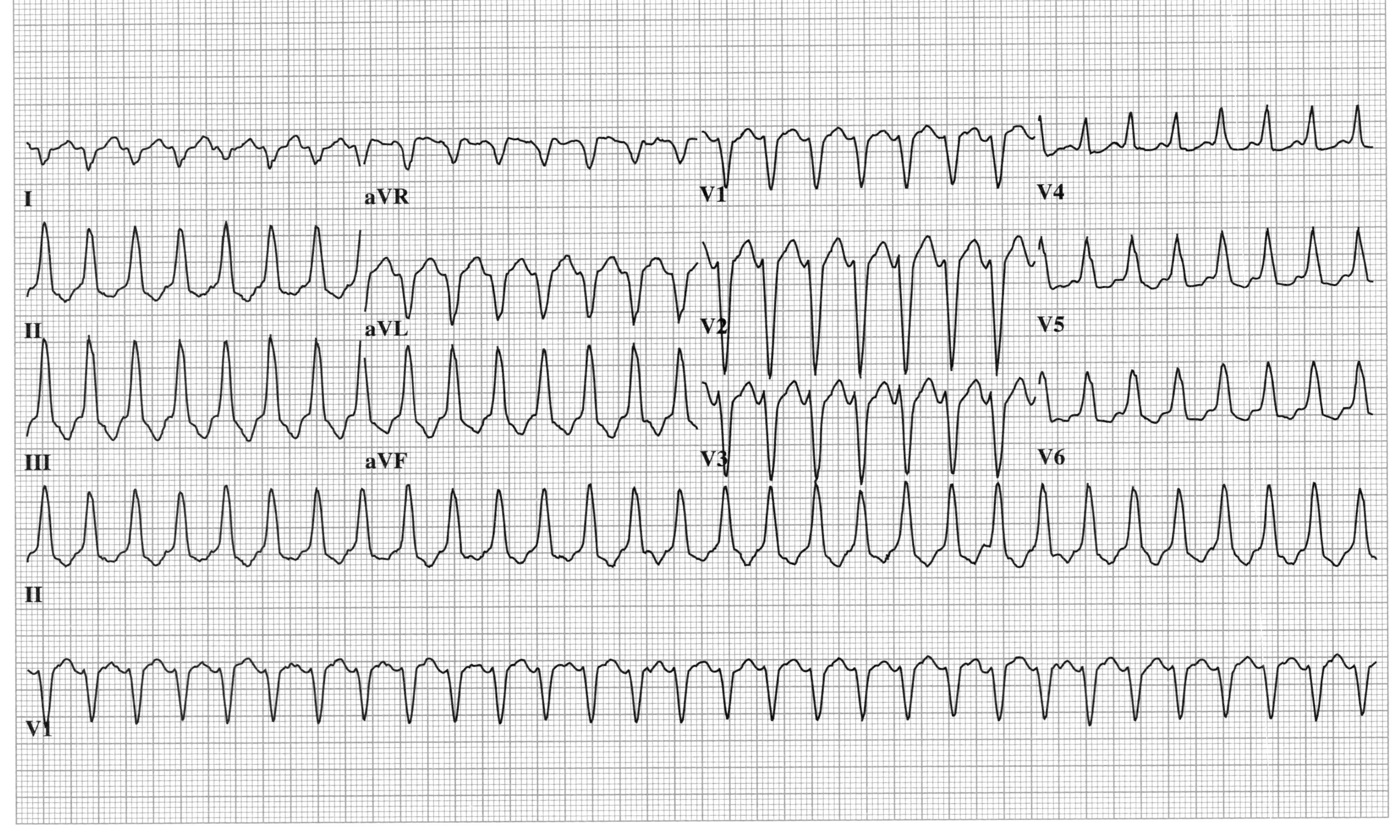

1. GENERAL FEATURES

☐ a. Normal ECG
☐ b. Borderline normal ECG or normal variant
☐ c. Incorrect electrode placement
☐ d. Artifact due to tremor

2. ATRIAL RHYTHMS

☐ a. Sinus rhythm
☐ b. Sinus arrhythmia
☐ c. Sinus bradycardia (< 60)
☐ d. Sinus tachycardia (> 100)
☐ e. Sinus pause or arrest
☐ f. Sinoatrial exit block
☐ g. Ecoptic atrial rhythm
☐ h. Wandering atrial pacemaker
☐ i. Atrial premature complexes, normally conducted
☐ j. Atrial premature complexes, nonconducted
☐ k. Atrial premature complexes with aberrant intraventricular conduction
☐ l. Atrial tachycardia (regular, sustained, 1:1 conduction)
☐ m. Atrial tachycardia, repetitive (short paroxysms)
☐ n. Atrial tachycardia, multifocal
☐ o. Atrial tachycardia with AV block
☐ p. Supraventricular tachycardia, unspecific
☐ q. Supraventricular tachycardia, paroxysmal
☐ r. Atrial flutter
☐ s. Atrial fibrillation
☐ t. Retrograde atrial activation

3. AV JUNCTIONAL RHYTHMS

☐ a. AV junctional premature complexes
☐ b. AV junctional escape complexes
☐ c. AV junctional rhythm, accelerated
☐ d. AV junctional rhythm

4. VENTRICULAR RHYTHMS

☐ a. Ventricular premature complex(es), uniform, fixed coupling
☐ b. Ventricular premature complex(es), uniform, nonfixed coupling
☐ c. Ventricular premature complexes(es), multiform
☐ d. Ventricular premature complexes, in pairs
☐ e. Ventricular parasystole
☐ f. Ventricular tachycardia (≥ 3 consecutive complexes)
☐ g. Accelerated idioventricular rhythm
☐ h. Ventricular escape complexes or rhythm
☐ i. Ventricular fibrillation

5. ATRIAL-VENTRICULAR INTERACTIONS IN ARRHYTHMIAS

☐ a. Fusion complexes
☐ b. Reciprocal (echo) complexes
☐ c. Ventricular capture complexes
☐ d. AV dissociation
☐ e. Ventriculophasic sinus arrhythmia

6. AV CONDUCTION ABNORMALITIES

☐ a. AV block. 1°
☐ b. AV block, 2° - Mobitz type I (Wenckebach)
☐ c. AV block, 2° - Mobitz type II
☐ d. AV block, 2:1
☐ e. AV block, 3°
☐ f. AV block, variable
☐ g. Short PR interval (with sinus rhythm and normal QRS duration)
☐ h. Wolff-Parkinson-White pattern

7. INTRAVENTRICULAR CONDUCTION DISTURBANCES

☐ a. RBBB, incomplete
☐ b. RBBB, complete
☐ c. Left anterior fascicular block
☐ d. Left posterior fascicular block
☐ e. LBBB, with ST-T wave suggestive of acute myocardial injury or infarction
☐ f. LBBB, complete
☐ g. LBBB, intermittent
☐ h. Intraventricular conduction disturbance, nonspecific
☐ i. Aberrant intraventricular conduction with supraventricular arrhythmia

8. P WAVE ABNORMALITIES

☐ a. Right atrial abnormality
☐ b. Left atrial abnormalities
☐ c. Nonspecific atrial abnormality

9. ABNORMALITIES OF QRS VOLTAGE OR AXIS

☐ a. Low voltage, limb leads only
☐ b. Low voltage, limb and precordial leads
☐ c. Left axis deviation (> - 30%)
☐ d. Right axis deviation (> + 100)
☐ e. Electrical alternans

10. VENTRICULAR HYPERTROPHY

☐ a. LVH by voltage only
☐ b. LVH by voltage and ST-T segment abnormalities
☐ c. RVH
☐ d. Combined ventricular hypertrophy

11. Q WAVE MYOCARDIAL INFARCTION

	Probably Acute or Recent	Probably Old or Age Indeterminate
Anterolateral	☐ a.	☐ g.
Anterior	☐ b.	☐ h.
Anteroseptal	☐ c.	☐ i.
Lateral/High lateral	☐ d.	☐ j.
Inferior	☐ e.	☐ k.
Posterior	☐ f.	☐ l.

☐ m. Probably ventricular aneurysm

12. ST, T, U, WAVE ABNORMALITIES

☐ a. Normal variant, early repolarization
☐ b. Normal variant, juvenile T waves
☐ c. Nonspecific ST and/or T wave abnormalities
☐ d. ST and/or T wave abnormalities suggesting myocardial ischemia
☐ e. ST and/or T wave abnormalities suggesting myocardial injury
☐ f. ST and/or T wave abnormalities suggesting acute pericarditis
☐ g. ST-T segment abnormalities secondary to intraventricular conduction disturbance or hypertrophy
☐ h. Post-extrasystolic T wave abnormality
☐ i. Isolated J point depression
☐ j. Peaked T waves
☐ k. Prolonged QT interval
☐ l. Prominent U waves

13. PACEMAKER FUNCTION AND RHYTHM

☐ a. Atrial or coronary sinus pacing
☐ b. Ventricular demand pacing
☐ c. AV sequential pacing
☐ d. Ventricular pacing, complete control
☐ e. Dual chamber, atrial sensing pacemaker
☐ f. Pacemaker malfunction, not constantly capturing (atrium or ventricle)
☐ g. Pacemaker malfunction, not constantly sensing (atrium or ventricle)
☐ h. Pacemaker malfunction, not firing
☐ i. Pacemaker malfunction, slowing

14. SUGGESTED OR PROBABLE CLINICAL DISORDERS

☐ a. Digitalis effect
☐ b. Digitalis toxicity
☐ c. Antiarrhythmic drug effect
☐ d. Antiarrhythmic drug toxicity
☐ e. Hyperkalemia
☐ f. Hypokalemia
☐ g. Hypercalcemia
☐ h. Hypocalcemia
☐ i. Atrial septal defect, secundum
☐ j. Atrial septal defect, primum
☐ k. Dextrocardia, mirror image
☐ l. Mitral valve disease
☐ m. Chronic lung disease
☐ n. Acute cor pulmonale, including pulmonary embolus
☐ o. Pericardial effusion
☐ p. Acute pericarditis
☐ q. Hypertrophic cardiomyopathy
☐ r. Coronary artery disease
☐ s. Central nervous system disorder
☐ t. Myxedema
☐ u. Hypothermia
☐ v. Sick sinus syndrome

ECG 19 was obtained in a 24-year-old female with post-partum cardiomyopathy currently being evaluated for palpitations. The ECG shows an underlying sinus rhythm at 90 beats/minute (arrows mark the P waves) and a wide complex tachycardia at 178 beats/minute consistent with ventricular tachycardia with AV dissociation. The ventricular tachycardia morphology shows a LBBB pattern with right axis deviation, localizing the site of origin of the VT to the right ventricular outflow tract. (Note: Right-sided VT results in a LBBB *pattern*, not a true LBBB).

Codes:

4f	Ventricular tachycardia (≥ 3 consecutive complexes)
5d	AV dissociation
9d	Right axis deviation (> + 100°)

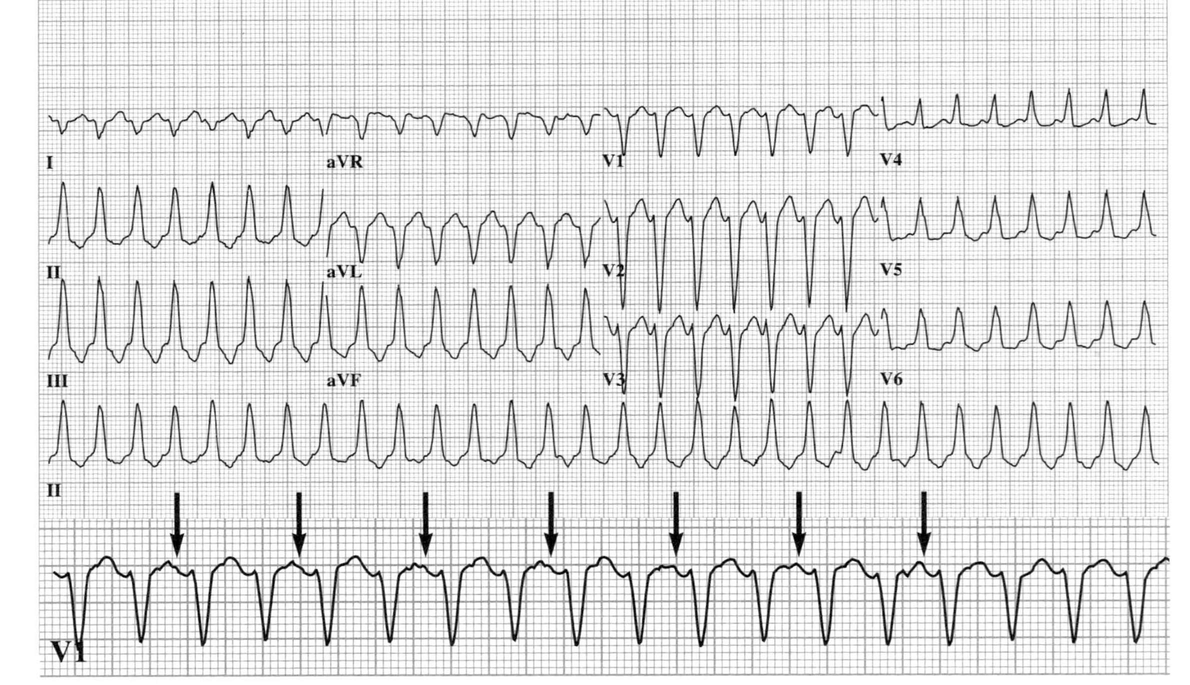

Questions: ECG 19

1. ECG findings in the setting of a wide QRS tachycardia that favor the diagnosis of ventricular tachycardia over SVT with aberrancy include:

   a. AV dissociation
   b. Capture beats
   c. QRS duration of 0.14 seconds if LBBB morphology is present (assuming the QRS is narrow during sinus rhythm)
   d. Some positive and some negative QRS deflections in the precordial leads
   e. R' is taller than the R wave when an RSR' complex is present in V_1

2. Ventricular tachycardia always manifests a QRS duration >0.11 seconds:

   a. True
   b. False

Answers: ECG 19

1. Ventricular tachycardia is favored when the QRS morphology is similar to VPCs seen in an earlier tracing; when the tachycardia is initiated by VPCs; when AV dissociation, capture beats, and/or fusion beats are present; when the QRS duration exceeds 0.14 seconds if RBBB morphology is present or 0.16 seconds if LBBB morphology is present; when the QRS deflections in the precordial leads are all positive or all negative (concordance); and when the R wave is taller than the R' wave in V_1. (Answer: a, b)

2. Although rare, if the ventricular focus is high in the septum (i.e., immediately below the bundle of His), ventricular tachycardia can present with a relatively narrow QRS complex. (Answer: b)

— Quick Review 19 —

Ventricular tachycardia	
• Rapid succession of three or more premature ventricular beats at a rate > ____ per minute	100
• RR intervals are usually regular but may be irregular (true/false)	true
• (Abrupt/gradual) onset and termination are evident	Abrupt
• AV ____ is common	dissociation
• Look for ventricular ____ complexes and ____ beats as markers for VT	capture, fusion
AV dissociation	
• Atrial and ventricular rhythms are ____ of each other	independent
• Ventricular rate is (</≥) than the atrial rate	≥

ECG 20. 37-year-old male with a lifelong systolic murmur:

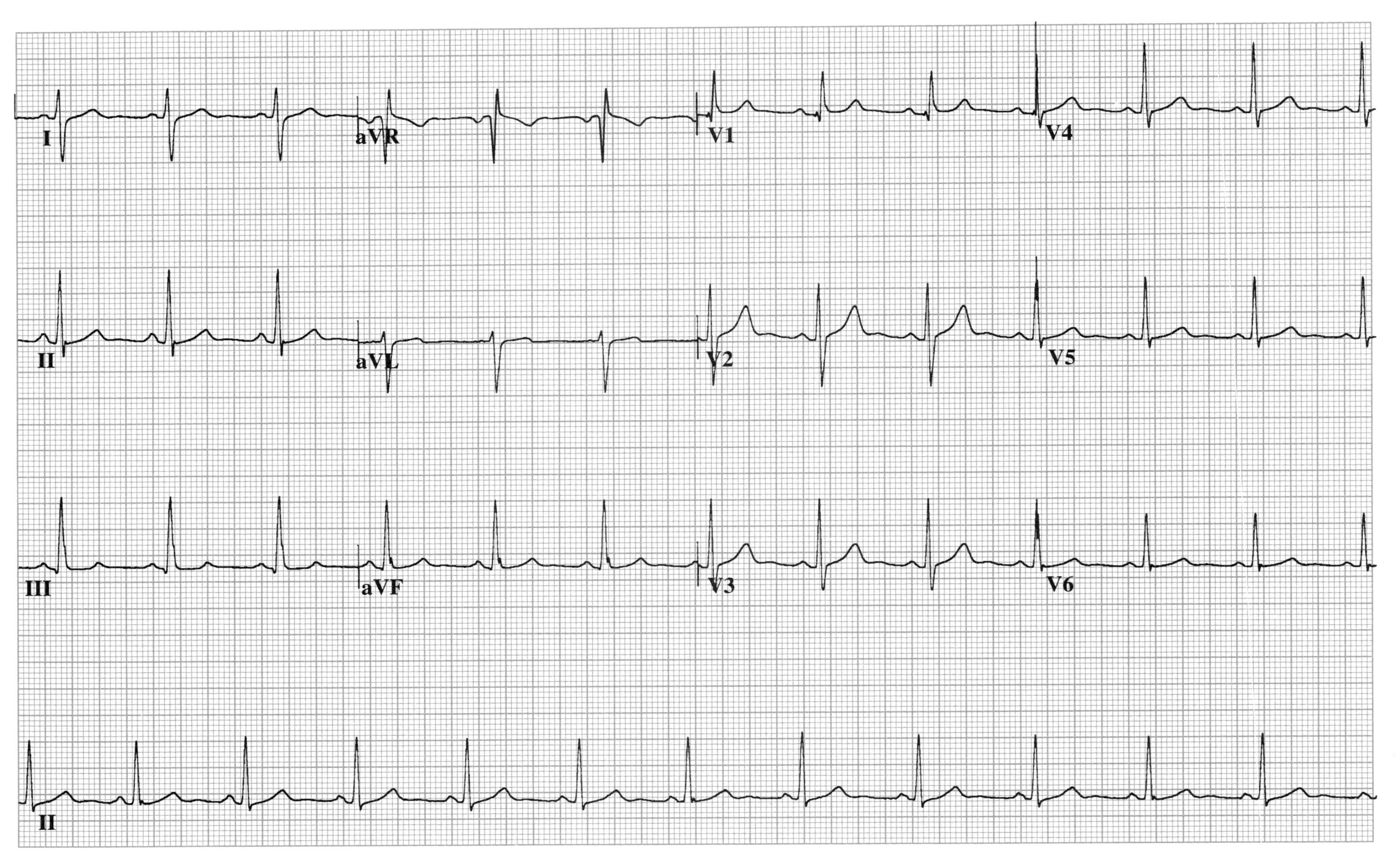

1. GENERAL FEATURES

- ☐ a. Normal ECG
- ☐ b. Borderline normal ECG or normal variant
- ☐ c. Incorrect electrode placement
- ☐ d. Artifact due to tremor

2. ATRIAL RHYTHMS

- ☐ a. Sinus rhythm
- ☐ b. Sinus arrhythmia
- ☐ c. Sinus bradycardia (< 60)
- ☐ d. Sinus tachycardia (> 100)
- ☐ e. Sinus pause or arrest
- ☐ f. Sinoatrial exit block
- ☐ g. Ecoptic atrial rhythm
- ☐ h. Wandering atrial pacemaker
- ☐ i. Atrial premature complexes, normally conducted
- ☐ j. Atrial premature complexes, nonconducted
- ☐ k. Atrial premature complexes with aberrant intraventricular conduction
- ☐ l. Atrial tachycardia (regular, sustained, 1:1 conduction)
- ☐ m. Atrial tachycardia, repetitive (short paroxysms)
- ☐ n. Atrial tachycardia, multifocal
- ☐ o. Atrial tachycardia with AV block
- ☐ p. Supraventricular tachycardia, unspecific
- ☐ q. Supraventricular tachycardia, paroxysmal
- ☐ r. Atrial flutter
- ☐ s. Atrial fibrillation
- ☐ t. Retrograde atrial activation

3. AV JUNCTIONAL RHYTHMS

- ☐ a. AV junctional premature complexes
- ☐ b. AV junctional escape complexes
- ☐ c. AV junctional rhythm, accelerated
- ☐ d. AV junctional rhythm

4. VENTRICULAR RHYTHMS

- ☐ a. Ventricular premature complex(es), uniform, fixed coupling
- ☐ b. Ventricular premature complex(es), uniform, nonfixed coupling
- ☐ c. Ventricular premature complexes(es), multiform
- ☐ d. Ventricular premature complexes, in pairs
- ☐ e. Ventricular parasystole
- ☐ f. Ventricular tachycardia (≥ 3 consecutive complexes)
- ☐ g. Accelerated idioventricular rhythm
- ☐ h. Ventricular escape complexes or rhythm
- ☐ i. Ventricular fibrillation

5. ATRIAL-VENTRICULAR INTERACTIONS IN ARRHYTHMIAS

- ☐ a. Fusion complexes
- ☐ b. Reciprocal (echo) complexes
- ☐ c. Ventricular capture complexes
- ☐ d. AV dissociation
- ☐ e. Ventriculophasic sinus arrhythmia

6. AV CONDUCTION ABNORMALITIES

- ☐ a. AV block, 1°
- ☐ b. AV block, 2° - Mobitz type I (Wenckebach)
- ☐ c. AV block, 2° - Mobitz type II
- ☐ d. AV block, 2:1
- ☐ e. AV block, 3°
- ☐ f. AV block, variable
- ☐ g. Short PR interval (with sinus rhythm and normal QRS duration)
- ☐ h. Wolff-Parkinson-White pattern

7. INTRAVENTRICULAR CONDUCTION DISTURBANCES

- ☐ a. RBBB, incomplete
- ☐ b. RBBB, complete
- ☐ c. Left anterior fascicular block
- ☐ d. Left posterior fascicular block
- ☐ e. LBBB, with ST-T wave suggestive of acute myocardial injury or infarction
- ☐ f. LBBB, complete
- ☐ g. LBBB, intermittent
- ☐ h. Intraventricular conduction disturbance, nonspecific
- ☐ i. Aberrant intraventricular conduction with supraventricular arrhythmia

8. P WAVE ABNORMALITIES

- ☐ a. Right atrial abnormality
- ☐ b. Left atrial abnormalities
- ☐ c. Nonspecific atrial abnormality

9. ABNORMALITIES OF QRS VOLTAGE OR AXIS

- ☐ a. Low voltage, limb leads only
- ☐ b. Low voltage, limb and precordial leads
- ☐ c. Left axis deviation (> - 30%)
- ☐ d. Right axis deviation (> + 100)
- ☐ e. Electrical alternans

10. VENTRICULAR HYPERTROPHY

- ☐ a. LVH by voltage only
- ☐ b. LVH by voltage and ST-T segment abnormalities
- ☐ c. RVH
- ☐ d. Combined ventricular hypertrophy

11. Q WAVE MYOCARDIAL INFARCTION

	Probably Acute or Recent	Probably Old or Age Indeterminate
Anterolateral	☐ a.	☐ g.
Anterior	☐ b.	☐ h.
Anteroseptal	☐ c.	☐ i.
Lateral/High lateral	☐ d.	☐ j.
Inferior	☐ e.	☐ k.
Posterior	☐ f.	☐ l.

- ☐ m. Probably ventricular aneurysm

12. ST, T, U, WAVE ABNORMALITIES

- ☐ a. Normal variant, early repolarization
- ☐ b. Normal variant, juvenile T waves
- ☐ c. Nonspecific ST and/or T wave abnormalities
- ☐ d. ST and/or T wave abnormalities suggesting myocardial ischemia
- ☐ e. ST and/or T wave abnormalities suggesting myocardial injury
- ☐ f. ST and/or T wave abnormalities suggesting acute pericarditis
- ☐ g. ST-T segment abnormalities secondary to intraventricular conduction disturbance or hypertrophy
- ☐ h. Post-extrasystolic T wave abnormality
- ☐ i. Isolated J point depression
- ☐ j. Peaked T waves
- ☐ k. Prolonged QT interval
- ☐ l. Prominent U waves

13. PACEMAKER FUNCTION AND RHYTHM

- ☐ a. Atrial or coronary sinus pacing
- ☐ b. Ventricular demand pacing
- ☐ c. AV sequential pacing
- ☐ d. Ventricular pacing, complete control
- ☐ e. Dual chamber, atrial sensing pacemaker
- ☐ f. Pacemaker malfunction, not constantly capturing (atrium or ventricle)
- ☐ g. Pacemaker malfunction, not constantly sensing (atrium or ventricle)
- ☐ h. Pacemaker malfunction, not firing
- ☐ i. Pacemaker malfunction, slowing

14. SUGGESTED OR PROBABLE CLINICAL DISORDERS

- ☐ a. Digitalis effect
- ☐ b. Digitalis toxicity
- ☐ c. Antiarrhythmic drug effect
- ☐ d. Antiarrhythmic drug toxicity
- ☐ e. Hyperkalemia
- ☐ f. Hypokalemia
- ☐ g. Hypercalcemia
- ☐ h. Hypocalcemia
- ☐ i. Atrial septal defect, secundum
- ☐ j. Atrial septal defect, primum
- ☐ k. Dextrocardia, mirror image
- ☐ l. Mitral valve disease
- ☐ m. Chronic lung disease
- ☐ n. Acute cor pulmonale, including pulmonary embolus
- ☐ o. Pericardial effusion
- ☐ p. Acute pericarditis
- ☐ q. Hypertrophic cardiomyopathy
- ☐ r. Coronary artery disease
- ☐ s. Central nervous system disorder
- ☐ t. Myxedema
- ☐ u. Hypothermia
- ☐ v. Sick sinus syndrome

ECG 20 was obtained from a 37-year-old male with a history of a lifelong systolic murmur. The tracing shows a sinus rhythm with right axis deviation and a prominent R wave in lead V_1 consistent with right ventricular hypertrophy (arrow). This patient was shown to have moderate stenosis of the pulmonary valve.

Codes:

2a	Sinus rhythm
9d	Right axis deviation (> +100°)
10c	Right ventricular hypertrophy

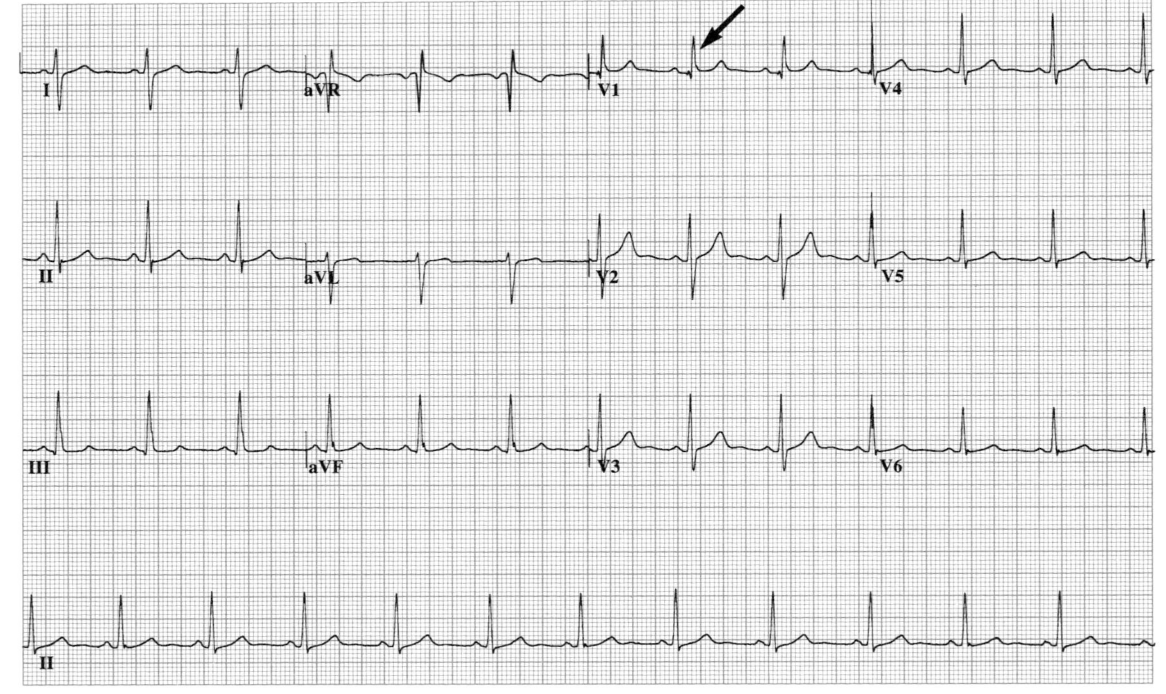

Questions: ECG 20

1. All of the following conditions can cause right axis deviation except:

   a. Right ventricular hypertrophy (RVH)
   b. COPD without pulmonary hypertension
   c. Lateral MI
   d. Posterior MI
   e. Left posterior fascicular block
   f. Ostium primum atrial septal defect
   g. Ostium secundum atrial septal defect
   h. Dextroposition

2. The differential diagnosis of a QRS duration < 0.12 sec with an RSR' pattern in lead V_1 includes:

   a. Right ventricular hypertrophy
   b. Posterior MI
   c. Incomplete right bundle branch block
   d. Normal variant
   e. Pectus excavatum

3. ECG findings that favor the diagnosis of posterior MI over RVH when a tall R wave is present in V_1 include:

   a. T wave inversion in lead V_1
   b. Upright T wave in lead V_1
   c. Right axis deviation
   d. Abnormal Q waves in leads II, III, and aVF

Answers: ECG 20

1. Causes of right axis deviation include right ventricular hypertrophy, COPD, lateral MI, left posterior fascicular block, ostium secundum ASD, and dextroposition. Posterior myocardial infarction per se does not induce a change in QRS axis (but left axis deviation may develop when the inferior wall is also involved). Ostium primum atrial septal defect is associated with left axis deviation, incomplete RBBB, and a prolonged PR interval. (Answer: d, f)

2. Causes of RSR' with a QRS duration < 0.12 seconds in lead V_1 may be seen in right ventricular hypertrophy, posterior MI, RBBB, chest wall deformities (e.g., pectus excavatum), and in up to 2% of normal individuals. (Answer: All)

3. When a tall R wave is present in lead V_1, other ECG findings can

help distinguish right ventricular hypertrophy (RVH) from posterior MI: T wave inversions in V_1V_2 and right axis deviation favors the diagnosis of RVH, while inferior Q waves suggestive of inferior MI favors the diagnosis of posterior MI. (Answer: b, d)

— Quick Review 20 —

Right axis deviation	
• Mean QRS axis between ____ and ____ degrees	101, 254
Right ventricular hypertrophy	
• Mean QRS axis ≥ ____ degrees	100
• Dominant ____ wave	R
▸ R/S ratio in V_1 or V_{3R} (<, =, >) 1, or R/S ratio in	>
V_5 or V_6 (≤, >) 1	≤
▸ R wave in V_1 ≥ ____ mm	7
▸ R wave in V_1 + S wave in V_5 or V_6 > ____ mm	10.5
▸ rSR' in V_1 with R' > ____ mm	10
• Secondary downsloping ST depression & T-wave inversion in the (right/left) precordial leads	right
• (Right/left) atrial abnormality	right

Differential Diagnosis

Peaked T Waves

(T wave amplitude > 6 mm in limb leads or > 10 mm in precordial leads)

- Acute MI (item 12e)
- Normal variant (item 1b); most common in mid-precordial leads
- Hyperkalemia (item 14e): QT normal
- Intracranial bleeding (item 14s): prolonged QT (item 12k); prominent U waves (item 12l)
- LVH (item 10b)
- LBBB (item 7f)

ECG 21. 78-year-old female being treated for paroxysmal atrial fibrillation:

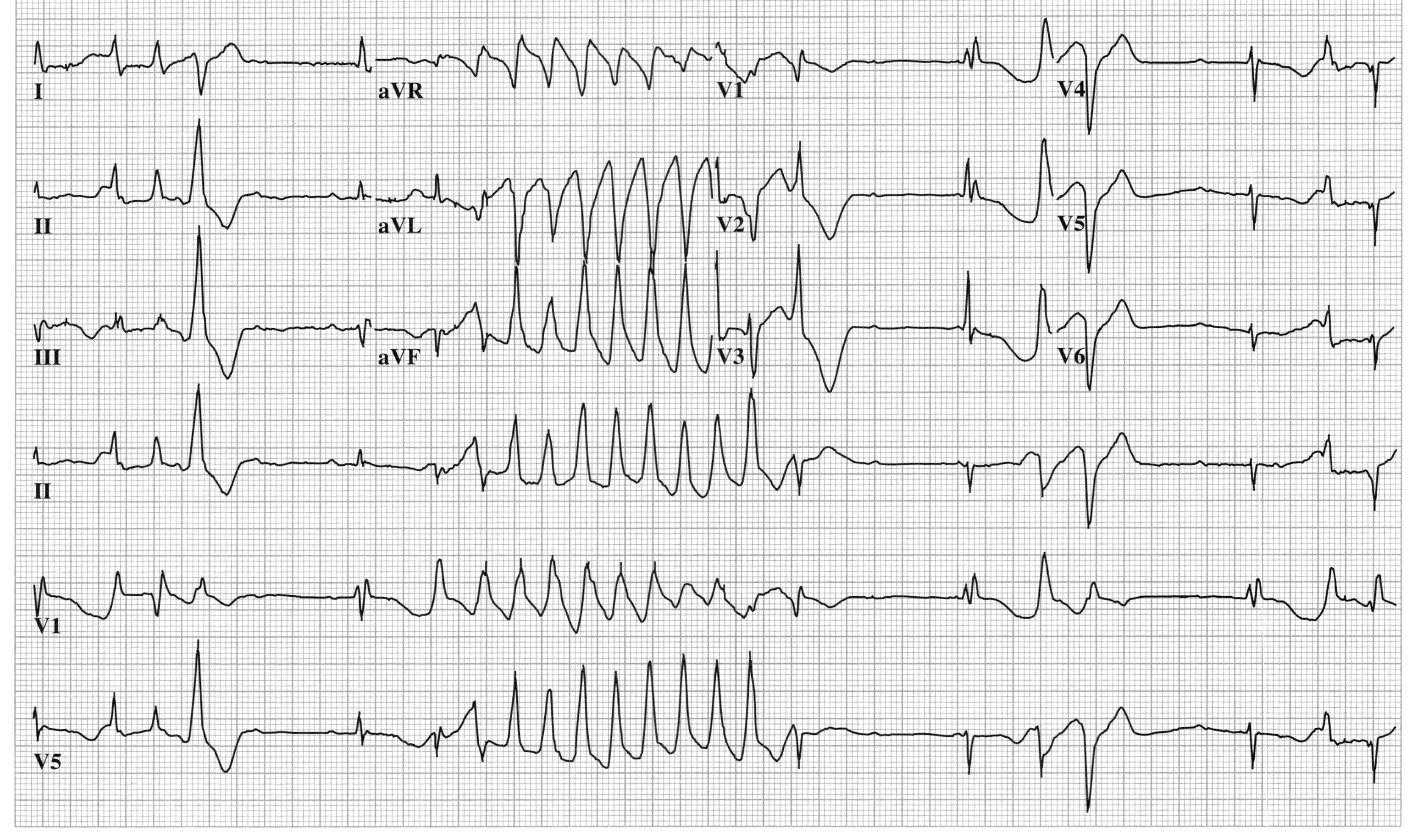

1. GENERAL FEATURES

- ☐ a. Normal ECG
- ☐ b. Borderline normal ECG or normal variant
- ☐ c. Incorrect electrode placement
- ☐ d. Artifact due to tremor

2. ATRIAL RHYTHMS

- ☐ a. Sinus rhythm
- ☐ b. Sinus arrhythmia
- ☐ c. Sinus bradycardia (< 60)
- ☐ d. Sinus tachycardia (> 100)
- ☐ e. Sinus pause or arrest
- ☐ f. Sinoatrial exit block
- ☐ g. Ecoptic atrial rhythm
- ☐ h. Wandering atrial pacemaker
- ☐ i. Atrial premature complexes, normally conducted
- ☐ j. Atrial premature complexes, nonconducted
- ☐ k. Atrial premature complexes with aberrant intraventricular conduction
- ☐ l. Atrial tachycardia (regular, sustained, 1:1 conduction)
- ☐ m. Atrial tachycardia, repetitive (short paroxysms)
- ☐ n. Atrial tachycardia, multifocal
- ☐ o. Atrial tachycardia with AV block
- ☐ p. Supraventricular tachycardia, unspecific
- ☐ q. Supraventricular tachycardia, paroxysmal
- ☐ r. Atrial flutter
- ☐ s. Atrial fibrillation
- ☐ t. Retrograde atrial activation

3. AV JUNCTIONAL RHYTHMS

- ☐ a. AV junctional premature complexes
- ☐ b. AV junctional escape complexes
- ☐ c. AV junctional rhythm, accelerated
- ☐ d. AV junctional rhythm

4. VENTRICULAR RHYTHMS

- ☐ a. Ventricular premature complex(es), uniform, fixed coupling
- ☐ b. Ventricular premature complex(es), uniform, nonfixed coupling
- ☐ c. Ventricular premature complexes(es), multiform
- ☐ d. Ventricular premature complexes, in pairs
- ☐ e. Ventricular parasystole
- ☐ f. Ventricular tachycardia (≥ 3 consecutive complexes)
- ☐ g. Accelerated idioventricular rhythm
- ☐ h. Ventricular escape complexes or rhythm
- ☐ i. Ventricular fibrillation

5. ATRIAL-VENTRICULAR INTERACTIONS IN ARRHYTHMIAS

- ☐ a. Fusion complexes
- ☐ b. Reciprocal (echo) complexes
- ☐ c. Ventricular capture complexes
- ☐ d. AV dissociation
- ☐ e. Ventriculophasic sinus arrhythmia

6. AV CONDUCTION ABNORMALITIES

- ☐ a. AV block, 1°
- ☐ b. AV block, 2° - Mobitz type I (Wenckebach)
- ☐ c. AV block, 2° - Mobitz type II
- ☐ d. AV block, 2:1
- ☐ e. AV block, 3°
- ☐ f. AV block, variable
- ☐ g. Short PR interval (with sinus rhythm and normal QRS duration)
- ☐ h. Wolff-Parkinson-White pattern

7. INTRAVENTRICULAR CONDUCTION DISTURBANCES

- ☐ a. RBBB, incomplete
- ☐ b. RBBB, complete
- ☐ c. Left anterior fascicular block
- ☐ d. Left posterior fascicular block
- ☐ e. LBBB, with ST-T wave suggestive of acute myocardial injury or infarction
- ☐ f. LBBB, complete
- ☐ g. LBBB, intermittent
- ☐ h. Intraventricular conduction disturbance, nonspecific
- ☐ i. Aberrant intraventricular conduction with supraventricular arrhythmia

8. P WAVE ABNORMALITIES

- ☐ a. Right atrial abnormality
- ☐ b. Left atrial abnormalities
- ☐ c. Nonspecific atrial abnormality

9. ABNORMALITIES OF QRS VOLTAGE OR AXIS

- ☐ a. Low voltage, limb leads only
- ☐ b. Low voltage, limb and precordial leads
- ☐ c. Left axis deviation (> - 30%)
- ☐ d. Right axis deviation (> + 100)
- ☐ e. Electrical alternans

10. VENTRICULAR HYPERTROPHY

- ☐ a. LVH by voltage only
- ☐ b. LVH by voltage and ST-T segment abnormalities
- ☐ c. RVH
- ☐ d. Combined ventricular hypertrophy

11. Q WAVE MYOCARDIAL INFARCTION

	Probably Acute or Recent	Probably Old or Age Indeterminate
Anterolateral	☐ a.	☐ g.
Anterior	☐ b.	☐ h.
Anteroseptal	☐ c.	☐ i.
Lateral/High lateral	☐ d.	☐ j.
Inferior	☐ e.	☐ k.
Posterior	☐ f.	☐ l.

- ☐ m. Probably ventricular aneurysm

12. ST, T, U, WAVE ABNORMALITIES

- ☐ a. Normal variant, early repolarization
- ☐ b. Normal variant, juvenile T waves
- ☐ c. Nonspecific ST and/or T wave abnormalities
- ☐ d. ST and/or T wave abnormalities suggesting myocardial ischemia
- ☐ e. ST and/or T wave abnormalities suggesting myocardial injury
- ☐ f. ST and/or T wave abnormalities suggesting acute pericarditis
- ☐ g. ST-T segment abnormalities secondary to intraventricular conduction disturbance or hypertrophy
- ☐ h. Post-extrasystolic T wave abnormality
- ☐ i. Isolated J point depression
- ☐ j. Peaked T waves
- ☐ k. Prolonged QT interval
- ☐ l. Prominent U waves

13. PACEMAKER FUNCTION AND RHYTHM

- ☐ a. Atrial or coronary sinus pacing
- ☐ b. Ventricular demand pacing
- ☐ c. AV sequential pacing
- ☐ d. Ventricular pacing, complete control
- ☐ e. Dual chamber, atrial sensing pacemaker
- ☐ f. Pacemaker malfunction, not constantly capturing (atrium or ventricle)
- ☐ g. Pacemaker malfunction, not constantly sensing (atrium or ventricle)
- ☐ h. Pacemaker malfunction, not firing
- ☐ i. Pacemaker malfunction, slowing

14. SUGGESTED OR PROBABLE CLINICAL DISORDERS

- ☐ a. Digitalis effect
- ☐ b. Digitalis toxicity
- ☐ c. Antiarrhythmic drug effect
- ☐ d. Antiarrhythmic drug toxicity
- ☐ e. Hyperkalemia
- ☐ f. Hypokalemia
- ☐ g. Hypercalcemia
- ☐ h. Hypocalcemia
- ☐ i. Atrial septal defect, secundum
- ☐ j. Atrial septal defect, primum
- ☐ k. Dextrocardia, mirror image
- ☐ l. Mitral valve disease
- ☐ m. Chronic lung disease
- ☐ n. Acute cor pulmonale, including pulmonary embolus
- ☐ o. Pericardial effusion
- ☐ p. Acute pericarditis
- ☐ q. Hypertrophic cardiomyopathy
- ☐ r. Coronary artery disease
- ☐ s. Central nervous system disorder
- ☐ t. Myxedema
- ☐ u. Hypothermia
- ☐ v. Sick sinus syndrome

ECG 21 was obtained in a 78-year-old female who is being treated for paroxysmal atrial fibrillation. The ECG shows a sinus rhythm at just under 100 beats/minute (arrows mark sinus P waves) with third-degree AV block and a run of nonsustained polymorphic ventricular tachycardia (asterisk). The run of VT is followed by a junctional escape (arrowhead) with RBBB morphology and a long QT interval. This constellation of findings is typical for Torsade de Pointes due to antiarrhythmic drug toxicity. This patient was receiving quinidine at the time of admission; within 24 hours of drug discontinuation, the QT interval shortened and the ventricular tachycardia resolved.

Codes:

2a	Sinus rhythm
3b	AV junctional escape complexes
4f	Ventricular tachycardia (≥ 3 consecutive complexes)
6e	AV block, 3°
7b	RBBB, complete
12k	Prolonged QT interval
14d	Antiarrhythmic drug toxicity

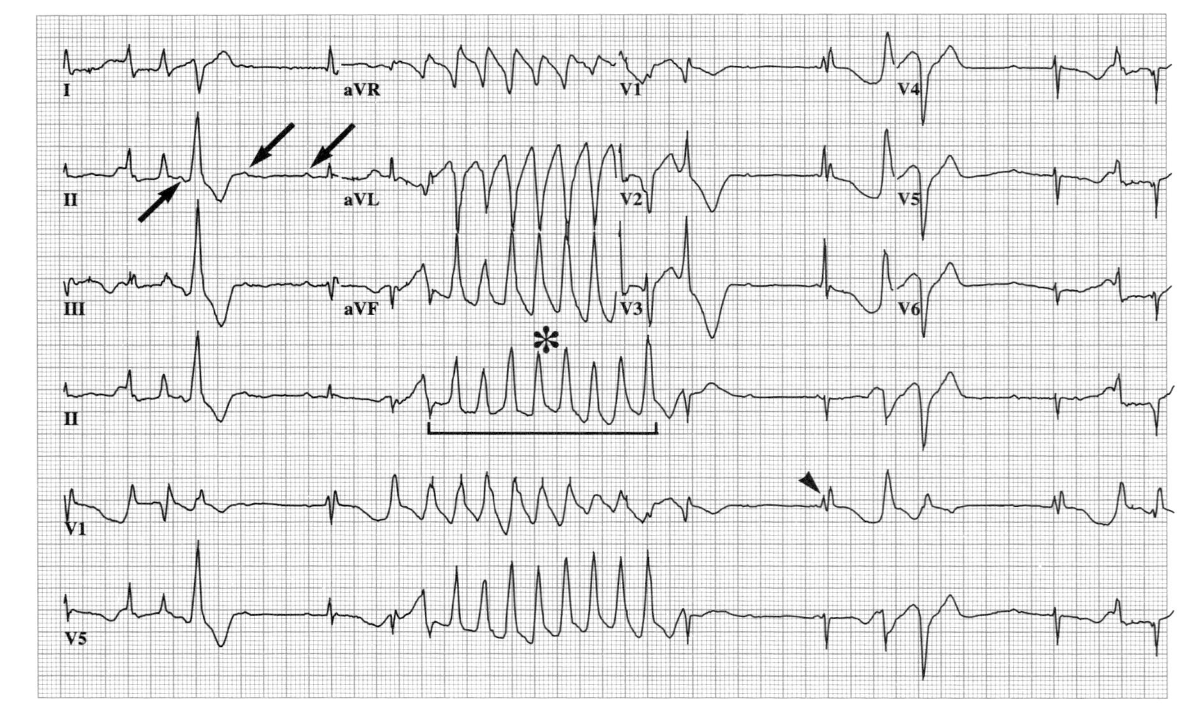

Questions: ECG 21

1. ECG features consistent with antiarrhythmic drug toxicity include:

   a. Polymorphic VT
   b. Long QT
   c. Narrowing of QRS
   d. SA or AV block

2. At a heart rate of 90, the normal QT interval should be ___ ± 0.07 seconds:

   a. 0.38
   b. 0.44
   c. 0.42
   d. 0.36

Answers: ECG 21

1. Antiarrhythmic drugs can have a variety of effects on the 12-lead ECG. The most serious effect, proarrhythmia, manifests as worsening ventricular ectopy, including frequent ventricular premature complexes, pairs, and/or polymorphic ventricular tachycardia (Torsade de Pointes). Other findings seen with antiarrhythmic drug therapy can include a prominent U wave; prolongation of the QT interval; widening, flattening, notching, or inversion of the T wave; prolongation of the PR interval; and SA or AV nodal block. Some antiarrhythmic drugs can cause QRS widening (especially when toxic levels are present). Narrowing of the QRS complex is not a feature of antiarrhythmic drug toxicity. (Answer: a, b, d)

2. Prolongation of the QT interval is a common finding in antiarrhythmic drug toxicity. The normal QT interval varies inversely with the heart rate. At a heart rate of 90, the QT interval should be 0.36 ± .07 seconds. The QT interval is prolonged in this tracing, and is most apparent in the beat prior to the initiation of the polymorphic ventricular tachycardia. (Answer: d)

— Quick Review 21 —

Ventricular tachycardia	
• Rapid succession of three or more premature ventricular beats at a rate > ____ per minute	100
• RR intervals are usually regular but may be irregular (true/false)	true
• (Abrupt/gradual) onset and termination are evident	Abrupt
• AV ____ is common	dissociation
• Look for ventricular ____ complexes and ____ beats as markers for VT	capture, fusion
AV block, 3°	
• Atrial and ventricular rhythms are ____ of each other	independent
• Atrial rate is (faster/slower) than the ventricular rate	faster
Prolonged QT interval	
• Corrected QT interval (QTc) ≥ ____ seconds, where QTc = QT interval divided by the square root of the preceding ____ interval	0.42-0.46 RR
• QT interval varies (directly/inversely) with heart rate	inversely
• The normal QT interval should be (less than/greater than) 50% of the RR interval	less than
Antiarrhythmic drug toxicity	
• Widening of the ____ complex and ____ interval	QRS, QT
• Various degrees of ____ block	AV

— ECG CROSSWORD PUZZLE —

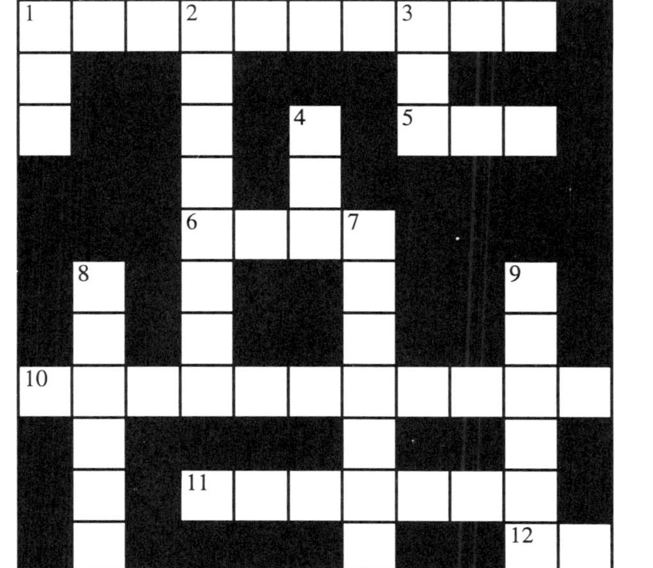

ACROSS

1. "Group beating" can result from this type of AV block
5. A type of AV sequential pacemaker
6. The type of complex that occurs when an impulse activates a chamber, returns to the site of origin, and reactivates the same chamber again
10. Associated with fusion beats and VPCs with nonfixed coupling
11. The type of complex that occurs when an atrial impulse stimulates the ventricle during VT
12. Multifocal atrial tachycardia is associated with varying PR, RP and _____ intervals

DOWN

1. Associated with atrial fibrillation or flutter with a QRS that varies in width (generally wide) and a ventricular response rate > 200 per minute
2. Hypo_____ results in a prolonged QT interval due to ST segment prolongation
3. Associated with an RSR' complex in V_1, left or right axis deviation, and a murmur
4. R wave in aVL > 12 mm
7. Can cause left axis deviation and low voltage
8. _____ T waves can be caused by hypekalemia, acute MI, intracranial bleeding
9. In the setting of a wide QRS tachycardia, the presence of an R' wave in V_1 that is _____ than the R wave is suggestive of SVT with aberrancy

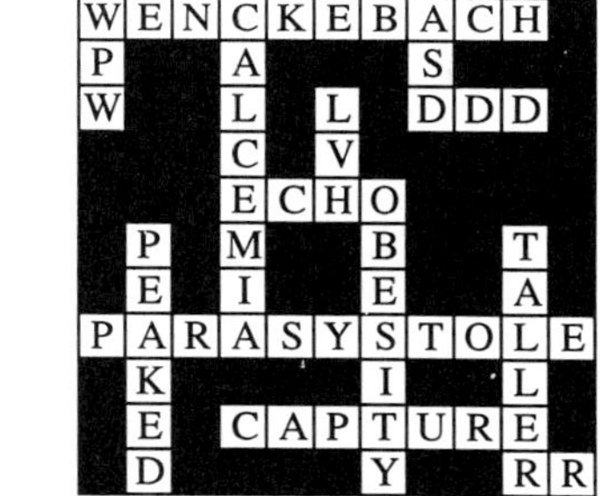

ECG 22. 49-year-old male with chest tightness and nausea:

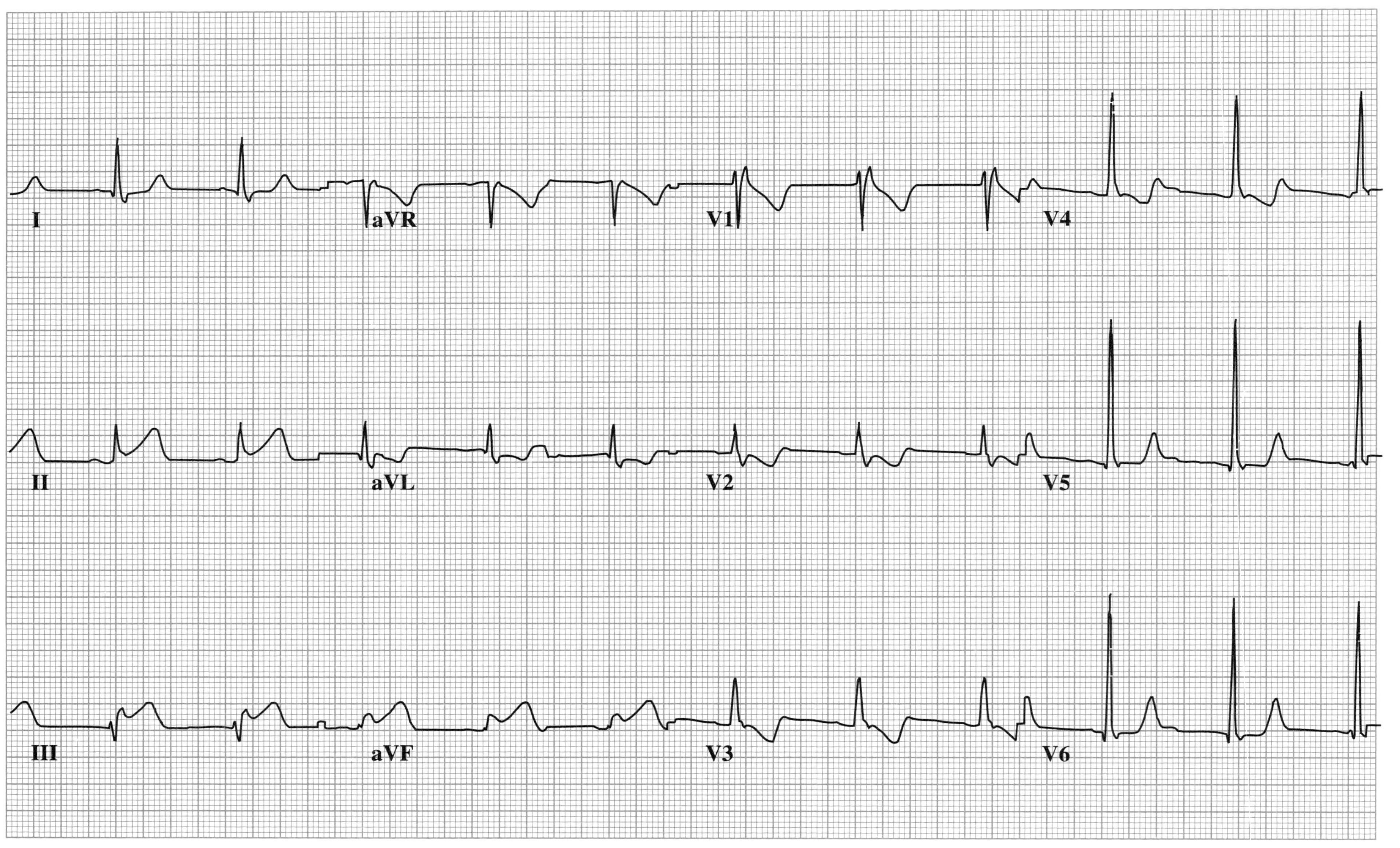

1. GENERAL FEATURES
- ☐ a. Normal ECG
- ☐ b. Borderline normal ECG or normal variant
- ☐ c. Incorrect electrode placement
- ☐ d. Artifact due to tremor

2. ATRIAL RHYTHMS
- ☐ a. Sinus rhythm
- ☐ b. Sinus arrhythmia
- ☐ c. Sinus bradycardia (< 60)
- ☐ d. Sinus tachycardia (> 100)
- ☐ e. Sinus pause or arrest
- ☐ f. Sinoatrial exit block
- ☐ g. Ecoptic atrial rhythm
- ☐ h. Wandering atrial pacemaker
- ☐ i. Atrial premature complexes, normally conducted
- ☐ j. Atrial premature complexes, nonconducted
- ☐ k. Atrial premature complexes with aberrant intraventricular conduction
- ☐ l. Atrial tachycardia (regular, sustained, 1:1 conduction)
- ☐ m. Atrial tachycardia, repetitive (short paroxysms)
- ☐ n. Atrial tachycardia, multifocal
- ☐ o. Atrial tachycardia with AV block
- ☐ p. Supraventricular tachycardia, unspecific
- ☐ q. Supraventricular tachycardia, paroxysmal
- ☐ r. Atrial flutter
- ☐ s. Atrial fibrillation
- ☐ t. Retrograde atrial activation

3. AV JUNCTIONAL RHYTHMS
- ☐ a. AV junctional premature complexes
- ☐ b. AV junctional escape complexes
- ☐ c. AV junctional rhythm, accelerated
- ☐ d. AV junctional rhythm

4. VENTRICULAR RHYTHMS
- ☐ a. Ventricular premature complex(es), uniform, fixed coupling
- ☐ b. Ventricular premature complex(es), uniform, nonfixed coupling
- ☐ c. Ventricular premature complexes(es), multiform
- ☐ d. Ventricular premature complexes, in pairs
- ☐ e. Ventricular parasystole
- ☐ f. Ventricular tachycardia (≥ 3 consecutive complexes)
- ☐ g. Accelerated idioventricular rhythm
- ☐ h. Ventricular escape complexes or rhythm
- ☐ i. Ventricular fibrillation

5. ATRIAL-VENTRICULAR INTERACTIONS IN ARRHYTHMIAS
- ☐ a. Fusion complexes
- ☐ b. Reciprocal (echo) complexes
- ☐ c. Ventricular capture complexes
- ☐ d. AV dissociation
- ☐ e. Ventriculophasic sinus arrhythmia

6. AV CONDUCTION ABNORMALITIES
- ☐ a. AV block, 1°
- ☐ b. AV block, 2° - Mobitz type I (Wenckebach)
- ☐ c. AV block, 2° - Mobitz type II
- ☐ d. AV block, 2:1
- ☐ e. AV block, 3°
- ☐ f. AV block, variable
- ☐ g. Short PR interval (with sinus rhythm and normal QRS duration)
- ☐ h. Wolff-Parkinson-White pattern

7. INTRAVENTRICULAR CONDUCTION DISTURBANCES
- ☐ a. RBBB, incomplete
- ☐ b. RBBB, complete
- ☐ c. Left anterior fascicular block
- ☐ d. Left posterior fascicular block
- ☐ e. LBBB, with ST-T wave suggestive of acute myocardial injury or infarction
- ☐ f. LBBB, complete
- ☐ g. LBBB, intermittent
- ☐ h. Intraventricular conduction disturbance, nonspecific
- ☐ i. Aberrant intraventricular conduction with supraventricular arrhythmia

8. P WAVE ABNORMALITIES
- ☐ a. Right atrial abnormality
- ☐ b. Left atrial abnormalities
- ☐ c. Nonspecific atrial abnormality

9. ABNORMALITIES OF QRS VOLTAGE OR AXIS
- ☐ a. Low voltage, limb leads only
- ☐ b. Low voltage, limb and precordial leads
- ☐ c. Left axis deviation (> - 30%)
- ☐ d. Right axis deviation (> + 100)
- ☐ e. Electrical alternans

10. VENTRICULAR HYPERTROPHY
- ☐ a. LVH by voltage only
- ☐ b. LVH by voltage and ST-T segment abnormalities
- ☐ c. RVH
- ☐ d. Combined ventricular hypertrophy

11. Q WAVE MYOCARDIAL INFARCTION

	Probably Acute or Recent	Probably Old or Age Indeterminate
Anterolateral	☐ a.	☐ g.
Anterior	☐ b.	☐ h.
Anteroseptal	☐ c.	☐ i.
Lateral/High lateral	☐ d.	☐ j.
Inferior	☐ e.	☐ k.
Posterior	☐ f.	☐ l.

- ☐ m. Probably ventricular aneurysm

12. ST, T, U, WAVE ABNORMALITIES
- ☐ a. Normal variant, early repolarization
- ☐ b. Normal variant, juvenile T waves
- ☐ c. Nonspecific ST and/or T wave abnormalities
- ☐ d. ST and/or T wave abnormalities suggesting myocardial ischemia
- ☐ e. ST and/or T wave abnormalities suggesting myocardial injury
- ☐ f. ST and/or T wave abnormalities suggesting acute pericarditis
- ☐ g. ST-T segment abnormalities secondary to intraventricular conduction disturbance or hypertrophy
- ☐ h. Post-extrasystolic T wave abnormality
- ☐ i. Isolated J point depression
- ☐ j. Peaked T waves
- ☐ k. Prolonged QT interval
- ☐ l. Prominent U waves

13. PACEMAKER FUNCTION AND RHYTHM
- ☐ a. Atrial or coronary sinus pacing
- ☐ b. Ventricular demand pacing
- ☐ c. AV sequential pacing
- ☐ d. Ventricular pacing, complete control
- ☐ e. Dual chamber, atrial sensing pacemaker
- ☐ f. Pacemaker malfunction, not constantly capturing (atrium or ventricle)
- ☐ g. Pacemaker malfunction, not constantly sensing (atrium or ventricle)
- ☐ h. Pacemaker malfunction, not firing
- ☐ i. Pacemaker malfunction, slowing

14. SUGGESTED OR PROBABLE CLINICAL DISORDERS
- ☐ a. Digitalis effect
- ☐ b. Digitalis toxicity
- ☐ c. Antiarrhythmic drug effect
- ☐ d. Antiarrhythmic drug toxicity
- ☐ e. Hyperkalemia
- ☐ f. Hypokalemia
- ☐ g. Hypercalcemia
- ☐ h. Hypocalcemia
- ☐ i. Atrial septal defect, secundum
- ☐ j. Atrial septal defect, primum
- ☐ k. Dextrocardia, mirror image
- ☐ l. Mitral valve disease
- ☐ m. Chronic lung disease
- ☐ n. Acute cor pulmonale, including pulmonary embolus
- ☐ o. Pericardial effusion
- ☐ p. Acute pericarditis
- ☐ q. Hypertrophic cardiomyopathy
- ☐ r. Coronary artery disease
- ☐ s. Central nervous system disorder
- ☐ t. Myxedema
- ☐ u. Hypothermia
- ☐ v. Sick sinus syndrome

ECG 22 was obtained in a 49-year-old male with chest tightness and nausea. The tracing shows a sinus rhythm at 66 beats/minute with RBBB and secondary ST-T changes (asterisk). A current of injury is present in leads II, III and aVF (arrowheads) without pathological Q waves (inferoposterior myocardial infarction may be present, but formal criteria are not yet met). LVH by voltage criteria (R wave in $V_6 > 20$ mm) and coronary artery disease should also be coded.

Codes:

2a	Sinus rhythm
7b	RBBB, complete
10a	Left ventricular hypertrophy by voltage only
12e	ST and/or T-wave abnormalities suggesting myocardial injury
12g	ST-T segment abnormalities secondary to IVCD or hypertrophy
14r	Coronary artery disease

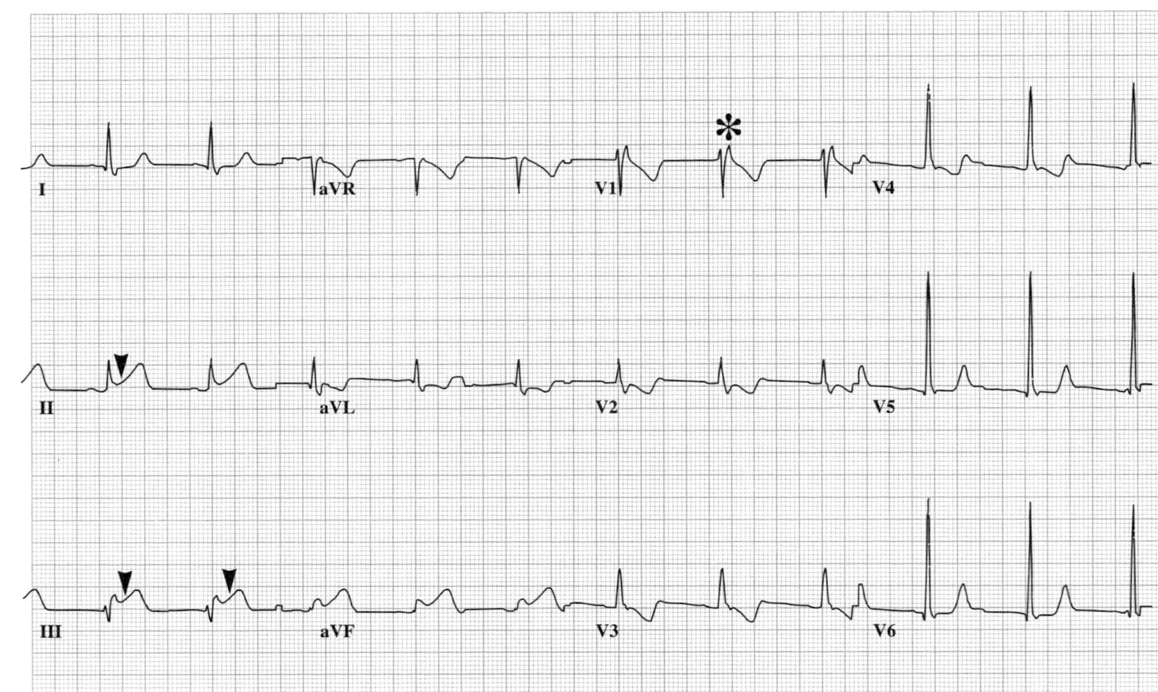

Questions: ECG 22

1. Causes of an RSR' complex in lead V_1 include right ventricular hypertrophy, posterior MI, Wolff-Parkinson-White syndrome, and right bundle branch block. Which of these diagnoses is most likely if the following additional ECG findings were present:

   a. Right axis deviation
   b. Inferior myocardial infarction
   c. Right atrial abnormality
   d. T wave inversion in V_1 - V_3
   e. Upright T wave in V_1 - V_3
   f. QRS duration > 0.12 seconds
   g. Short PR interval

2. The differential diagnosis of inferior ST elevation includes:

   a. Coronary artery spasm of the right coronary artery
   b. Acute inferior MI
   c. Early repolarization
   d. Pericarditis
   e. Ventricular aneurysm

Answers: ECG 22

1. Coexistent ECG findings can be used to discern the cause of an RSR' in lead V_1. RVH should be suspected in the presence of right axis deviation, right atrial abnormality, an R' in V_1 > 10 mm, and/or ST depression and T wave inversions in V_1-V_3; QRS duration may be normal or slightly prolonged, and the onset of intrinsicoid deflection may be delayed. Posterior MI is likely when inferior MI, upright T waves in the right precordial leads, and an initial R wave ≥ 0.04 seconds are present. Features favoring right bundle branch block include a QRS ≥ 0.12 seconds, T wave inversions in V_1V_2, and wide S waves in I, V_5, V_6. Finally, WPW should be suspected in the presence of a short PR, wide QRS, delta waves & secondary ST & T wave changes. [Answer: a (RVH); b (Posterior MI); c (RVH); d (RVH, RBBB); e (Posterior MI); f (RBBB, WPW); g (WPW)]

2. Inferior wall myocardial injury, ischemia, or aneurysm can present with ST segment elevation in leads II, III, and aVF. Early repolarization may be associated with elevated take-off of the ST segment at the terminal portion (J junction) of the QRS complex and upwardly concave ST segments, but more commonly involves the precordial leads (V_2-V_6). The degree of ST elevation in this syndrome may vary from one ECG to another, and may diminish or resolve with age. Other ECG features include tall upright T waves (in leads with tall R waves), and a notch in the descending limb of the R wave. Pericarditis

may be localized (e.g., post-CABG), but is more commonly associated with diffuse ST segment elevation. (Answer: All)

— Quick Review 22 —

RBBB, complete	
• QRS duration ≥ ____ seconds	0.12
• Secondary R wave (R') in lead ____ is usually (shorter/taller) than the initial R wave	V_1 taller
• Onset of intrinsicoid deflection in leads V_1 and V_2 > ____ seconds	0.05
• ST segment ____ and T wave ____ in V_1, V_2	depression inversion
• Wide slurred S wave in leads ____	I, V_5, V_6
• QRS axis is usually (normal/leftward/rightward)	normal
• RBBB (does/does not) interfere with the ECG diagnosis of ventricular hypertrophy or Q wave MI	does not
ST and/or T wave changes suggesting myocardial injury	
• Acute ST segment (elevation/depression) with upward (convexity/concavity) in the leads representing the area of infarction	elevation convexity
• T waves invert (before/after) ST segments return to baseline	before
• Associated ST (elevation/depression) in the noninfarct leads is common	depression
• Acute ____ wall injury often has horizontal or downsloping ST segment depression with upright T waves in V_1-V_3, with or without a prominent R wave in these same leads	posterior

— Quick Review 22 —

LVH by voltage only	
• **Cornell Criteria** (most accurate): R wave in aVL + S wave in V_3 > ____ mm in males or > ____ mm in females	24, 20
• **Other commonly used voltage-based criteria**	
▸ Precordial leads (one or more)	
(1) R wave in V_5 or V_6 + S wave in V_1	
▸ > ____ mm if age > 30 years	35
▸ > ____ mm if age 20-30 years	40
▸ > ____ mm if age 16-19 years	60
(2) Maximum R wave + S wave in precordial leads > ____ mm	45
(3) R wave in V_5 > ____ mm	26
(4) R wave in V_6 > ____ mm	20
▸ Limb leads (one or more)	
(1) R wave in lead I + S wave in lead II ≥ ____ mm	26
(2) R wave in lead I ≥ ____ mm	14
(3) S wave in aVR ≥ ____ mm	15
(4) R wave in aVL ≥ ____ mm	12
(5) R wave in aVF ≥ ____ mm	21

Don't Forget!

- Atrial flutter waves can deform QRS, ST and/or T to mimic intraventricular conduction delay and/or myocardial ischemia
- Think digoxin toxicity when regularization of the QRS is present during atrial fibrillation — this is usually due to complete heart block with junctional tachycardia
- Think Wolff-Parkinson-White (item 6h) in a patient with atrial fibrillation when the ventricular rate is >200 per minute and the QRS is > 0.12 seconds.
- Look for retrograde P waves after ventricular premature complexes and other junctional, ventricular, or low ectopic atrial rhythms
- In junctional premature complexes, the P wave may precede the QRS by ≤ 0.11 seconds (retrograde atrial activation, item 2t), be buried in the QRS (and not visualized), or follow the QRS complex
- Although multiform VPCs are usually multifocal in origin (i.e., originate from more than one ventricular focus), a single ventricular focus can produce VPCs of varying morphology

ECG 23. 31-year-old male with palpitations:

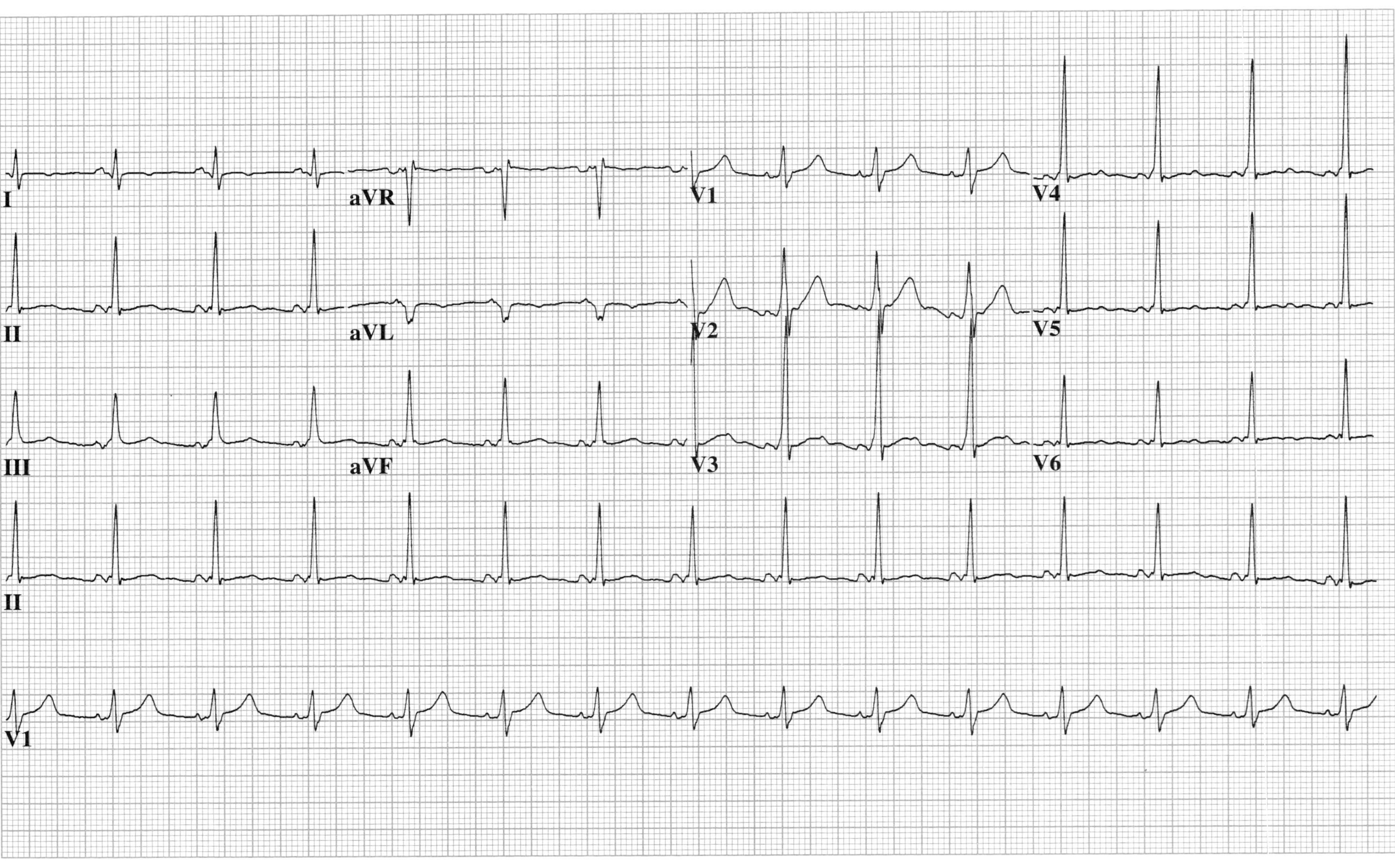

1. GENERAL FEATURES

- ☐ a. Normal ECG
- ☐ b. Borderline normal ECG or normal variant
- ☐ c. Incorrect electrode placement
- ☐ d. Artifact due to tremor

2. ATRIAL RHYTHMS

- ☐ a. Sinus rhythm
- ☐ b. Sinus arrhythmia
- ☐ c. Sinus bradycardia (< 60)
- ☐ d. Sinus tachycardia (> 100)
- ☐ e. Sinus pause or arrest
- ☐ f. Sinoatrial exit block
- ☐ g. Ecoptic atrial rhythm
- ☐ h. Wandering atrial pacemaker
- ☐ i. Atrial premature complexes, normally conducted
- ☐ j. Atrial premature complexes, nonconducted
- ☐ k. Atrial premature complexes with aberrant intraventricular conduction
- ☐ l. Atrial tachycardia (regular, sustained, 1:1 conduction)
- ☐ m. Atrial tachycardia, repetitive (short paroxysms)
- ☐ n. Atrial tachycardia, multifocal
- ☐ o. Atrial tachycardia with AV block
- ☐ p. Supraventricular tachycardia, unspecific
- ☐ q. Supraventricular tachycardia, paroxysmal
- ☐ r. Atrial flutter
- ☐ s. Atrial fibrillation
- ☐ t. Retrograde atrial activation

3. AV JUNCTIONAL RHYTHMS

- ☐ a. AV junctional premature complexes
- ☐ b. AV junctional escape complexes
- ☐ c. AV junctional rhythm, accelerated
- ☐ d. AV junctional rhythm

4. VENTRICULAR RHYTHMS

- ☐ a. Ventricular premature complex(es), uniform, fixed coupling
- ☐ b. Ventricular premature complex(es), uniform, nonfixed coupling
- ☐ c. Ventricular premature complexes(es), multiform
- ☐ d. Ventricular premature complexes, in pairs
- ☐ e. Ventricular parasystole
- ☐ f. Ventricular tachycardia (≥ 3 consecutive complexes)
- ☐ g. Accelerated idioventricular rhythm
- ☐ h. Ventricular escape complexes or rhythm
- ☐ i. Ventricular fibrillation

5. ATRIAL-VENTRICULAR INTERACTIONS IN ARRHYTHMIAS

- ☐ a. Fusion complexes
- ☐ b. Reciprocal (echo) complexes
- ☐ c. Ventricular capture complexes
- ☐ d. AV dissociation
- ☐ e. Ventriculophasic sinus arrhythmia

6. AV CONDUCTION ABNORMALITIES

- ☐ a. AV block, 1°
- ☐ b. AV block, 2° - Mobitz type I (Wenckebach)
- ☐ c. AV block, 2° - Mobitz type II
- ☐ d. AV block, 2:1
- ☐ e. AV block, 3°
- ☐ f. AV block, variable
- ☐ g. Short PR interval (with sinus rhythm and normal QRS duration)
- ☐ h. Wolff-Parkinson-White pattern

7. INTRAVENTRICULAR CONDUCTION DISTURBANCES

- ☐ a. RBBB, incomplete
- ☐ b. RBBB, complete
- ☐ c. Left anterior fascicular block
- ☐ d. Left posterior fascicular block
- ☐ e. LBBB, with ST-T wave suggestive of acute myocardial injury or infarction
- ☐ f. LBBB, complete
- ☐ g. LBBB, intermittent
- ☐ h. Intraventricular conduction disturbance, nonspecific
- ☐ i. Aberrant intraventricular conduction with supraventricular arrhythmia

8. P WAVE ABNORMALITIES

- ☐ a. Right atrial abnormality
- ☐ b. Left atrial abnormalities
- ☐ c. Nonspecific atrial abnormality

9. ABNORMALITIES OF QRS VOLTAGE OR AXIS

- ☐ a. Low voltage, limb leads only
- ☐ b. Low voltage, limb and precordial leads
- ☐ c. Left axis deviation (> - 30%)
- ☐ d. Right axis deviation (> + 100)
- ☐ e. Electrical alternans

10. VENTRICULAR HYPERTROPHY

- ☐ a. LVH by voltage only
- ☐ b. LVH by voltage and ST-T segment abnormalities
- ☐ c. RVH
- ☐ d. Combined ventricular hypertrophy

11. Q WAVE MYOCARDIAL INFARCTION

	Probably Acute or Recent	Probably Old or Age Indeterminate
Anterolateral	☐ a.	☐ g.
Anterior	☐ b.	☐ h.
Anteroseptal	☐ c.	☐ i.
Lateral/High lateral	☐ d.	☐ j.
Inferior	☐ e.	☐ k.
Posterior	☐ f.	☐ l.

- ☐ m. Probably ventricular aneurysm

12. ST, T, U, WAVE ABNORMALITIES

- ☐ a. Normal variant, early repolarization
- ☐ b. Normal variant, juvenile T waves
- ☐ c. Nonspecific ST and/or T wave abnormalities
- ☐ d. ST and/or T wave abnormalities suggesting myocardial ischemia
- ☐ e. ST and/or T wave abnormalities suggesting myocardial injury
- ☐ f. ST and/or T wave abnormalities suggesting acute pericarditis
- ☐ g. ST-T segment abnormalities secondary to intraventricular conduction disturbance or hypertrophy
- ☐ h. Post-extrasystolic T wave abnormality
- ☐ i. Isolated J point depression
- ☐ j. Peaked T waves
- ☐ k. Prolonged QT interval
- ☐ l. Prominent U waves

13. PACEMAKER FUNCTION AND RHYTHM

- ☐ a. Atrial or coronary sinus pacing
- ☐ b. Ventricular demand pacing
- ☐ c. AV sequential pacing
- ☐ d. Ventricular pacing, complete control
- ☐ e. Dual chamber, atrial sensing pacemaker
- ☐ f. Pacemaker malfunction, not constantly capturing (atrium or ventricle)
- ☐ g. Pacemaker malfunction, not constantly sensing (atrium or ventricle)
- ☐ h. Pacemaker malfunction, not firing
- ☐ i. Pacemaker malfunction, slowing

14. SUGGESTED OR PROBABLE CLINICAL DISORDERS

- ☐ a. Digitalis effect
- ☐ b. Digitalis toxicity
- ☐ c. Antiarrhythmic drug effect
- ☐ d. Antiarrhythmic drug toxicity
- ☐ e. Hyperkalemia
- ☐ f. Hypokalemia
- ☐ g. Hypercalcemia
- ☐ h. Hypocalcemia
- ☐ i. Atrial septal defect, secundum
- ☐ j. Atrial septal defect, primum
- ☐ k. Dextrocardia, mirror image
- ☐ l. Mitral valve disease
- ☐ m. Chronic lung disease
- ☐ n. Acute cor pulmonale, including pulmonary embolus
- ☐ o. Pericardial effusion
- ☐ p. Acute pericarditis
- ☐ q. Hypertrophic cardiomyopathy
- ☐ r. Coronary artery disease
- ☐ s. Central nervous system disorder
- ☐ t. Myxedema
- ☐ u. Hypothermia
- ☐ v. Sick sinus syndrome

ECG 23 was obtained in a 31-year-old male with palpitations. The tracing shows sinus rhythm with a short PR interval, delta waves (arrows), and a prolonged QRS (> 0.10 seconds), consistent with Wolff-Parkinson-White pattern. Fusion complexes and ST-T abnormalities secondary to IVCD should be coded as well.

Codes:

2a	Sinus rhythm
5a	Fusion complexes
6h	Wolff-Parkinson-White pattern
12g	ST-T segment abnormalities secondary to IVCD or hypertrophy

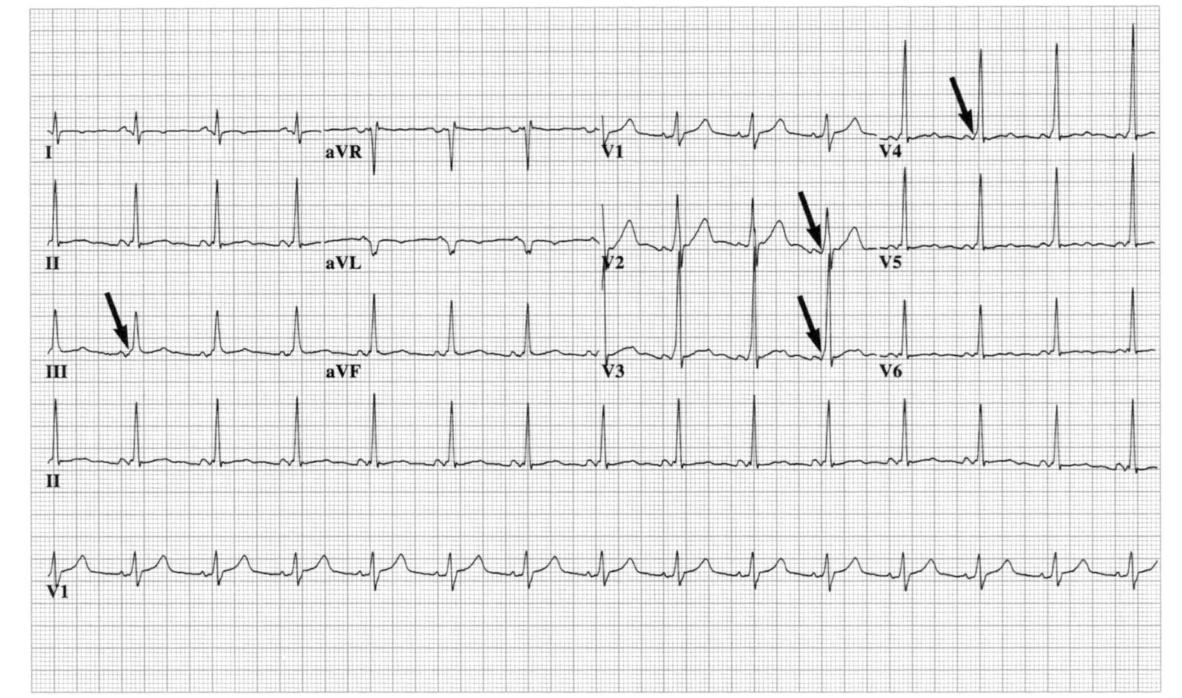

Questions: ECG 23

1. Fusion complexes can be seen with any of the following except:

   a. Wolff-Parkinson-White syndrome
   b. Atrial premature complexes
   c. Paced beats
   d. Ventricular tachycardia

2. Supraventricular tachycardia is needed to make the diagnosis of Wolff-Parkinson-White pattern:

   a. True
   b. False

Answers: ECG 23

1. Fusion complexes can be seen with Wolff-Parkinson-White, paced beats, ventricular tachycardia, or isolated VPCs. Atrial premature complexes do not result in fusion complexes. (Answer: b)

2. Wolff-Parkinson-White ***pattern*** differs from Wolff-Parkinson-White ***syndrome***: the former requires delta waves and a short PR interval; the latter requires delta waves, a short PR, *and* a history of supraventricular tachycardia or atrial fibrillation. (Answer: b)

— Quick Review 23 —	
Fusion complexes	
• Due to simultaneous activation of the ventricle from ____ sources, resulting in a QRS complex that is ____ in morphology between each source	2 intermediate
Wolff-Parkinson-White pattern	
• (Sinus/nonsinus) P wave	sinus
• PR interval < ____ seconds	0.12
• Initial slurring of QRS (____ wave) resulting in QRS duration > ____ seconds	delta 0.10
• Secondary ST-T wave changes occur (true/false)	true
• PJ interval (beginning of P wave to end of QRS) (is constant/varies)	is constant

ECG 24. 63-year-old female with sudden onset of rapid heart beating:

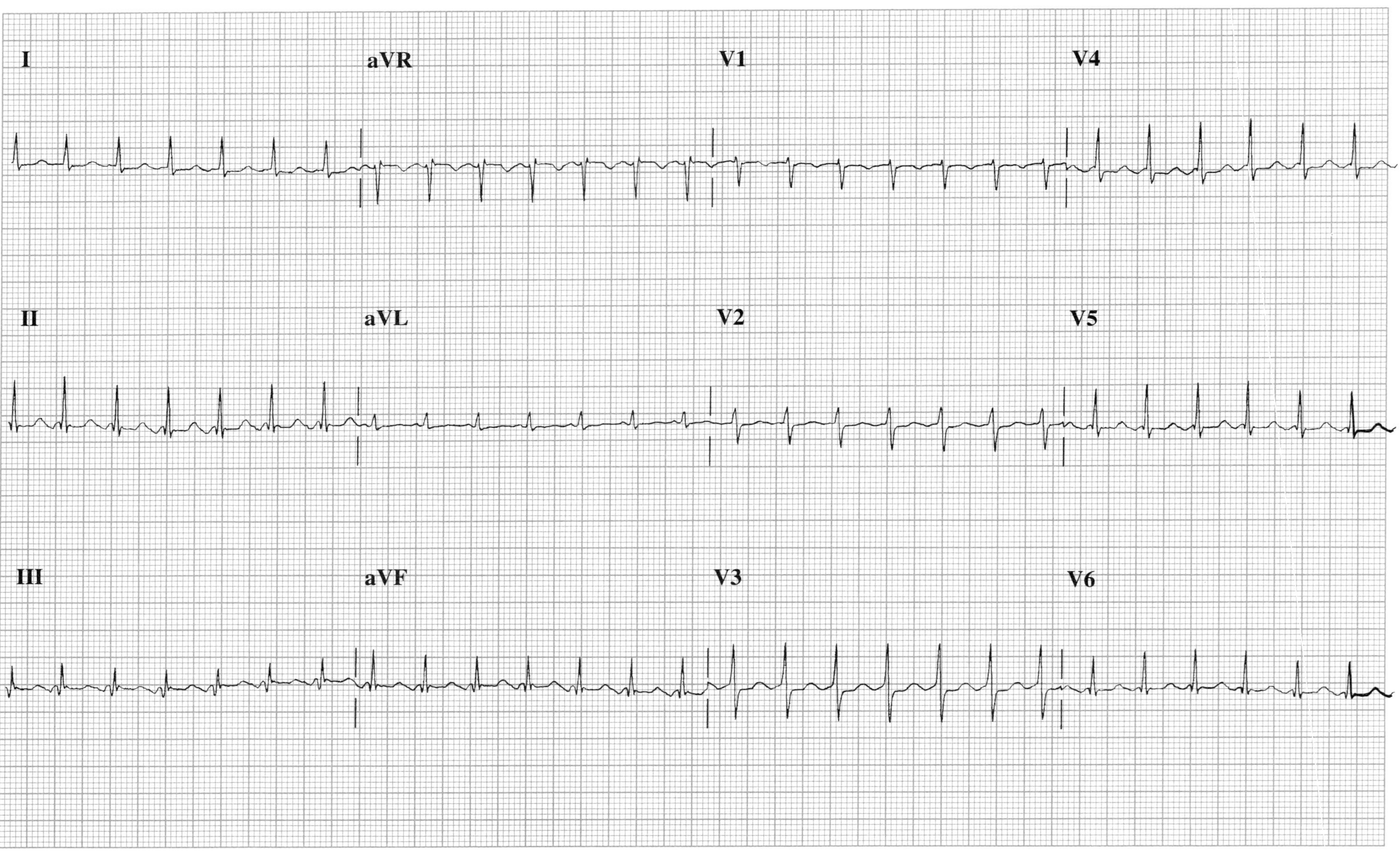

1. GENERAL FEATURES
☐ a. Normal ECG
☐ b. Borderline normal ECG or normal variant
☐ c. Incorrect electrode placement
☐ d. Artifact due to tremor

2. ATRIAL RHYTHMS
☐ a. Sinus rhythm
☐ b. Sinus arrhythmia
☐ c. Sinus bradycardia (< 60)
☐ d. Sinus tachycardia (> 100)
☐ e. Sinus pause or arrest
☐ f. Sinoatrial exit block
☐ g. Ecoptic atrial rhythm
☐ h. Wandering atrial pacemaker
☐ i. Atrial premature complexes, normally conducted
☐ j. Atrial premature complexes, nonconducted
☐ k. Atrial premature complexes with aberrant intraventricular conduction
☐ l. Atrial tachycardia (regular, sustained, 1:1 conduction)
☐ m. Atrial tachycardia, repetitive (short paroxysms)
☐ n. Atrial tachycardia, multifocal
☐ o. Atrial tachycardia with AV block
☐ p. Supraventricular tachycardia, unspecific
☐ q. Supraventricular tachycardia, paroxysmal
☐ r. Atrial flutter
☐ s. Atrial fibrillation
☐ t. Retrograde atrial activation

3. AV JUNCTIONAL RHYTHMS
☐ a. AV junctional premature complexes
☐ b. AV junctional escape complexes
☐ c. AV junctional rhythm, accelerated
☐ d. AV junctional rhythm

4. VENTRICULAR RHYTHMS
☐ a. Ventricular premature complex(es), uniform, fixed coupling
☐ b. Ventricular premature complex(es), uniform, nonfixed coupling
☐ c. Ventricular premature complexes(es), multiform
☐ d. Ventricular premature complexes, in pairs
☐ e. Ventricular parasystole
☐ f. Ventricular tachycardia (≥ 3 consecutive complexes)
☐ g. Accelerated idioventricular rhythm
☐ h. Ventricular escape complexes or rhythm
☐ i. Ventricular fibrillation

5. ATRIAL-VENTRICULAR INTERACTIONS IN ARRHYTHMIAS
☐ a. Fusion complexes
☐ b. Reciprocal (echo) complexes
☐ c. Ventricular capture complexes
☐ d. AV dissociation
☐ e. Ventriculophasic sinus arrhythmia

6. AV CONDUCTION ABNORMALITIES
☐ a. AV block, 1°
☐ b. AV block, 2° - Mobitz type I (Wenckebach)
☐ c. AV block, 2° - Mobitz type II
☐ d. AV block, 2:1
☐ e. AV block, 3°
☐ f. AV block, variable
☐ g. Short PR interval (with sinus rhythm and normal QRS duration)
☐ h. Wolff-Parkinson-White pattern

7. INTRAVENTRICULAR CONDUCTION DISTURBANCES
☐ a. RBBB, incomplete
☐ b. RBBB, complete
☐ c. Left anterior fascicular block
☐ d. Left posterior fascicular block
☐ e. LBBB, with ST-T wave suggestive of acute myocardial injury or infarction
☐ f. LBBB, complete
☐ g. LBBB, intermittent
☐ h. Intraventricular conduction disturbance, nonspecific
☐ i. Aberrant intraventricular conduction with supraventricular arrhythmia

8. P WAVE ABNORMALITIES
☐ a. Right atrial abnormality
☐ b. Left atrial abnormalities
☐ c. Nonspecific atrial abnormality

9. ABNORMALITIES OF QRS VOLTAGE OR AXIS
☐ a. Low voltage, limb leads only
☐ b. Low voltage, limb and precordial leads
☐ c. Left axis deviation (> - 30%)
☐ d. Right axis deviation (> + 100)
☐ e. Electrical alternans

10. VENTRICULAR HYPERTROPHY
☐ a. LVH by voltage only
☐ b. LVH by voltage and ST-T segment abnormalities
☐ c. RVH
☐ d. Combined ventricular hypertrophy

11. Q WAVE MYOCARDIAL INFARCTION

	Probably Acute or Recent	Probably Old or Age Indeterminate
Anterolateral	☐ a.	☐ g.
Anterior	☐ b.	☐ h.
Anteroseptal	☐ c.	☐ i.
Lateral/High lateral	☐ d.	☐ j.
Inferior	☐ e.	☐ k.
Posterior	☐ f.	☐ l.

☐ m. Probably ventricular aneurysm

12. ST, T, U, WAVE ABNORMALITIES
☐ a. Normal variant, early repolarization
☐ b. Normal variant, juvenile T waves
☐ c. Nonspecific ST and/or T wave abnormalities
☐ d. ST and/or T wave abnormalities suggesting myocardial ischemia
☐ e. ST and/or T wave abnormalities suggesting myocardial injury
☐ f. ST and/or T wave abnormalities suggesting acute pericarditis
☐ g. ST-T segment abnormalities secondary to intraventricular conduction disturbance or hypertrophy
☐ h. Post-extrasystolic T wave abnormality
☐ i. Isolated J point depression
☐ j. Peaked T waves
☐ k. Prolonged QT interval
☐ l. Prominent U waves

13. PACEMAKER FUNCTION AND RHYTHM
☐ a. Atrial or coronary sinus pacing
☐ b. Ventricular demand pacing
☐ c. AV sequential pacing
☐ d. Ventricular pacing, complete control
☐ e. Dual chamber, atrial sensing pacemaker
☐ f. Pacemaker malfunction, not constantly capturing (atrium or ventricle)
☐ g. Pacemaker malfunction, not constantly sensing (atrium or ventricle)
☐ h. Pacemaker malfunction, not firing
☐ i. Pacemaker malfunction, slowing

14. SUGGESTED OR PROBABLE CLINICAL DISORDERS
☐ a. Digitalis effect
☐ b. Digitalis toxicity
☐ c. Antiarrhythmic drug effect
☐ d. Antiarrhythmic drug toxicity
☐ e. Hyperkalemia
☐ f. Hypokalemia
☐ g. Hypercalcemia
☐ h. Hypocalcemia
☐ i. Atrial septal defect, secundum
☐ j. Atrial septal defect, primum
☐ k. Dextrocardia, mirror image
☐ l. Mitral valve disease
☐ m. Chronic lung disease
☐ n. Acute cor pulmonale, including pulmonary embolus
☐ o. Pericardial effusion
☐ p. Acute pericarditis
☐ q. Hypertrophic cardiomyopathy
☐ r. Coronary artery disease
☐ s. Central nervous system disorder
☐ t. Myxedema
☐ u. Hypothermia
☐ v. Sick sinus syndrome

ECG 24 was obtained in a 63-year-old female complaining of sudden onset of rapid heart beating. This tracing shows a narrow complex tachycardia at 162 beats/minute. This rhythm is most appropriately coded as a supraventricular tachycardia, unspecified. Minor nonspecific repolarization abnormalities are present.

Codes:

2p	Supraventricular tachycardia, unspecified
12c	Nonspecific ST and/or T wave abnormalities

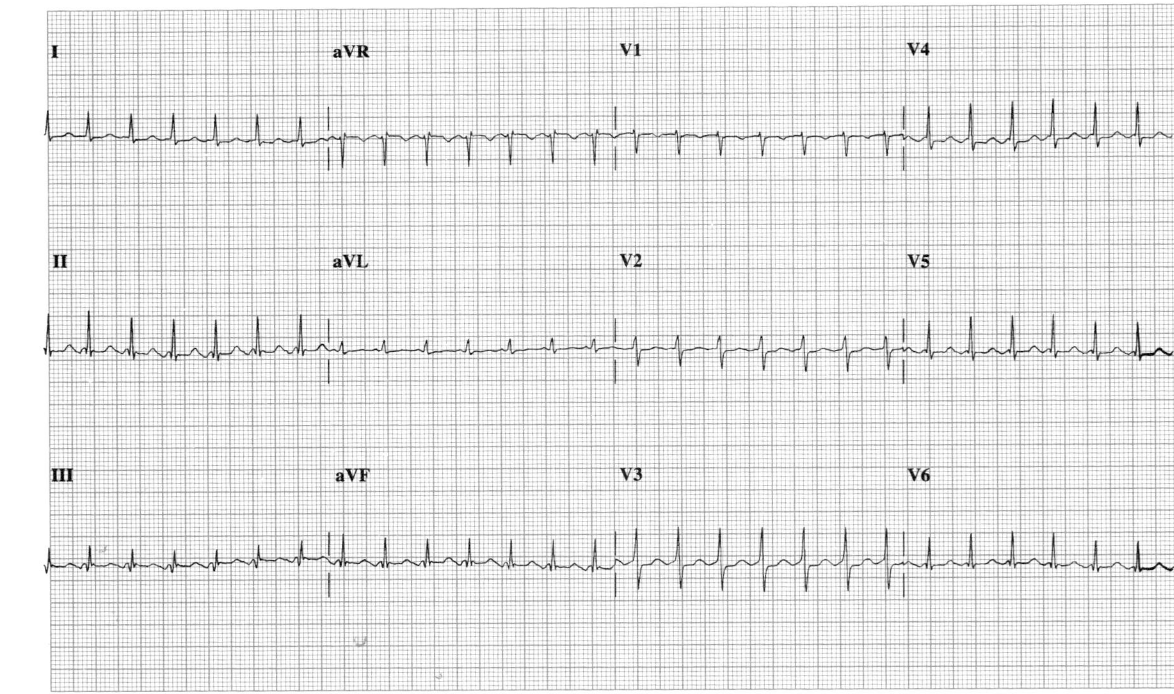

Questions: ECG 24

1. This ECG is consistent with each of the following arrhythmias except:

   a. Atrial flutter with 2:1 AV block
   b. Sinus tachycardia
   c. Atrial fibrillation
   d. Junctional tachycardia
   e. Multifocal atrial tachycardia
   f. Sinus node reentrant tachycardia
   g. Intra-atrial reentrant tachycardia
   h. Automatic atrial tachycardia
   i. AV nodal reentrant tachycardia
   j AV reentrant tachycardia (orthodromic)
   k. AV reentrant tachycardia (antidromic)

2. Match the clinical situations below to the arrhythmia(s) in question 1 (list all that apply):

   a. Digitalis toxicity
   b. Healthy female without structural heart disease (most likely diagnosis only)
   c. Abrupt onset of arrhythmia initiated by atrial premature contraction
   d. Warmup period during initiation of tachycardia
   e. Carotid sinus massage has no effect
   f. Carotid sinus massage results in gradual slowing then return to normal rate
   g. Carotid sinus massage terminates the arrhythmia
   h. A short RP interval (< 0.09 sec) is present

Answers: ECG 24

1. The ability to distinguish between mechanisms of supraventricular tachycardia (SVT) based solely on the ECG is often very difficult. Sometimes the mechanism can be inferred from the RP interval, presence of a warm-up period, initiation by premature atrial contraction, and the response to carotid sinus massage; however, the definitive mechanism is best elucidated by electrophysiological testing. The present ECG is consistent with the diagnosis of atrial flutter with 2:1 block, sinus tachycardia, junctional tachycardia, sinus node reentry tachycardia, intra-atrial reentry tachycardia, automatic atrial tachycardia, AV nodal reentry tachycardia, and orthodromic AV reentry tachycardia. The regular RR interval makes the diagnosis of atrial fibrillation highly unlikely, although fine atrial fibrillation with complete heart block and junctional tachycardia secondary to digitalis toxicity cannot be definitively excluded. The present ECG is also inconsistent with multifocal atrial tachycardia, which manifests as an irregular rhythm with ≥ 3

distinct P wave morphologies and varying T-P, P-R, and R-R intervals. Finally, antidromic AV reentrant tachycardia is excluded as a possible diagnosis, since antegrade conduction down the accessory pathway (and retrograde conduction via the AV node) presents as a wide QRS complex tachycardia. (Answer: c, e, k)

2. Answer:
   a: d, h (with block)
   b: i
   c: f, g, i, j
   d: d, h, b
   e: d
   f: b
   g: f, i, j, k
   h: i, j

— Quick Review 24 —

SVT, unspecified	
• (Regular/irregular) rhythm	Regular
• Rate > ____ per minute	100
• P waves (easily/not easily) identified	not easily
• QRS complex is usually (narrow/wide)	narrow
• If rate is 150 per minute, consider ____	atrial flutter with 2:1 block
Nonspecific ST and/or T wave abnormalities	
• Slight ____ segment depression or elevation	ST
• Slightly inverted or flat ____ wave	T

— POP QUIZ —

Find The Mistake

__Instructions__: Identify the incorrect ECG feature(s) for each of the ECG diagnoses listed below

ECG Features	Answer
Ventriculophasic sinus arrhythmia • PP interval containing a QRS complex is less than the PP interval without a QRS complex • Seen with 3° but not 2° heart block	Can be seen in the setting of 2° or 3° heart block
2° AV block, Mobitz Type I (Wenkebach) • Progressive prolongation of the PR and RR intervals until a P wave is blocked • RR interval containing the nonconducted P wave is less than the sum of two PP intervals • Results in group beating due to the presence of nonconducted P waves	Progressive shortening (not prolongation) of the RR interval occurs until a P wave is blocked
2° AV block, Mobitz Type II • Regular sinus or atrial rhythm with intermittent nonconducted P waves without evidence for atrial prematurity • PR interval in the conducted beats is constant • RR interval containing the nonconducted P wave is less than or equal to the sum of two PP intervals	RR interval with nonconducted P wave is equal to (not $\leq$) two PP intervals
Wolff-Parkinson-White pattern • Non-sinus P wave • PR interval < 0.12 seconds • Initial slurring of QRS (delta wave) resulting in QRS duration > 0.10 seconds • Secondary ST-T wave changes • PJ interval (beginning of P wave to end of QRS) varies	Sinus P wave is present; PJ interval is constant (not variable)

ECG 25. Asymptomatic 19-year-old male athlete:

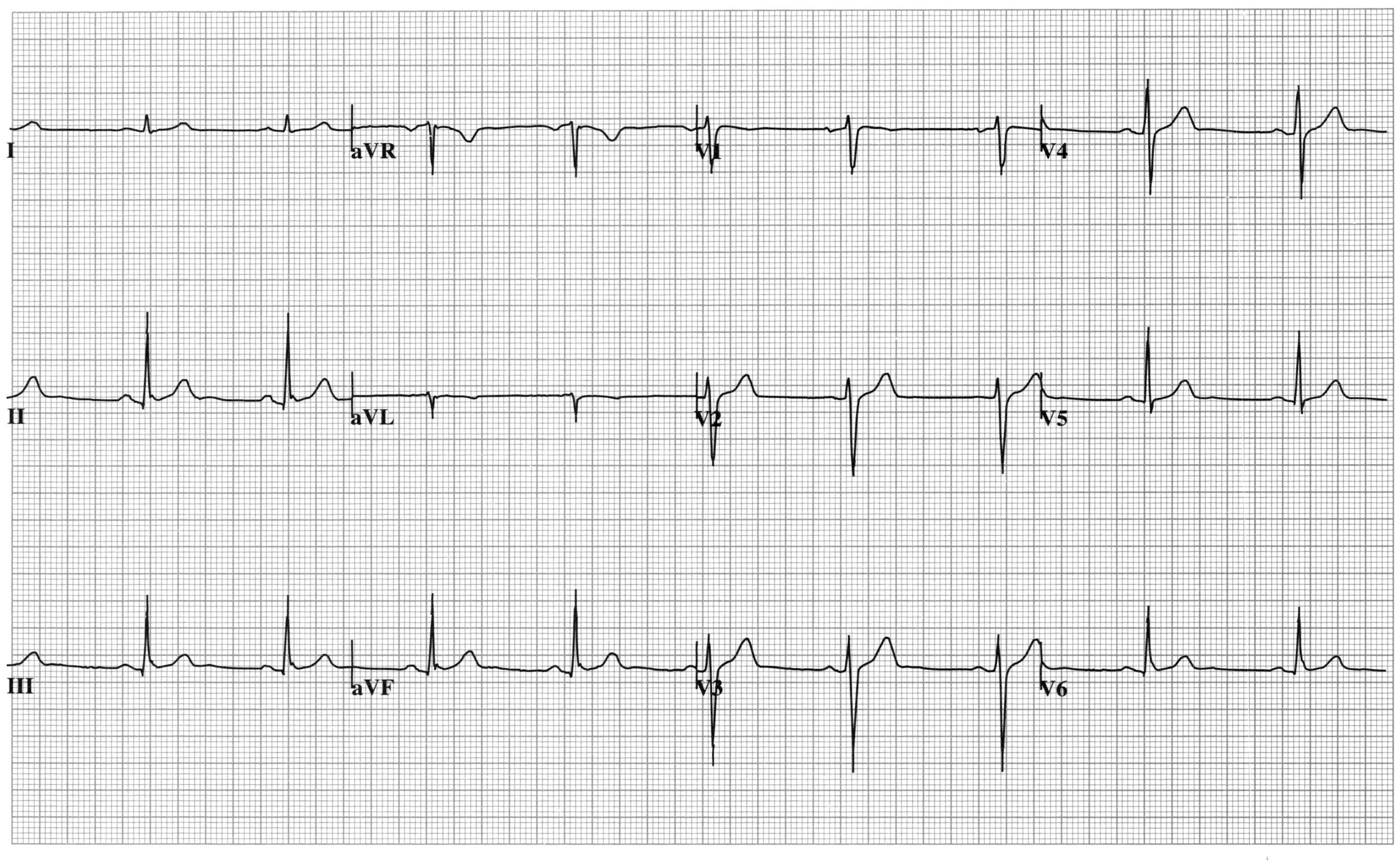

1. GENERAL FEATURES

- ☐ a. Normal ECG
- ☐ b. Borderline normal ECG or normal variant
- ☐ c. Incorrect electrode placement
- ☐ d. Artifact due to tremor

2. ATRIAL RHYTHMS

- ☐ a. Sinus rhythm
- ☐ b. Sinus arrhythmia
- ☐ c. Sinus bradycardia (< 60)
- ☐ d. Sinus tachycardia (> 100)
- ☐ e. Sinus pause or arrest
- ☐ f. Sinoatrial exit block
- ☐ g. Ecoptic atrial rhythm
- ☐ h. Wandering atrial pacemaker
- ☐ i. Atrial premature complexes, normally conducted
- ☐ j. Atrial premature complexes, nonconducted
- ☐ k. Atrial premature complexes with aberrant intraventricular conduction
- ☐ l. Atrial tachycardia (regular, sustained, 1:1 conduction)
- ☐ m. Atrial tachycardia, repetitive (short paroxysms)
- ☐ n. Atrial tachycardia, multifocal
- ☐ o. Atrial tachycardia with AV block
- ☐ p. Supraventricular tachycardia, unspecific
- ☐ q. Supraventricular tachycardia, paroxysmal
- ☐ r. Atrial flutter
- ☐ s. Atrial fibrillation
- ☐ t. Retrograde atrial activation

3. AV JUNCTIONAL RHYTHMS

- ☐ a. AV junctional premature complexes
- ☐ b. AV junctional escape complexes
- ☐ c. AV junctional rhythm, accelerated
- ☐ d. AV junctional rhythm

4. VENTRICULAR RHYTHMS

- ☐ a. Ventricular premature complex(es), uniform, fixed coupling
- ☐ b. Ventricular premature complex(es), uniform, nonfixed coupling
- ☐ c. Ventricular premature complexes(es), multiform
- ☐ d. Ventricular premature complexes, in pairs
- ☐ e. Ventricular parasystole
- ☐ f. Ventricular tachycardia (≥ 3 consecutive complexes)
- ☐ g. Accelerated idioventricular rhythm
- ☐ h. Ventricular escape complexes or rhythm
- ☐ i. Ventricular fibrillation

5. ATRIAL-VENTRICULAR INTERACTIONS IN ARRHYTHMIAS

- ☐ a. Fusion complexes
- ☐ b. Reciprocal (echo) complexes
- ☐ c. Ventricular capture complexes
- ☐ d. AV dissociation
- ☐ e. Ventriculophasic sinus arrhythmia

6. AV CONDUCTION ABNORMALITIES

- ☐ a. AV block, 1°
- ☐ b. AV block, 2° - Mobitz type I (Wenckebach)
- ☐ c. AV block, 2° - Mobitz type II
- ☐ d. AV block, 2:1
- ☐ e. AV block, 3°
- ☐ f. AV block, variable
- ☐ g. Short PR interval (with sinus rhythm and normal QRS duration)
- ☐ h. Wolff-Parkinson-White pattern

7. INTRAVENTRICULAR CONDUCTION DISTURBANCES

- ☐ a. RBBB, incomplete
- ☐ b. RBBB, complete
- ☐ c. Left anterior fascicular block
- ☐ d. Left posterior fascicular block
- ☐ e. LBBB, with ST-T wave suggestive of acute myocardial injury or infarction
- ☐ f. LBBB, complete
- ☐ g. LBBB, intermittent
- ☐ h. Intraventricular conduction disturbance, nonspecific
- ☐ i. Aberrant intraventricular conduction with supraventricular arrhythmia

8. P WAVE ABNORMALITIES

- ☐ a. Right atrial abnormality
- ☐ b. Left atrial abnormalities
- ☐ c. Nonspecific atrial abnormality

9. ABNORMALITIES OF QRS VOLTAGE OR AXIS

- ☐ a. Low voltage, limb leads only
- ☐ b. Low voltage, limb and precordial leads
- ☐ c. Left axis deviation (> - 30%)
- ☐ d. Right axis deviation (> + 100)
- ☐ e. Electrical alternans

10. VENTRICULAR HYPERTROPHY

- ☐ a. LVH by voltage only
- ☐ b. LVH by voltage and ST-T segment abnormalities
- ☐ c. RVH
- ☐ d. Combined ventricular hypertrophy

11. Q WAVE MYOCARDIAL INFARCTION

	Probably Acute or Recent	Probably Old or Age Indeterminate
Anterolateral	☐ a.	☐ g.
Anterior	☐ b.	☐ h.
Anteroseptal	☐ c.	☐ i.
Lateral/High lateral	☐ d.	☐ j.
Inferior	☐ e.	☐ k.
Posterior	☐ f.	☐ l.

☐ m. Probably ventricular aneurysm

12. ST, T, U, WAVE ABNORMALITIES

- ☐ a. Normal variant, early repolarization
- ☐ b. Normal variant, juvenile T waves
- ☐ c. Nonspecific ST and/or T wave abnormalities
- ☐ d. ST and/or T wave abnormalities suggesting myocardial ischemia
- ☐ e. ST and/or T wave abnormalities suggesting myocardial injury
- ☐ f. ST and/or T wave abnormalities suggesting acute pericarditis
- ☐ g. ST-T segment abnormalities secondary to intraventricular conduction disturbance or hypertrophy
- ☐ h. Post-extrasystolic T wave abnormality
- ☐ i. Isolated J point depression
- ☐ j. Peaked T waves
- ☐ k. Prolonged QT interval
- ☐ l. Prominent U waves

13. PACEMAKER FUNCTION AND RHYTHM

- ☐ a. Atrial or coronary sinus pacing
- ☐ b. Ventricular demand pacing
- ☐ c. AV sequential pacing
- ☐ d. Ventricular pacing, complete control
- ☐ e. Dual chamber, atrial sensing pacemaker
- ☐ f. Pacemaker malfunction, not constantly capturing (atrium or ventricle)
- ☐ g. Pacemaker malfunction, not constantly sensing (atrium or ventricle)
- ☐ h. Pacemaker malfunction, not firing
- ☐ i. Pacemaker malfunction, slowing

14. SUGGESTED OR PROBABLE CLINICAL DISORDERS

- ☐ a. Digitalis effect
- ☐ b. Digitalis toxicity
- ☐ c. Antiarrhythmic drug effect
- ☐ d. Antiarrhythmic drug toxicity
- ☐ e. Hyperkalemia
- ☐ f. Hypokalemia
- ☐ g. Hypercalcemia
- ☐ h. Hypocalcemia
- ☐ i. Atrial septal defect, secundum
- ☐ j. Atrial septal defect, primum
- ☐ k. Dextrocardia, mirror image
- ☐ l. Mitral valve disease
- ☐ m. Chronic lung disease
- ☐ n. Acute cor pulmonale, including pulmonary embolus
- ☐ o. Pericardial effusion
- ☐ p. Acute pericarditis
- ☐ q. Hypertrophic cardiomyopathy
- ☐ r. Coronary artery disease
- ☐ s. Central nervous system disorder
- ☐ t. Myxedema
- ☐ u. Hypothermia
- ☐ v. Sick sinus syndrome

ECG 25 was obtained in an asymptomatic 19-year-old male athlete. The tracing shows sinus bradycardia with notching of the J point (arrows) and subtle ST segment elevation in the inferior and lateral precordial leads. These findings are compatible with a borderline normal ECG or normal variant. Although subtle fluctuations in the RR intervals are present, this does not meet criteria for sinus arrhythmia.

Codes:

1b	Borderline normal ECG or normal variant
2c	Sinus bradycardia
12a	Normal variant, early repolarization

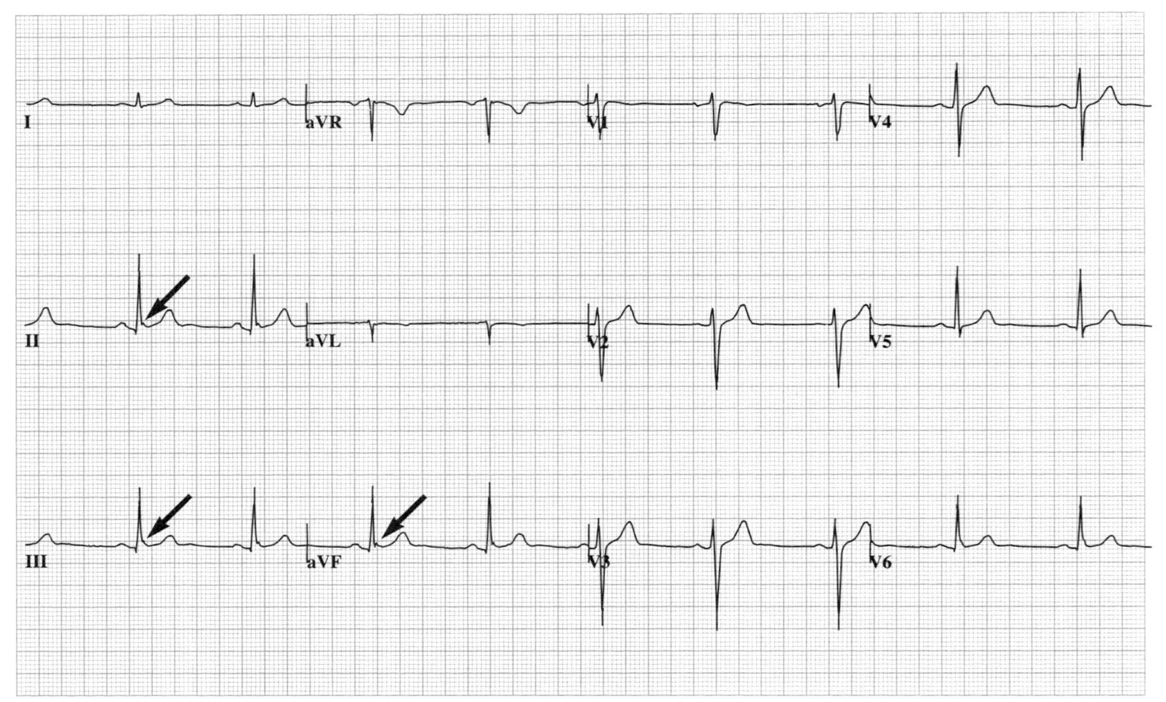

Questions: ECG 25

1. Some degree of ST elevation is present on the resting ECG of many young healthy adults:

   a. True
   b. False

2. Normal variant ECG findings include:

   a. Left axis deviation
   b. Peaked T waves
   c. Shallow T wave inversion in V_1-V_3
   d. Upwardly concave ST elevation

3. Juvenile T waves (normal variant) are characterized by shallow T wave inversions most often seen in leads:

   a. V_4-V_6
   b. V_1-V_3
   c. II, III, F
   d. I, aVL

Answers: ECG 25

1. Many, if not most, young healthy individuals below the age of 20 have some degree of ST segment elevation on their resting ECG. The ST elevation of normal variant early repolarization abnormality is typically concave upward, is often associated with subtle notching of the J-point, and has no pathological significance. (Answer: a)

2. Normal variant ECG findings include peaked T waves, shallow T wave inversion (especially in leads V_1-V_3), upwardly concave ST segment elevation, and right axis deviation. Left axis deviation is not a normal ECG variant. (Answer: All except a)

3. Juvenile T waves are a common normal variant ECG finding characterized by shallow T wave inversions in leads V_1-V_3. Juvenile T waves are commonly seen in children, occasionally seen as a normal variant in adult women, but only rarely seen as a normal variant in adult men. (Answer: b)

— Quick Review 25 —

Normal variant, early repolarization	
• Elevated ____ of the ST segment at the J junction	take-off
• (Concave/convex) upward ST elevation ending with a symmetrical upright T wave, which is often of large amplitude	Concave
• Distinct notch or slur on downstroke of ____ wave	R
• Most commonly involves leads ____	V_2-V_5
• Reciprocal ST segment depression is present (true/false)	false
• Some degree of ST elevation is present in the majority of young healthy individuals, especially in the precordial leads (true/false)	true

Differential Diagnosis

PP Pause Greater Than 1.6-2.0 Seconds

- Sinus pause/arrest: Due to transient failure of impulse formation at the SA node; sinus rhythm resumes at a PP interval that is not a multiple of the basic sinus PP interval
- Sinus arrhythmia (item 2b): Phasic, gradual change in PP interval
- Second-degree sinoatrial exit block, Mobitz I (Wenckebach) (item 2f): Progressive shortening of PP interval until a P wave fails to appear
- Second-degree sinoatrial exit block, Mobitz II (item 2f): Resumption of sinus rhythm at a PP interval that is a multiple (e.g., 2x, 3x, etc.) of the basic sinus rhythm
- Third-degree sinoatrial exit block (item 2f): Complete failure of sinoatrial conduction; cannot be differentiated from complete sinus arrest on surface ECG
- Abrupt change in autonomic tone
- "Pseudo" sinus pause due to nonconducted APCs (item 2j): P wave appears to be absent but is actually buried in the T wave — look for subtle deformity of the T wave just preceding the pause to detect nonconducted atrial premature complexes

ECG 26. 50-year-old male with chest pain and pulmonary edema:

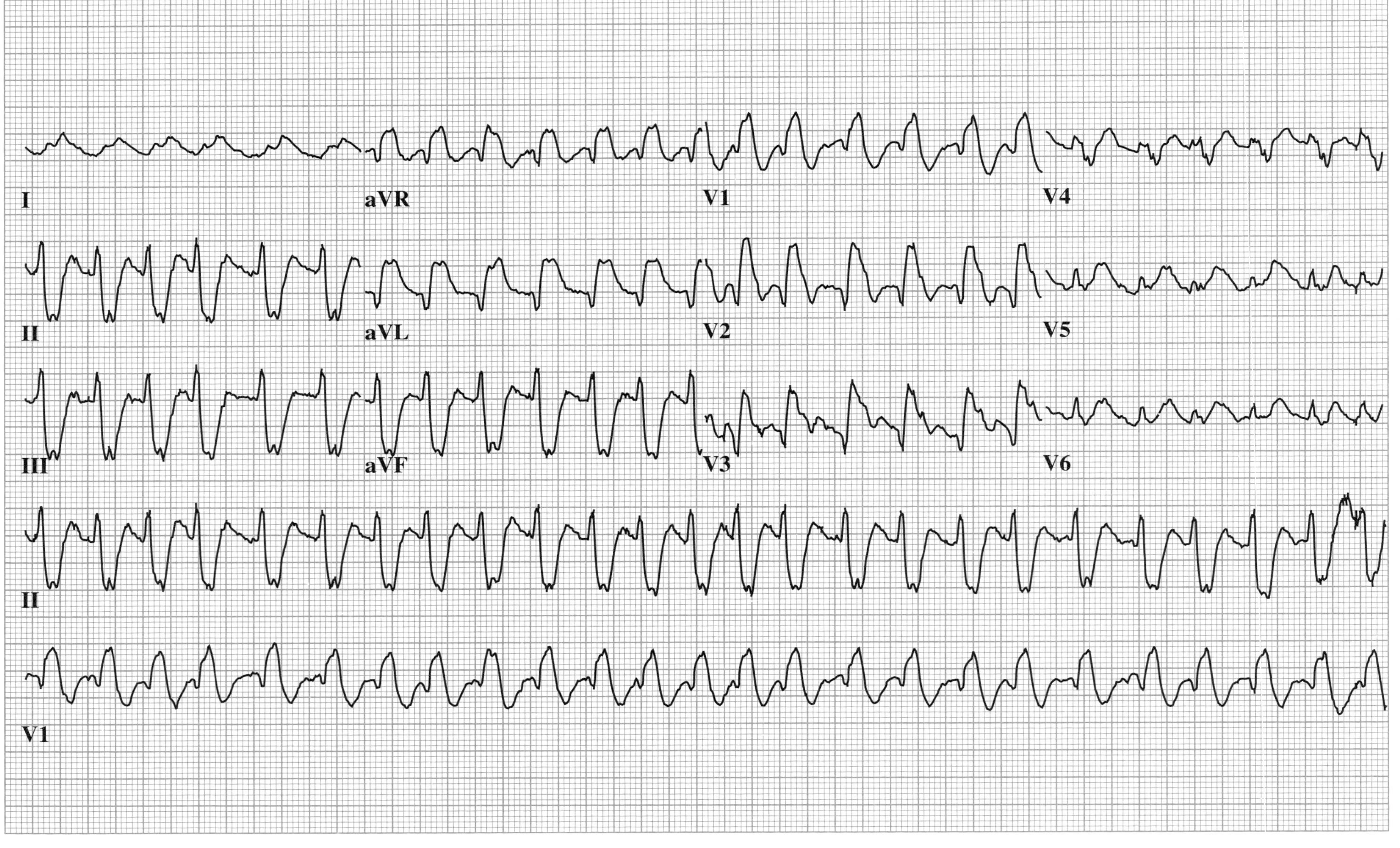

1. GENERAL FEATURES
- ☐ a. Normal ECG
- ☐ b. Borderline normal ECG or normal variant
- ☐ c. Incorrect electrode placement
- ☐ d. Artifact due to tremor

2. ATRIAL RHYTHMS
- ☐ a. Sinus rhythm
- ☐ b. Sinus arrhythmia
- ☐ c. Sinus bradycardia (< 60)
- ☐ d. Sinus tachycardia (> 100)
- ☐ e. Sinus pause or arrest
- ☐ f. Sinoatrial exit block
- ☐ g. Ecoptic atrial rhythm
- ☐ h. Wandering atrial pacemaker
- ☐ i. Atrial premature complexes, normally conducted
- ☐ j. Atrial premature complexes, nonconducted
- ☐ k. Atrial premature complexes with aberrant intraventricular conduction
- ☐ l. Atrial tachycardia (regular, sustained, 1:1 conduction)
- ☐ m. Atrial tachycardia, repetitive (short paroxysms)
- ☐ n. Atrial tachycardia, multifocal
- ☐ o. Atrial tachycardia with AV block
- ☐ p. Supraventricular tachycardia, unspecific
- ☐ q. Supraventricular tachycardia, paroxysmal
- ☐ r. Atrial flutter
- ☐ s. Atrial fibrillation
- ☐ t. Retrograde atrial activation

3. AV JUNCTIONAL RHYTHMS
- ☐ a. AV junctional premature complexes
- ☐ b. AV junctional escape complexes
- ☐ c. AV junctional rhythm, accelerated
- ☐ d. AV junctional rhythm

4. VENTRICULAR RHYTHMS
- ☐ a. Ventricular premature complex(es), uniform, fixed coupling
- ☐ b. Ventricular premature complex(es), uniform, nonfixed coupling
- ☐ c. Ventricular premature complexes(es), multiform
- ☐ d. Ventricular premature complexes, in pairs
- ☐ e. Ventricular parasystole
- ☐ f. Ventricular tachycardia (≥ 3 consecutive complexes)
- ☐ g. Accelerated idioventricular rhythm
- ☐ h. Ventricular escape complexes or rhythm
- ☐ i. Ventricular fibrillation

5. ATRIAL-VENTRICULAR INTERACTIONS IN ARRHYTHMIAS
- ☐ a. Fusion complexes
- ☐ b. Reciprocal (echo) complexes
- ☐ c. Ventricular capture complexes
- ☐ d. AV dissociation
- ☐ e. Ventriculophasic sinus arrhythmia

6. AV CONDUCTION ABNORMALITIES
- ☐ a. AV block, 1°
- ☐ b. AV block, 2° - Mobitz type I (Wenckebach)
- ☐ c. AV block, 2° - Mobitz type II
- ☐ d. AV block, 2:1
- ☐ e. AV block, 3°
- ☐ f. AV block, variable
- ☐ g. Short PR interval (with sinus rhythm and normal QRS duration)
- ☐ h. Wolff-Parkinson-White pattern

7. INTRAVENTRICULAR CONDUCTION DISTURBANCES
- ☐ a. RBBB, incomplete
- ☐ b. RBBB, complete
- ☐ c. Left anterior fascicular block
- ☐ d. Left posterior fascicular block
- ☐ e. LBBB, with ST-T wave suggestive of acute myocardial injury or infarction
- ☐ f. LBBB, complete
- ☐ g. LBBB, intermittent
- ☐ h. Intraventricular conduction disturbance, nonspecific
- ☐ i. Aberrant intraventricular conduction with supraventricular arrhythmia

8. P WAVE ABNORMALITIES
- ☐ a. Right atrial abnormality
- ☐ b. Left atrial abnormalities
- ☐ c. Nonspecific atrial abnormality

9. ABNORMALITIES OF QRS VOLTAGE OR AXIS
- ☐ a. Low voltage, limb leads only
- ☐ b. Low voltage, limb and precordial leads
- ☐ c. Left axis deviation (> - 30%)
- ☐ d. Right axis deviation (> + 100)
- ☐ e. Electrical alternans

10. VENTRICULAR HYPERTROPHY
- ☐ a. LVH by voltage only
- ☐ b. LVH by voltage and ST-T segment abnormalities
- ☐ c. RVH
- ☐ d. Combined ventricular hypertrophy

11. Q WAVE MYOCARDIAL INFARCTION

	Probably Acute or Recent	Probably Old or Age Indeterminate
Anterolateral	☐ a.	☐ g.
Anterior	☐ b.	☐ h.
Anteroseptal	☐ c.	☐ i.
Lateral/High lateral	☐ d.	☐ j.
Inferior	☐ e.	☐ k.
Posterior	☐ f.	☐ l.

- ☐ m. Probably ventricular aneurysm

12. ST, T, U, WAVE ABNORMALITIES
- ☐ a. Normal variant, early repolarization
- ☐ b. Normal variant, juvenile T waves
- ☐ c. Nonspecific ST and/or T wave abnormalities
- ☐ d. ST and/or T wave abnormalities suggesting myocardial ischemia
- ☐ e. ST and/or T wave abnormalities suggesting myocardial injury
- ☐ f. ST and/or T wave abnormalities suggesting acute pericarditis
- ☐ g. ST-T segment abnormalities secondary to intraventricular conduction disturbance or hypertrophy
- ☐ h. Post-extrasystolic T wave abnormality
- ☐ i. Isolated J point depression
- ☐ j. Peaked T waves
- ☐ k. Prolonged QT interval
- ☐ l. Prominent U waves

13. PACEMAKER FUNCTION AND RHYTHM
- ☐ a. Atrial or coronary sinus pacing
- ☐ b. Ventricular demand pacing
- ☐ c. AV sequential pacing
- ☐ d. Ventricular pacing, complete control
- ☐ e. Dual chamber, atrial sensing pacemaker
- ☐ f. Pacemaker malfunction, not constantly capturing (atrium or ventricle)
- ☐ g. Pacemaker malfunction, not constantly sensing (atrium or ventricle)
- ☐ h. Pacemaker malfunction, not firing
- ☐ i. Pacemaker malfunction, slowing

14. SUGGESTED OR PROBABLE CLINICAL DISORDERS
- ☐ a. Digitalis effect
- ☐ b. Digitalis toxicity
- ☐ c. Antiarrhythmic drug effect
- ☐ d. Antiarrhythmic drug toxicity
- ☐ e. Hyperkalemia
- ☐ f. Hypokalemia
- ☐ g. Hypercalcemia
- ☐ h. Hypocalcemia
- ☐ i. Atrial septal defect, secundum
- ☐ j. Atrial septal defect, primum
- ☐ k. Dextrocardia, mirror image
- ☐ l. Mitral valve disease
- ☐ m. Chronic lung disease
- ☐ n. Acute cor pulmonale, including pulmonary embolus
- ☐ o. Pericardial effusion
- ☐ p. Acute pericarditis
- ☐ q. Hypertrophic cardiomyopathy
- ☐ r. Coronary artery disease
- ☐ s. Central nervous system disorder
- ☐ t. Myxedema
- ☐ u. Hypothermia
- ☐ v. Sick sinus syndrome

ECG 26 was obtained in a 50-year-old male with chest pain and pulmonary edema. The tracing shows atrial fibrillation with a rapid ventricular response of 148 beats/minute. Left axis deviation is also present. Acute anteroseptal myocardial infarction and high lateral myocardial injury are evident (Q waves and ST elevation are marked by arrows and asterisks, respectively); the Q wave in aVL is insufficient for the diagnosis of high lateral infarction. Although the exact QRS duration is difficult to ascertain due to the current of injury, a nonspecific intraventricular defect is probably present (or an atypical RBBB with LAFB). These findings are compatible with coronary artery disease. The patient was taken to the catheterization laboratory where left main occlusion was discovered.

Codes:

2s	Atrial fibrillation
7h	IVCD, nonspecific type
9c	Left axis deviation (>-30°)
11c	Anteroseptal Q wave MI, probably acute or recent
12e	ST and/or T wave abnormalities suggesting myocardial injury
14r	Coronary artery disease

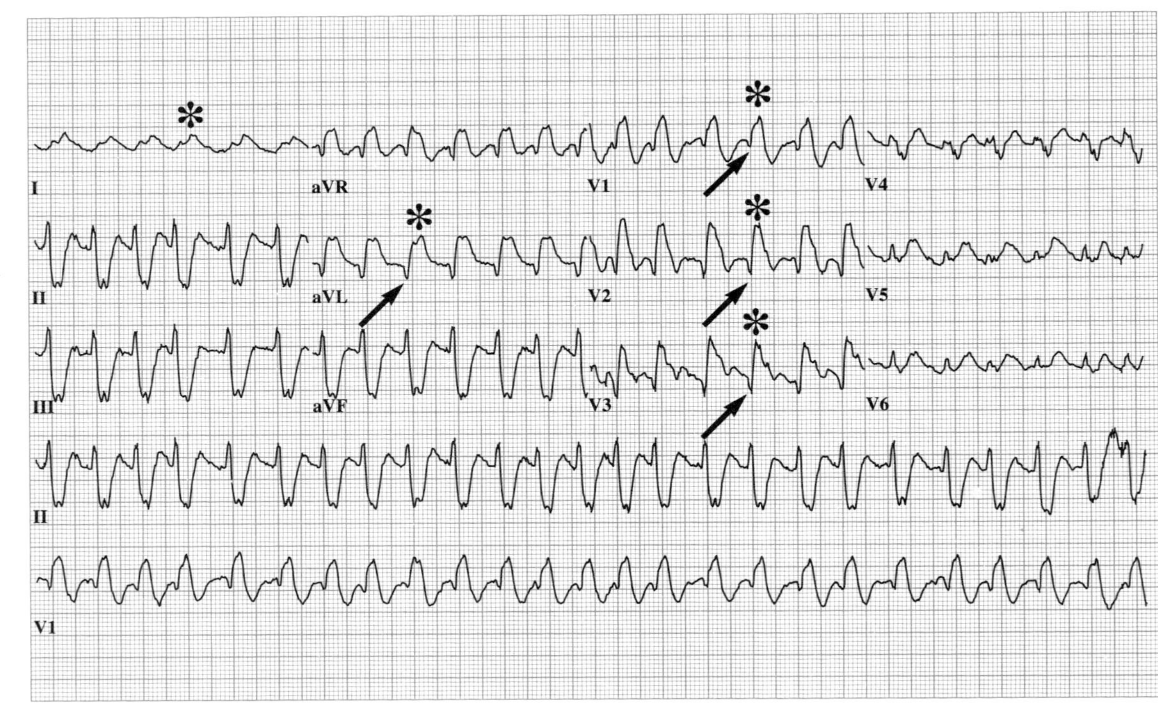

Questions: ECG 26

1. Could the rhythm in this tracing be ventricular tachycardia?

   a. Yes
   b. No

2. Is the rhythm in this tracing consistent with atrial fibrillation in a patient with Wolff-Parkinson-White syndrome?

   a. Yes
   b. No

Answers: ECG 26

1. Although ventricular tachycardia may be somewhat irregular, the irregularly irregular rhythm on this tracing excludes VT. (Answer: b)

2. The absence of delta waves excludes the diagnosis of WPW. In addition, patients with WPW and atrial fibrillation usually have ventricular response rates > 180-200. (Answer: b)

— Quick Review 26 —

Atrial fibrillation	
• ____ waves are absent	P
• Atrial activity is totally ____ and represented by fibrillatory (f) waves of varying amplitudes, duration and morphology	irregular
• Atrial activity is best seen in the ____ and ____ leads	right precordial, inferior
• Ventricular rhythm is (regularly/irregularly) irregular	irregularly
• ____ toxicity may result in regularization of the RR interval due to complete heart block with junctional tachycardia	Digitalis
• Ventricular rate is usually ____ per minute in the absence of drugs	100-180
▸ Think ____ if the ventricular rate is > 200 per minute and the QRS is > 0.12 seconds	Wolff-Parkinson-White
Anteroseptal MI, recent or probably acute	
• Abnormal Q or QS deflection and ST elevation in leads ____ (and sometimes V_4)	V_1-V_3
• The presence of a Q wave in lead ____ distinguishes anteroseptal from anterior infarction	V_1
Lateral or high lateral MI, recent or probably acute	
• Abnormal Q waves and ST elevation in leads I and ____	aVL
• An isolated Q wave in aVL (does/does not) qualify as a lateral MI	does not

ECG 27. 59-year-old male with chest pain of several days duration and a cough:

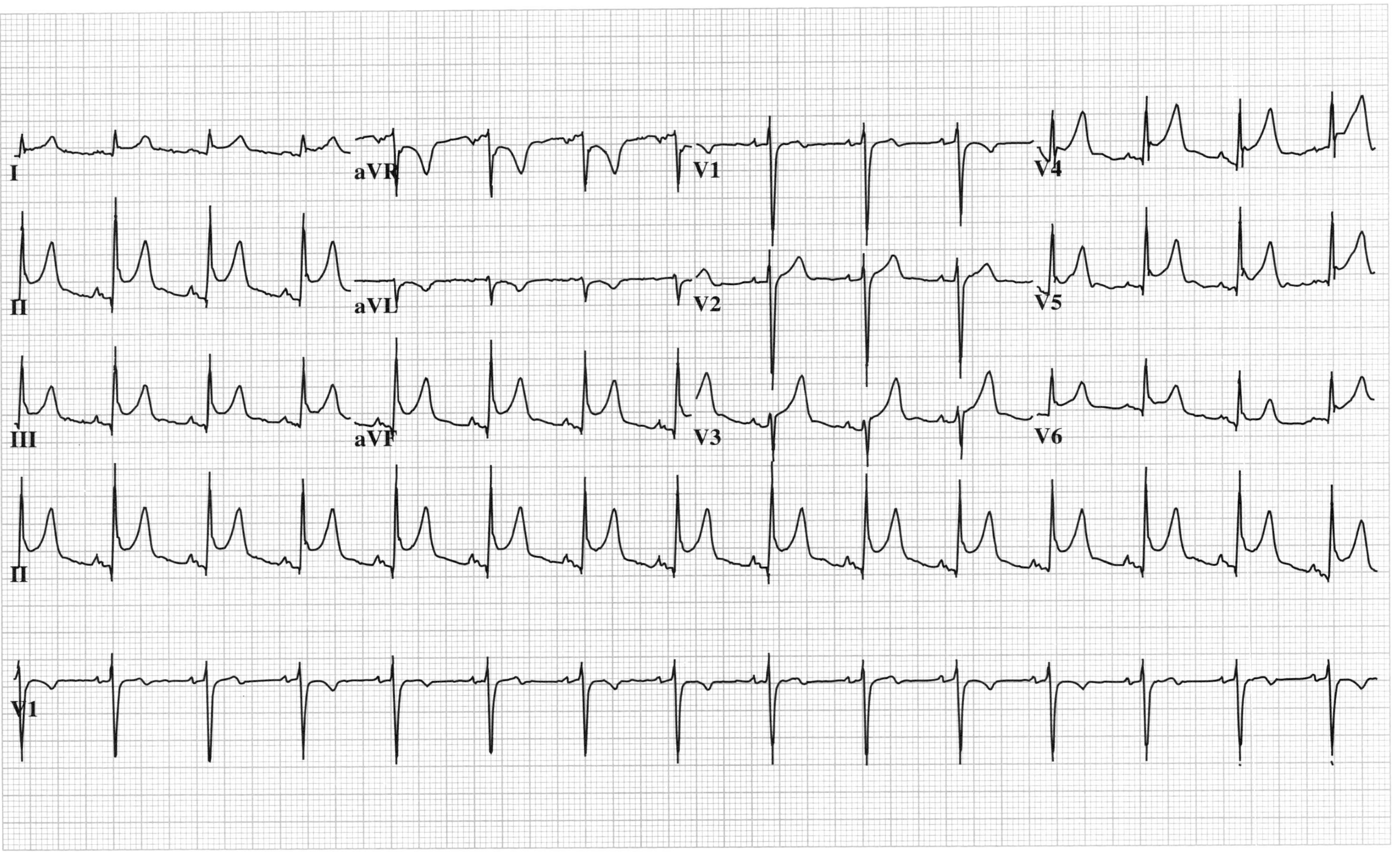

1. GENERAL FEATURES

- ☐ a. Normal ECG
- ☐ b. Borderline normal ECG or normal variant
- ☐ c. Incorrect electrode placement
- ☐ d. Artifact due to tremor

2. ATRIAL RHYTHMS

- ☐ a. Sinus rhythm
- ☐ b. Sinus arrhythmia
- ☐ c. Sinus bradycardia (< 60)
- ☐ d. Sinus tachycardia (> 100)
- ☐ e. Sinus pause or arrest
- ☐ f. Sinoatrial exit block
- ☐ g. Ecoptic atrial rhythm
- ☐ h. Wandering atrial pacemaker
- ☐ i. Atrial premature complexes, normally conducted
- ☐ j. Atrial premature complexes, nonconducted
- ☐ k. Atrial premature complexes with aberrant intraventricular conduction
- ☐ l. Atrial tachycardia (regular, sustained, 1:1 conduction)
- ☐ m. Atrial tachycardia, repetitive (short paroxysms)
- ☐ n. Atrial tachycardia, multifocal
- ☐ o. Atrial tachycardia with AV block
- ☐ p. Supraventricular tachycardia, unspecific
- ☐ q. Supraventricular tachycardia, paroxysmal
- ☐ r. Atrial flutter
- ☐ s. Atrial fibrillation
- ☐ t. Retrograde atrial activation

3. AV JUNCTIONAL RHYTHMS

- ☐ a. AV junctional premature complexes
- ☐ b. AV junctional escape complexes
- ☐ c. AV junctional rhythm, accelerated
- ☐ d. AV junctional rhythm

4. VENTRICULAR RHYTHMS

- ☐ a. Ventricular premature complex(es), uniform, fixed coupling
- ☐ b. Ventricular premature complex(es), uniform, nonfixed coupling
- ☐ c. Ventricular premature complexes(es), multiform
- ☐ d. Ventricular premature complexes, in pairs
- ☐ e. Ventricular parasystole
- ☐ f. Ventricular tachycardia (≥ 3 consecutive complexes)
- ☐ g. Accelerated idioventricular rhythm
- ☐ h. Ventricular escape complexes or rhythm
- ☐ i. Ventricular fibrillation

5. ATRIAL-VENTRICULAR INTERACTIONS IN ARRHYTHMIAS

- ☐ a. Fusion complexes
- ☐ b. Reciprocal (echo) complexes
- ☐ c. Ventricular capture complexes
- ☐ d. AV dissociation
- ☐ e. Ventriculophasic sinus arrhythmia

6. AV CONDUCTION ABNORMALITIES

- ☐ a. AV block, 1°
- ☐ b. AV block, 2° - Mobitz type I (Wenckebach)
- ☐ c. AV block, 2° - Mobitz type II
- ☐ d. AV block, 2:1
- ☐ e. AV block, 3°
- ☐ f. AV block, variable
- ☐ g. Short PR interval (with sinus rhythm and normal QRS duration)
- ☐ h. Wolff-Parkinson-White pattern

7. INTRAVENTRICULAR CONDUCTION DISTURBANCES

- ☐ a. RBBB, incomplete
- ☐ b. RBBB, complete
- ☐ c. Left anterior fascicular block
- ☐ d. Left posterior fascicular block
- ☐ e. LBBB, with ST-T wave suggestive of acute myocardial injury or infarction
- ☐ f. LBBB, complete
- ☐ g. LBBB, intermittent
- ☐ h. Intraventricular conduction disturbance, nonspecific
- ☐ i. Aberrant intraventricular conduction with supraventricular arrhythmia

8. P WAVE ABNORMALITIES

- ☐ a. Right atrial abnormality
- ☐ b. Left atrial abnormalities
- ☐ c. Nonspecific atrial abnormality

9. ABNORMALITIES OF QRS VOLTAGE OR AXIS

- ☐ a. Low voltage, limb leads only
- ☐ b. Low voltage, limb and precordial leads
- ☐ c. Left axis deviation (> - 30%)
- ☐ d. Right axis deviation (> + 100)
- ☐ e. Electrical alternans

10. VENTRICULAR HYPERTROPHY

- ☐ a. LVH by voltage only
- ☐ b. LVH by voltage and ST-T segment abnormalities
- ☐ c. RVH
- ☐ d. Combined ventricular hypertrophy

11. Q WAVE MYOCARDIAL INFARCTION

	Probably Acute or Recent	Probably Old or Age Indeterminate
Anterolateral	☐ a.	☐ g.
Anterior	☐ b.	☐ h.
Anteroseptal	☐ c.	☐ i.
Lateral/High lateral	☐ d.	☐ j.
Inferior	☐ e.	☐ k.
Posterior	☐ f.	☐ l.

- ☐ m. Probably ventricular aneurysm

12. ST, T, U, WAVE ABNORMALITIES

- ☐ a. Normal variant, early repolarization
- ☐ b. Normal variant, juvenile T waves
- ☐ c. Nonspecific ST and/or T wave abnormalities
- ☐ d. ST and/or T wave abnormalities suggesting myocardial ischemia
- ☐ e. ST and/or T wave abnormalities suggesting myocardial injury
- ☐ f. ST and/or T wave abnormalities suggesting acute pericarditis
- ☐ g. ST-T segment abnormalities secondary to intraventricular conduction disturbance or hypertrophy
- ☐ h. Post-extrasystolic T wave abnormality
- ☐ i. Isolated J point depression
- ☐ j. Peaked T waves
- ☐ k. Prolonged QT interval
- ☐ l. Prominent U waves

13. PACEMAKER FUNCTION AND RHYTHM

- ☐ a. Atrial or coronary sinus pacing
- ☐ b. Ventricular demand pacing
- ☐ c. AV sequential pacing
- ☐ d. Ventricular pacing, complete control
- ☐ e. Dual chamber, atrial sensing pacemaker
- ☐ f. Pacemaker malfunction, not constantly capturing (atrium or ventricle)
- ☐ g. Pacemaker malfunction, not constantly sensing (atrium or ventricle)
- ☐ h. Pacemaker malfunction, not firing
- ☐ i. Pacemaker malfunction, slowing

14. SUGGESTED OR PROBABLE CLINICAL DISORDERS

- ☐ a. Digitalis effect
- ☐ b. Digitalis toxicity
- ☐ c. Antiarrhythmic drug effect
- ☐ d. Antiarrhythmic drug toxicity
- ☐ e. Hyperkalemia
- ☐ f. Hypokalemia
- ☐ g. Hypercalcemia
- ☐ h. Hypocalcemia
- ☐ i. Atrial septal defect, secundum
- ☐ j. Atrial septal defect, primum
- ☐ k. Dextrocardia, mirror image
- ☐ l. Mitral valve disease
- ☐ m. Chronic lung disease
- ☐ n. Acute cor pulmonale, including pulmonary embolus
- ☐ o. Pericardial effusion
- ☐ p. Acute pericarditis
- ☐ q. Hypertrophic cardiomyopathy
- ☐ r. Coronary artery disease
- ☐ s. Central nervous system disorder
- ☐ t. Myxedema
- ☐ u. Hypothermia
- ☐ v. Sick sinus syndrome

ECG 27 was obtained in a 59-year-old male with chest pain of several days duration and a cough. The ECG showed a sinus rhythm at 87 beats/minute. Diffuse ST segment elevation that is upwardly concave (arrows) is noted in nearly all leads. Some PR depression is apparent in leads II, III, aVF, and V_3 (arrowheads). Electrical alternans is present in the rhythm strip on lead II. Peaked T waves (> 6 mm in height) are also noted in the inferior leads (asterisks). These findings are consistent with acute pericarditis. While this tracing is also consistent with extensive myocardial infarction (left main or dominant left circumflex occlusion), the several day history of chest pain makes this diagnosis unlikely.

Codes:

2a	Sinus rhythm
9e	Electrical alternans
12f	ST and/or T wave abnormalities suggesting acute pericarditis
12j	Peaked T waves
14p	Acute pericarditis

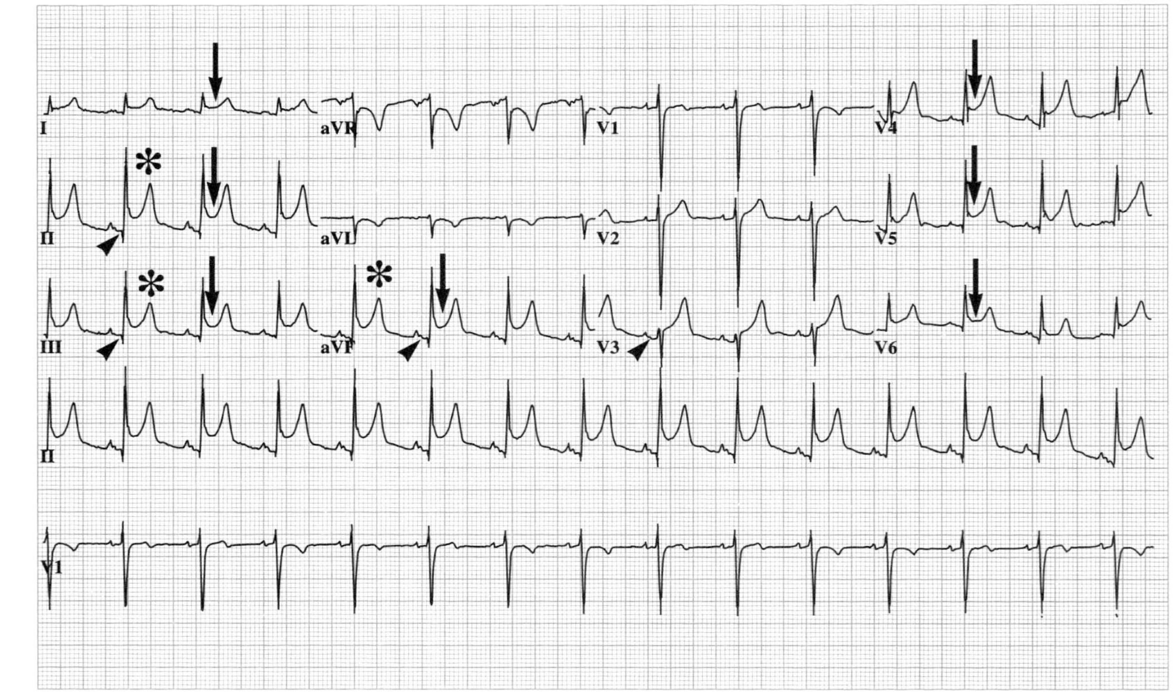

Questions: ECG 27

1. ST elevation can be seen in pericarditis in all leads except:
   a. aVR
   b. aVF
   c. III
   d. V_1

2. Diffuse loss of QRS voltage in the setting of pericarditis suggests:

   a. Associated myocardial infarction
   b. Obesity
   c. Pericardial effusion
   d. Amyloidosis

Answers: ECG 27

1. ST segment elevation associated with acute pericarditis is typically diffuse and upwardly concave. All leads can (and often do) show ST elevation except aVR, which typically shows ST depression. (Answer: a)

2. Amyloidosis, obesity, and diffuse myocardial disease related to previous infarction can cause loss of QRS voltage. However, in the setting of pericarditis, the most likely cause is the development of a pericardial effusion. (Answer: c)

— Quick Review 27 —

Electrical alternans	
• Alteration in the ____ and/or ____ of the P, QRS and/or T waves	amplitude, direction
ST and/or T wave changes suggesting acute pericarditis	
• Classic evolutionary pattern consists of ____ stages	4
▸ Stage 1: Upwardly concave ST segment ____ in almost all leads	elevation
▸ Stage 2: ST junction (J point) returns to baseline and T wave amplitude begins to (increase/decrease)	decrease
▸ Stage 3: T waves (invert/remain upright)	invert
▸ Stage 4: ECG (does/does not) return to normal	does
• Other clues to acute pericarditis:	
▸ Sinus ____	tachycardia
▸ PR ____ early (PR elevation in aVR)	depression
▸ (High/low) voltage QRS	low
▸ Electrical alternans if pericardial ____ is present	effusion
Peaked T waves	
• T wave > ____ mm in the limb leads or > ____ mm in the precordial leads	6, 10

ECG 28. 76-year-old asymptomatic female:

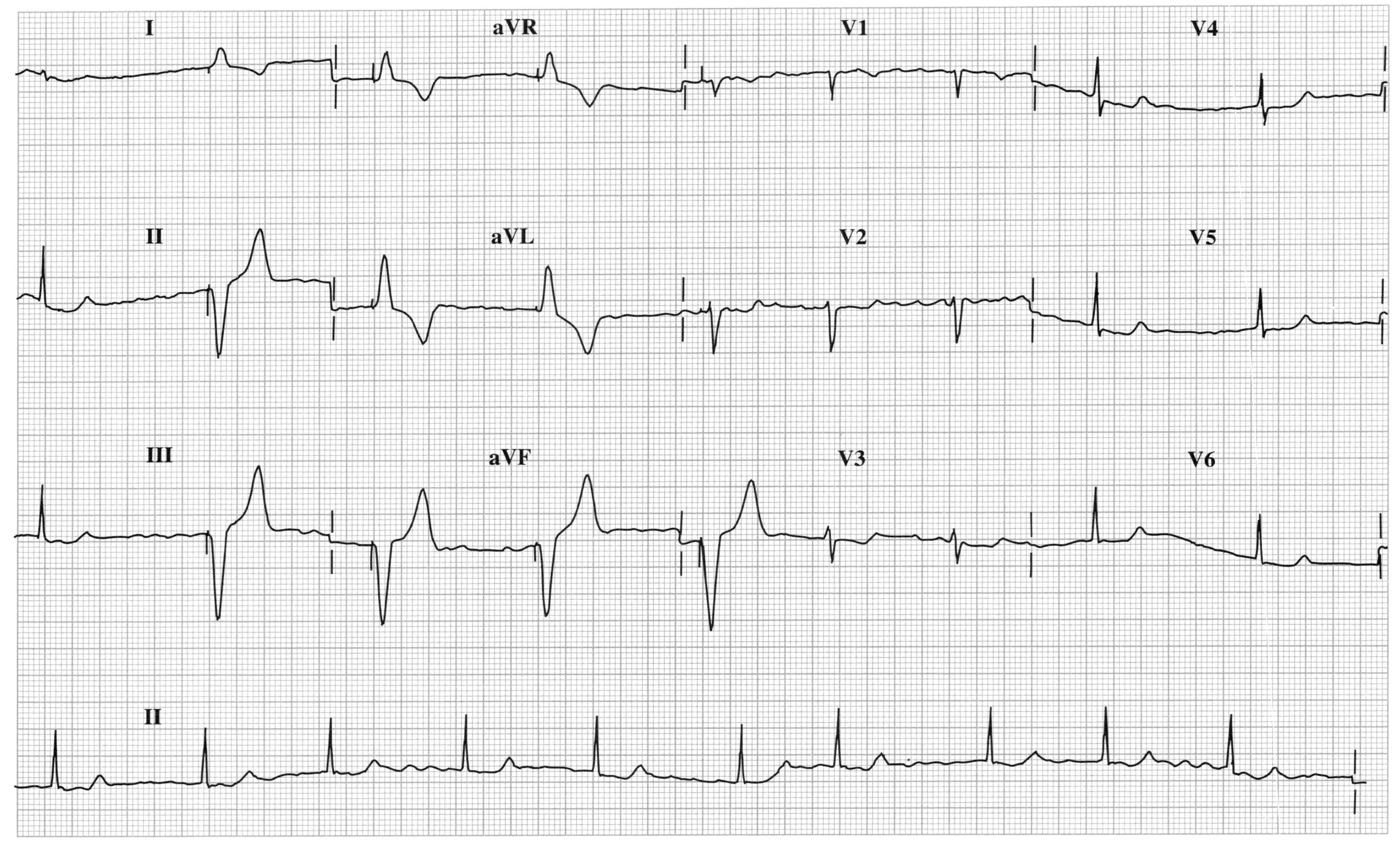

1. GENERAL FEATURES

- ☐ a. Normal ECG
- ☐ b. Borderline normal ECG or normal variant
- ☐ c. Incorrect electrode placement
- ☐ d. Artifact due to tremor

2. ATRIAL RHYTHMS

- ☐ a. Sinus rhythm
- ☐ b. Sinus arrhythmia
- ☐ c. Sinus bradycardia (< 60)
- ☐ d. Sinus tachycardia (> 100)
- ☐ e. Sinus pause or arrest
- ☐ f. Sinoatrial exit block
- ☐ g. Ecoptic atrial rhythm
- ☐ h. Wandering atrial pacemaker
- ☐ i. Atrial premature complexes, normally conducted
- ☐ j. Atrial premature complexes, nonconducted
- ☐ k. Atrial premature complexes with aberrant intraventricular conduction
- ☐ l. Atrial tachycardia (regular, sustained, 1:1 conduction)
- ☐ m. Atrial tachycardia, repetitive (short paroxysms)
- ☐ n. Atrial tachycardia, multifocal
- ☐ o. Atrial tachycardia with AV block
- ☐ p. Supraventricular tachycardia, unspecific
- ☐ q. Supraventricular tachycardia, paroxysmal
- ☐ r. Atrial flutter
- ☐ s. Atrial fibrillation
- ☐ t. Retrograde atrial activation

3. AV JUNCTIONAL RHYTHMS

- ☐ a. AV junctional premature complexes
- ☐ b. AV junctional escape complexes
- ☐ c. AV junctional rhythm, accelerated
- ☐ d. AV junctional rhythm

4. VENTRICULAR RHYTHMS

- ☐ a. Ventricular premature complex(es), uniform, fixed coupling
- ☐ b. Ventricular premature complex(es), uniform, nonfixed coupling
- ☐ c. Ventricular premature complexes(es), multiform
- ☐ d. Ventricular premature complexes, in pairs
- ☐ e. Ventricular parasystole
- ☐ f. Ventricular tachycardia (≥ 3 consecutive complexes)
- ☐ g. Accelerated idioventricular rhythm
- ☐ h. Ventricular escape complexes or rhythm
- ☐ i. Ventricular fibrillation

5. ATRIAL-VENTRICULAR INTERACTIONS IN ARRHYTHMIAS

- ☐ a. Fusion complexes
- ☐ b. Reciprocal (echo) complexes
- ☐ c. Ventricular capture complexes
- ☐ d. AV dissociation
- ☐ e. Ventriculophasic sinus arrhythmia

6. AV CONDUCTION ABNORMALITIES

- ☐ a. AV block, 1°
- ☐ b. AV block, 2° - Mobitz type I (Wenckebach)
- ☐ c. AV block, 2° - Mobitz type II
- ☐ d. AV block, 2:1
- ☐ e. AV block, 3°
- ☐ f. AV block, variable
- ☐ g. Short PR interval (with sinus rhythm and normal QRS duration)
- ☐ h. Wolff-Parkinson-White pattern

7. INTRAVENTRICULAR CONDUCTION DISTURBANCES

- ☐ a. RBBB, incomplete
- ☐ b. RBBB, complete
- ☐ c. Left anterior fascicular block
- ☐ d. Left posterior fascicular block
- ☐ e. LBBB, with ST-T wave suggestive of acute myocardial injury or infarction
- ☐ f. LBBB, complete
- ☐ g. LBBB, intermittent
- ☐ h. Intraventricular conduction disturbance, nonspecific
- ☐ i. Aberrant intraventricular conduction with supraventricular arrhythmia

8. P WAVE ABNORMALITIES

- ☐ a. Right atrial abnormality
- ☐ b. Left atrial abnormalities
- ☐ c. Nonspecific atrial abnormality

9. ABNORMALITIES OF QRS VOLTAGE OR AXIS

- ☐ a. Low voltage, limb leads only
- ☐ b. Low voltage, limb and precordial leads
- ☐ c. Left axis deviation (> - 30%)
- ☐ d. Right axis deviation (> + 100)
- ☐ e. Electrical alternans

10. VENTRICULAR HYPERTROPHY

- ☐ a. LVH by voltage only
- ☐ b. LVH by voltage and ST-T segment abnormalities
- ☐ c. RVH
- ☐ d. Combined ventricular hypertrophy

11. Q WAVE MYOCARDIAL INFARCTION

	Probably Acute or Recent	Probably Old or Age Indeterminate
Anterolateral	☐ a.	☐ g.
Anterior	☐ b.	☐ h.
Anteroseptal	☐ c.	☐ i.
Lateral/High lateral	☐ d.	☐ j.
Inferior	☐ e.	☐ k.
Posterior	☐ f.	☐ l.

☐ m. Probably ventricular aneurysm

12. ST, T, U, WAVE ABNORMALITIES

- ☐ a. Normal variant, early repolarization
- ☐ b. Normal variant, juvenile T waves
- ☐ c. Nonspecific ST and/or T wave abnormalities
- ☐ d. ST and/or T wave abnormalities suggesting myocardial ischemia
- ☐ e. ST and/or T wave abnormalities suggesting myocardial injury
- ☐ f. ST and/or T wave abnormalities suggesting acute pericarditis
- ☐ g. ST-T segment abnormalities secondary to intraventricular conduction disturbance or hypertrophy
- ☐ h. Post-extrasystolic T wave abnormality
- ☐ i. Isolated J point depression
- ☐ j. Peaked T waves
- ☐ k. Prolonged QT interval
- ☐ l. Prominent U waves

13. PACEMAKER FUNCTION AND RHYTHM

- ☐ a. Atrial or coronary sinus pacing
- ☐ b. Ventricular demand pacing
- ☐ c. AV sequential pacing
- ☐ d. Ventricular pacing, complete control
- ☐ e. Dual chamber, atrial sensing pacemaker
- ☐ f. Pacemaker malfunction, not constantly capturing (atrium or ventricle)
- ☐ g. Pacemaker malfunction, not constantly sensing (atrium or ventricle)
- ☐ h. Pacemaker malfunction, not firing
- ☐ i. Pacemaker malfunction, slowing

14. SUGGESTED OR PROBABLE CLINICAL DISORDERS

- ☐ a. Digitalis effect
- ☐ b. Digitalis toxicity
- ☐ c. Antiarrhythmic drug effect
- ☐ d. Antiarrhythmic drug toxicity
- ☐ e. Hyperkalemia
- ☐ f. Hypokalemia
- ☐ g. Hypercalcemia
- ☐ h. Hypocalcemia
- ☐ i. Atrial septal defect, secundum
- ☐ j. Atrial septal defect, primum
- ☐ k. Dextrocardia, mirror image
- ☐ l. Mitral valve disease
- ☐ m. Chronic lung disease
- ☐ n. Acute cor pulmonale, including pulmonary embolus
- ☐ o. Pericardial effusion
- ☐ p. Acute pericarditis
- ☐ q. Hypertrophic cardiomyopathy
- ☐ r. Coronary artery disease
- ☐ s. Central nervous system disorder
- ☐ t. Myxedema
- ☐ u. Hypothermia
- ☐ v. Sick sinus syndrome

ECG 28 was obtained in a 76-year-old asymptomatic female. Atrial fibrillation is noted with appropriate ventricular demand pacing (asterisks) at 50 beats/minute. Nonspecific repolarization abnormalities are noted with sagging ST segment depression consistent with digitalis effect (arrows).

Codes:

2s	Atrial fibrillation
12c	Nonspecific ST and/or T wave abnormalities
13b	Ventricular demand pacing
14a	Digitalis effect

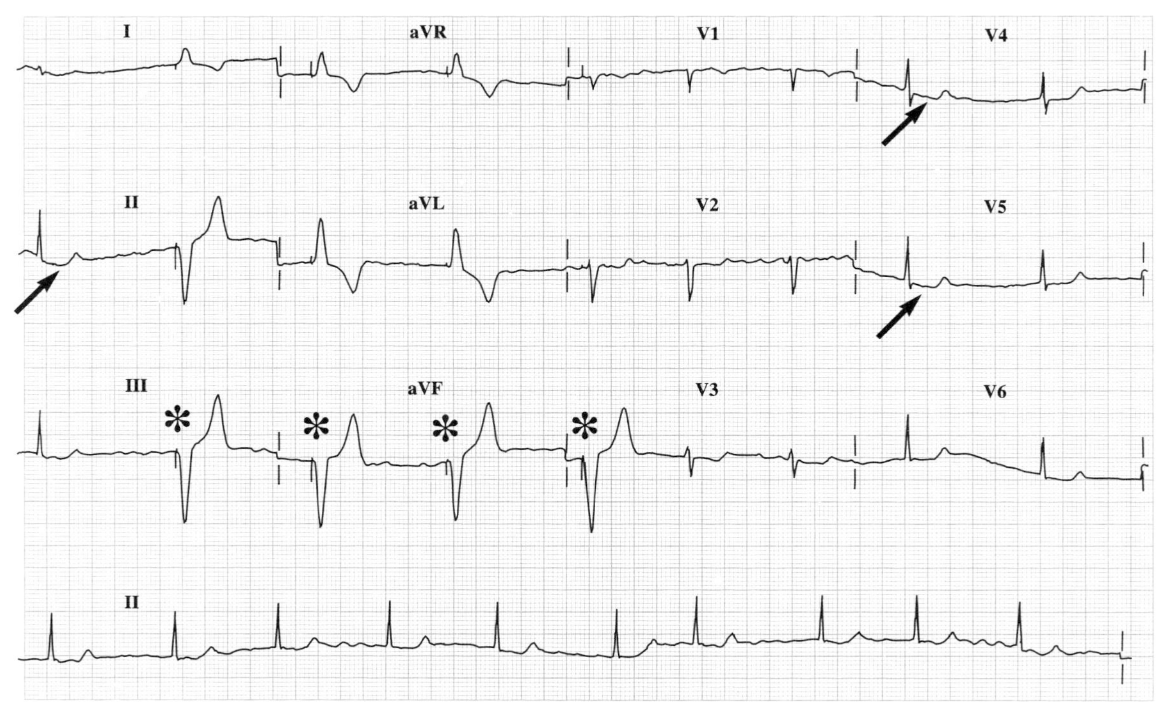

Questions: ECG 28

1. To make a diagnosis of ventricular demand (VVI) pacing, you should see:

   a. Inhibition of atrial output in response to native atrial activity
   b. Inhibition of ventricular output in response to an intrinsic QRS
   c. Retrograde VA conduction
   d. Variable pacing rates

— Quick Review 28 —

Ventricular demand pacing	
• Pacemaker stimulus followed by a QRS complex that has (the same/different) morphology compared to the intrinsic QRS	different
• Must demonstrate ____ of pacemaker output in response to intrinsic QRS	inhibition
Digitalis effect	
• ____ ST segment depression with upward (concavity/convexity)	Sagging concavity
• T wave flat, inverted, or ____	biphasic
• QT interval (shortened/prolonged)	shortened
• U wave amplitude (increased/decreased)	increased
• PR interval (shortened/lengthened)	lengthened

Answers: ECG 28

1. A ventricular demand (VVI) pacemaker senses and paces only in the ventricle and is oblivious to native atrial activity. If constant ventricular pacing is noted throughout the tracing, it is impossible to distinguish ventricular demand from asynchronous ventricular pacing. Thus, the diagnosis of ventricular demand pacing requires evidence of appropriate inhibition of pacemaker output in response to a native QRS (at least one). The pacing rate of a VVI pacemaker is generally constant at the programmed pacing rate; in contrast, VVI-R pacing allows for variable pacing rates in response to physiologic needs. (Answer: b)

ECG 29. 86-year-old male with palpitations and shortness of breath:

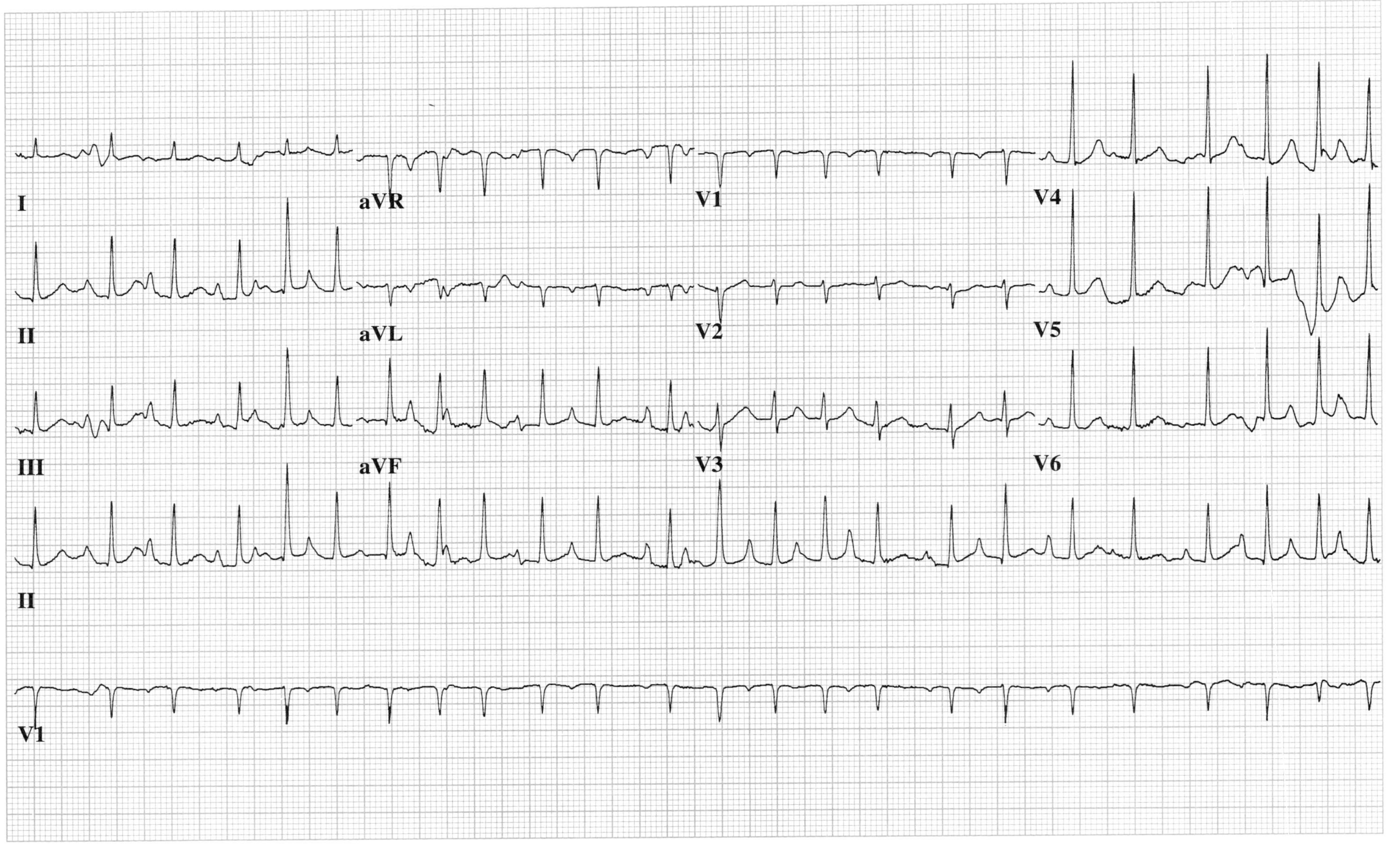

1. GENERAL FEATURES
- ☐ a. Normal ECG
- ☐ b. Borderline normal ECG or normal variant
- ☐ c. Incorrect electrode placement
- ☐ d. Artifact due to tremor

2. ATRIAL RHYTHMS
- ☐ a. Sinus rhythm
- ☐ b. Sinus arrhythmia
- ☐ c. Sinus bradycardia (< 60)
- ☐ d. Sinus tachycardia (> 100)
- ☐ e. Sinus pause or arrest
- ☐ f. Sinoatrial exit block
- ☐ g. Ecoptic atrial rhythm
- ☐ h. Wandering atrial pacemaker
- ☐ i. Atrial premature complexes, normally conducted
- ☐ j. Atrial premature complexes, nonconducted
- ☐ k. Atrial premature complexes with aberrant intraventricular conduction
- ☐ l. Atrial tachycardia (regular, sustained, 1:1 conduction)
- ☐ m. Atrial tachycardia, repetitive (short paroxysms)
- ☐ n. Atrial tachycardia, multifocal
- ☐ o. Atrial tachycardia with AV block
- ☐ p. Supraventricular tachycardia, unspecific
- ☐ q. Supraventricular tachycardia, paroxysmal
- ☐ r. Atrial flutter
- ☐ s. Atrial fibrillation
- ☐ t. Retrograde atrial activation

3. AV JUNCTIONAL RHYTHMS
- ☐ a. AV junctional premature complexes
- ☐ b. AV junctional escape complexes
- ☐ c. AV junctional rhythm, accelerated
- ☐ d. AV junctional rhythm

4. VENTRICULAR RHYTHMS
- ☐ a. Ventricular premature complex(es), uniform, fixed coupling
- ☐ b. Ventricular premature complex(es), uniform, nonfixed coupling
- ☐ c. Ventricular premature complexes(es), multiform
- ☐ d. Ventricular premature complexes, in pairs
- ☐ e. Ventricular parasystole
- ☐ f. Ventricular tachycardia (≥ 3 consecutive complexes)
- ☐ g. Accelerated idioventricular rhythm
- ☐ h. Ventricular escape complexes or rhythm
- ☐ i. Ventricular fibrillation

5. ATRIAL-VENTRICULAR INTERACTIONS IN ARRHYTHMIAS
- ☐ a. Fusion complexes
- ☐ b. Reciprocal (echo) complexes
- ☐ c. Ventricular capture complexes
- ☐ d. AV dissociation
- ☐ e. Ventriculophasic sinus arrhythmia

6. AV CONDUCTION ABNORMALITIES
- ☐ a. AV block, 1°
- ☐ b. AV block, 2° - Mobitz type I (Wenckebach)
- ☐ c. AV block, 2° - Mobitz type II
- ☐ d. AV block, 2:1
- ☐ e. AV block, 3°
- ☐ f. AV block, variable
- ☐ g. Short PR interval (with sinus rhythm and normal QRS duration)
- ☐ h. Wolff-Parkinson-White pattern

7. INTRAVENTRICULAR CONDUCTION DISTURBANCES
- ☐ a. RBBB, incomplete
- ☐ b. RBBB, complete
- ☐ c. Left anterior fascicular block
- ☐ d. Left posterior fascicular block
- ☐ e. LBBB, with ST-T wave suggestive of acute myocardial injury or infarction
- ☐ f. LBBB, complete
- ☐ g. LBBB, intermittent
- ☐ h. Intraventricular conduction disturbance, nonspecific
- ☐ i. Aberrant intraventricular conduction with supraventricular arrhythmia

8. P WAVE ABNORMALITIES
- ☐ a. Right atrial abnormality
- ☐ b. Left atrial abnormalities
- ☐ c. Nonspecific atrial abnormality

9. ABNORMALITIES OF QRS VOLTAGE OR AXIS
- ☐ a. Low voltage, limb leads only
- ☐ b. Low voltage, limb and precordial leads
- ☐ c. Left axis deviation (> - 30%)
- ☐ d. Right axis deviation (> + 100)
- ☐ e. Electrical alternans

10. VENTRICULAR HYPERTROPHY
- ☐ a. LVH by voltage only
- ☐ b. LVH by voltage and ST-T segment abnormalities
- ☐ c. RVH
- ☐ d. Combined ventricular hypertrophy

11. Q WAVE MYOCARDIAL INFARCTION

	Probably Acute or Recent	Probably Old or Age Indeterminate
Anterolateral	☐ a.	☐ g.
Anterior	☐ b.	☐ h.
Anteroseptal	☐ c.	☐ i.
Lateral/High lateral	☐ d.	☐ j.
Inferior	☐ e.	☐ k.
Posterior	☐ f.	☐ l.

- ☐ m. Probably ventricular aneurysm

12. ST, T, U, WAVE ABNORMALITIES
- ☐ a. Normal variant, early repolarization
- ☐ b. Normal variant, juvenile T waves
- ☐ c. Nonspecific ST and/or T wave abnormalities
- ☐ d. ST and/or T wave abnormalities suggesting myocardial ischemia
- ☐ e. ST and/or T wave abnormalities suggesting myocardial injury
- ☐ f. ST and/or T wave abnormalities suggesting acute pericarditis
- ☐ g. ST-T segment abnormalities secondary to intraventricular conduction disturbance or hypertrophy
- ☐ h. Post-extrasystolic T wave abnormality
- ☐ i. Isolated J point depression
- ☐ j. Peaked T waves
- ☐ k. Prolonged QT interval
- ☐ l. Prominent U waves

13. PACEMAKER FUNCTION AND RHYTHM
- ☐ a. Atrial or coronary sinus pacing
- ☐ b. Ventricular demand pacing
- ☐ c. AV sequential pacing
- ☐ d. Ventricular pacing, complete control
- ☐ e. Dual chamber, atrial sensing pacemaker
- ☐ f. Pacemaker malfunction, not constantly capturing (atrium or ventricle)
- ☐ g. Pacemaker malfunction, not constantly sensing (atrium or ventricle)
- ☐ h. Pacemaker malfunction, not firing
- ☐ i. Pacemaker malfunction, slowing

14. SUGGESTED OR PROBABLE CLINICAL DISORDERS
- ☐ a. Digitalis effect
- ☐ b. Digitalis toxicity
- ☐ c. Antiarrhythmic drug effect
- ☐ d. Antiarrhythmic drug toxicity
- ☐ e. Hyperkalemia
- ☐ f. Hypokalemia
- ☐ g. Hypercalcemia
- ☐ h. Hypocalcemia
- ☐ i. Atrial septal defect, secundum
- ☐ j. Atrial septal defect, primum
- ☐ k. Dextrocardia, mirror image
- ☐ l. Mitral valve disease
- ☐ m. Chronic lung disease
- ☐ n. Acute cor pulmonale, including pulmonary embolus
- ☐ o. Pericardial effusion
- ☐ p. Acute pericarditis
- ☐ q. Hypertrophic cardiomyopathy
- ☐ r. Coronary artery disease
- ☐ s. Central nervous system disorder
- ☐ t. Myxedema
- ☐ u. Hypothermia
- ☐ v. Sick sinus syndrome

ECG 29 was obtained in this 86-year-old male with palpitations and shortness of breath. The ECG shows multifocal atrial tachycardia and nonspecific ST and/or T wave changes. The arrows in the rhythm strip (lead II) mark several of the different P wave morphologies present in this tracing.

Codes:

2n	Atrial tachycardia, multifocal
12c	Nonspecific ST and/or T wave abnormalities

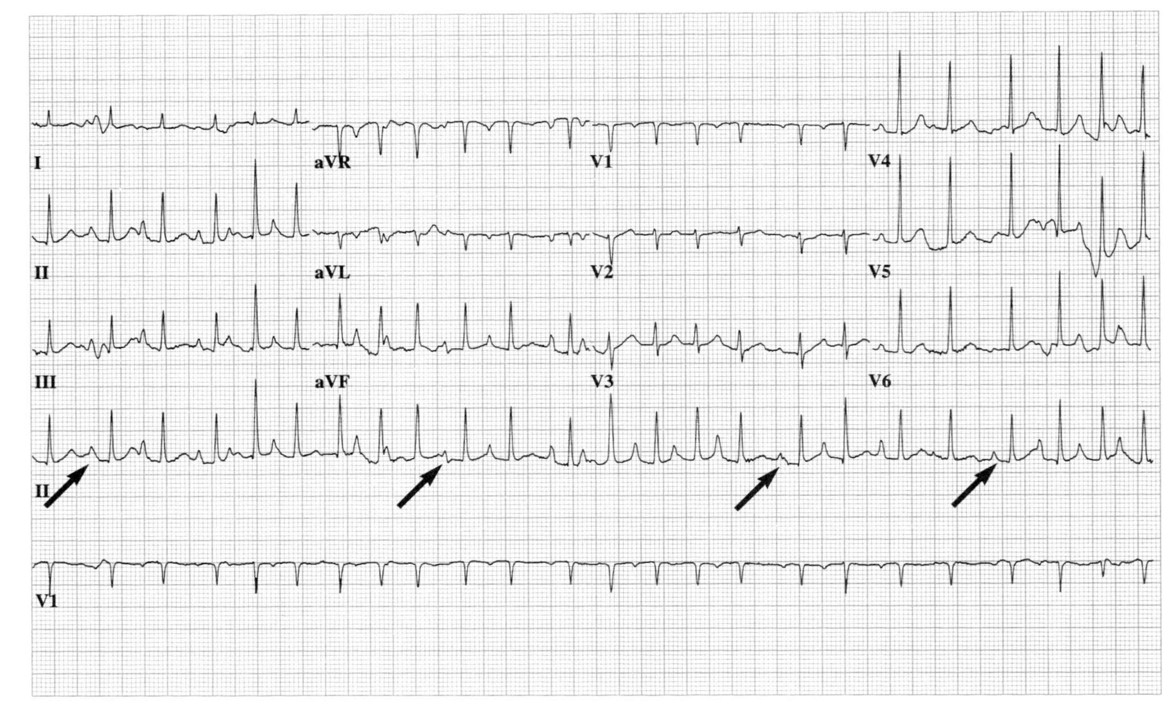

Questions: ECG 29

1. ECG features of multifocal atrial tachycardia include:

   a. Atrial rate > 100/minute
   b. Variable PR and RR intervals
   c. Absence of one dominant atrial pacemaker
   d. Normal AV conduction
   e. P waves of at least three morphologies
   f. Isoelectric baseline between P waves

2. Irregularly irregular rhythms include:

   a. Atrial fibrillation
   b. Multifocal atrial tachycardia
   c. Ventricular trigeminy
   d. Sinus tachycardia with frequent atrial premature complexes
   e. Atrial flutter with 4:1 AV conduction

Answers: ECG 29

1. Multifocal atrial tachycardia (MAT) is diagnosed when the atrial rate exceeds than 100 beats/minutes and there are at least 3 different P wave morphologies, each originating from a separate atrial focus . The absence of one dominant atrial pacemaker distinguishes MAT from sinus tachycardia with frequent multifocal atrial premature complexes. MAT is also characterized by the presence of an isoelectric baseline between P waves (as opposed to coarse atrial fibrillation), and rhythm irregularity, resulting in variable PR and RP intervals. MAT does not effect or require AV conduction and can persist during AV block. (Answer: All except d)

2. Irregularly irregular rhythms include atrial fibrillation, multifocal atrial tachycardia, and sinus tachycardia with frequent APCs (unless they are in a regular pattern such as bigeminy or trigeminy). Ventricular trigeminy (two normal QRS complexes followed by a ventricular premature complex in a repeating pattern) results in a regularly irregular rhythm. Atrial flutter with 4:1 AV conduction presents as a regular rhythm. (Answer: a, b, d)

— Quick Review 29 —

Atrial tachycardia, multifocal	
• Atrial rate > _____ per minute	100
• P waves with ≥ _____ morphologies	3
• PR, RR and RP intervals (are constant/vary)	vary
• May be confused with sinus tachycardia with multifocal APCs, or atrial fibrillation/flutter with a rapid ventricular response, but:	
▸ Unlike sinus tachycardia with multifocal APCs, multifocal atrial tachycardia (does/does not) manifest a dominant P wave morphology	does not
▸ Unlike atrial fibrillation/flutter, multifocal atrial tachycardia has a distinct ____ baseline	isoelectric
• P waves may be blocked or conducted with a narrow or aberrant QRS complex (true/false)	true
Nonspecific ST and/or T wave abnormalities	
• Slight ____ segment depression or elevation	ST
• Slightly inverted or flat ____ wave	T

Differential Diagnosis

NONSPECIFIC ST AND/OR T WAVE ABNORMALITIES

(Slight [< 1mm] ST depression or elevation, *and/or* T wave flat or slightly inverted)

- Organic heart disease
- Drugs (e.g., quinidine)
- Electrolyte disorders (e.g., hypokalemia, item 14f)
- Hyperventilation
- Hypothyroidism (item 14t)
- Stress
- Pancreatitis
- Pericarditis (item 14p)
- CNS disorders (item 14s)
- LVH (item 10b)
- RVH (item 10c)
- Bundle branch block (items 7a, f)
- Healthy adults (normal variant) (item 1b)

ECG 30. 49-year-old woman with dry skin, weakness, cold intolerance, constipation & weight gain:

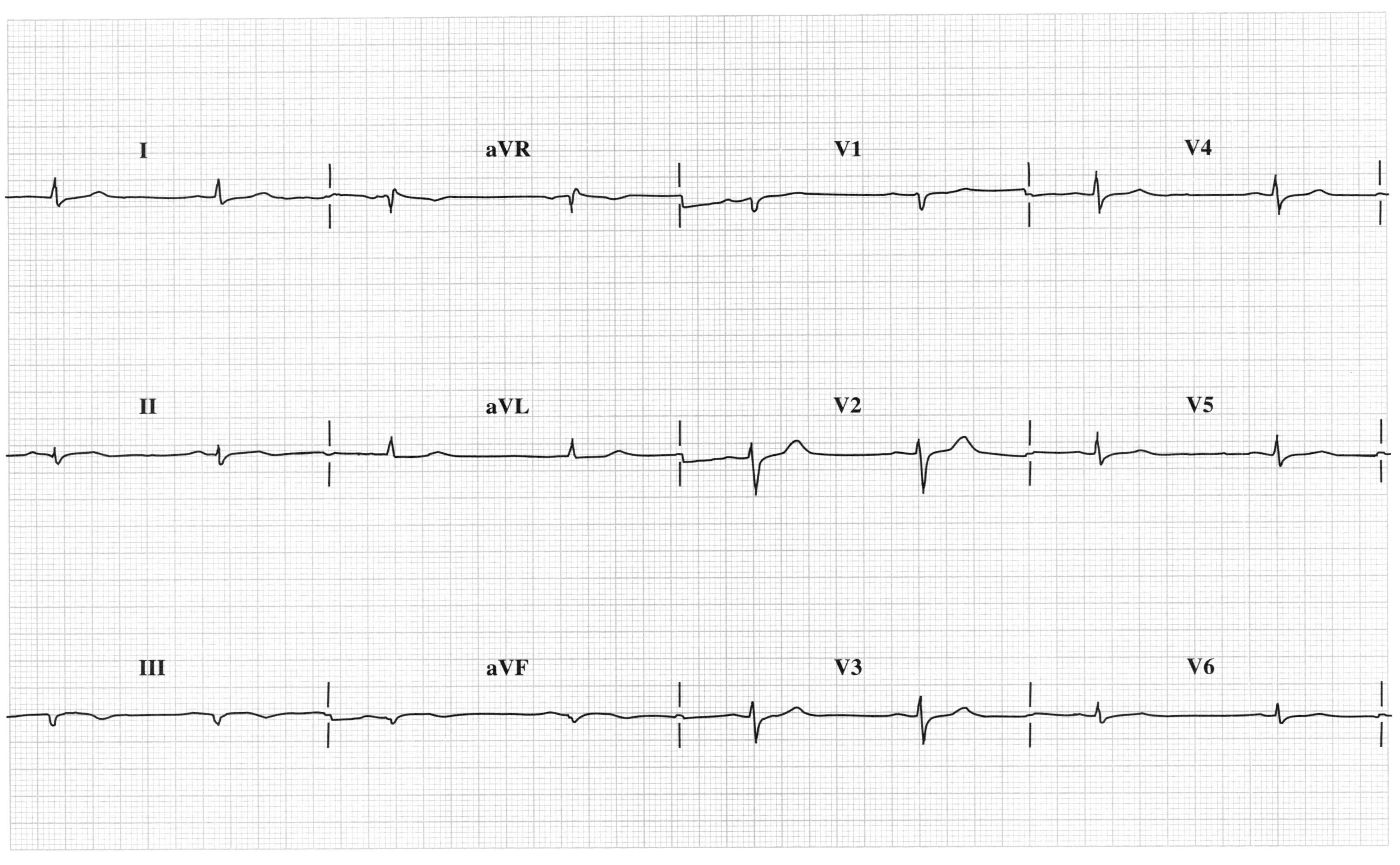

1. GENERAL FEATURES
- ☐ a. Normal ECG
- ☐ b. Borderline normal ECG or normal variant
- ☐ c. Incorrect electrode placement
- ☐ d. Artifact due to tremor

2. ATRIAL RHYTHMS
- ☐ a. Sinus rhythm
- ☐ b. Sinus arrhythmia
- ☐ c. Sinus bradycardia (< 60)
- ☐ d. Sinus tachycardia (> 100)
- ☐ e. Sinus pause or arrest
- ☐ f. Sinoatrial exit block
- ☐ g. Ecoptic atrial rhythm
- ☐ h. Wandering atrial pacemaker
- ☐ i. Atrial premature complexes, normally conducted
- ☐ j. Atrial premature complexes, nonconducted
- ☐ k. Atrial premature complexes with aberrant intraventricular conduction
- ☐ l. Atrial tachycardia (regular, sustained, 1:1 conduction)
- ☐ m. Atrial tachycardia, repetitive (short paroxysms)
- ☐ n. Atrial tachycardia, multifocal
- ☐ o. Atrial tachycardia with AV block
- ☐ p. Supraventricular tachycardia, unspecific
- ☐ q. Supraventricular tachycardia, paroxysmal
- ☐ r. Atrial flutter
- ☐ s. Atrial fibrillation
- ☐ t. Retrograde atrial activation

3. AV JUNCTIONAL RHYTHMS
- ☐ a. AV junctional premature complexes
- ☐ b. AV junctional escape complexes
- ☐ c. AV junctional rhythm, accelerated
- ☐ d. AV junctional rhythm

4. VENTRICULAR RHYTHMS
- ☐ a. Ventricular premature complex(es), uniform, fixed coupling
- ☐ b. Ventricular premature complex(es), uniform, nonfixed coupling
- ☐ c. Ventricular premature complexes(es), multiform
- ☐ d. Ventricular premature complexes, in pairs
- ☐ e. Ventricular parasystole
- ☐ f. Ventricular tachycardia (≥ 3 consecutive complexes)
- ☐ g. Accelerated idioventricular rhythm
- ☐ h. Ventricular escape complexes or rhythm
- ☐ i. Ventricular fibrillation

5. ATRIAL-VENTRICULAR INTERACTIONS IN ARRHYTHMIAS
- ☐ a. Fusion complexes
- ☐ b. Reciprocal (echo) complexes
- ☐ c. Ventricular capture complexes
- ☐ d. AV dissociation
- ☐ e. Ventriculophasic sinus arrhythmia

6. AV CONDUCTION ABNORMALITIES
- ☐ a. AV block, 1°
- ☐ b. AV block, 2° - Mobitz type I (Wenckebach)
- ☐ c. AV block, 2° - Mobitz type II
- ☐ d. AV block, 2:1
- ☐ e. AV block, 3°
- ☐ f. AV block, variable
- ☐ g. Short PR interval (with sinus rhythm and normal QRS duration)
- ☐ h. Wolff-Parkinson-White pattern

7. INTRAVENTRICULAR CONDUCTION DISTURBANCES
- ☐ a. RBBB, incomplete
- ☐ b. RBBB, complete
- ☐ c. Left anterior fascicular block
- ☐ d. Left posterior fascicular block
- ☐ e. LBBB, with ST-T wave suggestive of acute myocardial injury or infarction
- ☐ f. LBBB, complete
- ☐ g. LBBB, intermittent
- ☐ h. Intraventricular conduction disturbance, nonspecific
- ☐ i. Aberrant intraventricular conduction with supraventricular arrhythmia

8. P WAVE ABNORMALITIES
- ☐ a. Right atrial abnormality
- ☐ b. Left atrial abnormalities
- ☐ c. Nonspecific atrial abnormality

9. ABNORMALITIES OF QRS VOLTAGE OR AXIS
- ☐ a. Low voltage, limb leads only
- ☐ b. Low voltage, limb and precordial leads
- ☐ c. Left axis deviation (> - 30%)
- ☐ d. Right axis deviation (> + 100)
- ☐ e. Electrical alternans

10. VENTRICULAR HYPERTROPHY
- ☐ a. LVH by voltage only
- ☐ b. LVH by voltage and ST-T segment abnormalities
- ☐ c. RVH
- ☐ d. Combined ventricular hypertrophy

11. Q WAVE MYOCARDIAL INFARCTION

	Probably Acute or Recent	Probably Old or Age Indeterminate
Anterolateral	☐ a.	☐ g.
Anterior	☐ b.	☐ h.
Anteroseptal	☐ c.	☐ i.
Lateral/High lateral	☐ d.	☐ j.
Inferior	☐ e.	☐ k.
Posterior	☐ f.	☐ l.

- ☐ m. Probably ventricular aneurysm

12. ST, T, U, WAVE ABNORMALITIES
- ☐ a. Normal variant, early repolarization
- ☐ b. Normal variant, juvenile T waves
- ☐ c. Nonspecific ST and/or T wave abnormalities
- ☐ d. ST and/or T wave abnormalities suggesting myocardial ischemia
- ☐ e. ST and/or T wave abnormalities suggesting myocardial injury
- ☐ f. ST and/or T wave abnormalities suggesting acute pericarditis
- ☐ g. ST-T segment abnormalities secondary to intraventricular conduction disturbance or hypertrophy
- ☐ h. Post-extrasystolic T wave abnormality
- ☐ i. Isolated J point depression
- ☐ j. Peaked T waves
- ☐ k. Prolonged QT interval
- ☐ l. Prominent U waves

13. PACEMAKER FUNCTION AND RHYTHM
- ☐ a. Atrial or coronary sinus pacing
- ☐ b. Ventricular demand pacing
- ☐ c. AV sequential pacing
- ☐ d. Ventricular pacing, complete control
- ☐ e. Dual chamber, atrial sensing pacemaker
- ☐ f. Pacemaker malfunction, not constantly capturing (atrium or ventricle)
- ☐ g. Pacemaker malfunction, not constantly sensing (atrium or ventricle)
- ☐ h. Pacemaker malfunction, not firing
- ☐ i. Pacemaker malfunction, slowing

14. SUGGESTED OR PROBABLE CLINICAL DISORDERS
- ☐ a. Digitalis effect
- ☐ b. Digitalis toxicity
- ☐ c. Antiarrhythmic drug effect
- ☐ d. Antiarrhythmic drug toxicity
- ☐ e. Hyperkalemia
- ☐ f. Hypokalemia
- ☐ g. Hypercalcemia
- ☐ h. Hypocalcemia
- ☐ i. Atrial septal defect, secundum
- ☐ j. Atrial septal defect, primum
- ☐ k. Dextrocardia, mirror image
- ☐ l. Mitral valve disease
- ☐ m. Chronic lung disease
- ☐ n. Acute cor pulmonale, including pulmonary embolus
- ☐ o. Pericardial effusion
- ☐ p. Acute pericarditis
- ☐ q. Hypertrophic cardiomyopathy
- ☐ r. Coronary artery disease
- ☐ s. Central nervous system disorder
- ☐ t. Myxedema
- ☐ u. Hypothermia
- ☐ v. Sick sinus syndrome

ECG 30 was obtained from a 49-year-old woman with complaints of dry skin, weakness, cold intolerance, constipation, and weight gain. The ECG shows sinus bradycardia with left axis deviation, relatively low voltage QRS complexes (which do not quite meet criteria for formal coding of low voltage), old or age indeterminate inferior myocardial infarction, and minor nonspecific ST-T abnormalities. The ECG findings, especially when considered in context of the clinical presentation, are consistent with a diagnosis of hypothyroidism/myxedema. This woman had a past history of an inferior MI and was documented to be profoundly hypothyroid.

Codes:

2c	Sinus bradycardia
11k	Inferior Q wave MI, probably old or age indeterminate
14r	Coronary artery disease
14t	Myxedema

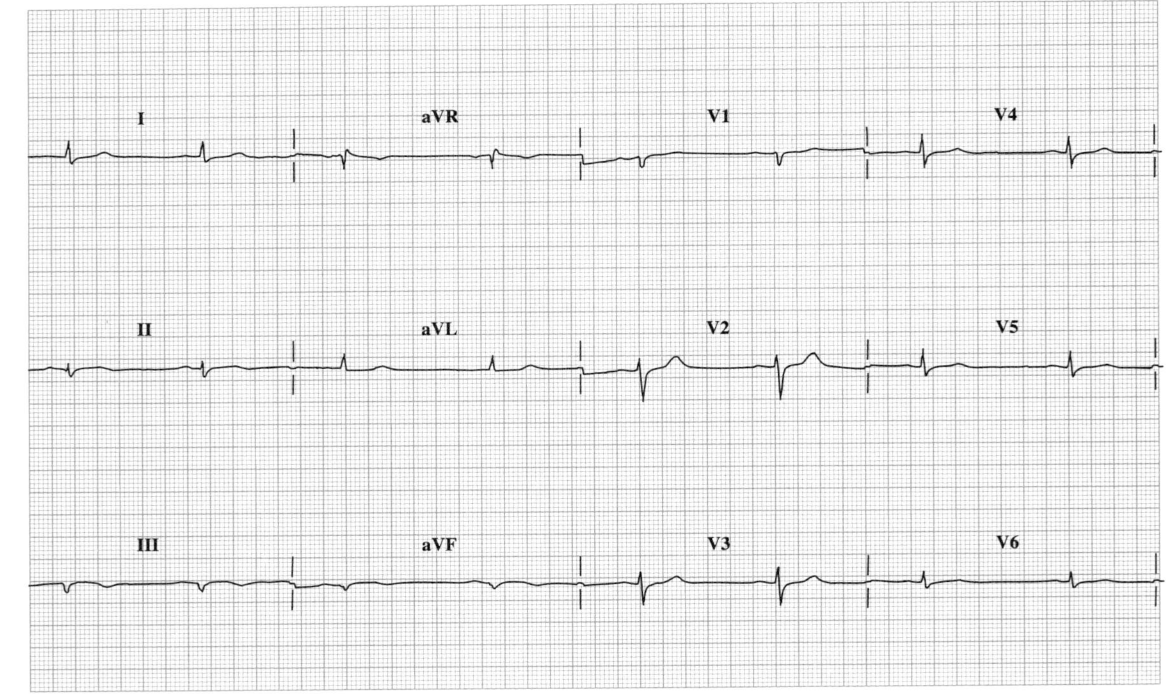

Questions: ECG 30

1. The differential diagnosis for low voltage ECG includes:

   a. COPD
   b. Myxedema
   c. Obesity
   d. Pericardial effusion
   e. Pleural effusion
   f. Amyloid heart
   g. Sarcoidosis of the heart
   h. Diffuse coronary artery disease
   i. Congestive heart failure

— Quick Review 30 —

Low voltage, limb and precordial leads	
• Amplitude of the entire QRS complex (R+S) < ____ mm in all precordial leads and < ____ mm in all limb leads	10 5
Inferior MI, age indeterminate or probably old	
• Abnormal Q waves (with/without) ST elevation in at least two of leads ____	without II, III, aVF
Myxedema	
• (High/low) QRS voltage in all leads	Low
• Sinus (tachycardia/bradycardia)	bradycardia
• T wave flattened or (upright/inverted)	inverted
• PR interval may be (shortened/prolonged)	prolonged
• Frequently associated with pericardial ____	effusion
• Electrical alternans may occur (true/false)	true

Answers: ECG 30

1. The amplitude of the QRS complex is often decreased by conditions that increase the amount of body tissue (obesity), air (COPD, pneumothorax), fluid (pericardial or plural effusion), fibrous tissue (coronary artery disease) or other infiltrative substances (sarcoid, amyloid, myxedema) between the myocardium and the surface ECG electrodes. (Answer: All)

ECG 31. 80-year-old female with chronic renal failure:

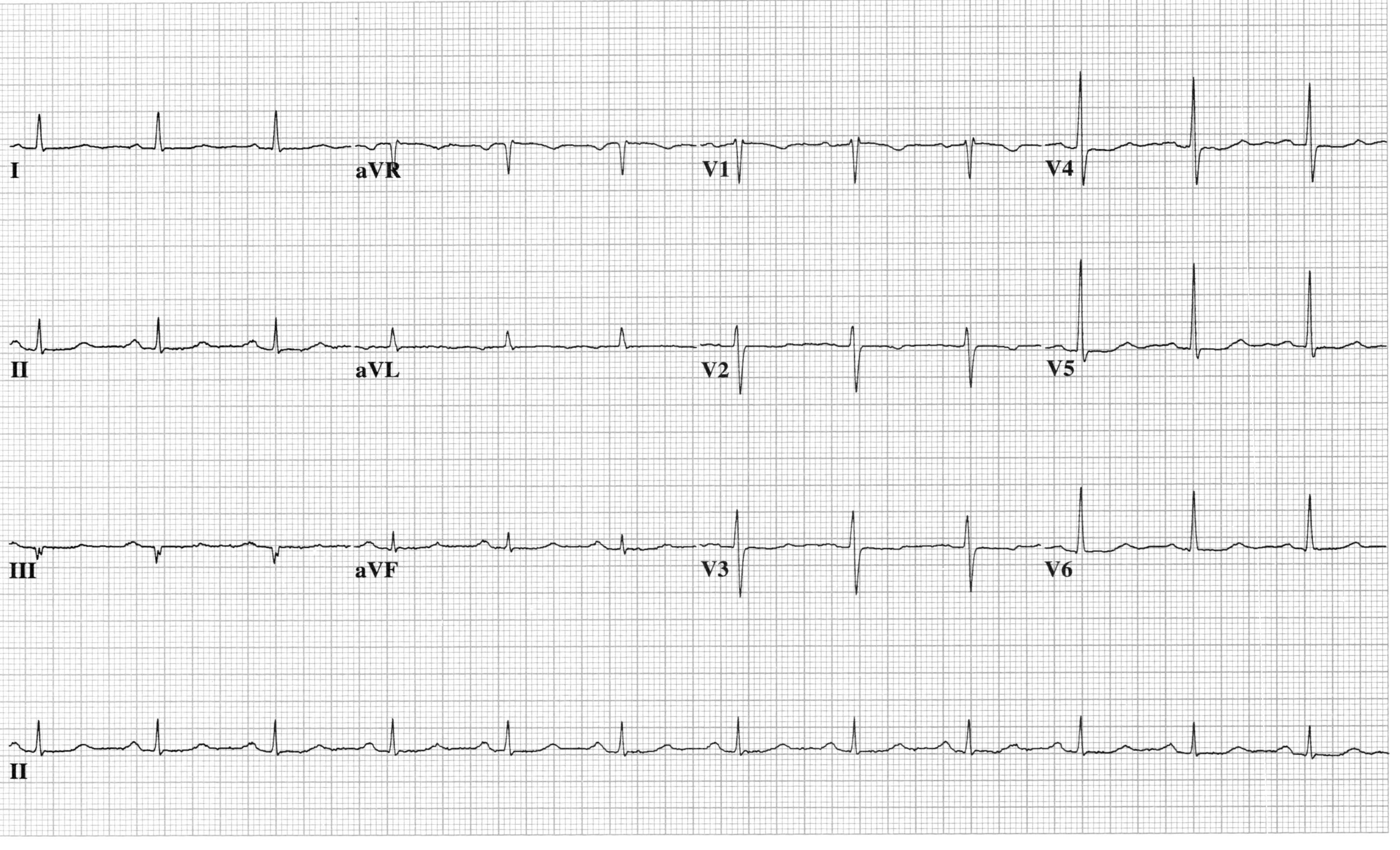

1. GENERAL FEATURES

☐ a. Normal ECG
☐ b. Borderline normal ECG or normal variant
☐ c. Incorrect electrode placement
☐ d. Artifact due to tremor

2. ATRIAL RHYTHMS

☐ a. Sinus rhythm
☐ b. Sinus arrhythmia
☐ c. Sinus bradycardia (< 60)
☐ d. Sinus tachycardia (> 100)
☐ e. Sinus pause or arrest
☐ f. Sinoatrial exit block
☐ g. Ecoptic atrial rhythm
☐ h. Wandering atrial pacemaker
☐ i. Atrial premature complexes, normally conducted
☐ j. Atrial premature complexes, nonconducted
☐ k. Atrial premature complexes with aberrant intraventricular conduction
☐ l. Atrial tachycardia (regular, sustained, 1:1 conduction)
☐ m. Atrial tachycardia, repetitive (short paroxysms)
☐ n. Atrial tachycardia, multifocal
☐ o. Atrial tachycardia with AV block
☐ p. Supraventricular tachycardia, unspecific
☐ q. Supraventricular tachycardia, paroxysmal
☐ r. Atrial flutter
☐ s. Atrial fibrillation
☐ t. Retrograde atrial activation

3. AV JUNCTIONAL RHYTHMS

☐ a. AV junctional premature complexes
☐ b. AV junctional escape complexes
☐ c. AV junctional rhythm, accelerated
☐ d. AV junctional rhythm

4. VENTRICULAR RHYTHMS

☐ a. Ventricular premature complex(es), uniform, fixed coupling
☐ b. Ventricular premature complex(es), uniform, nonfixed coupling
☐ c. Ventricular premature complexes(es), multiform
☐ d. Ventricular premature complexes, in pairs
☐ e. Ventricular parasystole
☐ f. Ventricular tachycardia (≥ 3 consecutive complexes)
☐ g. Accelerated idioventricular rhythm
☐ h. Ventricular escape complexes or rhythm
☐ i. Ventricular fibrillation

5. ATRIAL-VENTRICULAR INTERACTIONS IN ARRHYTHMIAS

☐ a. Fusion complexes
☐ b. Reciprocal (echo) complexes
☐ c. Ventricular capture complexes
☐ d. AV dissociation
☐ e. Ventriculophasic sinus arrhythmia

6. AV CONDUCTION ABNORMALITIES

☐ a. AV block, 1°
☐ b. AV block, 2° - Mobitz type I (Wenckebach)
☐ c. AV block, 2° - Mobitz type II
☐ d. AV block, 2:1
☐ e. AV block, 3°
☐ f. AV block, variable
☐ g. Short PR interval (with sinus rhythm and normal QRS duration)
☐ h. Wolff-Parkinson-White pattern

7. INTRAVENTRICULAR CONDUCTION DISTURBANCES

☐ a. RBBB, incomplete
☐ b. RBBB, complete
☐ c. Left anterior fascicular block
☐ d. Left posterior fascicular block
☐ e. LBBB, with ST-T wave suggestive of acute myocardial injury or infarction
☐ f. LBBB, complete
☐ g. LBBB, intermittent
☐ h. Intraventricular conduction disturbance, nonspecific
☐ i. Aberrant intraventricular conduction with supraventricular arrhythmia

8. P WAVE ABNORMALITIES

☐ a. Right atrial abnormality
☐ b. Left atrial abnormalities
☐ c. Nonspecific atrial abnormality

9. ABNORMALITIES OF QRS VOLTAGE OR AXIS

☐ a. Low voltage, limb leads only
☐ b. Low voltage, limb and precordial leads
☐ c. Left axis deviation (> - 30%)
☐ d. Right axis deviation (> + 100)
☐ e. Electrical alternans

10. VENTRICULAR HYPERTROPHY

☐ a. LVH by voltage only
☐ b. LVH by voltage and ST-T segment abnormalities
☐ c. RVH
☐ d. Combined ventricular hypertrophy

11. Q WAVE MYOCARDIAL INFARCTION

	Probably Acute or Recent	Probably Old or Age Indeterminate
Anterolateral	☐ a.	☐ g.
Anterior	☐ b.	☐ h.
Anteroseptal	☐ c.	☐ i.
Lateral/High lateral	☐ d.	☐ j.
Inferior	☐ e.	☐ k.
Posterior	☐ f.	☐ l.

☐ m. Probably ventricular aneurysm

12. ST, T, U, WAVE ABNORMALITIES

☐ a. Normal variant, early repolarization
☐ b. Normal variant, juvenile T waves
☐ c. Nonspecific ST and/or T wave abnormalities
☐ d. ST and/or T wave abnormalities suggesting myocardial ischemia
☐ e. ST and/or T wave abnormalities suggesting myocardial injury
☐ f. ST and/or T wave abnormalities suggesting acute pericarditis
☐ g. ST-T segment abnormalities secondary to intraventricular conduction disturbance or hypertrophy
☐ h. Post-extrasystolic T wave abnormality
☐ i. Isolated J point depression
☐ j. Peaked T waves
☐ k. Prolonged QT interval
☐ l. Prominent U waves

13. PACEMAKER FUNCTION AND RHYTHM

☐ a. Atrial or coronary sinus pacing
☐ b. Ventricular demand pacing
☐ c. AV sequential pacing
☐ d. Ventricular pacing, complete control
☐ e. Dual chamber, atrial sensing pacemaker
☐ f. Pacemaker malfunction, not constantly capturing (atrium or ventricle)
☐ g. Pacemaker malfunction, not constantly sensing (atrium or ventricle)
☐ h. Pacemaker malfunction, not firing
☐ i. Pacemaker malfunction, slowing

14. SUGGESTED OR PROBABLE CLINICAL DISORDERS

☐ a. Digitalis effect
☐ b. Digitalis toxicity
☐ c. Antiarrhythmic drug effect
☐ d. Antiarrhythmic drug toxicity
☐ e. Hyperkalemia
☐ f. Hypokalemia
☐ g. Hypercalcemia
☐ h. Hypocalcemia
☐ i. Atrial septal defect, secundum
☐ j. Atrial septal defect, primum
☐ k. Dextrocardia, mirror image
☐ l. Mitral valve disease
☐ m. Chronic lung disease
☐ n. Acute cor pulmonale, including pulmonary embolus
☐ o. Pericardial effusion
☐ p. Acute pericarditis
☐ q. Hypertrophic cardiomyopathy
☐ r. Coronary artery disease
☐ s. Central nervous system disorder
☐ t. Myxedema
☐ u. Hypothermia
☐ v. Sick sinus syndrome

ECG 31 was obtained in 80-year-old female with chronic renal failure. The ECG shows sinus rhythm with first-degree AV block, nonspecific ST-T wave abnormalities, and QT interval prolongation (corrected QT interval measures 0.50 seconds). The long QT interval is primarily due to prolongation of the ST segment rather than the T wave, a feature characteristic of hypocalcemia. This patient was shown to have a serum calcium level of 6.8 mg/dL.

Codes:

2a	Sinus rhythm
6a	AV block, 1°
12c	Nonspecific ST and/or T wave abnormality
12k	Prolonged QT interval
14h	Hypocalcemia

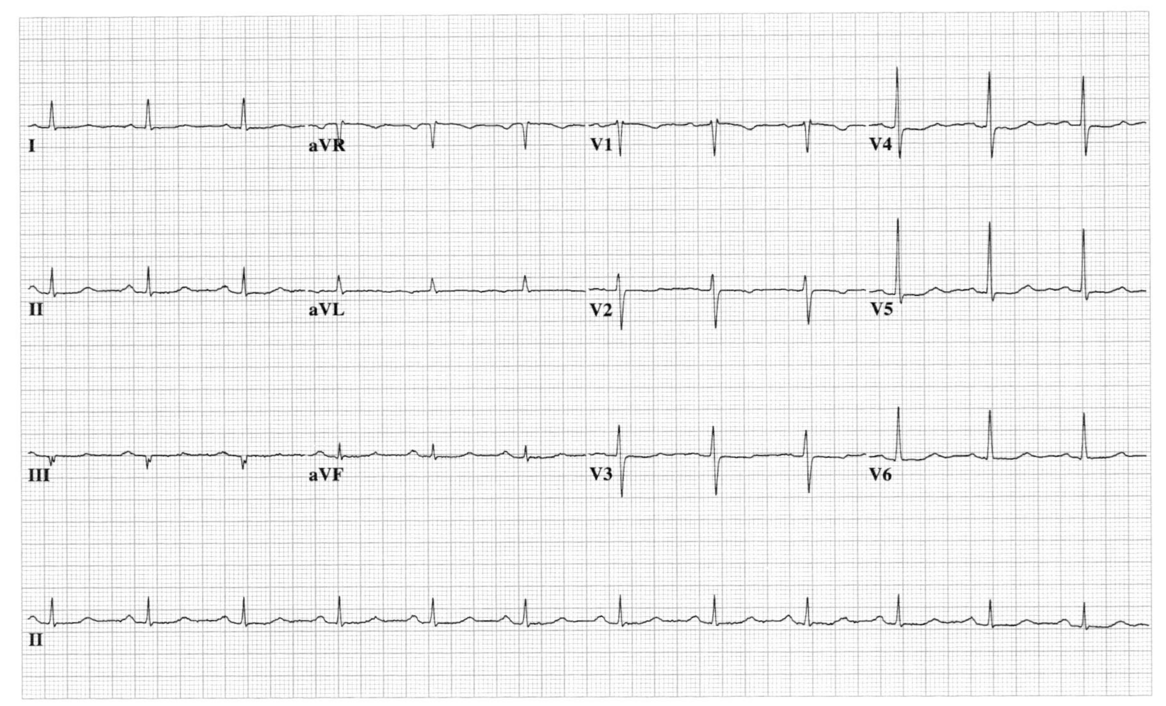

Questions: ECG 31

1. Electrolyte abnormalities associated with a prolonged QT interval include:

   a. Hypokalemia
   b. Hyperkalemia
   c. Hypocalcemia
   d. Hypercalcemia
   e. Hypomagnesemia
   f. Hypermagnesemia

2. Hypocalcemia is associated with:

   a. Prominent U waves
   b. Characteristic notching of the terminal QRS (Osborne wave)
   c. Normal T wave duration
   d. Flattened, peaked, or inverted T waves
   e. QT prolongation due to ST segment prolongation

Answers: ECG 31

1. When it comes to electrolyte disorders associated with a prolonged QT interval, think "hypo" — hypokalemia, hypocalcemia, and hypomagnesemia. (Answer: a, c, e)

2. Hypocalcemia prolongs the QT interval in a very characteristic way, namely, by prolonging the ST segment and not the T wave — the T wave can be mildly flattened, peaked, or inverted, but has a normal duration. Prominent U waves are typical of hypocalcemia (and other electrolyte disorders associated with a long QT, including hypokalemia and hypomagnesemia). Abnormal notching of the terminal QRS complex (Osborne wave) occurs in hypothermia, not hypocalcemia. (Answer: c, d, e)

— Quick Review 31 —

Prolonged QT interval	
• Corrected QT interval (QTc) ≥ ____ seconds, where QTc = QT interval divided by the square root of the preceding ____ interval	0.42-0.46 RR
• QT interval varies (directly/inversely) with heart rate	inversely
• The normal QT interval should be (less than/greater than) 50% of the RR interval	less than
Hypocalcemia	
• Earliest and most common finding is prolonged ____ interval	QT
• Occasional flattening, peaking, or inversion of ____ waves	T

ECG 32. 69-year-old male with orthopnea and pedal edema:

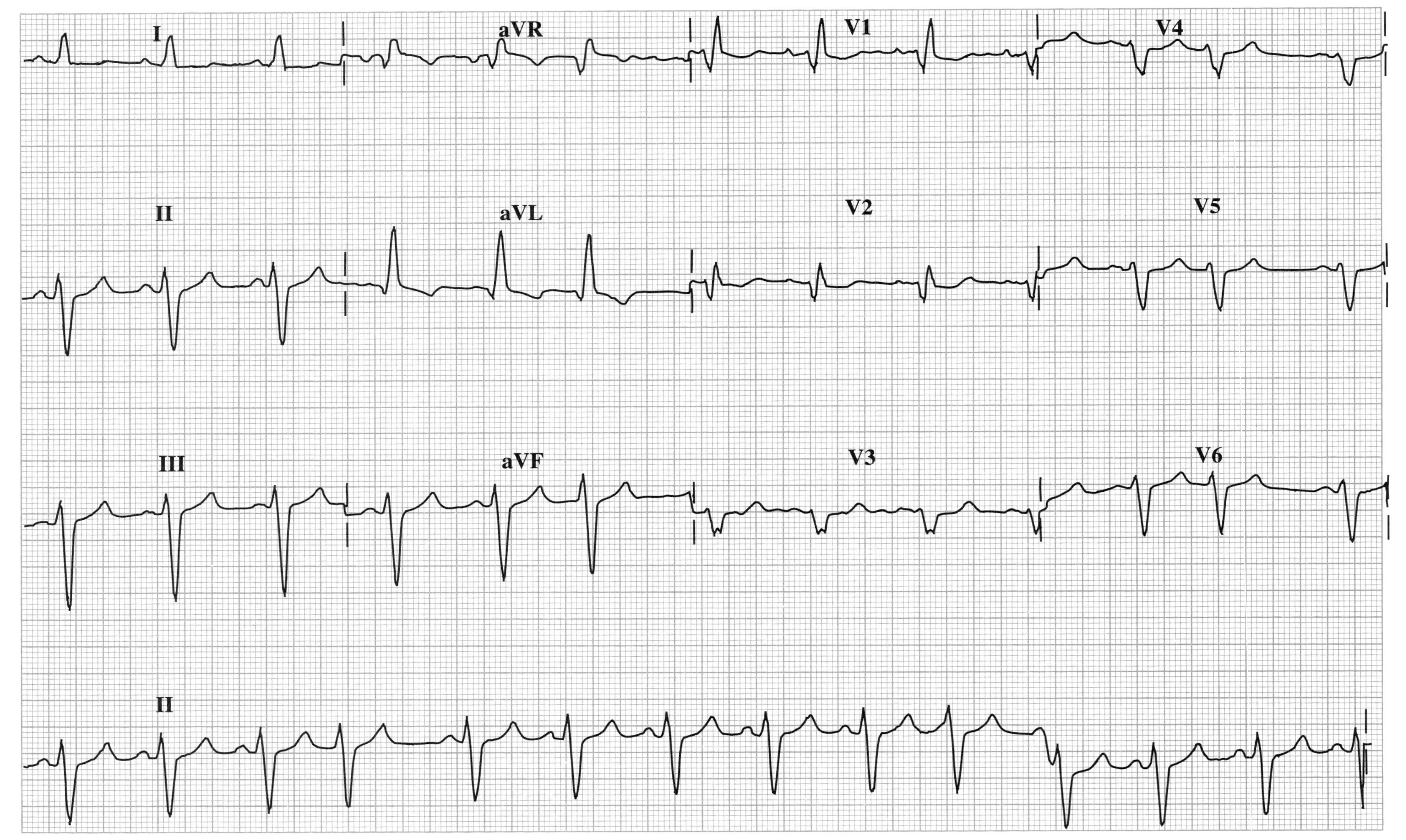

1. GENERAL FEATURES
- ☐ a. Normal ECG
- ☐ b. Borderline normal ECG or normal variant
- ☐ c. Incorrect electrode placement
- ☐ d. Artifact due to tremor

2. ATRIAL RHYTHMS
- ☐ a. Sinus rhythm
- ☐ b. Sinus arrhythmia
- ☐ c. Sinus bradycardia (< 60)
- ☐ d. Sinus tachycardia (> 100)
- ☐ e. Sinus pause or arrest
- ☐ f. Sinoatrial exit block
- ☐ g. Ecoptic atrial rhythm
- ☐ h. Wandering atrial pacemaker
- ☐ i. Atrial premature complexes, normally conducted
- ☐ j. Atrial premature complexes, nonconducted
- ☐ k. Atrial premature complexes with aberrant intraventricular conduction
- ☐ l. Atrial tachycardia (regular, sustained, 1:1 conduction)
- ☐ m. Atrial tachycardia, repetitive (short paroxysms)
- ☐ n. Atrial tachycardia, multifocal
- ☐ o. Atrial tachycardia with AV block
- ☐ p. Supraventricular tachycardia, unspecific
- ☐ q. Supraventricular tachycardia, paroxysmal
- ☐ r. Atrial flutter
- ☐ s. Atrial fibrillation
- ☐ t. Retrograde atrial activation

3. AV JUNCTIONAL RHYTHMS
- ☐ a. AV junctional premature complexes
- ☐ b. AV junctional escape complexes
- ☐ c. AV junctional rhythm, accelerated
- ☐ d. AV junctional rhythm

4. VENTRICULAR RHYTHMS
- ☐ a. Ventricular premature complex(es), uniform, fixed coupling
- ☐ b. Ventricular premature complex(es), uniform, nonfixed coupling
- ☐ c. Ventricular premature complexes(es), multiform
- ☐ d. Ventricular premature complexes, in pairs
- ☐ e. Ventricular parasystole
- ☐ f. Ventricular tachycardia (≥ 3 consecutive complexes)
- ☐ g. Accelerated idioventricular rhythm
- ☐ h. Ventricular escape complexes or rhythm
- ☐ i. Ventricular fibrillation

5. ATRIAL-VENTRICULAR INTERACTIONS IN ARRHYTHMIAS
- ☐ a. Fusion complexes
- ☐ b. Reciprocal (echo) complexes
- ☐ c. Ventricular capture complexes
- ☐ d. AV dissociation
- ☐ e. Ventriculophasic sinus arrhythmia

6. AV CONDUCTION ABNORMALITIES
- ☐ a. AV block, 1°
- ☐ b. AV block, 2° - Mobitz type I (Wenckebach)
- ☐ c. AV block, 2° - Mobitz type II
- ☐ d. AV block, 2:1
- ☐ e. AV block, 3°
- ☐ f. AV block, variable
- ☐ g. Short PR interval (with sinus rhythm and normal QRS duration)
- ☐ h. Wolff-Parkinson-White pattern

7. INTRAVENTRICULAR CONDUCTION DISTURBANCES
- ☐ a. RBBB, incomplete
- ☐ b. RBBB, complete
- ☐ c. Left anterior fascicular block
- ☐ d. Left posterior fascicular block
- ☐ e. LBBB, with ST-T wave suggestive of acute myocardial injury or infarction
- ☐ f. LBBB, complete
- ☐ g. LBBB, intermittent
- ☐ h. Intraventricular conduction disturbance, nonspecific
- ☐ i. Aberrant intraventricular conduction with supraventricular arrhythmia

8. P WAVE ABNORMALITIES
- ☐ a. Right atrial abnormality
- ☐ b. Left atrial abnormalities
- ☐ c. Nonspecific atrial abnormality

9. ABNORMALITIES OF QRS VOLTAGE OR AXIS
- ☐ a. Low voltage, limb leads only
- ☐ b. Low voltage, limb and precordial leads
- ☐ c. Left axis deviation (> - 30%)
- ☐ d. Right axis deviation (> + 100)
- ☐ e. Electrical alternans

10. VENTRICULAR HYPERTROPHY
- ☐ a. LVH by voltage only
- ☐ b. LVH by voltage and ST-T segment abnormalities
- ☐ c. RVH
- ☐ d. Combined ventricular hypertrophy

11. Q WAVE MYOCARDIAL INFARCTION

	Probably Acute or Recent	Probably Old or Age Indeterminate
Anterolateral	☐ a.	☐ g.
Anterior	☐ b.	☐ h.
Anteroseptal	☐ c.	☐ i.
Lateral/High lateral	☐ d.	☐ j.
Inferior	☐ e.	☐ k.
Posterior	☐ f.	☐ l.

- ☐ m. Probably ventricular aneurysm

12. ST, T, U, WAVE ABNORMALITIES
- ☐ a. Normal variant, early repolarization
- ☐ b. Normal variant, juvenile T waves
- ☐ c. Nonspecific ST and/or T wave abnormalities
- ☐ d. ST and/or T wave abnormalities suggesting myocardial ischemia
- ☐ e. ST and/or T wave abnormalities suggesting myocardial injury
- ☐ f. ST and/or T wave abnormalities suggesting acute pericarditis
- ☐ g. ST-T segment abnormalities secondary to intraventricular conduction disturbance or hypertrophy
- ☐ h. Post-extrasystolic T wave abnormality
- ☐ i. Isolated J point depression
- ☐ j. Peaked T waves
- ☐ k. Prolonged QT interval
- ☐ l. Prominent U waves

13. PACEMAKER FUNCTION AND RHYTHM
- ☐ a. Atrial or coronary sinus pacing
- ☐ b. Ventricular demand pacing
- ☐ c. AV sequential pacing
- ☐ d. Ventricular pacing, complete control
- ☐ e. Dual chamber, atrial sensing pacemaker
- ☐ f. Pacemaker malfunction, not constantly capturing (atrium or ventricle)
- ☐ g. Pacemaker malfunction, not constantly sensing (atrium or ventricle)
- ☐ h. Pacemaker malfunction, not firing
- ☐ i. Pacemaker malfunction, slowing

14. SUGGESTED OR PROBABLE CLINICAL DISORDERS
- ☐ a. Digitalis effect
- ☐ b. Digitalis toxicity
- ☐ c. Antiarrhythmic drug effect
- ☐ d. Antiarrhythmic drug toxicity
- ☐ e. Hyperkalemia
- ☐ f. Hypokalemia
- ☐ g. Hypercalcemia
- ☐ h. Hypocalcemia
- ☐ i. Atrial septal defect, secundum
- ☐ j. Atrial septal defect, primum
- ☐ k. Dextrocardia, mirror image
- ☐ l. Mitral valve disease
- ☐ m. Chronic lung disease
- ☐ n. Acute cor pulmonale, including pulmonary embolus
- ☐ o. Pericardial effusion
- ☐ p. Acute pericarditis
- ☐ q. Hypertrophic cardiomyopathy
- ☐ r. Coronary artery disease
- ☐ s. Central nervous system disorder
- ☐ t. Myxedema
- ☐ u. Hypothermia
- ☐ v. Sick sinus syndrome

ECG 32 was obtained from a 69-year-old male with orthopnea and pedal edema. The ECG shows a sinus rhythm with normally-conducted APCs (arrows mark the premature P waves, which are superimposed on the preceding T waves). The T wave following the first APC in the rhythm strip is slightly more peaked than the previous T waves, suggesting a post-extrasystolic T wave abnormality. RBBB with secondary ST-T abnormalities, left axis deviation, and left anterior fascicular block are also present.

Codes:

2a	Sinus rhythm
2i	Atrial premature complexes, normally conducted
7b	RBBB, complete
7c	Left anterior fascicular block
9c	Left axis deviation (> -30°)
12g	ST-T segment abnormalities secondary to IVCD or hypertrophy
12h	Post-extrasystolic T wave abnormality

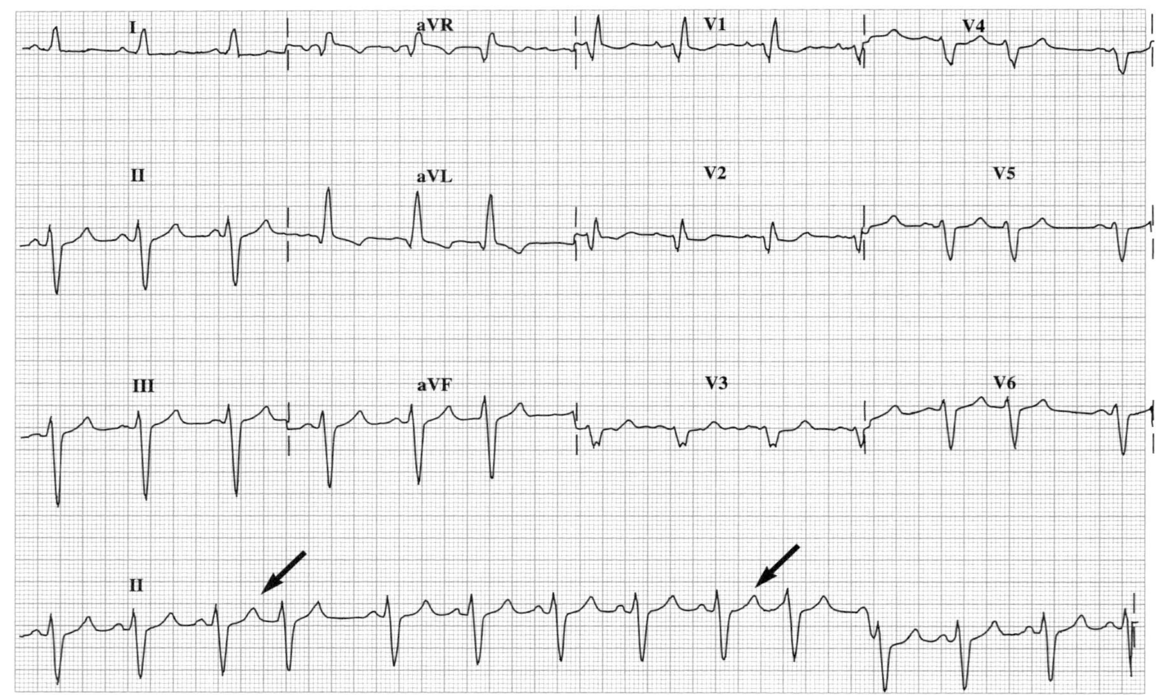

Questions: ECG 32

1. The tall R wave in aVL is highly specific for LVH:

   a. True
   b. False

2. Findings in this tracing that can be attributed to left anterior fascicular block include:

   a. qR in leads I and aVL
   b. rS in leads II, III and aVF
   c. Large S wave in leads V_4 - V_6
   d. Poor R wave progression

3. The most common cause of right bundle branch block and left anterior fascicular block is:

   a. Coronary artery disease
   b. Hypertensive heart disease
   c. Cardiomyopathy
   d. Lenegre's disease

4. The most common MI to present with RBBB and LAFB is:

   a. Inferior
   b. Anterior
   c. Lateral
   d. Posterior

5. What is the incidence of complete heart block when bifascicular block occurs during myocardial infarction?

   a. < 5%
   b. 5 - 10%
   c. 10 - 20%
   d. > 20%

6. Did the premature atrial contraction (4th beat in rhythm strip) reset the sinus node?

   a. Yes
   b. No

Answers: ECG 32

1. An R wave in lead aVL $\geq$ 12 mm lacks specificity for the diagnosis of LVH when left anterior fascicular block is present. (Answer: b)

2. ECG manifestations of left anterior fascicular block include left axis deviation, qR in leads I and aVL, and rS in leads II, III, and aVF. Large S waves in V_4 - V_6 and poor R wave progression may also be seen. (Answer: All)

3. The most common cause of bifascicular block (RBBB & LAFB) is coronary artery disease, responsible for up to 50% of cases. Other causes include hypertensive heart disease, calcific aortic valve disease (with extension of the calcification into the anterior interventricular septum), cardiomyopathy, Lev's disease, Lenegre's disease, surgical trauma, post cardiac transplant, and others. Complete heart block develops in 5-15% of patients with chronic bifascicular block and 25-40% of patients with bifascicular block secondary to acute MI. (Answer: a)

4. Anterior myocardial infarction secondary to occlusion of the proximal LAD coronary artery is the most common cause of acute bifascicular block (RBBB and LAFB). The right bundle branch and anterior division of the left bundle branch course together in the anterior portion of the interventricular septum, and receive their blood supply from septal perforators of the LAD. (Answer: b)

5. Since progression to complete heart block develops in more than 20% of patients who develop acute bifascicular block during MI; temporary transvenous pacing should be considered. When extensive anterior infarction is evident, mortality remains high despite the presence of a pacemaker; death is often due to pump failure rather than progression to complete heart block. (Answer: d)

6. The PP interval remains constant and the sinus node undisturbed by the premature atrial contraction in this tracing. (Answer: b)

— Quick Review 32 —	
Atrial premature complexes, normally conducted	
• P wave is (normal/abnormal) in configuration	abnormal
• QRS complex is (similar/different) in morphology to the QRS complex present during sinus rhythm	similar
• PR interval may be normal, increased, or decreased (true/false)	true
• The post-extrasystolic pause is usually (compensatory/noncompensatory)	noncompensatory

— Quick Review 32 —

RBBB, complete	
• QRS duration ≥ ____ seconds	0.12
• Secondary R wave (R') in lead ____ is usually (shorter/taller) than the initial R wave	V_1 taller
• Onset of intrinsicoid deflection in leads V_1 and V_2 > ____ seconds	0.05
• ST segment ____ and T wave ____ in V_1, V_2	depression inversion
• Wide slurred S wave in leads ____	I, V_5, V_6
• QRS axis is usually (normal/leftward/rightward)	normal
• RBBB (does/does not) interfere with the ECG diagnosis of ventricular hypertrophy or Q wave MI	does not
Left anterior fascicular block	
• ____ axis deviation with a mean QRS axis between ____ and ____ degrees	left -45, -90
• (qR/rS) complex in leads I and aVL	qR
• (qR/rS) complex in lead III	rS
• Normal or slightly prolonged QRS duration (true/false)	true
• No other cause for left axis deviation should be present (true/false)	true
• Poor R wave progression is (common/uncommon)	common

ECG 33. 66-year-old female with chest pain:

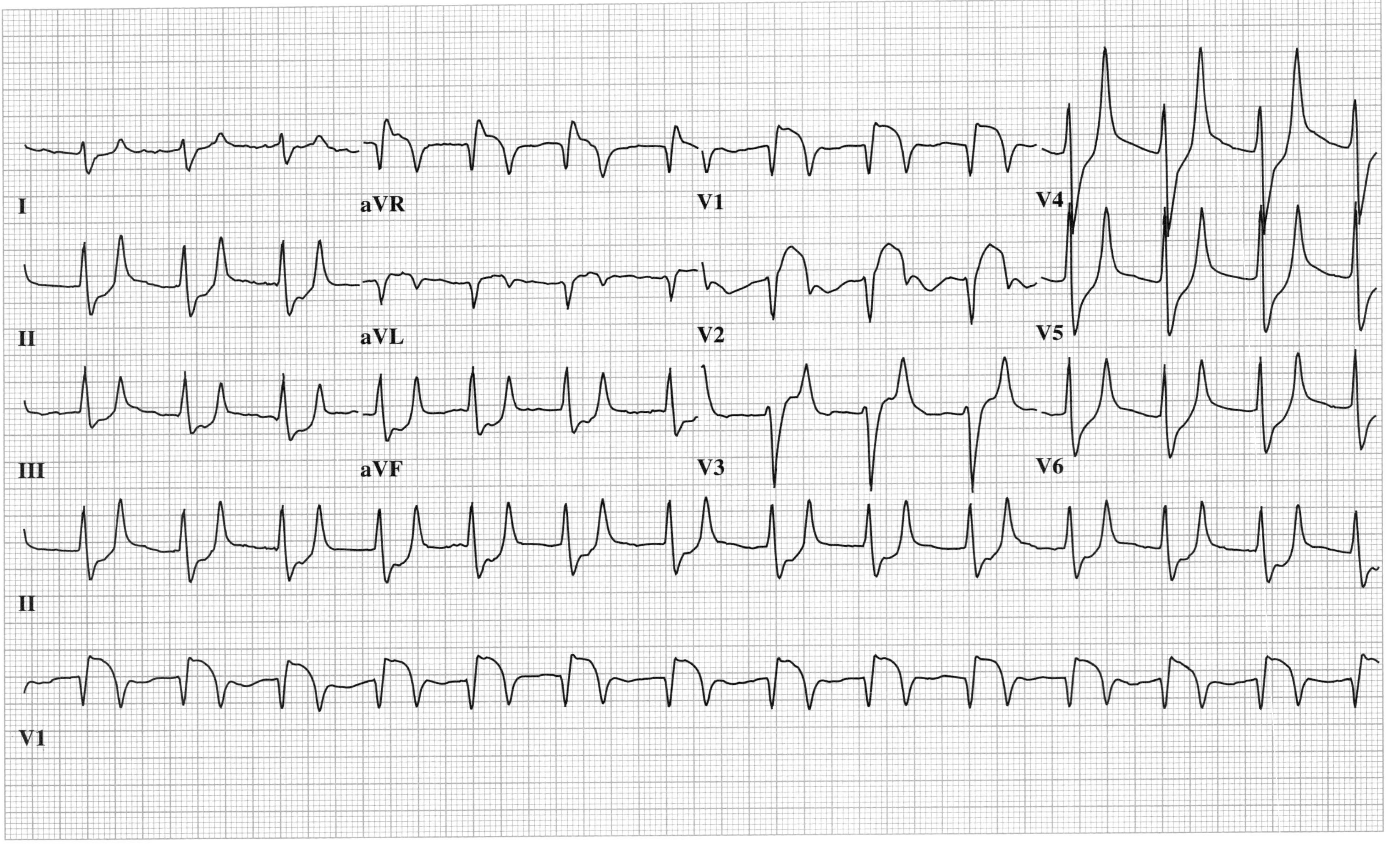

1. GENERAL FEATURES

☐ a. Normal ECG
☐ b. Borderline normal ECG or normal variant
☐ c. Incorrect electrode placement
☐ d. Artifact due to tremor

2. ATRIAL RHYTHMS

☐ a. Sinus rhythm
☐ b. Sinus arrhythmia
☐ c. Sinus bradycardia (< 60)
☐ d. Sinus tachycardia (> 100)
☐ e. Sinus pause or arrest
☐ f. Sinoatrial exit block
☐ g. Ecoptic atrial rhythm
☐ h. Wandering atrial pacemaker
☐ i. Atrial premature complexes, normally conducted
☐ j. Atrial premature complexes, nonconducted
☐ k. Atrial premature complexes with aberrant intraventricular conduction
☐ l. Atrial tachycardia (regular, sustained, 1:1 conduction)
☐ m. Atrial tachycardia, repetitive (short paroxysms)
☐ n. Atrial tachycardia, multifocal
☐ o. Atrial tachycardia with AV block
☐ p. Supraventricular tachycardia, unspecific
☐ q. Supraventricular tachycardia, paroxysmal
☐ r. Atrial flutter
☐ s. Atrial fibrillation
☐ t. Retrograde atrial activation

3. AV JUNCTIONAL RHYTHMS

☐ a. AV junctional premature complexes
☐ b. AV junctional escape complexes
☐ c. AV junctional rhythm, accelerated
☐ d. AV junctional rhythm

4. VENTRICULAR RHYTHMS

☐ a. Ventricular premature complex(es), uniform, fixed coupling
☐ b. Ventricular premature complex(es), uniform, nonfixed coupling
☐ c. Ventricular premature complexes(es), multiform
☐ d. Ventricular premature complexes, in pairs
☐ e. Ventricular parasystole
☐ f. Ventricular tachycardia (≥ 3 consecutive complexes)
☐ g. Accelerated idioventricular rhythm
☐ h. Ventricular escape complexes or rhythm
☐ i. Ventricular fibrillation

5. ATRIAL-VENTRICULAR INTERACTIONS IN ARRHYTHMIAS

☐ a. Fusion complexes
☐ b. Reciprocal (echo) complexes
☐ c. Ventricular capture complexes
☐ d. AV dissociation
☐ e. Ventriculophasic sinus arrhythmia

6. AV CONDUCTION ABNORMALITIES

☐ a. AV block, 1°
☐ b. AV block, 2° - Mobitz type I (Wenckebach)
☐ c. AV block, 2° - Mobitz type II
☐ d. AV block, 2:1
☐ e. AV block, 3°
☐ f. AV block, variable
☐ g. Short PR interval (with sinus rhythm and normal QRS duration)
☐ h. Wolff-Parkinson-White pattern

7. INTRAVENTRICULAR CONDUCTION DISTURBANCES

☐ a. RBBB, incomplete
☐ b. RBBB, complete
☐ c. Left anterior fascicular block
☐ d. Left posterior fascicular block
☐ e. LBBB, with ST-T wave suggestive of acute myocardial injury or infarction
☐ f. LBBB, complete
☐ g. LBBB, intermittent
☐ h. Intraventricular conduction disturbance, nonspecific
☐ i. Aberrant intraventricular conduction with supraventricular arrhythmia

8. P WAVE ABNORMALITIES

☐ a. Right atrial abnormality
☐ b. Left atrial abnormalities
☐ c. Nonspecific atrial abnormality

9. ABNORMALITIES OF QRS VOLTAGE OR AXIS

☐ a. Low voltage, limb leads only
☐ b. Low voltage, limb and precordial leads
☐ c. Left axis deviation (> - 30%)
☐ d. Right axis deviation (> + 100)
☐ e. Electrical alternans

10. VENTRICULAR HYPERTROPHY

☐ a. LVH by voltage only
☐ b. LVH by voltage and ST-T segment abnormalities
☐ c. RVH
☐ d. Combined ventricular hypertrophy

11. Q WAVE MYOCARDIAL INFARCTION

	Probably Acute or Recent	Probably Old or Age Indeterminate
Anterolateral	☐ a.	☐ g.
Anterior	☐ b.	☐ h.
Anteroseptal	☐ c.	☐ i.
Lateral/High lateral	☐ d.	☐ j.
Inferior	☐ e.	☐ k.
Posterior	☐ f.	☐ l.

☐ m. Probably ventricular aneurysm

12. ST, T, U, WAVE ABNORMALITIES

☐ a. Normal variant, early repolarization
☐ b. Normal variant, juvenile T waves
☐ c. Nonspecific ST and/or T wave abnormalities
☐ d. ST and/or T wave abnormalities suggesting myocardial ischemia
☐ e. ST and/or T wave abnormalities suggesting myocardial injury
☐ f. ST and/or T wave abnormalities suggesting acute pericarditis
☐ g. ST-T segment abnormalities secondary to intraventricular conduction disturbance or hypertrophy
☐ h. Post-extrasystolic T wave abnormality
☐ i. Isolated J point depression
☐ j. Peaked T waves
☐ k. Prolonged QT interval
☐ l. Prominent U waves

13. PACEMAKER FUNCTION AND RHYTHM

☐ a. Atrial or coronary sinus pacing
☐ b. Ventricular demand pacing
☐ c. AV sequential pacing
☐ d. Ventricular pacing, complete control
☐ e. Dual chamber, atrial sensing pacemaker
☐ f. Pacemaker malfunction, not constantly capturing (atrium or ventricle)
☐ g. Pacemaker malfunction, not constantly sensing (atrium or ventricle)
☐ h. Pacemaker malfunction, not firing
☐ i. Pacemaker malfunction, slowing

14. SUGGESTED OR PROBABLE CLINICAL DISORDERS

☐ a. Digitalis effect
☐ b. Digitalis toxicity
☐ c. Antiarrhythmic drug effect
☐ d. Antiarrhythmic drug toxicity
☐ e. Hyperkalemia
☐ f. Hypokalemia
☐ g. Hypercalcemia
☐ h. Hypocalcemia
☐ i. Atrial septal defect, secundum
☐ j. Atrial septal defect, primum
☐ k. Dextrocardia, mirror image
☐ l. Mitral valve disease
☐ m. Chronic lung disease
☐ n. Acute cor pulmonale, including pulmonary embolus
☐ o. Pericardial effusion
☐ p. Acute pericarditis
☐ q. Hypertrophic cardiomyopathy
☐ r. Coronary artery disease
☐ s. Central nervous system disorder
☐ t. Myxedema
☐ u. Hypothermia
☐ v. Sick sinus syndrome

ECG 33 was obtained in a 66-year-old female with chest pain. The ECG shows sinus rhythm, first-degree AV block, right axis deviation (due to left posterior fascicular block), and nonspecific atrial abnormality (arrowhead). The most striking features on this tracing include marked peaking of the T waves (arrows), and a myocardial injury pattern in leads V_1-V_3 and aVL (asterisks). Since a pathological Q wave is present in lead aVL only, acute myocardial infarction should not be coded. This woman was subsequently documented to have an occluded left anterior descending coronary artery and a potassium level of 8.0 mg/dL.

Codes:

2a	Sinus rhythm
6a	AV block, 1°
7h	IVCD, nonspecific type
8c	Nonspecific atrial abnormality
12e	ST and/or T wave abnormalities suggesting myocardial injury
12j	Peaked T waves
14e	Hyperkalemia
14r	Coronary artery disease

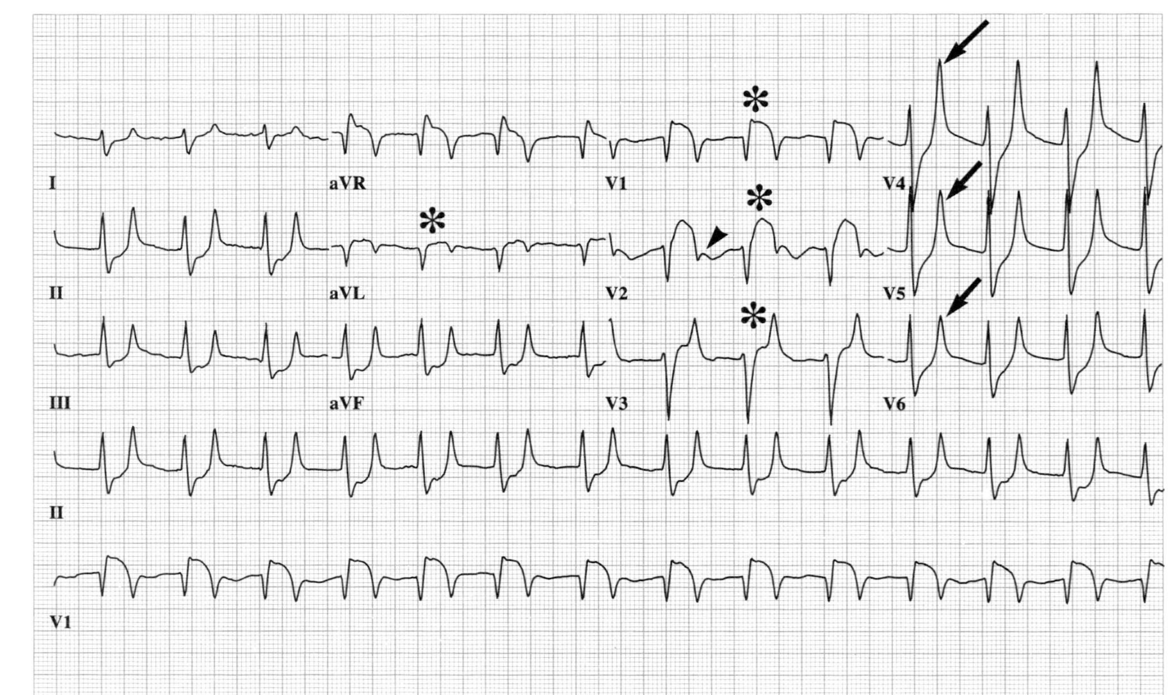

Questions: ECG 33

1. Peaked T waves can occur with:

   a. Hyperkalemia
   b. Acute myocardial infarction
   c. LVH
   d. Normal variant early repolarization abnormality
   e. Intracranial bleeding
   f. LBBB

2. Hyperkalemia can cause all of the following except:

   a. U waves
   b. PR prolongation
   c. QRS widening
   d. Left anterior fascicular block

Answers: ECG 33

1. Peaked T waves can be seen in hyperkalemia, acute myocardial infarction, intracranial bleeding, and normal variant early repolarization abnormalities. Peaked T waves may also be seen in marked LVH (usually in right precordial leads) and LBBB. (Answer: All)

2. Hyperkalemia can cause PR prolongation, QRS widening, peaked T waves, and left anterior fascicular block. Hypokalemia, not hyperkalemia, is associated with prominent U waves. (Answer: a)

— Quick Review 33 —

Peaked T waves	
• T wave > ____ mm in the limb leads or > ____ mm in the precordial leads	6, 10
Hyperkalemia	
• *K^+ = 5.5 - 6.5 mEq/L*	
▸ Tall, peaked, narrow based ____ waves	T
▸ QT interval (shortening/lengthening)	shortening
▸ (Reversible/irreversible) left anterior or posterior fascicular block	Reversible
• *K^+ = 6.5 - 7.5 mEq/L*	
▸ ____ degree AV block	First
▸ Flattening and widening of the ____ wave	P
▸ ST segment (depression/elevation)	depression
▸ ____widening	QRS
• *K^+ > 7.5 mEq/L*	
▸ Disappearance of ____ waves	P
▸ LBBB, RBBB, or markedly widened and diffuse intraventricular conduction delay resembling a ____ wave pattern	sine
▸ Arrhythmias and conduction disturbances including VT, VF, idioventricular rhythm, asystole (true/false)	true

ECG 34. 58-year-old female with chronic congestive heart failure:

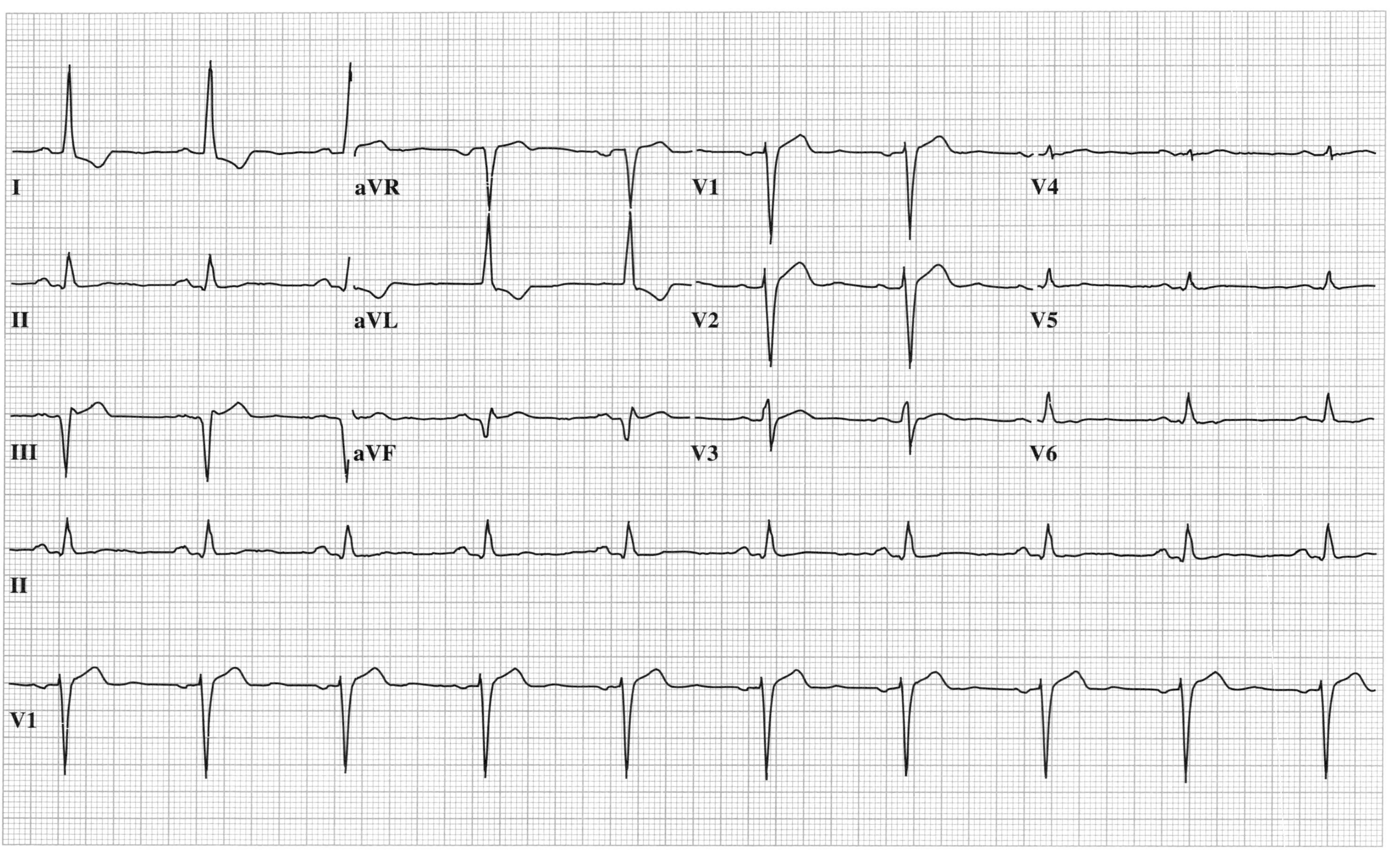

1. GENERAL FEATURES

- ☐ a. Normal ECG
- ☐ b. Borderline normal ECG or normal variant
- ☐ c. Incorrect electrode placement
- ☐ d. Artifact due to tremor

2. ATRIAL RHYTHMS

- ☐ a. Sinus rhythm
- ☐ b. Sinus arrhythmia
- ☐ c. Sinus bradycardia (< 60)
- ☐ d. Sinus tachycardia (> 100)
- ☐ e. Sinus pause or arrest
- ☐ f. Sinoatrial exit block
- ☐ g. Ecoptic atrial rhythm
- ☐ h. Wandering atrial pacemaker
- ☐ i. Atrial premature complexes, normally conducted
- ☐ j. Atrial premature complexes, nonconducted
- ☐ k. Atrial premature complexes with aberrant intraventricular conduction
- ☐ l. Atrial tachycardia (regular, sustained, 1:1 conduction)
- ☐ m. Atrial tachycardia, repetitive (short paroxysms)
- ☐ n. Atrial tachycardia, multifocal
- ☐ o. Atrial tachycardia with AV block
- ☐ p. Supraventricular tachycardia, unspecific
- ☐ q. Supraventricular tachycardia, paroxysmal
- ☐ r. Atrial flutter
- ☐ s. Atrial fibrillation
- ☐ t. Retrograde atrial activation

3. AV JUNCTIONAL RHYTHMS

- ☐ a. AV junctional premature complexes
- ☐ b. AV junctional escape complexes
- ☐ c. AV junctional rhythm, accelerated
- ☐ d. AV junctional rhythm

4. VENTRICULAR RHYTHMS

- ☐ a. Ventricular premature complex(es), uniform, fixed coupling
- ☐ b. Ventricular premature complex(es), uniform, nonfixed coupling
- ☐ c. Ventricular premature complexes(es), multiform
- ☐ d. Ventricular premature complexes, in pairs
- ☐ e. Ventricular parasystole
- ☐ f. Ventricular tachycardia (≥ 3 consecutive complexes)
- ☐ g. Accelerated idioventricular rhythm
- ☐ h. Ventricular escape complexes or rhythm
- ☐ i. Ventricular fibrillation

5. ATRIAL-VENTRICULAR INTERACTIONS IN ARRHYTHMIAS

- ☐ a. Fusion complexes
- ☐ b. Reciprocal (echo) complexes
- ☐ c. Ventricular capture complexes
- ☐ d. AV dissociation
- ☐ e. Ventriculophasic sinus arrhythmia

6. AV CONDUCTION ABNORMALITIES

- ☐ a. AV block, 1°
- ☐ b. AV block, 2° - Mobitz type I (Wenckebach)
- ☐ c. AV block, 2° - Mobitz type II
- ☐ d. AV block, 2:1
- ☐ e. AV block, 3°
- ☐ f. AV block, variable
- ☐ g. Short PR interval (with sinus rhythm and normal QRS duration)
- ☐ h. Wolff-Parkinson-White pattern

7. INTRAVENTRICULAR CONDUCTION DISTURBANCES

- ☐ a. RBBB, incomplete
- ☐ b. RBBB, complete
- ☐ c. Left anterior fascicular block
- ☐ d. Left posterior fascicular block
- ☐ e. LBBB, with ST-T wave suggestive of acute myocardial injury or infarction
- ☐ f. LBBB, complete
- ☐ g. LBBB, intermittent
- ☐ h. Intraventricular conduction disturbance, nonspecific
- ☐ i. Aberrant intraventricular conduction with supraventricular arrhythmia

8. P WAVE ABNORMALITIES

- ☐ a. Right atrial abnormality
- ☐ b. Left atrial abnormalities
- ☐ c. Nonspecific atrial abnormality

9. ABNORMALITIES OF QRS VOLTAGE OR AXIS

- ☐ a. Low voltage, limb leads only
- ☐ b. Low voltage, limb and precordial leads
- ☐ c. Left axis deviation (> - 30%)
- ☐ d. Right axis deviation (> + 100)
- ☐ e. Electrical alternans

10. VENTRICULAR HYPERTROPHY

- ☐ a. LVH by voltage only
- ☐ b. LVH by voltage and ST-T segment abnormalities
- ☐ c. RVH
- ☐ d. Combined ventricular hypertrophy

11. Q WAVE MYOCARDIAL INFARCTION

	Probably Acute or Recent	Probably Old or Age Indeterminate
Anterolateral	☐ a.	☐ g.
Anterior	☐ b.	☐ h.
Anteroseptal	☐ c.	☐ i.
Lateral/High lateral	☐ d.	☐ j.
Inferior	☐ e.	☐ k.
Posterior	☐ f.	☐ l.

☐ m. Probably ventricular aneurysm

12. ST, T, U, WAVE ABNORMALITIES

- ☐ a. Normal variant, early repolarization
- ☐ b. Normal variant, juvenile T waves
- ☐ c. Nonspecific ST and/or T wave abnormalities
- ☐ d. ST and/or T wave abnormalities suggesting myocardial ischemia
- ☐ e. ST and/or T wave abnormalities suggesting myocardial injury
- ☐ f. ST and/or T wave abnormalities suggesting acute pericarditis
- ☐ g. ST-T segment abnormalities secondary to intraventricular conduction disturbance or hypertrophy
- ☐ h. Post-extrasystolic T wave abnormality
- ☐ i. Isolated J point depression
- ☐ j. Peaked T waves
- ☐ k. Prolonged QT interval
- ☐ l. Prominent U waves

13. PACEMAKER FUNCTION AND RHYTHM

- ☐ a. Atrial or coronary sinus pacing
- ☐ b. Ventricular demand pacing
- ☐ c. AV sequential pacing
- ☐ d. Ventricular pacing, complete control
- ☐ e. Dual chamber, atrial sensing pacemaker
- ☐ f. Pacemaker malfunction, not constantly capturing (atrium or ventricle)
- ☐ g. Pacemaker malfunction, not constantly sensing (atrium or ventricle)
- ☐ h. Pacemaker malfunction, not firing
- ☐ i. Pacemaker malfunction, slowing

14. SUGGESTED OR PROBABLE CLINICAL DISORDERS

- ☐ a. Digitalis effect
- ☐ b. Digitalis toxicity
- ☐ c. Antiarrhythmic drug effect
- ☐ d. Antiarrhythmic drug toxicity
- ☐ e. Hyperkalemia
- ☐ f. Hypokalemia
- ☐ g. Hypercalcemia
- ☐ h. Hypocalcemia
- ☐ i. Atrial septal defect, secundum
- ☐ j. Atrial septal defect, primum
- ☐ k. Dextrocardia, mirror image
- ☐ l. Mitral valve disease
- ☐ m. Chronic lung disease
- ☐ n. Acute cor pulmonale, including pulmonary embolus
- ☐ o. Pericardial effusion
- ☐ p. Acute pericarditis
- ☐ q. Hypertrophic cardiomyopathy
- ☐ r. Coronary artery disease
- ☐ s. Central nervous system disorder
- ☐ t. Myxedema
- ☐ u. Hypothermia
- ☐ v. Sick sinus syndrome

ECG 34 was obtained in a 58-year-old female with chronic congestive heart failure. The ECG shows a sinus bradycardia at 58 beats/minute, and LVH with associated ST-T abnormalities (R wave in I ≥ 14 mm; R wave in aVL ≥ 12 mm; arrows). While some degree of QRS widening is often present with LVH, the QRS measures 120 msec, consistent with nonspecific IVCD. Evidence for an old inferior myocardial infarction (arrowheads) and coronary artery disease are present.

Codes:

2c	Sinus bradycardia
7h	IVCD, nonspecific type
10b	LVH by both voltage and ST-T segment abnormalities
11k	Inferior Q wave MI, probably old or age indeterminate
12g	ST-T segment abnormalities secondary to IVCD or hypertrophy
14r	Coronary artery disease

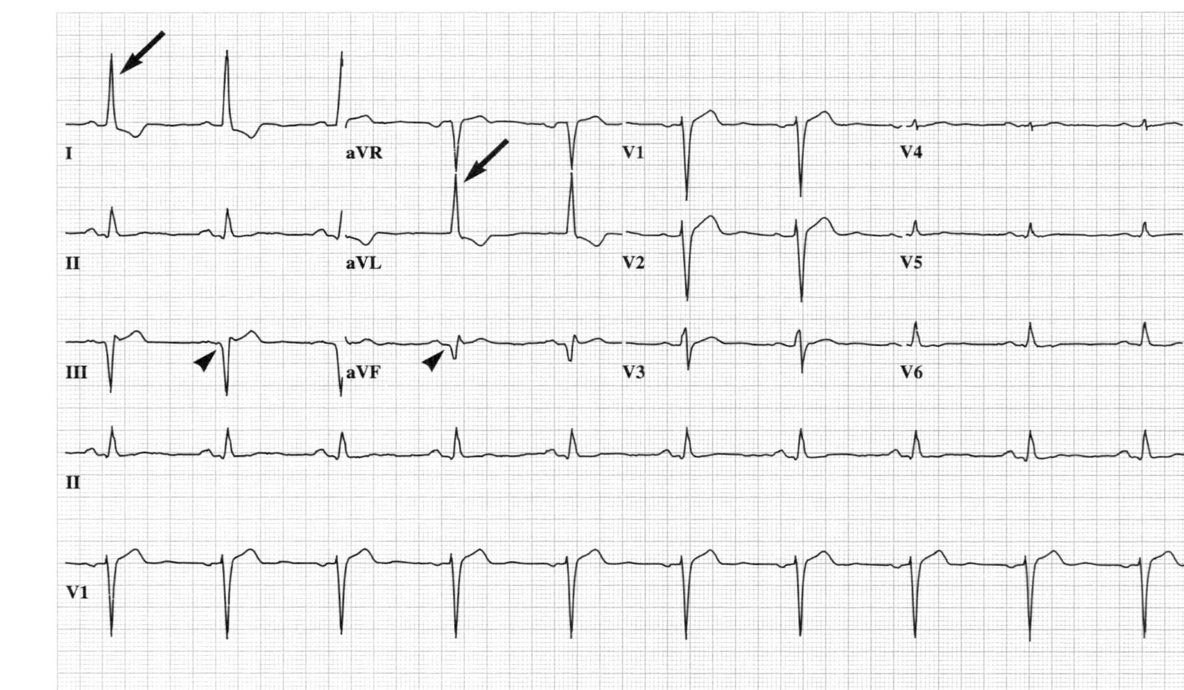

Questions: ECG 34

1. Which leads in the present tracing demonstrate LVH by voltage criteria?

   a. R wave in V_5 or V_6 + S wave in lead V_1
   b. R wave in I + S wave in II
   c. R wave in I
   d. S wave in aVR
   e. R wave in aVL
   f. R wave in aVF

2 Findings consistent with the diagnosis of LVH include:

   a. ST segment depression and T wave inversion in leads I, aVL, V_4 - V_6
   b. ST elevation in leads V_1 - V_3
   c. Prominent U waves

Answers: ECG 34

1. In the present tracing, voltage criteria for LVH is satisfied by the presence of R waves in leads I and aVL > 14 mm and 12 mm, respectively. Criteria not satisfied on this ECG include an R wave in lead V_5 or V_6 + S wave in lead I > 35 mm; an R wave in lead I + S wave in lead II > 26 mm; an S wave in aVR > 15 mm; and an R wave in aVF > 21 mm. (Answer: c, e)

2. Non-voltage criteria for LVH include ST segment depression and T wave inversion in leads V_5 and V_6, ST elevation in the right precordial leads (which may be misinterpreted as anteroseptal myocardial injury or infarction), and prominent U waves. Additional features that may be present include left atrial abnormality, left axis deviation, nonspecific intraventricular conduction delay, delayed intrinsicoid deflection, poor R wave progression, absent Q waves in the left precordial leads, and abnormal Q waves in the inferior leads (due to left axis deviation). (Answer: All)

— Quick Review 34 —

Intraventricular conduction disturbance, nonspecific type	
• QRS ≥ ____ seconds in duration but morphology does not meet criteria for LBBB or RBBB, *or* abnormal ____ without widening of the QRS complex	0.11 notching
LVH by both voltage and ST-T segment abnormalities	
• Voltage criteria for LVH and one or more ST-T abnormalities:	
▸ ST segment and T wave deviation in (same/opposite) direction to the major deflection of QRS	opposite
▸ ST segment (elevation/depression) in leads I, aVL, III, aVF, and/or V_4-V_6	depression
▸ Subtle (< 1-2 mm) ST (elevation/depression) in leads V_1-V_3	elevation
▸ Inverted ____ waves in leads I, aVL, V_4-V_6	T
▸ (Absent/prominent) U waves	prominent

Common Dilemmas in ECG Interpretation

Problem

Acute myocardial infarction is present with ST elevation in one portion of the tracing and ST segment depression in another. Is it necessary to code both ST-T changes suggesting myocardial injury and ST-T changes suggesting myocardial ischemia?

Recommendation

Yes. Many acute myocardial infarctions have significant ST segment elevation in some leads and significant ST segment depression in others. The ST segment depression is usually a manifestation of ischemia adjacent to a remote from the infarct zone. Thus, correct coding for this situation should include item 12d (ST-T abnormalities suggesting myocardial ischemia) and item 12e (ST-T abnormalities suggesting myocardial injury).

ECG 35. 55-year-old woman with a history of dilated cardiomyopathy:

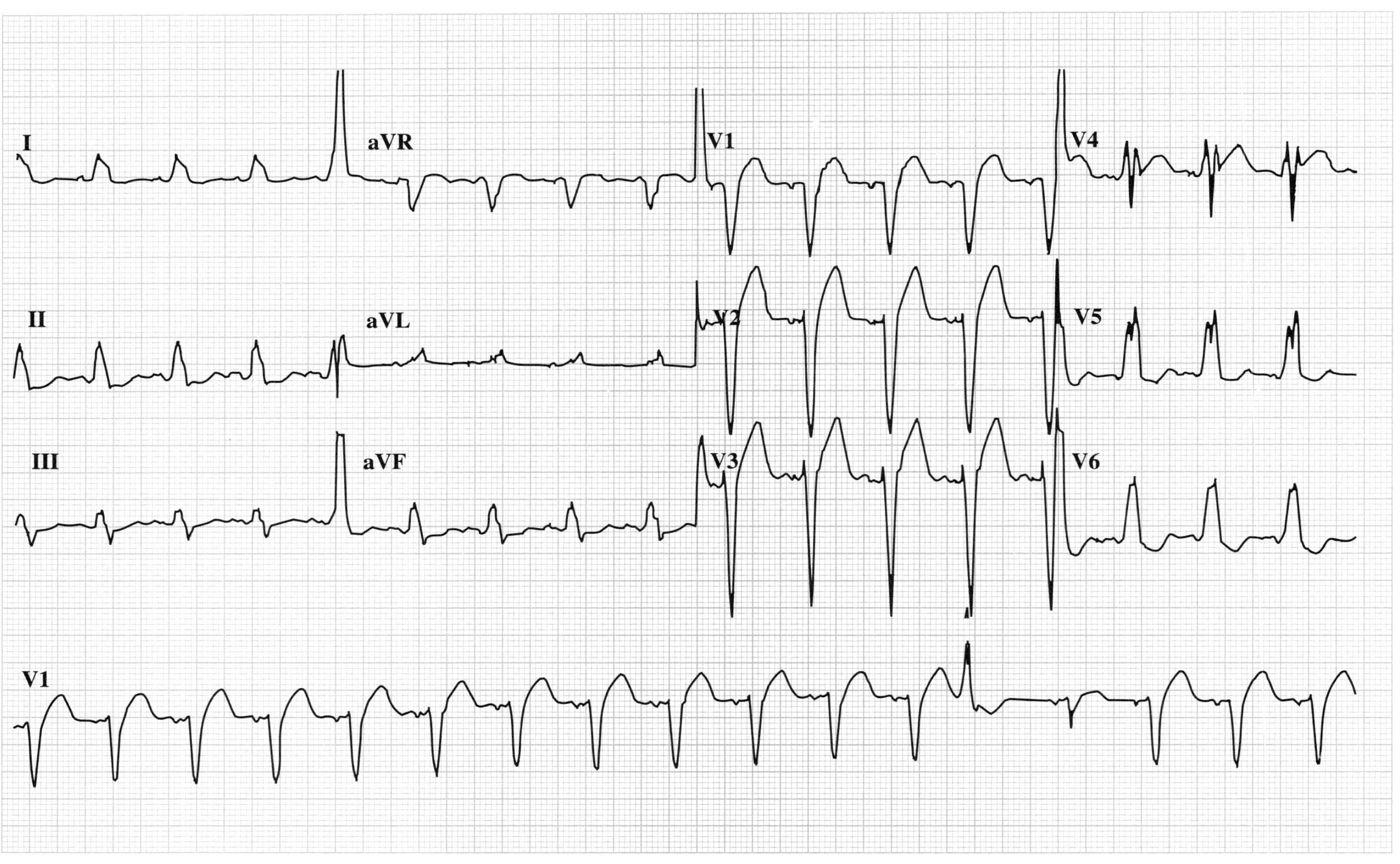

1. GENERAL FEATURES

- ☐ a. Normal ECG
- ☐ b. Borderline normal ECG or normal variant
- ☐ c. Incorrect electrode placement
- ☐ d. Artifact due to tremor

2. ATRIAL RHYTHMS

- ☐ a. Sinus rhythm
- ☐ b. Sinus arrhythmia
- ☐ c. Sinus bradycardia (< 60)
- ☐ d. Sinus tachycardia (> 100)
- ☐ e. Sinus pause or arrest
- ☐ f. Sinoatrial exit block
- ☐ g. Ecoptic atrial rhythm
- ☐ h. Wandering atrial pacemaker
- ☐ i. Atrial premature complexes, normally conducted
- ☐ j. Atrial premature complexes, nonconducted
- ☐ k. Atrial premature complexes with aberrant intraventricular conduction
- ☐ l. Atrial tachycardia (regular, sustained, 1:1 conduction)
- ☐ m. Atrial tachycardia, repetitive (short paroxysms)
- ☐ n. Atrial tachycardia, multifocal
- ☐ o. Atrial tachycardia with AV block
- ☐ p. Supraventricular tachycardia, unspecific
- ☐ q. Supraventricular tachycardia, paroxysmal
- ☐ r. Atrial flutter
- ☐ s. Atrial fibrillation
- ☐ t. Retrograde atrial activation

3. AV JUNCTIONAL RHYTHMS

- ☐ a. AV junctional premature complexes
- ☐ b. AV junctional escape complexes
- ☐ c. AV junctional rhythm, accelerated
- ☐ d. AV junctional rhythm

4. VENTRICULAR RHYTHMS

- ☐ a. Ventricular premature complex(es), uniform, fixed coupling
- ☐ b. Ventricular premature complex(es), uniform, nonfixed coupling
- ☐ c. Ventricular premature complexes(es), multiform
- ☐ d. Ventricular premature complexes, in pairs
- ☐ e. Ventricular parasystole
- ☐ f. Ventricular tachycardia (≥ 3 consecutive complexes)
- ☐ g. Accelerated idioventricular rhythm
- ☐ h. Ventricular escape complexes or rhythm
- ☐ i. Ventricular fibrillation

5. ATRIAL-VENTRICULAR INTERACTIONS IN ARRHYTHMIAS

- ☐ a. Fusion complexes
- ☐ b. Reciprocal (echo) complexes
- ☐ c. Ventricular capture complexes
- ☐ d. AV dissociation
- ☐ e. Ventriculophasic sinus arrhythmia

6. AV CONDUCTION ABNORMALITIES

- ☐ a. AV block, 1°
- ☐ b. AV block, 2° - Mobitz type I (Wenckebach)
- ☐ c. AV block, 2° - Mobitz type II
- ☐ d. AV block, 2:1
- ☐ e. AV block, 3°
- ☐ f. AV block, variable
- ☐ g. Short PR interval (with sinus rhythm and normal QRS duration)
- ☐ h. Wolff-Parkinson-White pattern

7. INTRAVENTRICULAR CONDUCTION DISTURBANCES

- ☐ a. RBBB, incomplete
- ☐ b. RBBB, complete
- ☐ c. Left anterior fascicular block
- ☐ d. Left posterior fascicular block
- ☐ e. LBBB, with ST-T wave suggestive of acute myocardial injury or infarction
- ☐ f. LBBB, complete
- ☐ g. LBBB, intermittent
- ☐ h. Intraventricular conduction disturbance, nonspecific
- ☐ i. Aberrant intraventricular conduction with supraventricular arrhythmia

8. P WAVE ABNORMALITIES

- ☐ a. Right atrial abnormality
- ☐ b. Left atrial abnormalities
- ☐ c. Nonspecific atrial abnormality

9. ABNORMALITIES OF QRS VOLTAGE OR AXIS

- ☐ a. Low voltage, limb leads only
- ☐ b. Low voltage, limb and precordial leads
- ☐ c. Left axis deviation (> - 30%)
- ☐ d. Right axis deviation (> + 100)
- ☐ e. Electrical alternans

10. VENTRICULAR HYPERTROPHY

- ☐ a. LVH by voltage only
- ☐ b. LVH by voltage and ST-T segment abnormalities
- ☐ c. RVH
- ☐ d. Combined ventricular hypertrophy

11. Q WAVE MYOCARDIAL INFARCTION

	Probably Acute or Recent	Probably Old or Age Indeterminate
Anterolateral	☐ a.	☐ g.
Anterior	☐ b.	☐ h.
Anteroseptal	☐ c.	☐ i.
Lateral/High lateral	☐ d.	☐ j.
Inferior	☐ e.	☐ k.
Posterior	☐ f.	☐ l.

☐ m. Probably ventricular aneurysm

12. ST, T, U, WAVE ABNORMALITIES

- ☐ a. Normal variant, early repolarization
- ☐ b. Normal variant, juvenile T waves
- ☐ c. Nonspecific ST and/or T wave abnormalities
- ☐ d. ST and/or T wave abnormalities suggesting myocardial ischemia
- ☐ e. ST and/or T wave abnormalities suggesting myocardial injury
- ☐ f. ST and/or T wave abnormalities suggesting acute pericarditis
- ☐ g. ST-T segment abnormalities secondary to intraventricular conduction disturbance or hypertrophy
- ☐ h. Post-extrasystolic T wave abnormality
- ☐ i. Isolated J point depression
- ☐ j. Peaked T waves
- ☐ k. Prolonged QT interval
- ☐ l. Prominent U waves

13. PACEMAKER FUNCTION AND RHYTHM

- ☐ a. Atrial or coronary sinus pacing
- ☐ b. Ventricular demand pacing
- ☐ c. AV sequential pacing
- ☐ d. Ventricular pacing, complete control
- ☐ e. Dual chamber, atrial sensing pacemaker
- ☐ f. Pacemaker malfunction, not constantly capturing (atrium or ventricle)
- ☐ g. Pacemaker malfunction, not constantly sensing (atrium or ventricle)
- ☐ h. Pacemaker malfunction, not firing
- ☐ i. Pacemaker malfunction, slowing

14. SUGGESTED OR PROBABLE CLINICAL DISORDERS

- ☐ a. Digitalis effect
- ☐ b. Digitalis toxicity
- ☐ c. Antiarrhythmic drug effect
- ☐ d. Antiarrhythmic drug toxicity
- ☐ e. Hyperkalemia
- ☐ f. Hypokalemia
- ☐ g. Hypercalcemia
- ☐ h. Hypocalcemia
- ☐ i. Atrial septal defect, secundum
- ☐ j. Atrial septal defect, primum
- ☐ k. Dextrocardia, mirror image
- ☐ l. Mitral valve disease
- ☐ m. Chronic lung disease
- ☐ n. Acute cor pulmonale, including pulmo
- ☐ o. Pericardial effusion
- ☐ p. Acute pericarditis
- ☐ q. Hypertrophic cardiomyopathy
- ☐ r. Coronary artery disease
- ☐ s. Central nervous system d
- ☐ t. Myxedema
- ☐ u. Hypothermia
- ☐ v. Sick sinus syndro

ECG 35 was obtained from a 55-year-old woman with a history of dilated cardiomyopathy. The ECG show: abnormality (arrowhead), and LBBB with secondary ST-T abnormalities. The rhythm strip at the bottom of th premature complex (arrow) followed by a compensatory pause; the first beat after the compensatory pause (asteris without LBBB, establishing the diagnosis of rate-related LBBB.

Codes:

2d	Sinus tachycardia
4a	Ventricular premature complex(es), uniform, fixed coupling
7g	LBBB, intermittent
8b	Left atrial abnormality
12g	ST-T segment abnormalities secondary to IVCD or hypertrophy

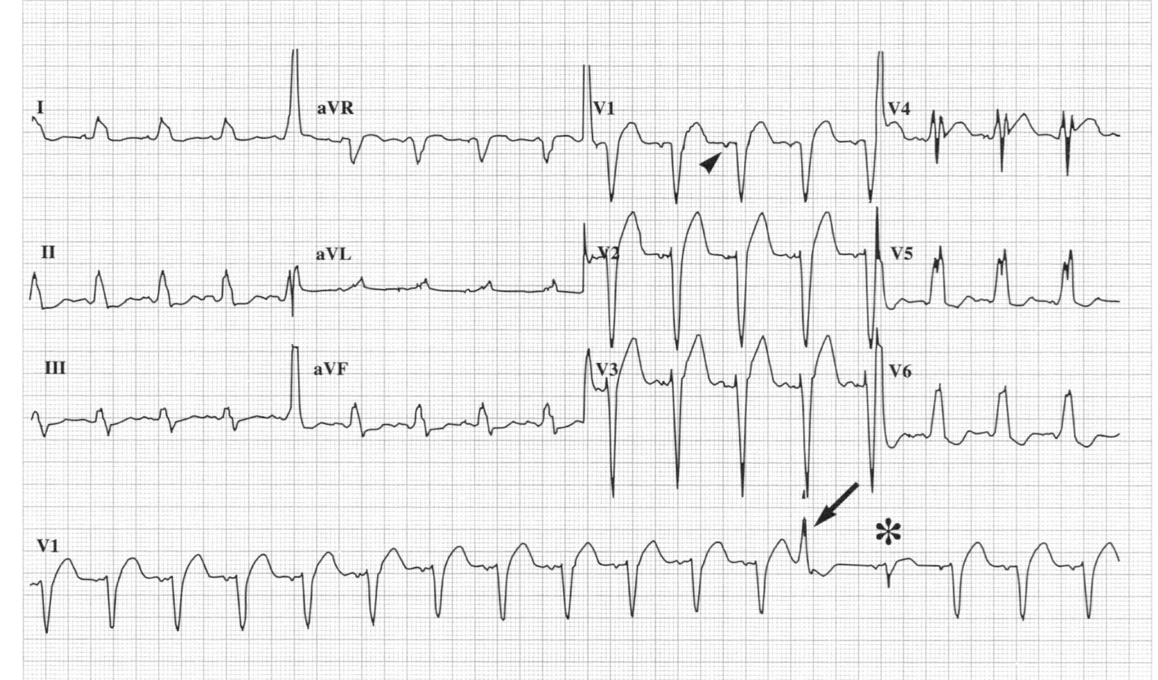

ne

sorder

ary embolus

Questions: ECG 35

1. Intermittent LBBB can be tachycardia- or bradycardia-dependent:

   a. True
   b. False

2. In the setting of LBBB, ___ mm of discordant ST segment elevation in leads V_1-V_4 suggests the presence of ischemia or infarction:

   a. 2
   b. 3
   c. 4
   d. 5

Answers: ECG 35

1. Rate-dependent LBBB most often develops during sinus tachycardia (as in the present tracing), but may be bradycardia-dependent as well. The ventricular premature complex results in a compensatory pause, allowing recovery of the refractory left bundle branch and resulting in normal QRS conduction for a single beat. Sinus tachycardia resumes on the following beat, resulting in a shorter cycle length and a refractory left bundle branch. (Answer: a)

2. In the setting of LBBB, discordant ST segment elevation (i.e., ST elevation in a direction opposite to the major QRS vector) needs to be ≥ 5 mm in height to be considered worrisome for ischemia. Concordant ST segment elevation (i.e., ST segment elevation in the same direction as the major QRS vector) ≥ 1 mm is a more specific finding for transmural ischemia. (Answer: d)

— Quick Review 35 —

Sinus tachycardia (>100)	
• Rate > ____ per minute	100
• P wave amplitude often (increases/decreases) and PR interval often (increases/decreases) with increasing heart rate	increases shortens
Left atrial abnormality	
• Notched P wave with a duration ≥ ____ seconds in leads II, III or aVF, *or*	0.12
• Terminal negative portion of the P wave in lead V_1 ≥ 1 mm deep and ≥ ____ seconds in duration	0.04

ECG 36. 26-year-old female with rapid heart beating:

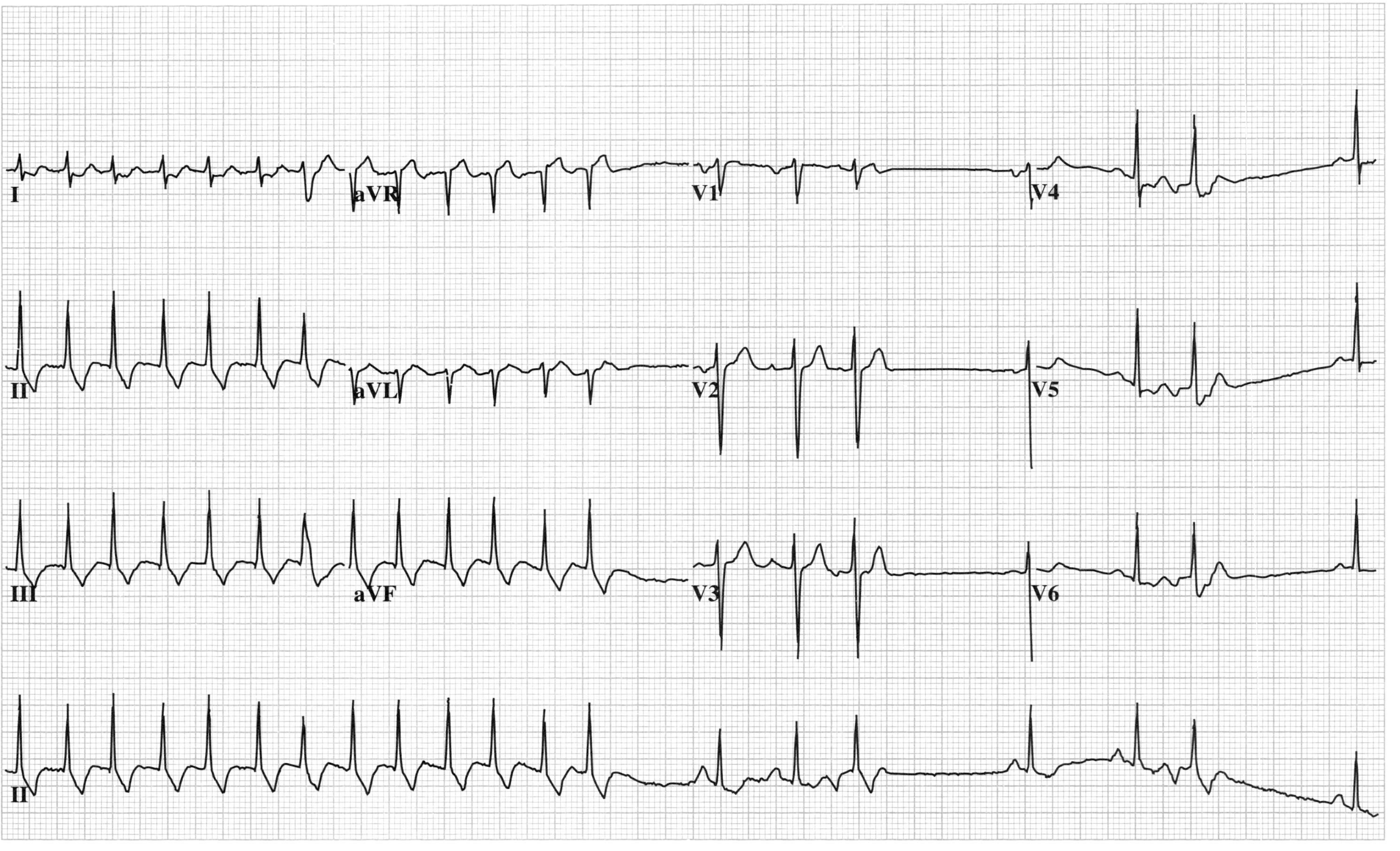

1. GENERAL FEATURES
☐ a. Normal ECG
☐ b. Borderline normal ECG or normal variant
☐ c. Incorrect electrode placement
☐ d. Artifact due to tremor

2. ATRIAL RHYTHMS
☐ a. Sinus rhythm
☐ b. Sinus arrhythmia
☐ c. Sinus bradycardia (< 60)
☐ d. Sinus tachycardia (> 100)
☐ e. Sinus pause or arrest
☐ f. Sinoatrial exit block
☐ g. Ecoptic atrial rhythm
☐ h. Wandering atrial pacemaker
☐ i. Atrial premature complexes, normally conducted
☐ j. Atrial premature complexes, nonconducted
☐ k. Atrial premature complexes with aberrant intraventricular conduction
☐ l. Atrial tachycardia (regular, sustained, 1:1 conduction)
☐ m. Atrial tachycardia, repetitive (short paroxysms)
☐ n. Atrial tachycardia, multifocal
☐ o. Atrial tachycardia with AV block
☐ p. Supraventricular tachycardia, unspecific
☐ q. Supraventricular tachycardia, paroxysmal
☐ r. Atrial flutter
☐ s. Atrial fibrillation
☐ t. Retrograde atrial activation

3. AV JUNCTIONAL RHYTHMS
☐ a. AV junctional premature complexes
☐ b. AV junctional escape complexes
☐ c. AV junctional rhythm, accelerated
☐ d. AV junctional rhythm

4. VENTRICULAR RHYTHMS
☐ a. Ventricular premature complex(es), uniform, fixed coupling
☐ b. Ventricular premature complex(es), uniform, nonfixed coupling
☐ c. Ventricular premature complexes(es), multiform
☐ d. Ventricular premature complexes, in pairs
☐ e. Ventricular parasystole
☐ f. Ventricular tachycardia (≥ 3 consecutive complexes)
☐ g. Accelerated idioventricular rhythm
☐ h. Ventricular escape complexes or rhythm
☐ i. Ventricular fibrillation

5. ATRIAL-VENTRICULAR INTERACTIONS IN ARRHYTHMIAS
☐ a. Fusion complexes
☐ b. Reciprocal (echo) complexes
☐ c. Ventricular capture complexes
☐ d. AV dissociation
☐ e. Ventriculophasic sinus arrhythmia

6. AV CONDUCTION ABNORMALITIES
☐ a. AV block, 1°
☐ b. AV block, 2° - Mobitz type I (Wenckebach)
☐ c. AV block, 2° - Mobitz type II
☐ d. AV block, 2:1
☐ e. AV block, 3°
☐ f. AV block, variable
☐ g. Short PR interval (with sinus rhythm and normal QRS duration)
☐ h. Wolff-Parkinson-White pattern

7. INTRAVENTRICULAR CONDUCTION DISTURBANCES
☐ a. RBBB, incomplete
☐ b. RBBB, complete
☐ c. Left anterior fascicular block
☐ d. Left posterior fascicular block
☐ e. LBBB, with ST-T wave suggestive of acute myocardial injury or infarction
☐ f. LBBB, complete
☐ g. LBBB, intermittent
☐ h. Intraventricular conduction disturbance, nonspecific
☐ i. Aberrant intraventricular conduction with supraventricular arrhythmia

8. P WAVE ABNORMALITIES
☐ a. Right atrial abnormality
☐ b. Left atrial abnormalities
☐ c. Nonspecific atrial abnormality

9. ABNORMALITIES OF QRS VOLTAGE OR AXIS
☐ a. Low voltage, limb leads only
☐ b. Low voltage, limb and precordial leads
☐ c. Left axis deviation (> - 30%)
☐ d. Right axis deviation (> + 100)
☐ e. Electrical alternans

10. VENTRICULAR HYPERTROPHY
☐ a. LVH by voltage only
☐ b. LVH by voltage and ST-T segment abnormalities
☐ c. RVH
☐ d. Combined ventricular hypertrophy

11. Q WAVE MYOCARDIAL INFARCTION

	Probably Acute or Recent	Probably Old or Age Indeterminate
Anterolateral	☐ a.	☐ g.
Anterior	☐ b.	☐ h.
Anteroseptal	☐ c.	☐ i.
Lateral/High lateral	☐ d.	☐ j.
Inferior	☐ e.	☐ k.
Posterior	☐ f.	☐ l.

☐ m. Probably ventricular aneurysm

12. ST, T, U, WAVE ABNORMALITIES
☐ a. Normal variant, early repolarization
☐ b. Normal variant, juvenile T waves
☐ c. Nonspecific ST and/or T wave abnormalities
☐ d. ST and/or T wave abnormalities suggesting myocardial ischemia
☐ e. ST and/or T wave abnormalities suggesting myocardial injury
☐ f. ST and/or T wave abnormalities suggesting acute pericarditis
☐ g. ST-T segment abnormalities secondary to intraventricular conduction disturbance or hypertrophy
☐ h. Post-extrasystolic T wave abnormality
☐ i. Isolated J point depression
☐ j. Peaked T waves
☐ k. Prolonged QT interval
☐ l. Prominent U waves

13. PACEMAKER FUNCTION AND RHYTHM
☐ a. Atrial or coronary sinus pacing
☐ b. Ventricular demand pacing
☐ c. AV sequential pacing
☐ d. Ventricular pacing, complete control
☐ e. Dual chamber, atrial sensing pacemaker
☐ f. Pacemaker malfunction, not constantly capturing (atrium or ventricle)
☐ g. Pacemaker malfunction, not constantly sensing (atrium or ventricle)
☐ h. Pacemaker malfunction, not firing
☐ i. Pacemaker malfunction, slowing

14. SUGGESTED OR PROBABLE CLIN
☐ a. Digitalis effect
☐ b. Digitalis toxicity
☐ c. Antiarrhythmic drug effec
☐ d. Antiarrhythmic drug to
☐ e. Hyperkalemia
☐ f. Hypokalemia
☐ g. Hypercalcemia
☐ h. Hypocalcemi
☐ i. Atrial sept
☐ j. Atrial s
☐ k. Dext
☐ l. Mi
☐ m.
☐
☐

ECG 36 was obtained from a 26-year-old female complaining of rapid heart beati
supraventricular tachycardia with electrical alternans (triple asterisk), and left atrial
marked "a" is shorter than the normal sinus PP interval marked "b" — is noted in th
subsequent retrograde atrial activation (arrowhead) results in an echo complex in
(double asterisk) is an aberrantly conducted supraventricular complex during the
concealed posteroseptal accessory pathway. Nonspecific (rate-related) ST-T abno

Codes:

2a	Sinus rhythm
2i	Atrial premature complexes, normally conducted
2q	Supraventricular tachycardia, paroxysmal
2t	Retrograde atrial activation
5b	Reciprocal (echo) complexes
7i	Aberrant intraventricular conduction with supraventri
8b	Left atrial abnormality
9e	Electrical alternans
12c	Nonspecific ST and/or T wave abnormalities

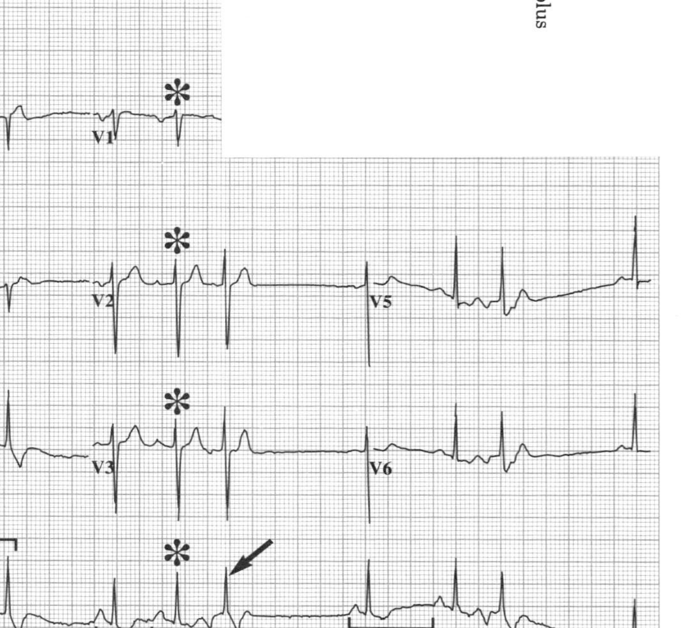

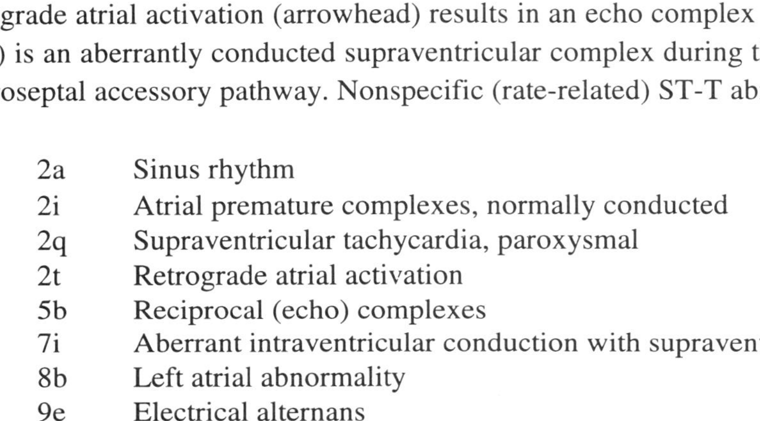

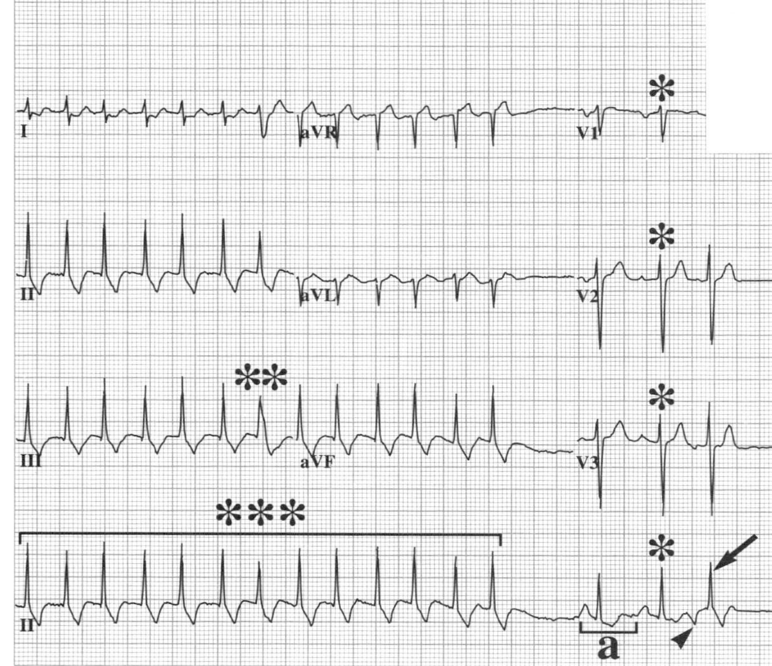

ICAL DISORDERS

[...]xicity

[...]al defect, secundum
[...]ptal defect, primum
[...]ocardia, mirror image
[...]ral valve disease
Chronic lung disease
[...] Acute cor pulmonale, including pulmonary embolus
- ☐ o. Pericardial effusion
- ☐ p. Acute pericarditis
- ☐ q. Hypertrophic cardiomyopathy
- ☐ r. Coronary artery disease
- ☐ s. Central nervous system disorder
- ☐ t. Myxedema
- ☐ u. Hypothermia
- ☐ v. Sick sinus syndrome

Questions: ECG 36

1. The most likely rhythm in this tracing is:

   a. Junctional tachycardia
   b. AV reentry tachycardia
   c. Automatic atrial tachycardia
   d. Atrial fibrillation with a rapid ventricular response

2. Could the tachycardia in this tracing be ventricular in origin?

   a. Yes
   b. No

3. Which of the following statements about electrical alternans are true?

   a. QRS alternans is highly specific for the diagnosis of pericardial effusion
   b. Total alternans is highly sensitive for the diagnosis of pericardial effusion
   c. Total alternans is highly specific for the diagnosis of pericardial effusion
   d. Electrical alternans occurs more commonly in pericardial effusion with tamponade than pericardial effusion without tamponade
   e. Causes of electrical alternans include pericardial effusion, supraventricular or ventricular tachycardia, hypertensive heart disease, cor pulmonale, coronary artery disease, and severe left ventricular failure

Answers: ECG 36

1. The different types of supraventricular complex tachycardia (SVT) are often difficult to distinguish based on the surface ECG. This tracing could represent junctional tachycardia or automatic atrial tachycardia. However, the most likely mechanism is AV reentry tachycardia (AVRT); the presence of atrial premature contractions (which often initiate AVNRT) and an echo beat (which is a form of reentry), lends further support for this diagnosis. (Answer: b)

2. Although rare, if the ventricular focus is high in the septum (i.e., immediately below the bundle of His), ventricular tachycardia can present with a relatively narrow QRS complex. (Answer: a)

3. Electrical alternans is identified as variation in the configuration and/or amplitude of the P, QRS, or T waves. Only one-third of patients with QRS alternans have a pericardial effusion, although the presence of total alternans (change in configuration or

amplitude of the P, QRS *and* T wave) substantially increases the likelihood that a pericardial effusion is present. Among patients with pericardial effusions, electrical alternans is more apt to be present if cardiac tamponade coexists. Other conditions associated with electrical alternans include supraventricular tachycardia (the most likely cause in the present tracing), ventricular tachycardia, hypertensive heart disease, cor pulmonale, coronary artery disease, and severe left ventricular failure. (Answer: c, d, e)

— Quick Review 36 —

Supraventricular tachycardia (paroxysmal)	
• Onset and termination of SVT is (gradual/sudden)	sudden
• SVT (does/does not) persist throughout the tracing	does not
• May see retrograde ____ activation	atrial
Retrograde atrial activation	
• Inverted P waves in leads ____	II, III and aVF

— Comic Relief —

If you're as hungry for interpretive pearls and pitfalls as the guy on the couch is for food, then you've come to the right book!

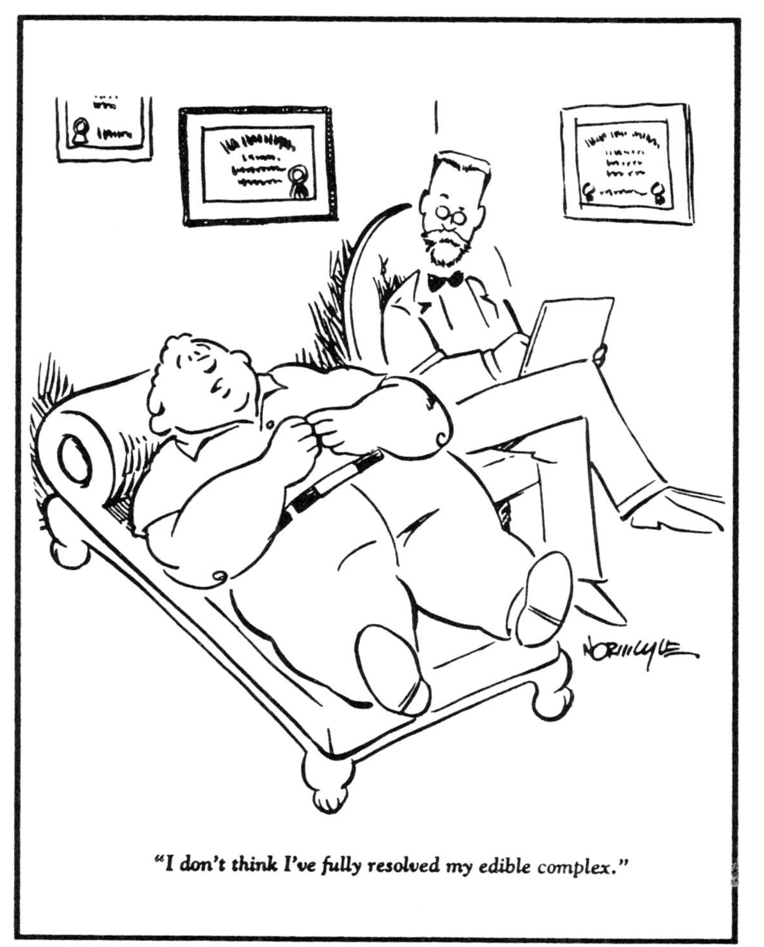

"I don't think I've fully resolved my edible complex."

ECG 37. 40-year-old asymptomatic female:

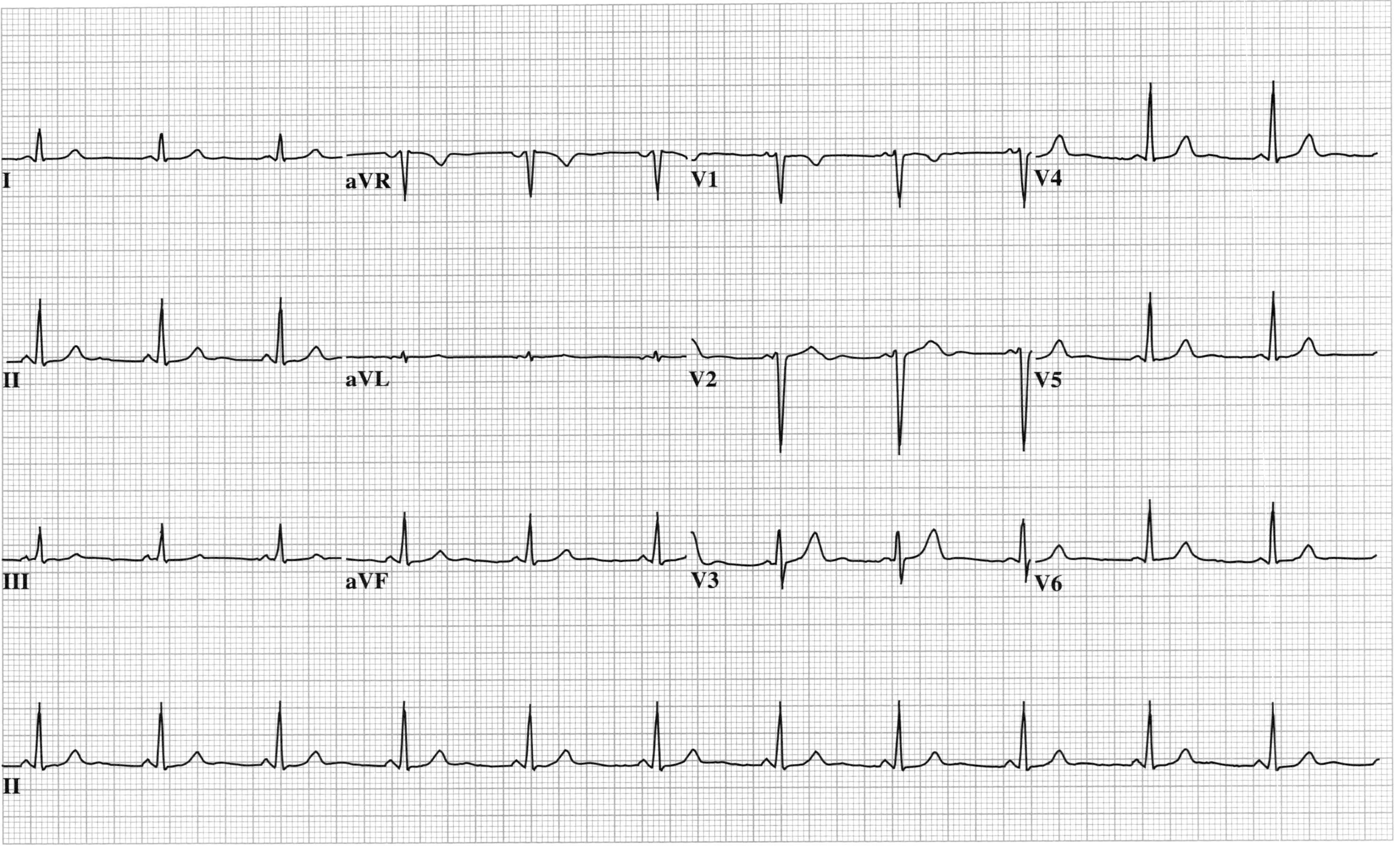

1. GENERAL FEATURES

- ☐ a. Normal ECG
- ☐ b. Borderline normal ECG or normal variant
- ☐ c. Incorrect electrode placement
- ☐ d. Artifact due to tremor

2. ATRIAL RHYTHMS

- ☐ a. Sinus rhythm
- ☐ b. Sinus arrhythmia
- ☐ c. Sinus bradycardia (< 60)
- ☐ d. Sinus tachycardia (> 100)
- ☐ e. Sinus pause or arrest
- ☐ f. Sinoatrial exit block
- ☐ g. Ecoptic atrial rhythm
- ☐ h. Wandering atrial pacemaker
- ☐ i. Atrial premature complexes, normally conducted
- ☐ j. Atrial premature complexes, nonconducted
- ☐ k. Atrial premature complexes with aberrant intraventricular conduction
- ☐ l. Atrial tachycardia (regular, sustained, 1:1 conduction)
- ☐ m. Atrial tachycardia, repetitive (short paroxysms)
- ☐ n. Atrial tachycardia, multifocal
- ☐ o. Atrial tachycardia with AV block
- ☐ p. Supraventricular tachycardia, unspecific
- ☐ q. Supraventricular tachycardia, paroxysmal
- ☐ r. Atrial flutter
- ☐ s. Atrial fibrillation
- ☐ t. Retrograde atrial activation

3. AV JUNCTIONAL RHYTHMS

- ☐ a. AV junctional premature complexes
- ☐ b. AV junctional escape complexes
- ☐ c. AV junctional rhythm, accelerated
- ☐ d. AV junctional rhythm

4. VENTRICULAR RHYTHMS

- ☐ a. Ventricular premature complex(es), uniform, fixed coupling
- ☐ b. Ventricular premature complex(es), uniform, nonfixed coupling
- ☐ c. Ventricular premature complexes(es), multiform
- ☐ d. Ventricular premature complexes, in pairs
- ☐ e. Ventricular parasystole
- ☐ f. Ventricular tachycardia (≥ 3 consecutive complexes)
- ☐ g. Accelerated idioventricular rhythm
- ☐ h. Ventricular escape complexes or rhythm
- ☐ i. Ventricular fibrillation

5. ATRIAL-VENTRICULAR INTERACTIONS IN ARRHYTHMIAS

- ☐ a. Fusion complexes
- ☐ b. Reciprocal (echo) complexes
- ☐ c. Ventricular capture complexes
- ☐ d. AV dissociation
- ☐ e. Ventriculophasic sinus arrhythmia

6. AV CONDUCTION ABNORMALITIES

- ☐ a. AV block, 1°
- ☐ b. AV block, 2° - Mobitz type I (Wenckebach)
- ☐ c. AV block, 2° - Mobitz type II
- ☐ d. AV block, 2:1
- ☐ e. AV block, 3°
- ☐ f. AV block, variable
- ☐ g. Short PR interval (with sinus rhythm and normal QRS duration)
- ☐ h. Wolff-Parkinson-White pattern

7. INTRAVENTRICULAR CONDUCTION DISTURBANCES

- ☐ a. RBBB, incomplete
- ☐ b. RBBB, complete
- ☐ c. Left anterior fascicular block
- ☐ d. Left posterior fascicular block
- ☐ e. LBBB, with ST-T wave suggestive of acute myocardial injury or infarction
- ☐ f. LBBB, complete
- ☐ g. LBBB, intermittent
- ☐ h. Intraventricular conduction disturbance, ncnspecific
- ☐ i. Aberrant intraventricular conduction with supraventricular arrhythmia

8. P WAVE ABNORMALITIES

- ☐ a. Right atrial abnormality
- ☐ b. Left atrial abnormalities
- ☐ c. Nonspecific atrial abnormality

9. ABNORMALITIES OF QRS VOLTAGE OR AXIS

- ☐ a. Low voltage, limb leads only
- ☐ b. Low voltage, limb and precordial leads
- ☐ c. Left axis deviation (> - 30%)
- ☐ d. Right axis deviation (> + 100)
- ☐ e. Electrical alternans

10. VENTRICULAR HYPERTROPHY

- ☐ a. LVH by voltage only
- ☐ b. LVH by voltage and ST-T segment abnormalities
- ☐ c. RVH
- ☐ d. Combined ventricular hypertrophy

11. Q WAVE MYOCARDIAL INFARCTION

	Probably Acute or Recent	Probably Old or Age Indeterminate
Anterolateral	☐ a.	☐ g.
Anterior	☐ b.	☐ h.
Anteroseptal	☐ c.	☐ i.
Lateral/High lateral	☐ d.	☐ j.
Inferior	☐ e.	☐ k.
Posterior	☐ f.	☐ l.

☐ m. Probably ventricular aneurysm

12. ST, T, U, WAVE ABNORMALITIES

- ☐ a. Normal variant, early repolarization
- ☐ b. Normal variant, juvenile T waves
- ☐ c. Nonspecific ST and/or T wave abnormalities
- ☐ d. ST and/or T wave abnormalities suggesting myocardial ischemia
- ☐ e. ST and/or T wave abnormalities suggesting myocardial injury
- ☐ f. ST and/or T wave abnormalities suggesting acute pericarditis
- ☐ g. ST-T segment abnormalities secondary to intraventricular conduction disturbance or hypertrophy
- ☐ h. Post-extrasystolic T wave abnormality
- ☐ i. Isolated J point depression
- ☐ j. Peaked T waves
- ☐ k. Prolonged QT interval
- ☐ l. Prominent U waves

13. PACEMAKER FUNCTION AND RHYTHM

- ☐ a. Atrial or coronary sinus pacing
- ☐ b. Ventricular demand pacing
- ☐ c. AV sequential pacing
- ☐ d. Ventricular pacing, complete control
- ☐ e. Dual chamber, atrial sensing pacemaker
- ☐ f. Pacemaker malfunction, not constantly capturing (atrium or ventricle)
- ☐ g. Pacemaker malfunction, not constantly sensing (atrium or ventricle)
- ☐ h. Pacemaker malfunction, not firing
- ☐ i. Pacemaker malfunction, slowing

14. SUGGESTED OR PROBABLE CLINICAL DISORDERS

- ☐ a. Digitalis effect
- ☐ b. Digitalis toxicity
- ☐ c. Antiarrhythmic drug effect
- ☐ d. Antiarrhythmic drug toxicity
- ☐ e. Hyperkalemia
- ☐ f. Hypokalemia
- ☐ g. Hypercalcemia
- ☐ h. Hypocalcemia
- ☐ i. Atrial septal defect, secundum
- ☐ j. Atrial septal defect, primum
- ☐ k. Dextrocardia, mirror image
- ☐ l. Mitral valve disease
- ☐ m. Chronic lung disease
- ☐ n. Acute cor pulmonale, including pulmonary embolus
- ☐ o. Pericardial effusion
- ☐ p. Acute pericarditis
- ☐ q. Hypertrophic cardiomyopathy
- ☐ r. Coronary artery disease
- ☐ s. Central nervous system disorder
- ☐ t. Myxedema
- ☐ u. Hypothermia
- ☐ v. Sick sinus syndrome

ECG 37 was obtained in this 40-year-old asymptomatic female. The tracing is normal except for a short PR interval (arrows).

Codes:

2a Sinus rhythm
6g Short PR interval

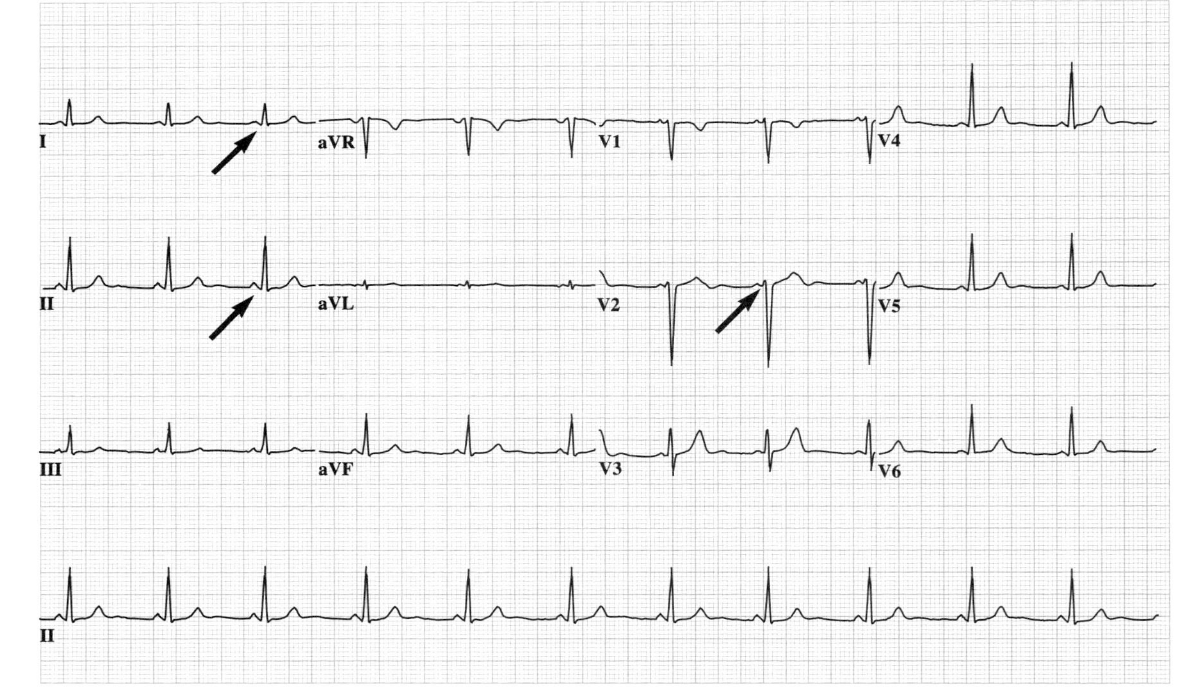

Questions: ECG 37

1. The ECG diagnosis of short PR interval requires:

   a. Sinus rhythm
   b. Initial slurring of the QRS (delta wave)
   c. PR interval less than 0.12 seconds
   d. Absence of AV dissociation

Answers: ECG 37

1. The diagnosis of short PR interval requires sinus rhythm, a PR interval less than 0.12 seconds, and absence of AV dissociation. Short PR interval with sinus rhythm and normal QRS duration (item 6g) should be distinguished from other conditions associated with a short PR interval: If initial slurring (delta wave) of a wide QRS is present, Wolff-Parkinson-White pattern should be coded. If the P waves are inverted in leads II, III, aVF, either AV junctional rhythm with retrograde atrial activation or low atrial rhythm should be coded. Finally, patients with isorhythmic dissociation may appear to have sinus rhythm with a short PR interval; however on close inspection, the P waves can be seen to merge in and out of (i.e., are dissociated from) the QRS complex without evidence of a short PR interval of fixed duration. (Answer: a, c, d)

— Quick Review 37 —	
Short PR interval (with sinus rhythm and normal QRS duration)	
• (Sinus/nonsinus) P wave	sinus
• PR interval < ____ seconds	0.12
• Delta wave is (present/absent)	absent

ECG 38. 51-year-old female receiving digitalis with complaints of "a racing heart":

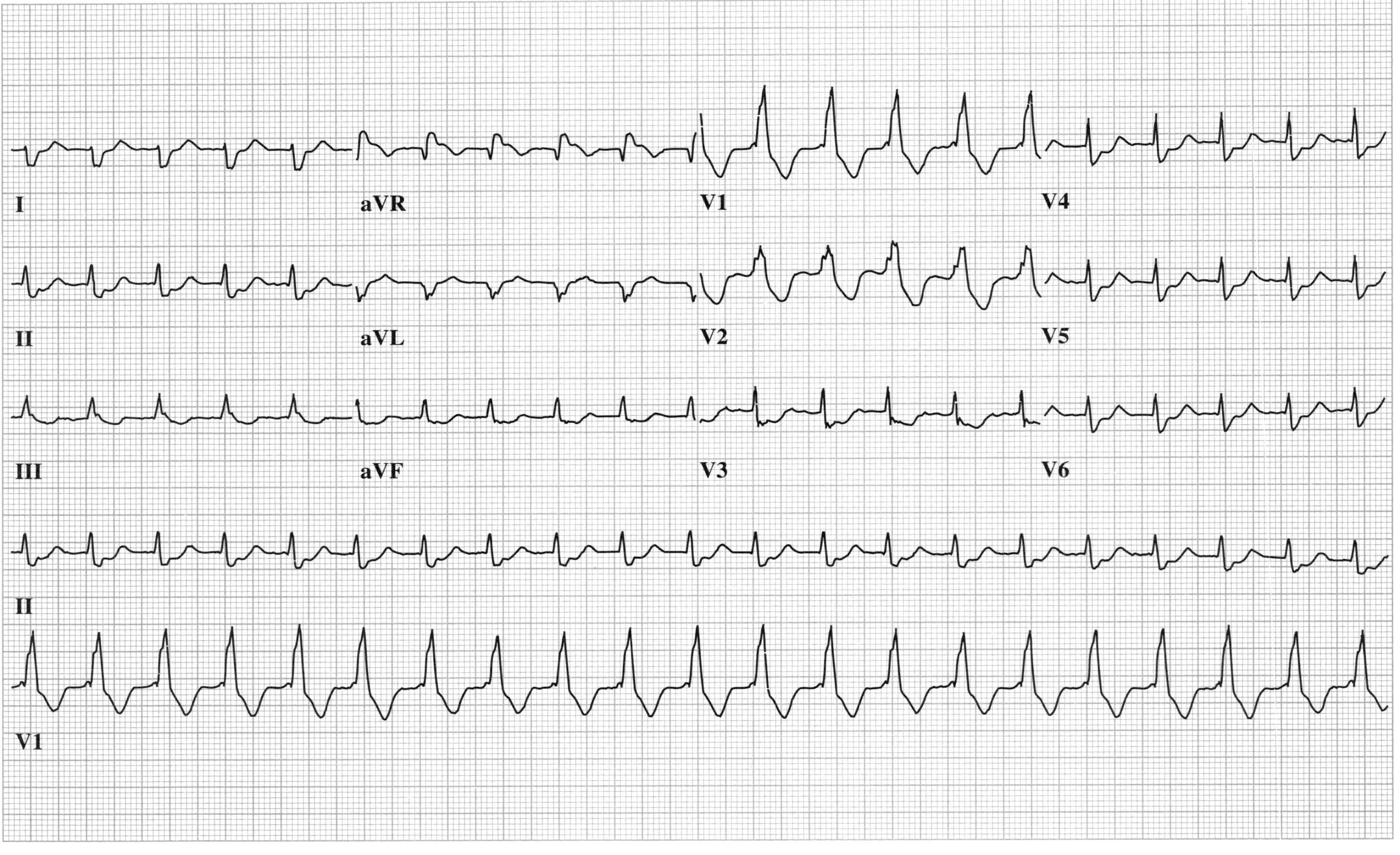

1. GENERAL FEATURES

☐ a. Normal ECG
☐ b. Borderline normal ECG or normal variant
☐ c. Incorrect electrode placement
☐ d. Artifact due to tremor

2. ATRIAL RHYTHMS

☐ a. Sinus rhythm
☐ b. Sinus arrhythmia
☐ c. Sinus bradycardia (< 60)
☐ d. Sinus tachycardia (> 100)
☐ e. Sinus pause or arrest
☐ f. Sinoatrial exit block
☐ g. Ecoptic atrial rhythm
☐ h. Wandering atrial pacemaker
☐ i. Atrial premature complexes, normally conducted
☐ j. Atrial premature complexes, nonconducted
☐ k. Atrial premature complexes with aberrant intraventricular conduction
☐ l. Atrial tachycardia (regular, sustained, 1:1 conduction)
☐ m. Atrial tachycardia, repetitive (short paroxysms)
☐ n. Atrial tachycardia, multifocal
☐ o. Atrial tachycardia with AV block
☐ p. Supraventricular tachycardia, unspecific
☐ q. Supraventricular tachycardia, paroxysmal
☐ r. Atrial flutter
☐ s. Atrial fibrillation
☐ t. Retrograde atrial activation

3. AV JUNCTIONAL RHYTHMS

☐ a. AV junctional premature complexes
☐ b. AV junctional escape complexes
☐ c. AV junctional rhythm, accelerated
☐ d. AV junctional rhythm

4. VENTRICULAR RHYTHMS

☐ a. Ventricular premature complex(es), uniform, fixed coupling
☐ b. Ventricular premature complex(es), uniform, nonfixed coupling
☐ c. Ventricular premature complexes(es), multiform
☐ d. Ventricular premature complexes, in pairs
☐ e. Ventricular parasystole
☐ f. Ventricular tachycardia (≥ 3 consecutive complexes)
☐ g. Accelerated idioventricular rhythm
☐ h. Ventricular escape complexes or rhythm
☐ i. Ventricular fibrillation

5. ATRIAL-VENTRICULAR INTERACTIONS IN ARRHYTHMIAS

☐ a. Fusion complexes
☐ b. Reciprocal (echo) complexes
☐ c. Ventricular capture complexes
☐ d. AV dissociation
☐ e. Ventriculophasic sinus arrhythmia

6. AV CONDUCTION ABNORMALITIES

☐ a. AV block, 1°
☐ b. AV block, 2° - Mobitz type I (Wenckebach)
☐ c. AV block, 2° - Mobitz type II
☐ d. AV block, 2:1
☐ e. AV block, 3°
☐ f. AV block, variable
☐ g. Short PR interval (with sinus rhythm and normal QRS duration)
☐ h. Wolff-Parkinson-White pattern

7. INTRAVENTRICULAR CONDUCTION DISTURBANCES

☐ a. RBBB, incomplete
☐ b. RBBB, complete
☐ c. Left anterior fascicular block
☐ d. Left posterior fascicular block
☐ e. LBBB, with ST-T wave suggestive of acute myocardial injury or infarction
☐ f. LBBB, complete
☐ g. LBBB, intermittent
☐ h. Intraventricular conduction disturbance, nonspecific
☐ i. Aberrant intraventricular conduction with supraventricular arrhythmia

8. P WAVE ABNORMALITIES

☐ a. Right atrial abnormality
☐ b. Left atrial abnormalities
☐ c. Nonspecific atrial abnormality

9. ABNORMALITIES OF QRS VOLTAGE OR AXIS

☐ a. Low voltage, limb leads only
☐ b. Low voltage, limb and precordial leads
☐ c. Left axis deviation (> - 30%)
☐ d. Right axis deviation (> + 100)
☐ e. Electrical alternans

10. VENTRICULAR HYPERTROPHY

☐ a. LVH by voltage only
☐ b. LVH by voltage and ST-T segment abnormalities
☐ c. RVH
☐ d. Combined ventricular hypertrophy

11. Q WAVE MYOCARDIAL INFARCTION

	Probably Acute or Recent	Probably Old or Age Indeterminate
Anterolateral	☐ a.	☐ g.
Anterior	☐ b.	☐ h.
Anteroseptal	☐ c.	☐ i.
Lateral/High lateral	☐ d.	☐ j.
Inferior	☐ e.	☐ k.
Posterior	☐ f.	☐ l.

☐ m. Probably ventricular aneurysm

12. ST, T, U, WAVE ABNORMALITIES

☐ a. Normal variant, early repolarization
☐ b. Normal variant, juvenile T waves
☐ c. Nonspecific ST and/or T wave abnormalities
☐ d. ST and/or T wave abnormalities suggesting myocardial ischemia
☐ e. ST and/or T wave abnormalities suggesting myocardial injury
☐ f. ST and/or T wave abnormalities suggesting acute pericarditis
☐ g. ST-T segment abnormalities secondary to intraventricular conduction disturbance or hypertrophy
☐ h. Post-extrasystolic T wave abnormality
☐ i. Isolated J point depression
☐ j. Peaked T waves
☐ k. Prolonged QT interval
☐ l. Prominent U waves

13. PACEMAKER FUNCTION AND RHYTHM

☐ a. Atrial or coronary sinus pacing
☐ b. Ventricular demand pacing
☐ c. AV sequential pacing
☐ d. Ventricular pacing, complete control
☐ e. Dual chamber, atrial sensing pacemaker
☐ f. Pacemaker malfunction, not constantly capturing (atrium or ventricle)
☐ g. Pacemaker malfunction, not constantly sensing (atrium or ventricle)
☐ h. Pacemaker malfunction, not firing
☐ i. Pacemaker malfunction, slowing

14. SUGGESTED OR PROBABLE CLINICAL DISORDERS

☐ a. Digitalis effect
☐ b. Digitalis toxicity
☐ c. Antiarrhythmic drug effect
☐ d. Antiarrhythmic drug toxicity
☐ e. Hyperkalemia
☐ f. Hypokalemia
☐ g. Hypercalcemia
☐ h. Hypocalcemia
☐ i. Atrial septal defect, secundum
☐ j. Atrial septal defect, primum
☐ k. Dextrocardia, mirror image
☐ l. Mitral valve disease
☐ m. Chronic lung disease
☐ n. Acute cor pulmonale, including pulmonary embolus
☐ o. Pericardial effusion
☐ p. Acute pericarditis
☐ q. Hypertrophic cardiomyopathy
☐ r. Coronary artery disease
☐ s. Central nervous system disorder
☐ t. Myxedema
☐ u. Hypothermia
☐ v. Sick sinus syndrome

ECG 38 was obtained from a 51-year-old female receiving digitalis who was being evaluated for complaints of a "racing heart." The tracing shows a wide complex tachycardia (QRS duration = 136 msec). This most likely represents junctional tachycardia with aberrancy (as opposed to VT), given the patient's history (digitalis toxicity can cause junctional tachycardia), the presence of an R' in V_1 taller than the R wave, lack of concordant QRS deflections in the precordial leads, right axis deviation, and QRS duration < 140 msec. The notch in the baseline during the early portion of the T wave (arrows) is also consistent with retrograde atrial activation from a junctional tachycardia (although VT can cause this as well). The aberrant intraventricular conduction manifests as RBBB with secondary ST-T changes, and left posterior fascicular block with right axis deviation. The patient's digoxin level on admission was 2.8 ng/mL.

Codes:

2t	Retrograde atrial activation
3c	AV junctional rhythm, accelerated
7b	RBBB, complete
7d	Left posterior fascicular block
7h	Aberrant intraventricular conduction with supraventricular arrhythmia
9d	Right axis deviation (> +100°)
12g	ST-T segment abnormalities secondary to IVCD or hypertrophy
14b	Digitalis toxicity

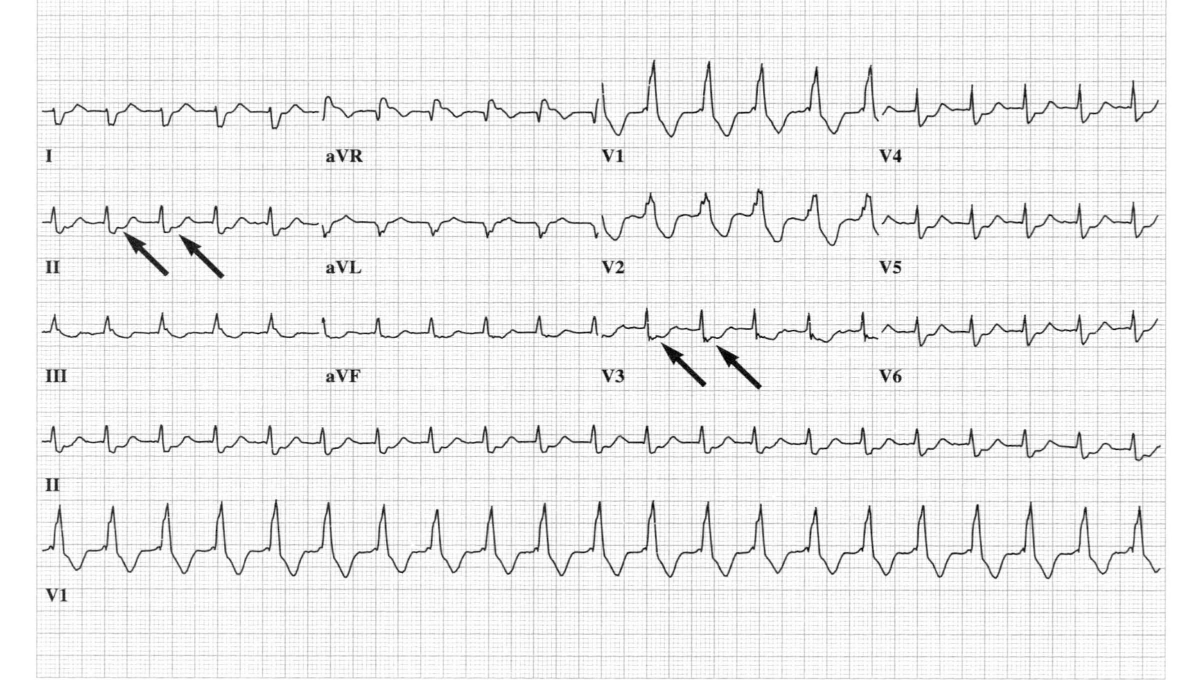

Questions: ECG 38

1. Retrograde atrial activation can be seen with:

   a. Atrial pacing
   b. Junctional rhythms
   c. Ventricular rhythms
   d. Ventricular pacing

2. Left posterior fascicular block results in:

   a. QRS prolongation greater than 0.10 seconds
   b. Left axis deviation greater than -45°
   c. Right axis deviation between + 100° and + 180°
   d. Pathological Q waves in leads II, III, and aVF

Answers: ECG 38

1. Retrograde atrial activation manifests as inverted P waves in leads II, III, and aVF, and can occur in association with junctional rhythms, and ventricular rhythms (e.g., VT, VPCs) and ventricular pacing (unless ventriculo-atrial block is present). Atrial pacing generally originates in the right atrial appendage and thus does not cause retrograde atrial activation. (Answer: b, c, d)

2. Left posterior fascicular block (LPFB) results in right axis deviation with a QRS axis between + 100° and + 180°. A deep S wave in lead I and a Q wave in lead III (S_1Q_3 pattern) is also typical of LPFB, although Q waves should not be seen in all the inferior leads. The QRS duration is normal to slightly prolonged and typically measures between 0.08-0.10 seconds. (Answer: c)

— Quick Review 38 —

AV junctional rhythm, accelerated	
• Regular QRS rhythm at rate > ____ per minute	60
• P wave may proceed, be buried in, or follow the QRS complex (true/false)	true
• QRS is usually narrow but may be wide if _____	aberrant or IVCD
• If retrograde block is present, the atria remain in sinus rhythm with ____	AV dissociation
• If retrograde atrial activation occurs, a (constant/inconstant) QRS-P interval will be present	constant
RBBB, complete	
• QRS duration ≥ ____ seconds	0.12
• Secondary R wave (R') in lead ____ is usually (shorter/taller) than the initial R wave	V_1 taller
• Onset of intrinsicoid deflection in leads V_1 and V_2 > ____ seconds	0.05
• ST segment ____ and T wave ____ in V_1, V_2	depression inversion
• Wide slurred S wave in leads ____	I, V_5, V_6
• QRS axis is usually (normal/leftward/rightward)	normal
• RBBB (does/does not) interfere with the ECG diagnosis of ventricular hypertrophy or Q wave MI	does not

— Quick Review 38 —

Left posterior fascicular block	
• ____ axis deviation with a mean QRS axis between ____ and ____ degrees	right +100, +180
• ____ wave in lead I and ____ wave in lead III	S, Q
• Normal or slightly prolonged QRS duration (true/false)	true
• No other cause for right axis deviation should be present (true/false)	true

— POP QUIZ —

Find The Mistake

Instructions: Identify the incorrect ECG feature(s) for each of the ECG diagnoses listed below

ECG Features	Answer
RBBB, complete • QRS duration ≥ 0.12 seconds • Secondary R wave (R') in lead V_1 is usually shorter than the initial R wave • Onset of intrinsicoid deflection in V_1 and V_2 > 0.05 sec • ST segment depression and T wave inversion in V_1, V_2 • Wide slurred S wave in leads I, V_5, V_6 • QRS axis is usually rightward	R' is usually taller (not shorter) than the initial R wave in V_1; QRS axis is usually normal (not rightward)
Left anterior fascicular block • Left axis deviation (-45 to -90 degrees) • qR complex in lead I, aVL, and III • Normal or slightly prolonged QRS duration • No other cause for left axis deviation present	There is an rS complex (not a qR complex) in lead III
Left posterior fascicular block • Right axis deviation (+100 to +180 degrees) • S wave in lead I and Q wave in lead III • Normal or slightly prolonged QRS duration • Other cause for right axis deviation may be present	LPFB should not be diagnosed when another cause for RAD exists
LBBB, complete • QRS duration ≥ 0.12 seconds • Onset of intrinsicoid deflection in I, V_5, V_6 > 0.05 sec • Broad monophasic R waves in leads I, V_5, V_6, which are usually notched or slurred • Secondary ST & T wave changes in same direction as the major QRS deflection • rS or QS complex in the right precordial leads	Secondary ST & T wave changes are in opposite (not the same) direction to the major QRS deflection

ECG 39. 18-year-old asymptomatic male:

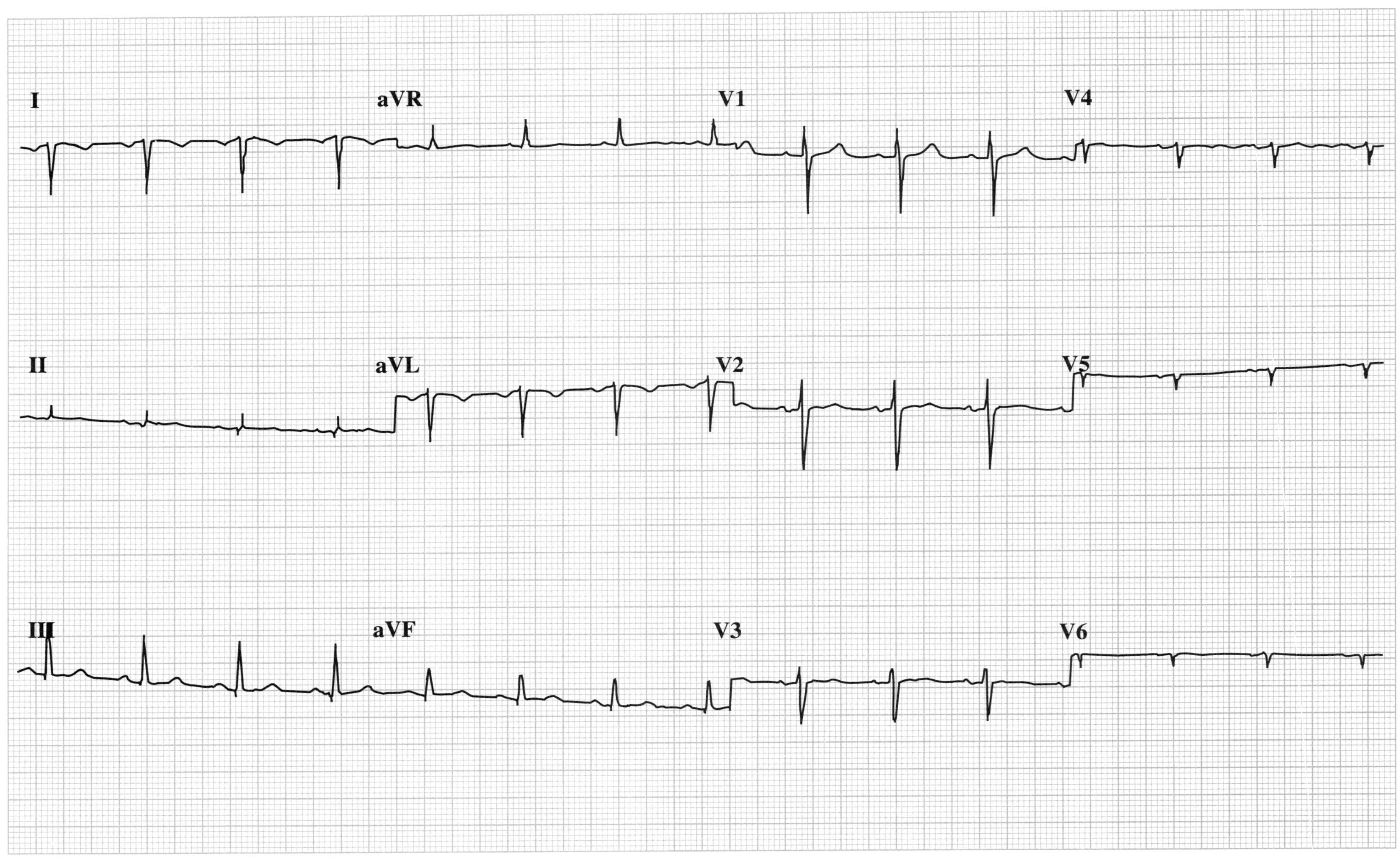

1. GENERAL FEATURES
- ☐ a. Normal ECG
- ☐ b. Borderline normal ECG or normal variant
- ☐ c. Incorrect electrode placement
- ☐ d. Artifact due to tremor

2. ATRIAL RHYTHMS
- ☐ a. Sinus rhythm
- ☐ b. Sinus arrhythmia
- ☐ c. Sinus bradycardia (< 60)
- ☐ d. Sinus tachycardia (> 100)
- ☐ e. Sinus pause or arrest
- ☐ f. Sinoatrial exit block
- ☐ g. Ecoptic atrial rhythm
- ☐ h. Wandering atrial pacemaker
- ☐ i. Atrial premature complexes, normally conducted
- ☐ j. Atrial premature complexes, nonconducted
- ☐ k. Atrial premature complexes with aberrant intraventricular conduction
- ☐ l. Atrial tachycardia (regular, sustained, 1:1 conduction)
- ☐ m. Atrial tachycardia, repetitive (short paroxysms)
- ☐ n. Atrial tachycardia, multifocal
- ☐ o. Atrial tachycardia with AV block
- ☐ p. Supraventricular tachycardia, unspecific
- ☐ q. Supraventricular tachycardia, paroxysmal
- ☐ r. Atrial flutter
- ☐ s. Atrial fibrillation
- ☐ t. Retrograde atrial activation

3. AV JUNCTIONAL RHYTHMS
- ☐ a. AV junctional premature complexes
- ☐ b. AV junctional escape complexes
- ☐ c. AV junctional rhythm, accelerated
- ☐ d. AV junctional rhythm

4. VENTRICULAR RHYTHMS
- ☐ a. Ventricular premature complex(es), uniform, fixed coupling
- ☐ b. Ventricular premature complex(es), uniform, nonfixed coupling
- ☐ c. Ventricular premature complexes(es), multiform
- ☐ d. Ventricular premature complexes, in pairs
- ☐ e. Ventricular parasystole
- ☐ f. Ventricular tachycardia (≥ 3 consecutive complexes)
- ☐ g. Accelerated idioventricular rhythm
- ☐ h. Ventricular escape complexes or rhythm
- ☐ i. Ventricular fibrillation

5. ATRIAL-VENTRICULAR INTERACTIONS IN ARRHYTHMIAS
- ☐ a. Fusion complexes
- ☐ b. Reciprocal (echo) complexes
- ☐ c. Ventricular capture complexes
- ☐ d. AV dissociation
- ☐ e. Ventriculophasic sinus arrhythmia

6. AV CONDUCTION ABNORMALITIES
- ☐ a. AV block, 1°
- ☐ b. AV block, 2° - Mobitz type I (Wenckebach)
- ☐ c. AV block, 2° - Mobitz type II
- ☐ d. AV block, 2:1
- ☐ e. AV block, 3°
- ☐ f. AV block, variable
- ☐ g. Short PR interval (with sinus rhythm and normal QRS duration)
- ☐ h. Wolff-Parkinson-White pattern

7. INTRAVENTRICULAR CONDUCTION DISTURBANCES
- ☐ a. RBBB, incomplete
- ☐ b. RBBB, complete
- ☐ c. Left anterior fascicular block
- ☐ d. Left posterior fascicular block
- ☐ e. LBBB, with ST-T wave suggestive of acute myocardial injury or infarction
- ☐ f. LBBB, complete
- ☐ g. LBBB, intermittent
- ☐ h. Intraventricular conduction disturbance, nonspecific
- ☐ i. Aberrant intraventricular conduction with supraventricular arrhythmia

8. P WAVE ABNORMALITIES
- ☐ a. Right atrial abnormality
- ☐ b. Left atrial abnormalities
- ☐ c. Nonspecific atrial abnormality

9. ABNORMALITIES OF QRS VOLTAGE OR AXIS
- ☐ a. Low voltage, limb leads only
- ☐ b. Low voltage, limb and precordial leads
- ☐ c. Left axis deviation (> - 30%)
- ☐ d. Right axis deviation (> + 100)
- ☐ e. Electrical alternans

10. VENTRICULAR HYPERTROPHY
- ☐ a. LVH by voltage only
- ☐ b. LVH by voltage and ST-T segment abnormalities
- ☐ c. RVH
- ☐ d. Combined ventricular hypertrophy

11. Q WAVE MYOCARDIAL INFARCTION

	Probably Acute or Recent	Probably Old or Age Indeterminate
Anterolateral	☐ a.	☐ g.
Anterior	☐ b.	☐ h.
Anteroseptal	☐ c.	☐ i.
Lateral/High lateral	☐ d.	☐ j.
Inferior	☐ e.	☐ k.
Posterior	☐ f.	☐ l.

- ☐ m. Probably ventricular aneurysm

12. ST, T, U, WAVE ABNORMALITIES
- ☐ a. Normal variant, early repolarization
- ☐ b. Normal variant, juvenile T waves
- ☐ c. Nonspecific ST and/or T wave abnormalities
- ☐ d. ST and/or T wave abnormalities suggesting myocardial ischemia
- ☐ e. ST and/or T wave abnormalities suggesting myocardial injury
- ☐ f. ST and/or T wave abnormalities suggesting acute pericarditis
- ☐ g. ST-T segment abnormalities secondary to intraventricular conduction disturbance or hypertrophy
- ☐ h. Post-extrasystolic T wave abnormality
- ☐ i. Isolated J point depression
- ☐ j. Peaked T waves
- ☐ k. Prolonged QT interval
- ☐ l. Prominent U waves

13. PACEMAKER FUNCTION AND RHYTHM
- ☐ a. Atrial or coronary sinus pacing
- ☐ b. Ventricular demand pacing
- ☐ c. AV sequential pacing
- ☐ d. Ventricular pacing, complete control
- ☐ e. Dual chamber, atrial sensing pacemaker
- ☐ f. Pacemaker malfunction, not constantly capturing (atrium or ventricle)
- ☐ g. Pacemaker malfunction, not constantly sensing (atrium or ventricle)
- ☐ h. Pacemaker malfunction, not firing
- ☐ i. Pacemaker malfunction, slowing

14. SUGGESTED OR PROBABLE CLINICAL DISORDERS
- ☐ a. Digitalis effect
- ☐ b. Digitalis toxicity
- ☐ c. Antiarrhythmic drug effect
- ☐ d. Antiarrhythmic drug toxicity
- ☐ e. Hyperkalemia
- ☐ f. Hypokalemia
- ☐ g. Hypercalcemia
- ☐ h. Hypocalcemia
- ☐ i. Atrial septal defect, secundum
- ☐ j. Atrial septal defect, primum
- ☐ k. Dextrocardia, mirror image
- ☐ l. Mitral valve disease
- ☐ m. Chronic lung disease
- ☐ n. Acute cor pulmonale, including pulmonary embolus
- ☐ o. Pericardial effusion
- ☐ p. Acute pericarditis
- ☐ q. Hypertrophic cardiomyopathy
- ☐ r. Coronary artery disease
- ☐ s. Central nervous system disorder
- ☐ t. Myxedema
- ☐ u. Hypothermia
- ☐ v. Sick sinus syndrome

ECG 39 was obtained in a 18-year-old asymptomatic male being screened for participation in high school basketball. The most notable feature of the ECG is the negative P-QRS-T in leads I and aVL (asterisks), which may be seen in dextrocardia and limb lead reversal. The diminishing R wave amplitude (arrows) across the precordium (V_1-V_6) confirms the diagnosis of dextrocardia. Right axis deviation and nonspecific ST-T abnormalities are also present.

Codes:

2a	Sinus rhythm
9d	Right axis deviation (> + 100°)
12c	Nonspecific ST and/or T wave abnormalities
14k	Dextrocardia, mirror image

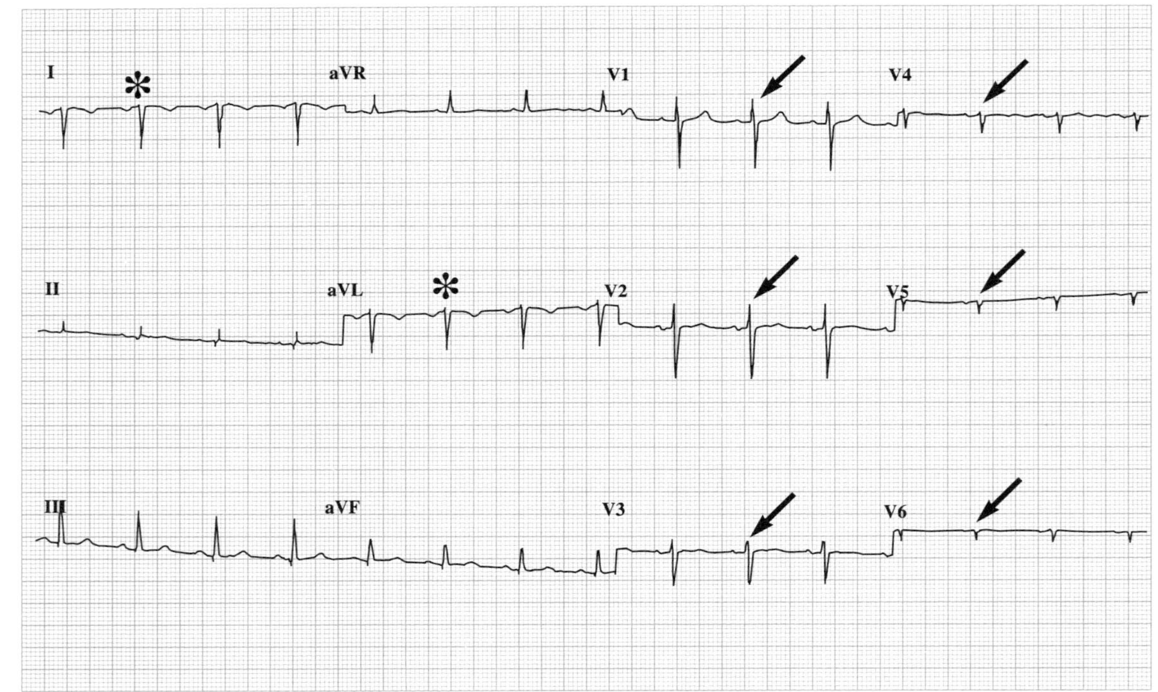

Questions: ECG 39

1. Dextrocardia is associated with:

   a. QT prolongation
   b. Low voltage in the limb leads
   c. Inverted P, QRS, and T waves in leads I and aVL
   d. Prominent R wave voltage in the left precordial leads (V_4-V_6)

2. Isolated dextrocardia (dextrocardia without inversion of other viscera) is almost invariably associated with other serious congenital cardiac malformations:

   a. True
   b. False

Answers: ECG 39

1. Dextrocardia is a rare condition characterized by congenital malpositioning of the heart in the right side of the chest. ECG features include inversion of the P-QRS-T in leads I and aVL, and decreasing R wave amplitude from leads V_1-V_6. (Answer: c)

2. In ***mirror-like dextrocardia***, the most common form of dextrocardia, the abdominal and thoracic viscera (in addition to the heart) are transposed to the side opposite their usual locations (dextrocardia with "situs inversus"). This form of dextrocardia is generally not associated with severe congenital cardiac abnormalities (other than the malposition, which does not affect cardiac function). In ***isolated dextrocardia***, the heart is rotated to the right side of the chest but other viscera remain in their usual locations. This type of dextrocardia is almost always associated with serious congenital cardiac abnormalities, resulting in clinical difficulties in infancy or early childhood. (Answer: a)

— Quick Review 39 —

Right axis deviation	
• Mean QRS axis between ____ and ____ degrees	101, 254
Dextrocardia, mirror image	
• P-QRS-T in leads ____ are inverted or "upside down"	I, aVL
• Decreasing ____ wave amplitude from leads V_1-V_6	R
• Dextrocardia and ____ can both produce an upside down P-QRS-T in leads I and aVL. To distinguish between these conditions, look at the R wave pattern in V_1 - V_6:	lead reversal
▸ Reverse R wave progression suggests (dextrocardia/lead reversal)	dextrocardia
▸ Normal R wave progression suggests (dextrocardia/lead reversal)	lead reversal

ECG 40. 53-year-old male with chest fluttering and dyspnea:

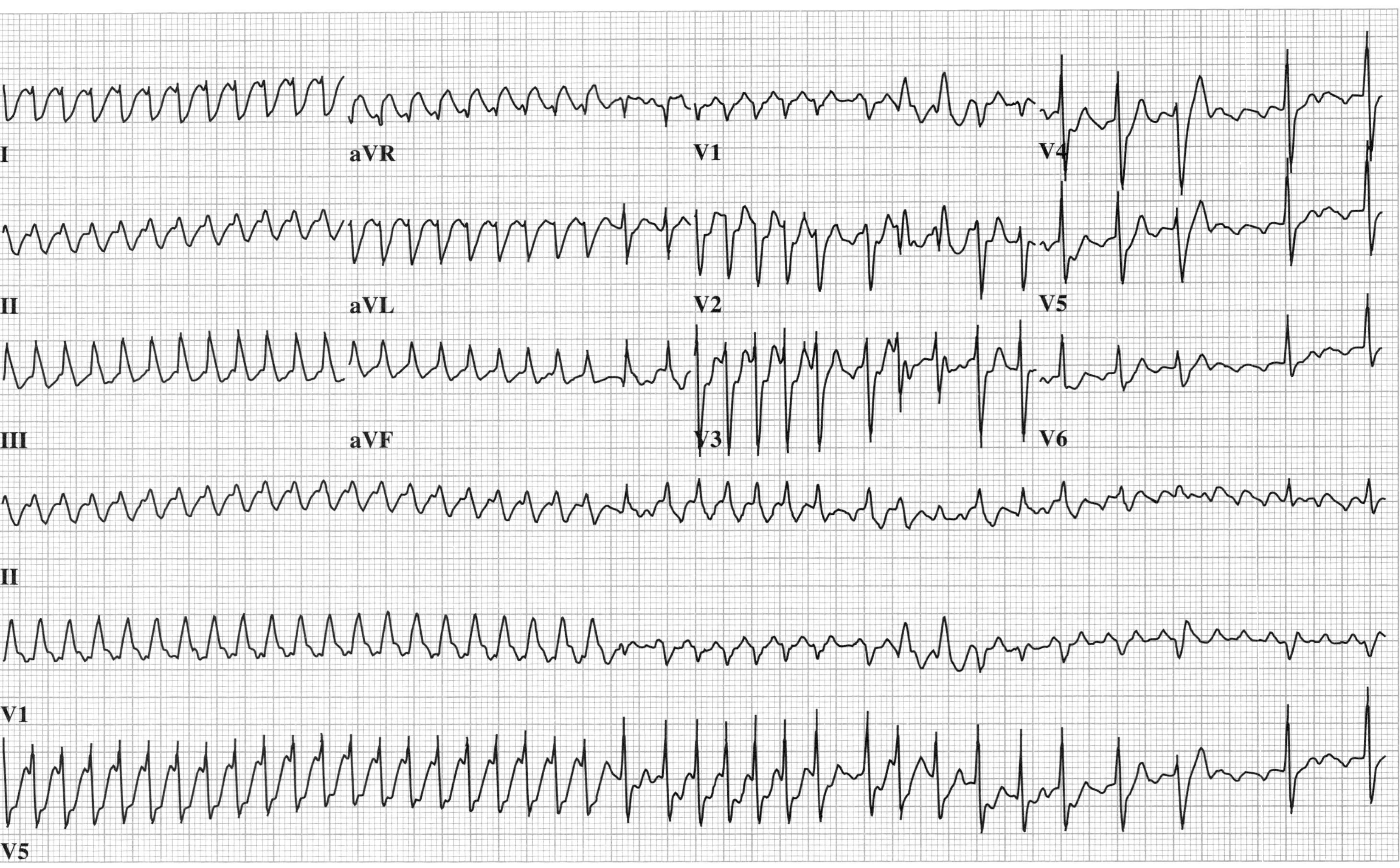

1. GENERAL FEATURES
- ☐ a. Normal ECG
- ☐ b. Borderline normal ECG or normal variant
- ☐ c. Incorrect electrode placement
- ☐ d. Artifact due to tremor

2. ATRIAL RHYTHMS
- ☐ a. Sinus rhythm
- ☐ b. Sinus arrhythmia
- ☐ c. Sinus bradycardia (< 60)
- ☐ d. Sinus tachycardia (> 100)
- ☐ e. Sinus pause or arrest
- ☐ f. Sinoatrial exit block
- ☐ g. Ecoptic atrial rhythm
- ☐ h. Wandering atrial pacemaker
- ☐ i. Atrial premature complexes, normally conducted
- ☐ j. Atrial premature complexes, nonconducted
- ☐ k. Atrial premature complexes with aberrant intraventricular conduction
- ☐ l. Atrial tachycardia (regular, sustained, 1:1 conduction)
- ☐ m. Atrial tachycardia, repetitive (short paroxysms)
- ☐ n. Atrial tachycardia, multifocal
- ☐ o. Atrial tachycardia with AV block
- ☐ p. Supraventricular tachycardia, unspecific
- ☐ q. Supraventricular tachycardia, paroxysmal
- ☐ r. Atrial flutter
- ☐ s. Atrial fibrillation
- ☐ t. Retrograde atrial activation

3. AV JUNCTIONAL RHYTHMS
- ☐ a. AV junctional premature complexes
- ☐ b. AV junctional escape complexes
- ☐ c. AV junctional rhythm, accelerated
- ☐ d. AV junctional rhythm

4. VENTRICULAR RHYTHMS
- ☐ a. Ventricular premature complex(es), uniform, fixed coupling
- ☐ b. Ventricular premature complex(es), uniform, nonfixed coupling
- ☐ c. Ventricular premature complexes(es), multiform
- ☐ d. Ventricular premature complexes, in pairs
- ☐ e. Ventricular parasystole
- ☐ f. Ventricular tachycardia (≥ 3 consecutive complexes)
- ☐ g. Accelerated idioventricular rhythm
- ☐ h. Ventricular escape complexes or rhythm
- ☐ i. Ventricular fibrillation

5. ATRIAL-VENTRICULAR INTERACTIONS IN ARRHYTHMIAS
- ☐ a. Fusion complexes
- ☐ b. Reciprocal (echo) complexes
- ☐ c. Ventricular capture complexes
- ☐ d. AV dissociation
- ☐ e. Ventriculophasic sinus arrhythmia

6. AV CONDUCTION ABNORMALITIES
- ☐ a. AV block, 1°
- ☐ b. AV block, 2° - Mobitz type I (Wenckebach)
- ☐ c. AV block, 2° - Mobitz type II
- ☐ d. AV block, 2:1
- ☐ e. AV block, 3°
- ☐ f. AV block, variable
- ☐ g. Short PR interval (with sinus rhythm and normal QRS duration)
- ☐ h. Wolff-Parkinson-White pattern

7. INTRAVENTRICULAR CONDUCTION DISTURBANCES
- ☐ a. RBBB, incomplete
- ☐ b. RBBB, complete
- ☐ c. Left anterior fascicular block
- ☐ d. Left posterior fascicular block
- ☐ e. LBBB, with ST-T wave suggestive of acute myocardial injury or infarction
- ☐ f. LBBB, complete
- ☐ g. LBBB, intermittent
- ☐ h. Intraventricular conduction disturbance, nonspecific
- ☐ i. Aberrant intraventricular conduction with supraventricular arrhythmia

8. P WAVE ABNORMALITIES
- ☐ a. Right atrial abnormality
- ☐ b. Left atrial abnormalities
- ☐ c. Nonspecific atrial abnormality

9. ABNORMALITIES OF QRS VOLTAGE OR AXIS
- ☐ a. Low voltage, limb leads only
- ☐ b. Low voltage, limb and precordial leads
- ☐ c. Left axis deviation (> - 30%)
- ☐ d. Right axis deviation (> + 100)
- ☐ e. Electrical alternans

10. VENTRICULAR HYPERTROPHY
- ☐ a. LVH by voltage only
- ☐ b. LVH by voltage and ST-T segment abnormalities
- ☐ c. RVH
- ☐ d. Combined ventricular hypertrophy

11. Q WAVE MYOCARDIAL INFARCTION

	Probably Acute or Recent	Probably Old or Age Indeterminate
Anterolateral	☐ a.	☐ g.
Anterior	☐ b.	☐ h.
Anteroseptal	☐ c.	☐ i.
Lateral/High lateral	☐ d.	☐ j.
Inferior	☐ e.	☐ k.
Posterior	☐ f.	☐ l.

- ☐ m. Probably ventricular aneurysm

12. ST, T, U, WAVE ABNORMALITIES
- ☐ a. Normal variant, early repolarization
- ☐ b. Normal variant, juvenile T waves
- ☐ c. Nonspecific ST and/or T wave abnormalities
- ☐ d. ST and/or T wave abnormalities suggesting myocardial ischemia
- ☐ e. ST and/or T wave abnormalities suggesting myocardial injury
- ☐ f. ST and/or T wave abnormalities suggesting acute pericarditis
- ☐ g. ST-T segment abnormalities secondary to intraventricular conduction disturbance or hypertrophy
- ☐ h. Post-extrasystolic T wave abnormality
- ☐ i. Isolated J point depression
- ☐ j. Peaked T waves
- ☐ k. Prolonged QT interval
- ☐ l. Prominent U waves

13. PACEMAKER FUNCTION AND RHYTHM
- ☐ a. Atrial or coronary sinus pacing
- ☐ b. Ventricular demand pacing
- ☐ c. AV sequential pacing
- ☐ d. Ventricular pacing, complete control
- ☐ e. Dual chamber, atrial sensing pacemaker
- ☐ f. Pacemaker malfunction, not constantly capturing (atrium or ventricle)
- ☐ g. Pacemaker malfunction, not constantly sensing (atrium or ventricle)
- ☐ h. Pacemaker malfunction, not firing
- ☐ i. Pacemaker malfunction, slowing

14. SUGGESTED OR PROBABLE CLINICAL DISORDERS
- ☐ a. Digitalis effect
- ☐ b. Digitalis toxicity
- ☐ c. Antiarrhythmic drug effect
- ☐ d. Antiarrhythmic drug toxicity
- ☐ e. Hyperkalemia
- ☐ f. Hypokalemia
- ☐ g. Hypercalcemia
- ☐ h. Hypocalcemia
- ☐ i. Atrial septal defect, secundum
- ☐ j. Atrial septal defect, primum
- ☐ k. Dextrocardia, mirror image
- ☐ l. Mitral valve disease
- ☐ m. Chronic lung disease
- ☐ n. Acute cor pulmonale, including pulmonary embolus
- ☐ o. Pericardial effusion
- ☐ p. Acute pericarditis
- ☐ q. Hypertrophic cardiomyopathy
- ☐ r. Coronary artery disease
- ☐ s. Central nervous system disorder
- ☐ t. Myxedema
- ☐ u. Hypothermia
- ☐ v. Sick sinus syndrome

ECG 40 was obtained in a 53-year-old male complaining of chest fluttering and dyspnea. The ECG shows atrial flutter, which is most apparent in the latter portion of the rhythm strip and in leads V_4-V_6 (arrows mark flutter waves). Variable AV block is noted, at times resulting in a rapid ventricular response and aberrant conduction (asterisk). During the tachycardia, the patient shows evidence for RBBB, right axis deviation, and left posterior fascicular block, which are transient findings related to the tachycardia and not essential for coding (although including these diagnoses would probably be given neutral credit).

Codes:

2r	Atrial flutter
6f	AV block, variable
7i	Aberrant intraventricular conduction with supraventricular arrhythmia

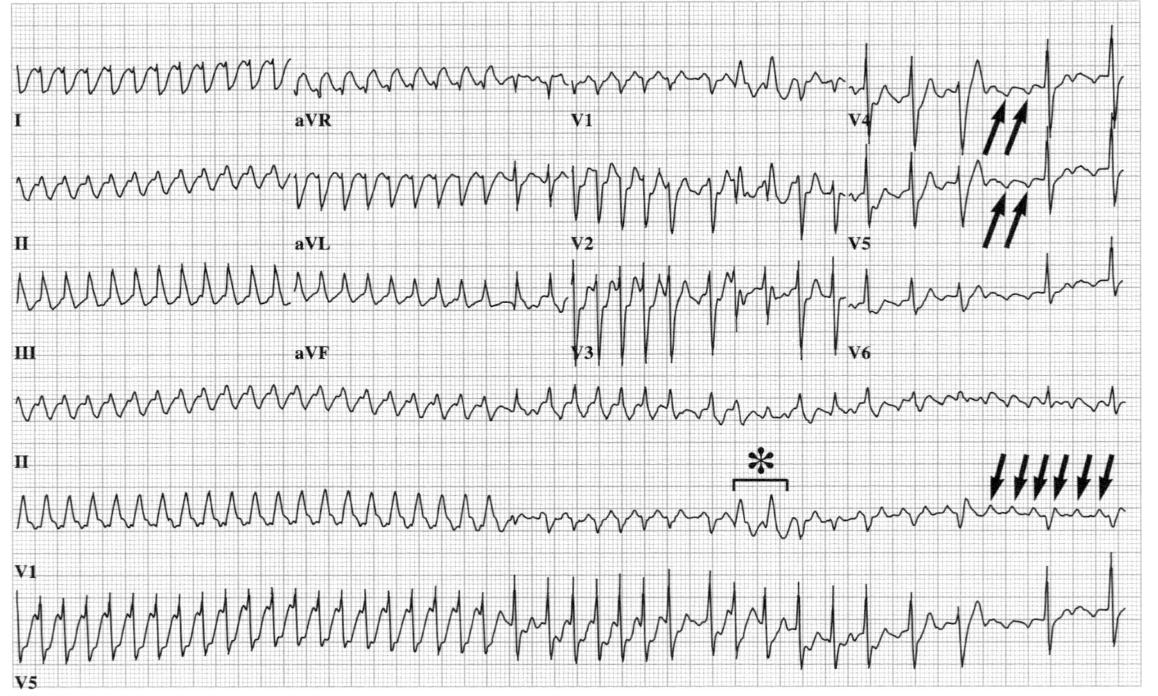

Questions: ECG 40

1. Which of the following statements about atrial flutter are true?

   a. Flutter rate is usually 240-340 bpm
   b. The interval between flutter waves may vary
   c. Ventricular response rates may vary
   d. Carotid sinus massage frequently restores normal sinus rhythm

2. The most common AV conduction rate in atrial flutter is:

   a. 1:1
   b. 2:1
   c. 3:1
   d. 4:1
   e. > 4:1

3. The QRS complexes of tachycardia-induced aberrancy are more likely to manifest:

   a. RBBB morphology
   b. LBBB morphology

Answers: ECG 40

1. Atrial flutter manifests as rapid regular atrial undulations (flutter or "F" waves) at a rate of 240-340 per minute. (In contrast, atrial fibrillation manifests totally irregular atrial fibrillatory (f) waves of varying amplitude, duration and morphology.) AV conduction ratio (ratio of flutter waves to QRS complexes) is usually fixed, but may vary, resulting in an irregular ventricular response, which is often due to two levels of block (e.g., 2:1 and 4:1 AV block) or concealed conduction. Atrial flutter typically responds to carotid sinus massage with a decrease in ventricular rate, which returns to baseline upon termination of this maneuver; restoration of normal sinus rhythm is rare. (Answer: a, c)

2. Atrial flutter most commonly manifests as 2:1 AV block. Conduction ratios of 1:1 and 3:1 are uncommon. In untreated patients, block ≥ 4:1 suggests the coexistence of AV conduction disease. (Answer: b)

3. Aberrant intrraventricular conduction occurs when a supraventricular impulse finds one of the bundle branches conductive and the other refractory. Since the right bundle typically has a longer action potential and refractory period than the left bundle, aberrancy usually manifests as a RBBB, especially in patients without structural heart disease. (Answer: a)

— Quick Review 40 —

Atrial flutter	
• Rapid (regular/irregular) atrial undulations ("F" waves) at a rate of ____ per minute	regular 240-340
• Flutter rate may (increase/decrease) in the presence of Types IA, IC or III antiarrhythmic drugs	decrease
• Flutter waves in leads II, III, AVF are typically (inverted/upright) (with/without) an isoelectric baseline	inverted,without
• Flutter waves in lead V_1 are typically small (positive/negative) deflections (with/without) a distinct isoelectric baseline	positive, with
• QRS complex may be normal or aberrant (true/false)	true
• AV conduction ratio (ratio of flutter waves to QRS complexes) is usually (fixed/variable)	fixed
▸ Conduction ratios of 1:1 and 3:1 are (common/uncommon)	uncommon
▸ In untreated patients, AV block ≥ ____ suggests the coexistence of AV conduction disease	4:1

— POP QUIZ —

VT or Not VT: That is the Question

Instructions: In the setting of a wide QRS tachycardia, decide whether the ECG findings below favor a diagnosis of ventricular tachycardia or SVT with aberrancy

ECG Feature	VT or SVT with Aberrancy
QRS morphology similar to sinus rhythm or aberrantly conducted APCs	SVT
Tachycardia initiated by VPCs	VT
AV dissociation present	VT
Capture beats absent	SVT
Fusion beats present	VT
QRS duration during tachycardia < 0.14 sec. if RBBB morphology (or < 0.16 sec. if LBBB morphology (assuming QRS is narrow during sinus rhythm)	SVT
Some QRS deflections in precordial leads are positive and some are negative (discordance)	SVT
RSR' V_1: R wave is taller than R'	VT

ECG 41. 23-year-old male with cyanosis:

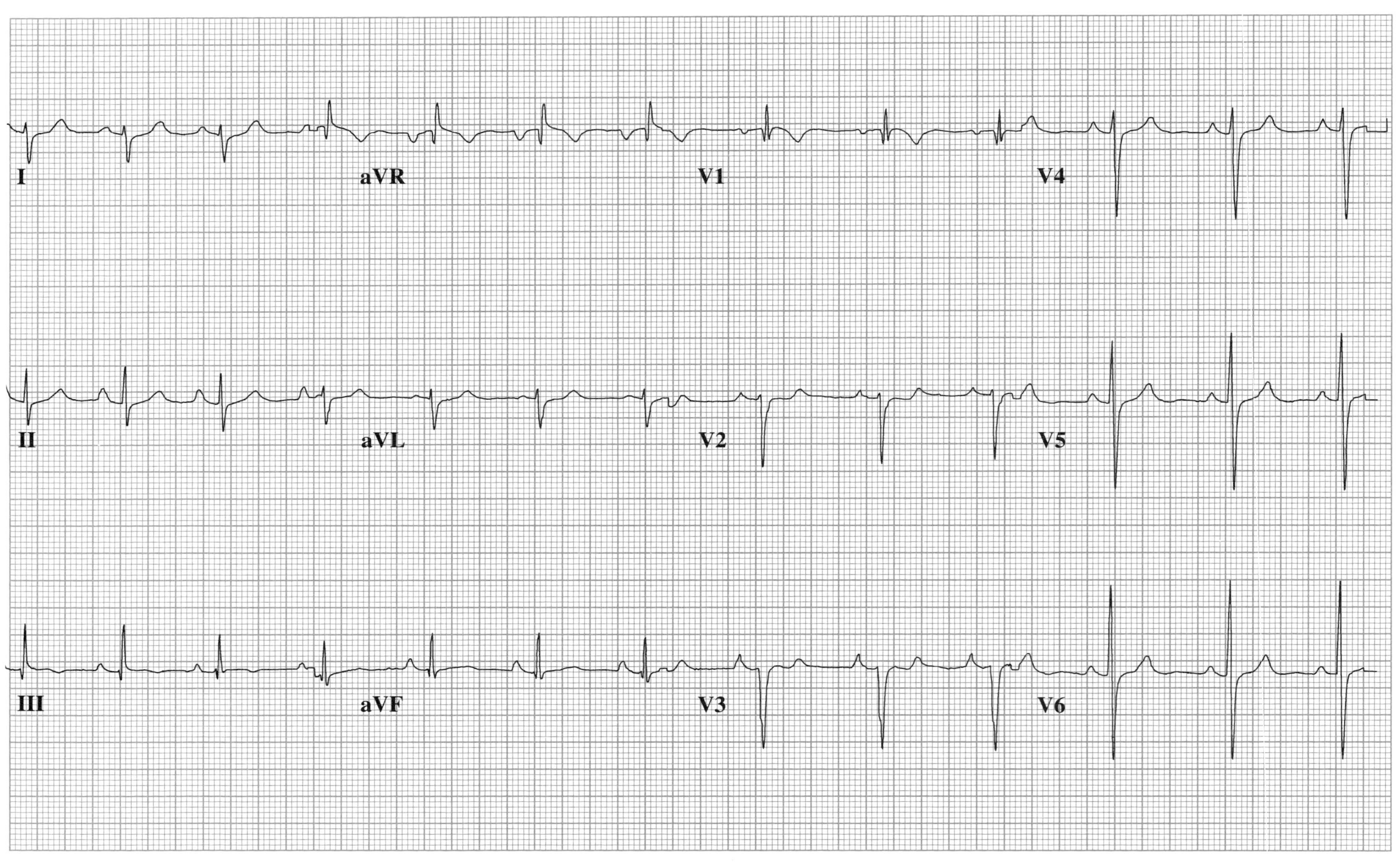

1. GENERAL FEATURES

☐ a. Normal ECG
☐ b. Borderline normal ECG or normal variant
☐ c. Incorrect electrode placement
☐ d. Artifact due to tremor

2. ATRIAL RHYTHMS

☐ a. Sinus rhythm
☐ b. Sinus arrhythmia
☐ c. Sinus bradycardia (< 60)
☐ d. Sinus tachycardia (> 100)
☐ e. Sinus pause or arrest
☐ f. Sinoatrial exit block
☐ g. Ecoptic atrial rhythm
☐ h. Wandering atrial pacemaker
☐ i. Atrial premature complexes, normally conducted
☐ j. Atrial premature complexes, nonconducted
☐ k. Atrial premature complexes with aberrant intraventricular conduction
☐ l. Atrial tachycardia (regular, sustained, 1:1 conduction)
☐ m. Atrial tachycardia, repetitive (short paroxysms)
☐ n. Atrial tachycardia, multifocal
☐ o. Atrial tachycardia with AV block
☐ p. Supraventricular tachycardia, unspecific
☐ q. Supraventricular tachycardia, paroxysmal
☐ r. Atrial flutter
☐ s. Atrial fibrillation
☐ t. Retrograde atrial activation

3. AV JUNCTIONAL RHYTHMS

☐ a. AV junctional premature complexes
☐ b. AV junctional escape complexes
☐ c. AV junctional rhythm, accelerated
☐ d. AV junctional rhythm

4. VENTRICULAR RHYTHMS

☐ a. Ventricular premature complex(es), uniform, fixed coupling
☐ b. Ventricular premature complex(es), uniform, nonfixed coupling
☐ c. Ventricular premature complexes(es), multiform
☐ d. Ventricular premature complexes, in pairs
☐ e. Ventricular parasystole
☐ f. Ventricular tachycardia (≥ 3 consecutive complexes)
☐ g. Accelerated idioventricular rhythm
☐ h. Ventricular escape complexes or rhythm
☐ i. Ventricular fibrillation

5. ATRIAL-VENTRICULAR INTERACTIONS IN ARRHYTHMIAS

☐ a. Fusion complexes
☐ b. Reciprocal (echo) complexes
☐ c. Ventricular capture complexes
☐ d. AV dissociation

☐ e. Ventriculophasic sinus arrhythmia

6. AV CONDUCTION ABNORMALITIES

☐ a. AV block, 1°
☐ b. AV block, 2° - Mobitz type I (Wenckebach)
☐ c. AV block, 2° - Mobitz type II
☐ d. AV block, 2:1
☐ e. AV block, 3°
☐ f. AV block, variable
☐ g. Short PR interval (with sinus rhythm and normal QRS duration)
☐ h. Wolff-Parkinson-White pattern

7. INTRAVENTRICULAR CONDUCTION DISTURBANCES

☐ a. RBBB, incomplete
☐ b. RBBB, complete
☐ c. Left anterior fascicular block
☐ d. Left posterior fascicular block
☐ e. LBBB, with ST-T wave suggestive of acute myocardial injury or infarction
☐ f. LBBB, complete
☐ g. LBBB, intermittent
☐ h. Intraventricular conduction disturbance, nonspecific
☐ i. Aberrant intraventricular conduction with supraventricular arrhythmia

8. P WAVE ABNORMALITIES

☐ a. Right atrial abnormality
☐ b. Left atrial abnormalities
☐ c. Nonspecific atrial abnormality

9. ABNORMALITIES OF QRS VOLTAGE OR AXIS

☐ a. Low voltage, limb leads only
☐ b. Low voltage, limb and precordial leads
☐ c. Left axis deviation (> - 30%)
☐ d. Right axis deviation (> + 100)
☐ e. Electrical alternans

10. VENTRICULAR HYPERTROPHY

☐ a. LVH by voltage only
☐ b. LVH by voltage and ST-T segment abnormalities
☐ c. RVH
☐ d. Combined ventricular hypertrophy

11. Q WAVE MYOCARDIAL INFARCTION

	Probably Acute or Recent	Probably Old or Age Indeterminate
Anterolateral	☐ a.	☐ g.
Anterior	☐ b.	☐ h.
Anteroseptal	☐ c.	☐ i.
Lateral/High lateral	☐ d.	☐ j.
Inferior	☐ e.	☐ k.
Posterior	☐ f.	☐ l.

☐ m. Probably ventricular aneurysm

12. ST, T, U, WAVE ABNORMALITIES

☐ a. Normal variant, early repolarization
☐ b. Normal variant, juvenile T waves
☐ c. Nonspecific ST and/or T wave abnormalities
☐ d. ST and/or T wave abnormalities suggesting myocardial ischemia
☐ e. ST and/or T wave abnormalities suggesting myocardial injury
☐ f. ST and/or T wave abnormalities suggesting acute pericarditis
☐ g. ST-T segment abnormalities secondary to intraventricular conduction disturbance or hypertrophy
☐ h. Post-extrasystolic T wave abnormality
☐ i. Isolated J point depression
☐ j. Peaked T waves
☐ k. Prolonged QT interval
☐ l. Prominent U waves

13. PACEMAKER FUNCTION AND RHYTHM

☐ a. Atrial or coronary sinus pacing
☐ b. Ventricular demand pacing
☐ c. AV sequential pacing
☐ d. Ventricular pacing, complete control
☐ e. Dual chamber, atrial sensing pacemaker
☐ f. Pacemaker malfunction, not constantly capturing (atrium or ventricle)
☐ g. Pacemaker malfunction, not constantly sensing (atrium or ventricle)
☐ h. Pacemaker malfunction, not firing
☐ i. Pacemaker malfunction, slowing

14. SUGGESTED OR PROBABLE CLINICAL DISORDERS

☐ a. Digitalis effect
☐ b. Digitalis toxicity
☐ c. Antiarrhythmic drug effect
☐ d. Antiarrhythmic drug toxicity
☐ e. Hyperkalemia
☐ f. Hypokalemia
☐ g. Hypercalcemia
☐ h. Hypocalcemia
☐ i. Atrial septal defect, secundum
☐ j. Atrial septal defect, primum
☐ k. Dextrocardia, mirror image
☐ l. Mitral valve disease
☐ m. Chronic lung disease
☐ n. Acute cor pulmonale, including pulmonary embolus
☐ o. Pericardial effusion
☐ p. Acute pericarditis
☐ q. Hypertrophic cardiomyopathy
☐ r. Coronary artery disease
☐ s. Central nervous system disorder
☐ t. Myxedema
☐ u. Hypothermia
☐ v. Sick sinus syndrome

ECG 41 was obtained in a 23-year-old male with cyanosis. The ECG shows a sinus rhythm at 76 beats/minute with right axis deviation, right atrial abnormality (arrowhead), an rSr' in V_1 (that does not meet duration criteria for incomplete RBBB), and right ventricular hypertrophy with secondary ST-T changes (asterisks). RVH is suggested by the finding of right axis deviation, a dominant R wave in V_1 with secondary ST-T changes, and right atrial abnormality.

Codes:

2a	Sinus rhythm
8a	Right atrial abnormality
9d	Right axis deviation (> +100°)
10c	Right ventricular hypertrophy
12g	ST-T segment abnormalities secondary to IVCD or hypertrophy

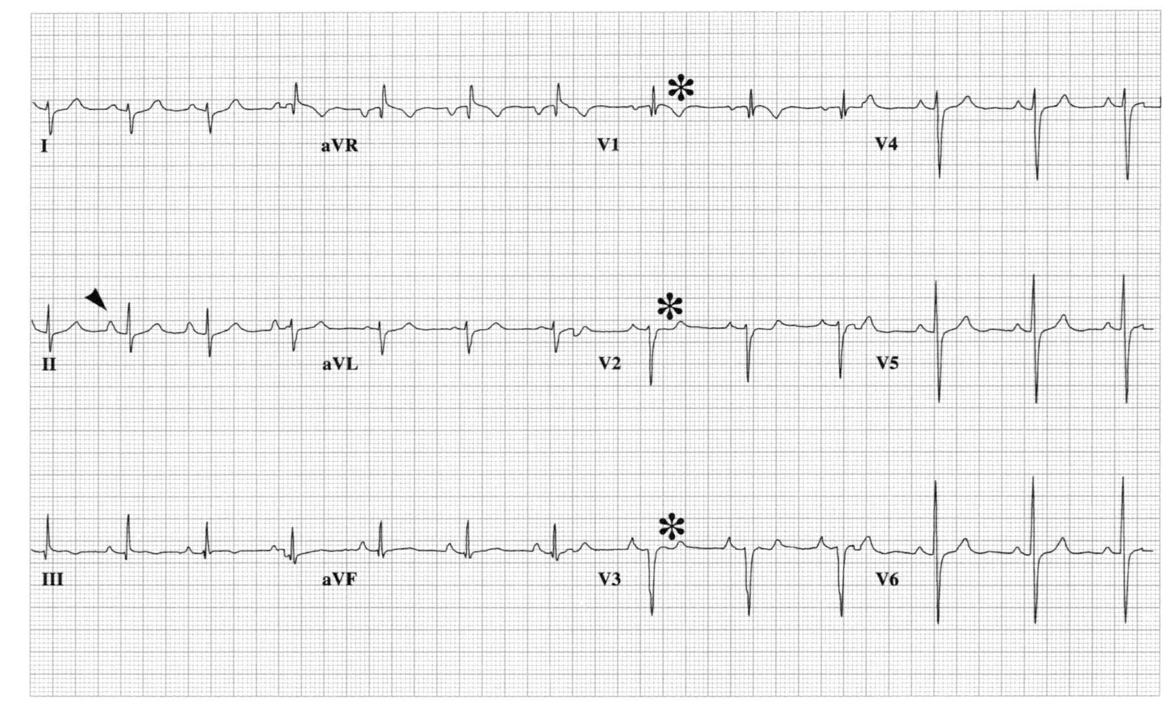

Questions: ECG 41

1. Repolarization abnormalities associated with RVH are typically most prominent in leads:

   a. V_4-V_6
   b. V_1-V_3
   c. I, aVL
   d. aVR, aVL

2. Conditions that can mimic RVH include:

   a. Wolff-Parkinson-White pattern
   b. Anterior myocardial infarction
   c. Posterior myocardial infarction
   d. RBBB

Answers: ECG 41

1. The "strain pattern" typically associated with right ventricular hypertrophy manifests as shallow T wave inversion in leads V_1-V_3. When RVH complicates COPD, ST segment depression in the inferior leads may also be seen. (Answer: b)

2. Many conditions are associated with a tall R wave in V_1 and right axis deviation, and can thus mimic right ventricular hypertrophy. These conditions include Wolff-Parkinson-White syndrome, posterior MI, and right bundle branch block. Anterior MI results in absent or diminished anterior forces. (Answer: a, c, d)

— Quick Review 41 —

Right atrial abnormality	
• Upright P wave > ____ mm in leads II, III and aVF	2.5
or > ____ mm in leads V_1 or V_2	1.5
• P wave axis ≥ ____ degrees	70
Right ventricular hypertrophy	
• Mean QRS axis ≥ ____ degrees	100
• Dominant ____ wave in V_1:	R
▸ R/S ratio in V_1 or V_{3R} (<, =, >) 1, or R/S ratio in	>
V_5 or V_6 (≤, >) 1	≤
▸ R wave in V_1 ≥ ____ mm	7
▸ R wave in V_1 + S wave in V_5 or V_6 > ____ mm	10.5
▸ rSR' in V_1 with R' > ____ mm	10
• Secondary downsloping ST depression & T-wave inversion in the (right/left) precordial leads	right
• (Right/left) atrial abnormality	right

ECG 42. 52-year-old male with chest pain:

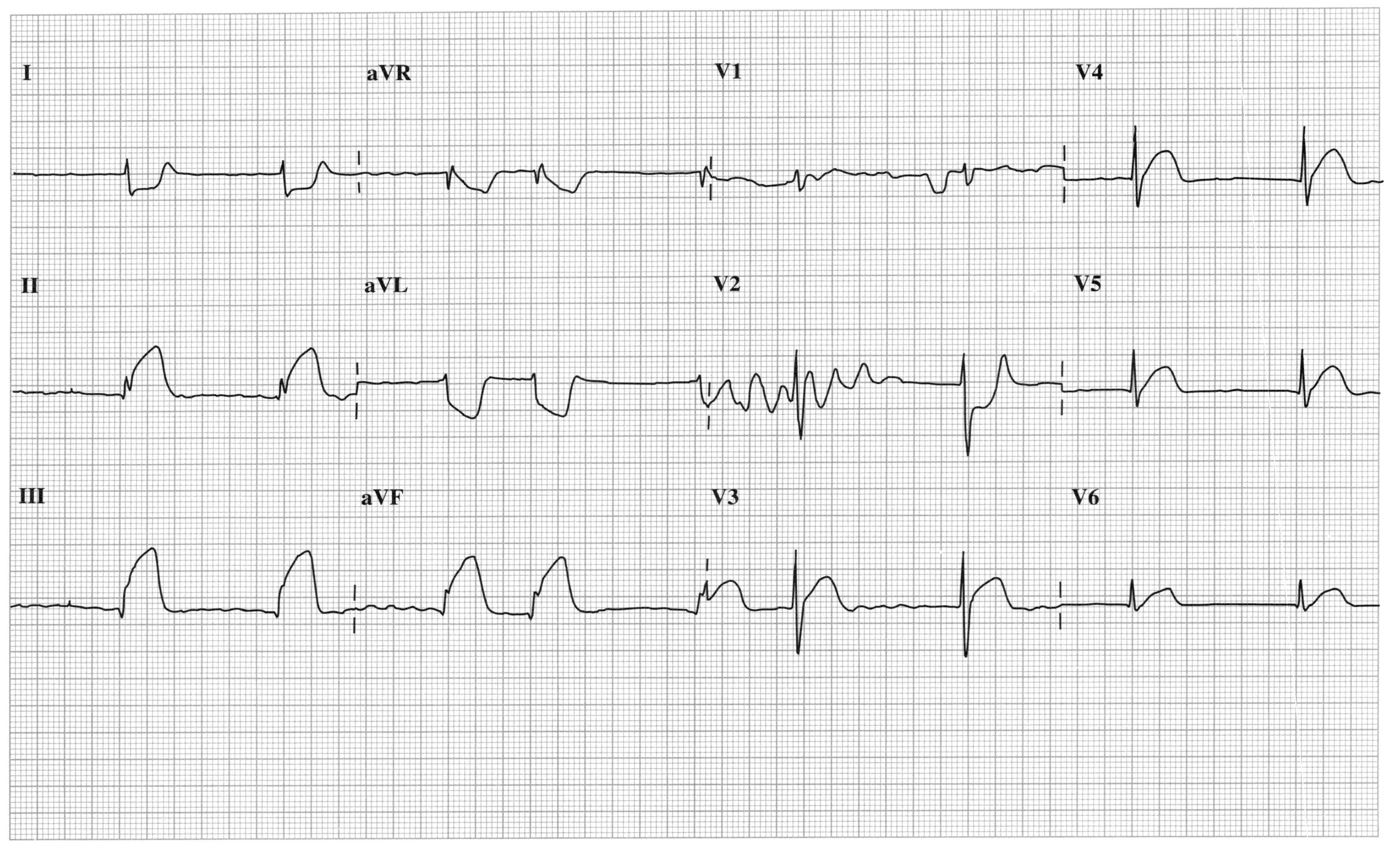

1. GENERAL FEATURES

- ☐ a. Normal ECG
- ☐ b. Borderline normal ECG or normal variant
- ☐ c. Incorrect electrode placement
- ☐ d. Artifact due to tremor

2. ATRIAL RHYTHMS

- ☐ a. Sinus rhythm
- ☐ b. Sinus arrhythmia
- ☐ c. Sinus bradycardia (< 60)
- ☐ d. Sinus tachycardia (> 100)
- ☐ e. Sinus pause or arrest
- ☐ f. Sinoatrial exit block
- ☐ g. Ecoptic atrial rhythm
- ☐ h. Wandering atrial pacemaker
- ☐ i. Atrial premature complexes, normally conducted
- ☐ j. Atrial premature complexes, nonconducted
- ☐ k. Atrial premature complexes with aberrant intraventricular conduction
- ☐ l. Atrial tachycardia (regular, sustained, 1:1 conduction)
- ☐ m. Atrial tachycardia, repetitive (short paroxysms)
- ☐ n. Atrial tachycardia, multifocal
- ☐ o. Atrial tachycardia with AV block
- ☐ p. Supraventricular tachycardia, unspecific
- ☐ q. Supraventricular tachycardia, paroxysmal
- ☐ r. Atrial flutter
- ☐ s. Atrial fibrillation
- ☐ t. Retrograde atrial activation

3. AV JUNCTIONAL RHYTHMS

- ☐ a. AV junctional premature complexes
- ☐ b. AV junctional escape complexes
- ☐ c. AV junctional rhythm, accelerated
- ☐ d. AV junctional rhythm

4. VENTRICULAR RHYTHMS

- ☐ a. Ventricular premature complex(es), uniform, fixed coupling
- ☐ b. Ventricular premature complex(es), uniform, nonfixed coupling
- ☐ c. Ventricular premature complexes(es), multiform
- ☐ d. Ventricular premature complexes, in pairs
- ☐ e. Ventricular parasystole
- ☐ f. Ventricular tachycardia (≥ 3 consecutive complexes)
- ☐ g. Accelerated idioventricular rhythm
- ☐ h. Ventricular escape complexes or rhythm
- ☐ i. Ventricular fibrillation

5. ATRIAL-VENTRICULAR INTERACTIONS IN ARRHYTHMIAS

- ☐ a. Fusion complexes
- ☐ b. Reciprocal (echo) complexes
- ☐ c. Ventricular capture complexes
- ☐ d. AV dissociation
- ☐ e. Ventriculophasic sinus arrhythmia

6. AV CONDUCTION ABNORMALITIES

- ☐ a. AV block, 1°
- ☐ b. AV block, 2° - Mobitz type I (Wenckebach)
- ☐ c. AV block, 2° - Mobitz type II
- ☐ d. AV block, 2:1
- ☐ e. AV block, 3°
- ☐ f. AV block, variable
- ☐ g. Short PR interval (with sinus rhythm and normal QRS duration)
- ☐ h. Wolff-Parkinson-White pattern

7. INTRAVENTRICULAR CONDUCTION DISTURBANCES

- ☐ a. RBBB, incomplete
- ☐ b. RBBB, complete
- ☐ c. Left anterior fascicular block
- ☐ d. Left posterior fascicular block
- ☐ e. LBBB, with ST-T wave suggestive of acute myocardial injury or infarction
- ☐ f. LBBB, complete
- ☐ g. LBBB, intermittent
- ☐ h. Intraventricular conduction disturbance, nonspecific
- ☐ i. Aberrant intraventricular conduction with supraventricular arrhythmia

8. P WAVE ABNORMALITIES

- ☐ a. Right atrial abnormality
- ☐ b. Left atrial abnormalities
- ☐ c. Nonspecific atrial abnormality

9. ABNORMALITIES OF QRS VOLTAGE OR AXIS

- ☐ a. Low voltage, limb leads only
- ☐ b. Low voltage, limb and precordial leads
- ☐ c. Left axis deviation (> - 30%)
- ☐ d. Right axis deviation (> + 100)
- ☐ e. Electrical alternans

10. VENTRICULAR HYPERTROPHY

- ☐ a. LVH by voltage only
- ☐ b. LVH by voltage and ST-T segment abnormalities
- ☐ c. RVH
- ☐ d. Combined ventricular hypertrophy

11. Q WAVE MYOCARDIAL INFARCTION

	Probably Acute or Recent	Probably Old or Age Indeterminate
Anterolateral	☐ a.	☐ g.
Anterior	☐ b.	☐ h.
Anteroseptal	☐ c.	☐ i.
Lateral/High lateral	☐ d.	☐ j.
Inferior	☐ e.	☐ k.
Posterior	☐ f.	☐ l.

☐ m. Probably ventricular aneurysm

12. ST, T, U, WAVE ABNORMALITIES

- ☐ a. Normal variant, early repolarization
- ☐ b. Normal variant, juvenile T waves
- ☐ c. Nonspecific ST and/or T wave abnormalities
- ☐ d. ST and/or T wave abnormalities suggesting myocardial ischemia
- ☐ e. ST and/or T wave abnormalities suggesting myocardial injury
- ☐ f. ST and/or T wave abnormalities suggesting acute pericarditis
- ☐ g. ST-T segment abnormalities secondary to intraventricular conduction disturbance or hypertrophy
- ☐ h. Post-extrasystolic T wave abnormality
- ☐ i. Isolated J point depression
- ☐ j. Peaked T waves
- ☐ k. Prolonged QT interval
- ☐ l. Prominent U waves

13. PACEMAKER FUNCTION AND RHYTHM

- ☐ a. Atrial or coronary sinus pacing
- ☐ b. Ventricular demand pacing
- ☐ c. AV sequential pacing
- ☐ d. Ventricular pacing, complete control
- ☐ e. Dual chamber, atrial sensing pacemaker
- ☐ f. Pacemaker malfunction, not constantly capturing (atrium or ventricle)
- ☐ g. Pacemaker malfunction, not constantly sensing (atrium or ventricle)
- ☐ h. Pacemaker malfunction, not firing
- ☐ i. Pacemaker malfunction, slowing

14. SUGGESTED OR PROBABLE CLINICAL DISORDERS

- ☐ a. Digitalis effect
- ☐ b. Digitalis toxicity
- ☐ c. Antiarrhythmic drug effect
- ☐ d. Antiarrhythmic drug toxicity
- ☐ e. Hyperkalemia
- ☐ f. Hypokalemia
- ☐ g. Hypercalcemia
- ☐ h. Hypocalcemia
- ☐ i. Atrial septal defect, secundum
- ☐ j. Atrial septal defect, primum
- ☐ k. Dextrocardia, mirror image
- ☐ l. Mitral valve disease
- ☐ m. Chronic lung disease
- ☐ n. Acute cor pulmonale, including pulmonary embolus
- ☐ o. Pericardial effusion
- ☐ p. Acute pericarditis
- ☐ q. Hypertrophic cardiomyopathy
- ☐ r. Coronary artery disease
- ☐ s. Central nervous system disorder
- ☐ t. Myxedema
- ☐ u. Hypothermia
- ☐ v. Sick sinus syndrome

ECG 42 was obtained from a 52-year-old male with chest pain. The ECG shows marked ST-T wave changes (arrows) consistent with acute myocardial injury to the inferior, posterior, and anterolateral walls (which will likely evolve into an extensive Q wave MI). Coarse baseline fluctuation noted in only V_2 is compatible with artifact (arrowhead). The rhythm is atrial fibrillation but becomes regular during the last half of the tracing suggesting AV block with an AV junctional escape rhythm (asterisk). Right axis deviation and ST-T abnormalities consistent with myocardial injury are noted (including peaked T waves). These findings are, of course, compatible with coronary artery disease.

Codes:

1d	Artifact due to tremor
2s	Atrial fibrillation
3b	AV junctional escape complexes
9d	Right axis deviation (> +100°)
12d	ST and/or T wave abnormalities suggesting myocardial ischemia
12e	ST and/or T wave abnormalities suggesting myocardial injury
12j	Peaked T waves
14r	Coronary artery disease

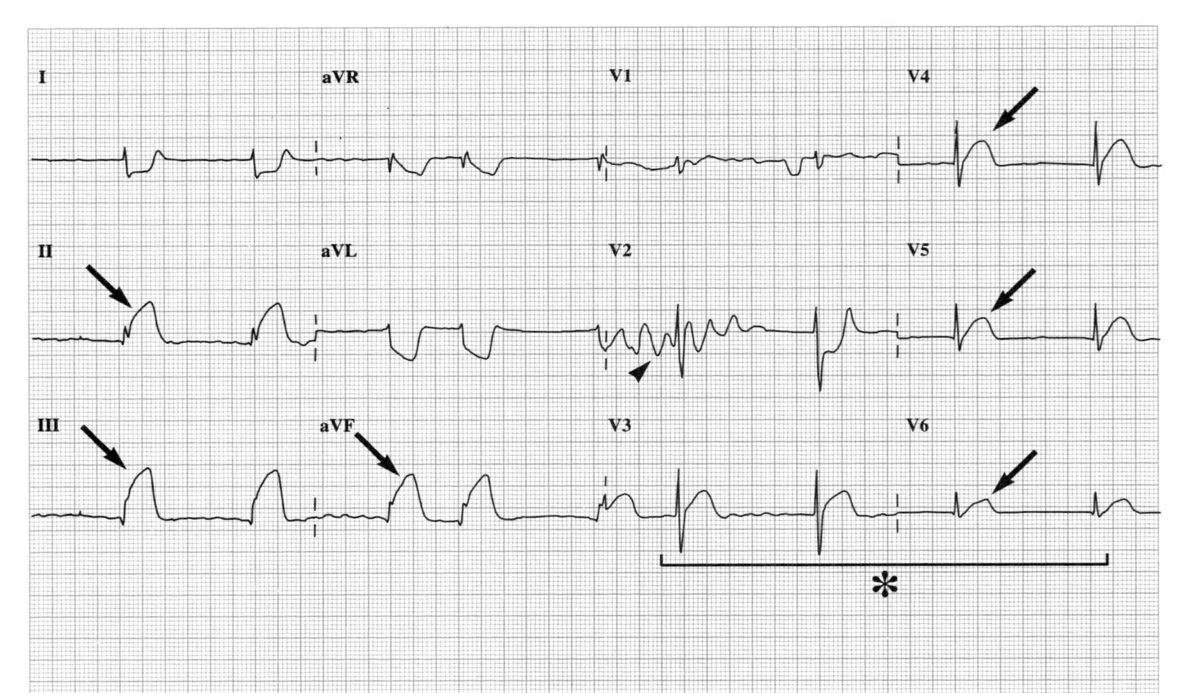

Questions: ECG 42

1. The most likely cause of the tall R wave in lead V_1 is:

   a. Right bundle branch block
   b. Right ventricular hypertrophy
   c. Normal variant
   d. Posterior MI

2. What is the likely age of the myocardial infarction on this ECG?

   a. Hours
   b. Days
   c. Weeks

3. What is responsible for the change in QRS morphology between the 4th and 5th beats in the bottom row of the ECG record?

4. The right axis deviation in this tracing is due to left posterior fascicular block:

   a. True
   b. False

5. Findings in this tracing consistent with hyperkalemia include:

   a. Atrial fibrillation
   b. Tall T waves
   c. ST elevation

6. The most likely cause for the ST depression in I and aVL is:

   a. Localized pericarditis
   b. Reciprocal changes secondary to acute myocardial infarction
   c. Ventricular aneurysm
   d. Lateral wall myocardial ischemia
   e. Digitalis effect

7. What is the cause of the baseline undulations in V_2?

   a. Coarse atrial fibrillation
   b. Flutter waves
   c. Artifact
   d. Tremor due to Parkinson's disease

Answers: ECG 42

1. Posterior MI is the most likely cause of the tall R wave in lead V_1 given the presence of acute inferior and lateral myocardial infarctions. Due to the loss of posterior QRS forces, unopposed anterior QRS forces manifest a prominent R wave in leads overlying the anterior wall, such as lead V_1. Right bundle branch block may also manifest in a tall R wave in lead V_1, but the normal QRS duration in the present ECG rules against this diagnosis. Right ventricular hypertrophy can manifest a tall R wave in V_1 (as well as right axis deviation, which is also present in this tracing) and cannot be definitively excluded. Finally, a tall R wave in V_1 may be considered a normal variant in adolescents, but this finding is considered abnormal in adults. (Answer: d)

2. The development of Q waves, and evolutionary changes in the T wave and ST segment can be used to approximate the age of myocardial infarction:

   - **T waves**: The development of large upright T waves is often the earliest manifestations of acute MI, occurring within minutes and lasting for minutes to hours. T wave inversion, which begins while ST segments are still elevated, may last for months to years, persist indefinitely, or regress to nonspecific T wave changes.

   - **ST segment**: ST elevation usually develops in the minutes to hours following acute MI. Resolution may occur within hours, but usually requires a few days for complete return to baseline. Persistence beyond 4 weeks should raise the suspicion of ventricular aneurysm.

   - **Q waves**: Abnormal Q waves usually develop in the first several hours to days following acute infarction. In most patients, they persist indefinitely, but may regress to no longer meet the criteria for abnormal Q waves; in some patients (< 15%), Q waves disappear entirely.

   In the present ECG, inferior and anterolateral Q waves accompanied by convex upward ST segment elevation suggest the myocardial infarction is acute. (Answer: a)

3. The abnormal QRS morphology seen in the fifth beat in the bottom row of the ECG record is due to lead change midway through the inscription of the QRS morphology; the first half of the QRS complex represents the recording from aVF, while the second half of the QRS complex represents the recording from V_3.

4. Other causes of right axis deviation must be excluded before right axis deviation can be attributed to left posterior fascicular block (LPFB), including lateral wall MI, right ventricular hypertrophy, and pulmonary emphysema. In the present ECG, lateral MI is the most likely explanation for the right axis deviation. (Answer: b)

5. Although this patient is not hyperkalemic, elevated potassium levels can induce ECG changes that mimic acute MI. Findings present on this ECG that can also be found in hyperkalemia include tall T waves and ST elevation. However, the T waves in hyperkalemia are usually peaked and narrow, and ST elevation is usually diffuse and does not show reciprocal ST segment depression, as seen here in leads I and aVL. (Answer: b, c)

6. The ST segment depression in leads I and aVL is most likely due to high lateral wall ischemia, although reciprocal changes are possible. In general, any ST depression associated with ST elevation in other leads is a marker for a larger region of jeopardized myocardium. Digitalis may cause ST depression, but it is typically diffuse and not confined to two leads as in the present tracing. Localized pericarditis and ventricular aneurysm cause ST segment elevation, not depression. (Answer: d)

7. The most likely cause of the baseline undulations in lead V_2 is artifact, probably due to a loose lead. Coarse atrial fibrillation is unlikely since fine atrial fibrillation is present throughout the rest of the tracing. Variability in the peak-to-peak intervals of the undulations and the lack of artifact in the limb leads make atrial fibrillation and tremor due to Parkinson's disease unlikely. (Answer: c)

— Quick Review 42 —

Atrial fibrillation	
• ____ waves are absent	P
• Atrial activity is totally ____ and represented by fibrillatory (f) waves of varying amplitudes, duration and morphology	irregular
• Atrial activity is best seen in the ____ and ____ leads	right precordial, inferior
• Ventricular rhythm is (regularly/irregularly) irregular	irregularly
• ____ toxicity may result in regularization of the RR interval due to complete heart block with junctional tachycardia	Digitalis
• Ventricular rate is usually ____ per minute in the absence of drugs	100-180
▸ Think ____ if the ventricular rate is > 200 per minute and the QRS is > 0.12 seconds	Wolff-Parkinson-White
AV junctional escape complexes	
• QRS complex occurs as a ____ phenomenon in response to decreased sinus impulse formation or conduction, or high-degree AV block	secondary
• Rate is typically ____ per minute	40-60
• Atrial mechanism may be sinus rhythm, paroxysmal atrial tachycardia, atrial flutter, or atrial fibrillation (true/false)	true
• QRS morphology is (similar to/different from) the sinus or supraventricular impulse	similar to

— Quick Review 42 —

Posterior MI, recent or probably acute	
• Initial R wave ≥ ____ seconds in leads ____ and ____ with:	0.04, V_1 V_2
▸ R wave amplitude (greater than/less than) S wave amplitude, *and* ST segment (elevation/depression) with (upright/inverted) T waves	greater than; depression, upright
• Posterior MI is usually seen in the setting of acute inferior MI (true/false)	true
• RVH, WPW and RBBB (do/do not) interfere with the ECG diagnosis of posterior MI	do
Peaked T waves	
• T wave > ____ mm in the limb leads or > ____ mm in the precordial leads	6, 10

— POP QUIZ —

Make The Diagnosis

Instructions: Determine the ECG diagnosis that best corresponds to the ECG features listed below (see score sheet for options)

ECG Features	Diagnosis
• QRS duration ≥ 0.12 seconds • Onset of intrinsicoid deflection in leads I, V_5, V_6 > 0.05 seconds • Broad monophasic R waves in leads I, V_5, V_6, which are usually notched or slurred • Secondary ST & T wave changes opposite in direction to the major QRS deflection • rS or QS complex in the right precordial leads	LBBB, complete
• Upright P wave > 2.5 mm in leads II, III and aVF *or* > 1.5 mm in leads V_1 or V_2 • P wave axis ≥ 70 degrees	Right atrial abnormality
• Notched P wave with a duration ≥ 0.12 seconds in leads II, III or aVF, *or* • Terminal negative portion of the P wave in lead V_1 ≥ 1 mm deep and ≥ 0.04 seconds in duration	Left atrial abnormality
• Amplitude of the entire QRS complex (R+S) < 10 mm in all precordial leads and < 5 mm in all limb leads	Low voltage, limb & precordial leads
• Alternation in the amplitude and/or direction of the P, QRS and/or T waves	Electrical alternans
• Mean QRS axis ≥ 100° • Dominant R wave V_1 • Secondary downsloping ST depression & T wave inversion in the right precordial leads • Right atrial abnormality	Right ventricular hypertrophy

ECG 43. 54-year-old male with dyspnea on exertion and hypertension:

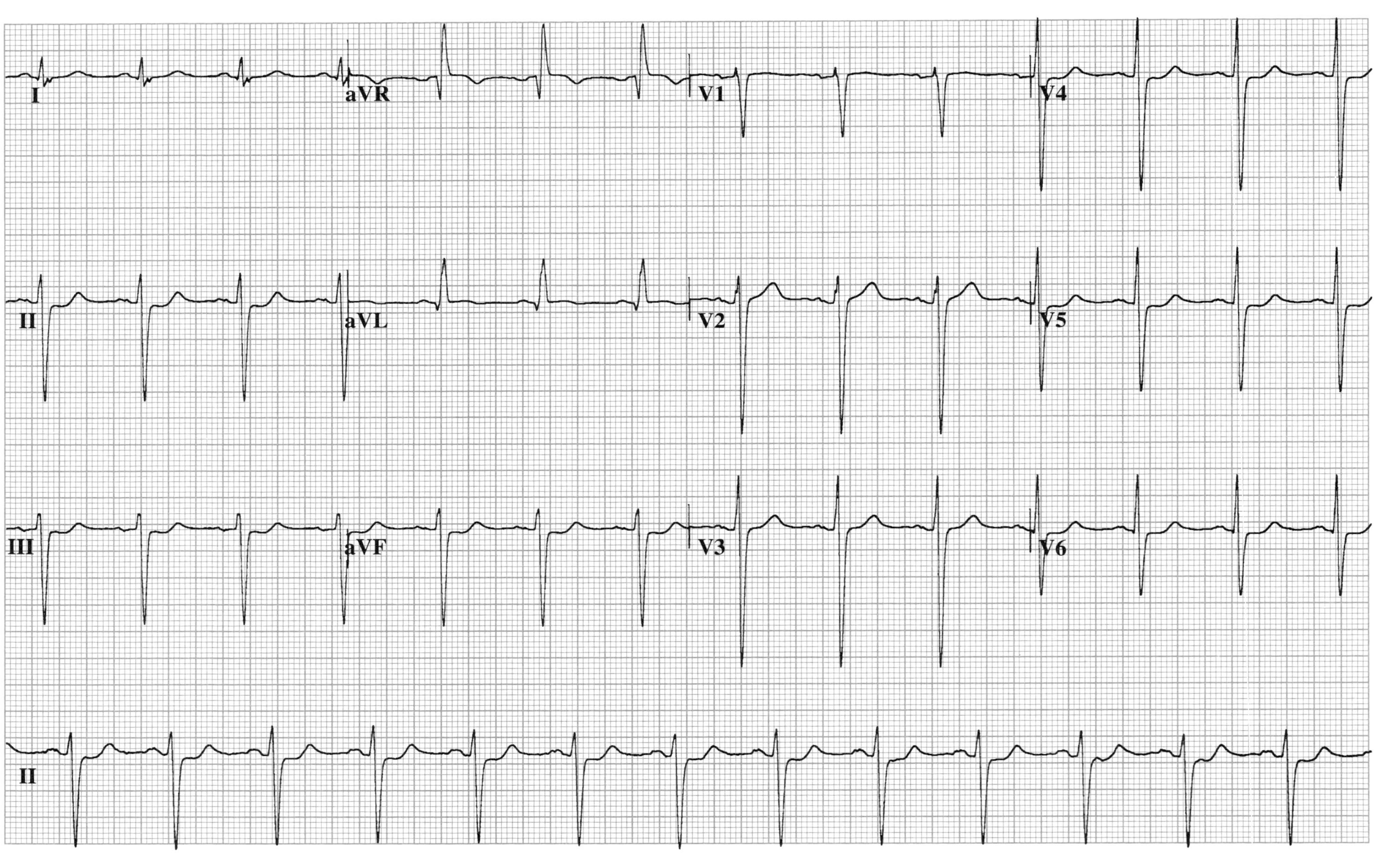

1. GENERAL FEATURES

- ☐ a. Normal ECG
- ☐ b. Borderline normal ECG or normal variant
- ☐ c. Incorrect electrode placement
- ☐ d. Artifact due to tremor

2. ATRIAL RHYTHMS

- ☐ a. Sinus rhythm
- ☐ b. Sinus arrhythmia
- ☐ c. Sinus bradycardia (< 60)
- ☐ d. Sinus tachycardia (> 100)
- ☐ e. Sinus pause or arrest
- ☐ f. Sinoatrial exit block
- ☐ g. Ecoptic atrial rhythm
- ☐ h. Wandering atrial pacemaker
- ☐ i. Atrial premature complexes, normally conducted
- ☐ j. Atrial premature complexes, nonconducted
- ☐ k. Atrial premature complexes with aberrant intraventricular conduction
- ☐ l. Atrial tachycardia (regular, sustained, 1:1 conduction)
- ☐ m. Atrial tachycardia, repetitive (short paroxysms)
- ☐ n. Atrial tachycardia, multifocal
- ☐ o. Atrial tachycardia with AV block
- ☐ p. Supraventricular tachycardia, unspecific
- ☐ q. Supraventricular tachycardia, paroxysmal
- ☐ r. Atrial flutter
- ☐ s. Atrial fibrillation
- ☐ t. Retrograde atrial activation

3. AV JUNCTIONAL RHYTHMS

- ☐ a. AV junctional premature complexes
- ☐ b. AV junctional escape complexes
- ☐ c. AV junctional rhythm, accelerated
- ☐ d. AV junctional rhythm

4. VENTRICULAR RHYTHMS

- ☐ a. Ventricular premature complex(es), uniform, fixed coupling
- ☐ b. Ventricular premature complex(es), uniform, nonfixed coupling
- ☐ c. Ventricular premature complexes(es), multiform
- ☐ d. Ventricular premature complexes, in pairs
- ☐ e. Ventricular parasystole
- ☐ f. Ventricular tachycardia (≥ 3 consecutive complexes)
- ☐ g. Accelerated idioventricular rhythm
- ☐ h. Ventricular escape complexes or rhythm
- ☐ i. Ventricular fibrillation

5. ATRIAL-VENTRICULAR INTERACTIONS IN ARRHYTHMIAS

- ☐ a. Fusion complexes
- ☐ b. Reciprocal (echo) complexes
- ☐ c. Ventricular capture complexes
- ☐ d. AV dissociation
- ☐ e. Ventriculophasic sinus arrhythmia

6. AV CONDUCTION ABNORMALITIES

- ☐ a. AV block, 1°
- ☐ b. AV block, 2° - Mobitz type I (Wenckebach)
- ☐ c. AV block, 2° - Mobitz type II
- ☐ d. AV block, 2:1
- ☐ e. AV block, 3°
- ☐ f. AV block, variable
- ☐ g. Short PR interval (with sinus rhythm and normal QRS duration)
- ☐ h. Wolff-Parkinson-White pattern

7. INTRAVENTRICULAR CONDUCTION DISTURBANCES

- ☐ a. RBBB, incomplete
- ☐ b. RBBB, complete
- ☐ c. Left anterior fascicular block
- ☐ d. Left posterior fascicular block
- ☐ e. LBBB, with ST-T wave suggestive of acute myocardial injury or infarction
- ☐ f. LBBB, complete
- ☐ g. LBBB, intermittent
- ☐ h. Intraventricular conduction disturbance, nonspecific
- ☐ i. Aberrant intraventricular conduction with supraventricular arrhythmia

8. P WAVE ABNORMALITIES

- ☐ a. Right atrial abnormality
- ☐ b. Left atrial abnormalities
- ☐ c. Nonspecific atrial abnormality

9. ABNORMALITIES OF QRS VOLTAGE OR AXIS

- ☐ a. Low voltage, limb leads only
- ☐ b. Low voltage, limb and precordial leads
- ☐ c. Left axis deviation (> - 30%)
- ☐ d. Right axis deviation (> + 100)
- ☐ e. Electrical alternans

10. VENTRICULAR HYPERTROPHY

- ☐ a. LVH by voltage only
- ☐ b. LVH by voltage and ST-T segment abnormalities
- ☐ c. RVH
- ☐ d. Combined ventricular hypertrophy

11. Q WAVE MYOCARDIAL INFARCTION

	Probably Acute or Recent	Probably Old or Age Indeterminate
Anterolateral	☐ a.	☐ g.
Anterior	☐ b.	☐ h.
Anteroseptal	☐ c.	☐ i.
Lateral/High lateral	☐ d.	☐ j.
Inferior	☐ e.	☐ k.
Posterior	☐ f.	☐ l.

☐ m. Probably ventricular aneurysm

12. ST, T, U, WAVE ABNORMALITIES

- ☐ a. Normal variant, early repolarization
- ☐ b. Normal variant, juvenile T waves
- ☐ c. Nonspecific ST and/or T wave abnormalities
- ☐ d. ST and/or T wave abnormalities suggesting myocardial ischemia
- ☐ e. ST and/or T wave abnormalities suggesting myocardial injury
- ☐ f. ST and/or T wave abnormalities suggesting acute pericarditis
- ☐ g. ST-T segment abnormalities secondary to intraventricular conduction disturbance or hypertrophy
- ☐ h. Post-extrasystolic T wave abnormality
- ☐ i. Isolated J point depression
- ☐ j. Peaked T waves
- ☐ k. Prolonged QT interval
- ☐ l. Prominent U waves

13. PACEMAKER FUNCTION AND RHYTHM

- ☐ a. Atrial or coronary sinus pacing
- ☐ b. Ventricular demand pacing
- ☐ c. AV sequential pacing
- ☐ d. Ventricular pacing, complete control
- ☐ e. Dual chamber, atrial sensing pacemaker
- ☐ f. Pacemaker malfunction, not constantly capturing (atrium or ventricle)
- ☐ g. Pacemaker malfunction, not constantly sensing (atrium or ventricle)
- ☐ h. Pacemaker malfunction, not firing
- ☐ i. Pacemaker malfunction, slowing

14. SUGGESTED OR PROBABLE CLINICAL DISORDERS

- ☐ a. Digitalis effect
- ☐ b. Digitalis toxicity
- ☐ c. Antiarrhythmic drug effect
- ☐ d. Antiarrhythmic drug toxicity
- ☐ e. Hyperkalemia
- ☐ f. Hypokalemia
- ☐ g. Hypercalcemia
- ☐ h. Hypocalcemia
- ☐ i. Atrial septal defect, secundum
- ☐ j. Atrial septal defect, primum
- ☐ k. Dextrocardia, mirror image
- ☐ l. Mitral valve disease
- ☐ m. Chronic lung disease
- ☐ n. Acute cor pulmonale, including pulmonary embolus
- ☐ o. Pericardial effusion
- ☐ p. Acute pericarditis
- ☐ q. Hypertrophic cardiomyopathy
- ☐ r. Coronary artery disease
- ☐ s. Central nervous system disorder
- ☐ t. Myxedema
- ☐ u. Hypothermia
- ☐ v. Sick sinus syndrome

ECG 43 was obtained in a 54-year-old male with dyspnea on exertion and hypertension. Normal sinus rhythm is present with voltage criteria for LVH (Cornell criteria: R wave in aVL + S wave in V_3 > 24 mm; arrows). The diffuse ST segment depression (arrowheads) is consistent with a strain pattern associated with LVH. Left axis deviation is present but left anterior fascicular block should not be coded in the presence of LVH, which may by itself cause left axis deviation. The QRS duration is 0.11 seconds and is consistent with nonspecific IVCD. Thus, in addition to the voltage criteria for LVH, several non-voltage-related LVH criteria are seen (left axis deviation, ST segment changes, intraventricular conduction delay).

Codes:

2a	Sinus rhythm
7h	IVCD, nonspecific type
9c	Left axis deviation (>-30°)
10b	LVH by both voltage and ST-T segment abnormalities
12g	ST-T segment abnormalities secondary to IVCD or hypertrophy

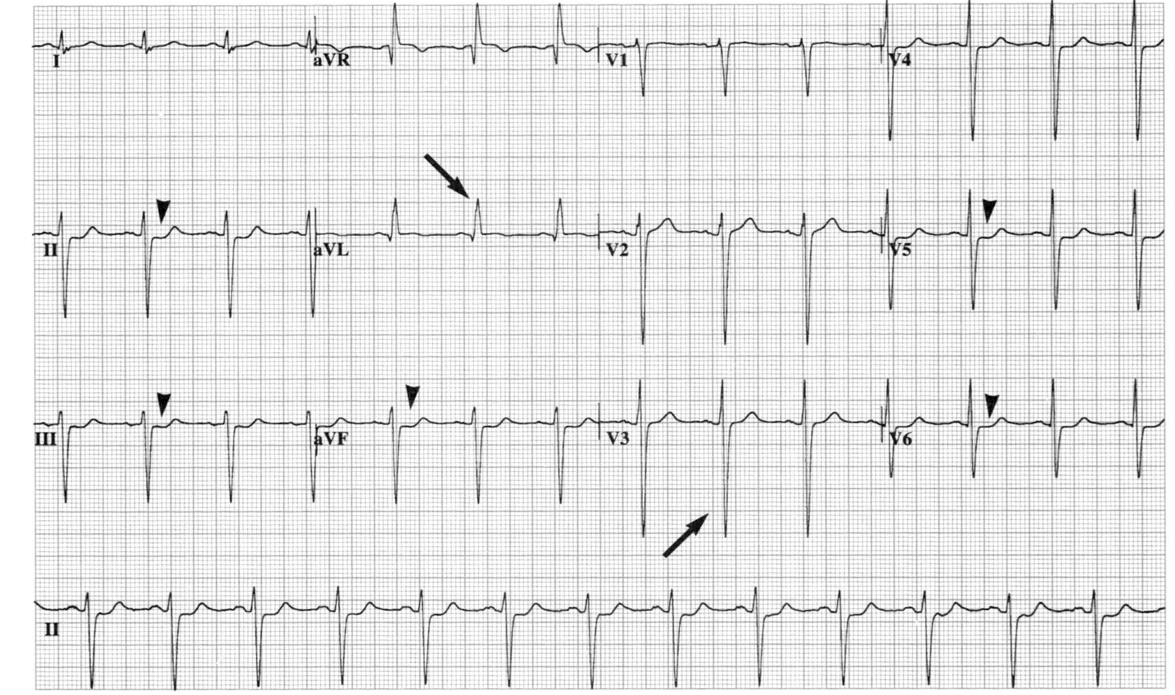

Questions: ECG 43

1. LVH by voltage criteria is present when the sum of the S wave in V_3 and the R wave in lead aVL exceeds ____ mm in males and ____ mm in females:

   a. 24 and 20
   b. 20 and 24
   c. 20 and 16
   d. 28 and 24

2. Non-voltage based criteria for LVH include:

   a. Left axis deviation
   b. Nonspecific intraventricular conduction disturbance
   c. First-degree AV block
   d. Left atrial abnormality

Answers: ECG 43

1. The Cornell criteria for LVH specify that the total amplitude of the S wave in V_3 and the R wave in aVL should be >24 mm in males and >20 mm in females. (Answer: a)

2. Left ventricular hypertrophy often manifests non-voltage-based findings on the ECG, including left atrial abnormality, left axis deviation, nonspecific IVCD, low anterior forces, prominent U waves, and abnormal Q waves in the inferior leads. First-degree AV block, however, is not a feature of left ventricular hypertrophy. (Answer: All except c)

— Quick Review 43 —

LVH by voltage only	
• **Cornell Criteria** (most accurate): R wave in aVL + S wave in V_3 > ____ mm in males or > ____ mm in females	24, 20
• **Other commonly used voltage-based criteria**	
▸ Precordial leads (one or more)	
(1) R wave in V_5 or V_6 + S wave in V_1	
▸ > ____ mm if age > 30 years	35
▸ > ____ mm if age 20-30 years	40
▸ > ____ mm if age 16-19 years	60
(2) Maximum R wave + S wave in precordial leads > ____ mm	45
(3) R wave in V_5 > ____ mm	26
(4) R wave in V_6 > ____ mm	20
▸ Limb leads (one or more)	
(1) R wave in lead I + S wave in lead II ≥ ____ mm	26
(2) R wave in lead I ≥ ____ mm	14
(3) S wave in aVR ≥ ____ mm	15
(4) R wave in aVL ≥ ____ mm	12
(5) R wave in aVF ≥ ____ mm	21
• **Non-voltage related criteria for LVH**	
▸ (Left/right) atrial abnormality	left
▸ (Left/right) axis deviation	left
▸ Onset of intrinsicoid deflection > ____ seconds	0.05
▸ Small or absent R waves in leads ____	V_1-V_3
▸ Absent ____ waves in leads I, V_5, V_6	Q
▸ Abnormal ____ waves in leads II, III, aVF	Q
▸ Prominent ____ waves, especially in leads with large R and T waves	U
▸ R wave amplitude in V_6 (greater than/less than) V_5, provided there are dominant R waves in these leads	greater than

Differential Diagnosis

"PSEUDOINFARCTS" (ECG pattern can mimic Q-wave myocardial infarction)	
• Wolff-Parkinson-White (item 6h) • Hypertrophic cardiomyopathy (item 14q) • LVH (items 10a, b) • RVH (item 10c) • Left anterior fascicular block (item 7c) • Chronic lung disease (item 14m) • Amyloid heart (or other infiltrative diseases) • Cardiomyopathy • Chest deformity (e.g., pectus excavatum) • Pulmonary embolism (item 14n) • Myocarditis • Myocardial tumors • Hyperkalemia (item 14g)	• Lead reversal (item 1c) • Corrected transposition • Dextrocardia (item 14k) • LBBB • Pancreatitis • Muscular dystrophy • Mitral valve prolapse • Myocardial contusion • Left/right atrial enlargement: Prominent atrial repolariztion wave (Ta) can depress the PR segment to mimic a Q wave • Pneumothorax

ECG 44. 52-year-old male with a history of heart disease:

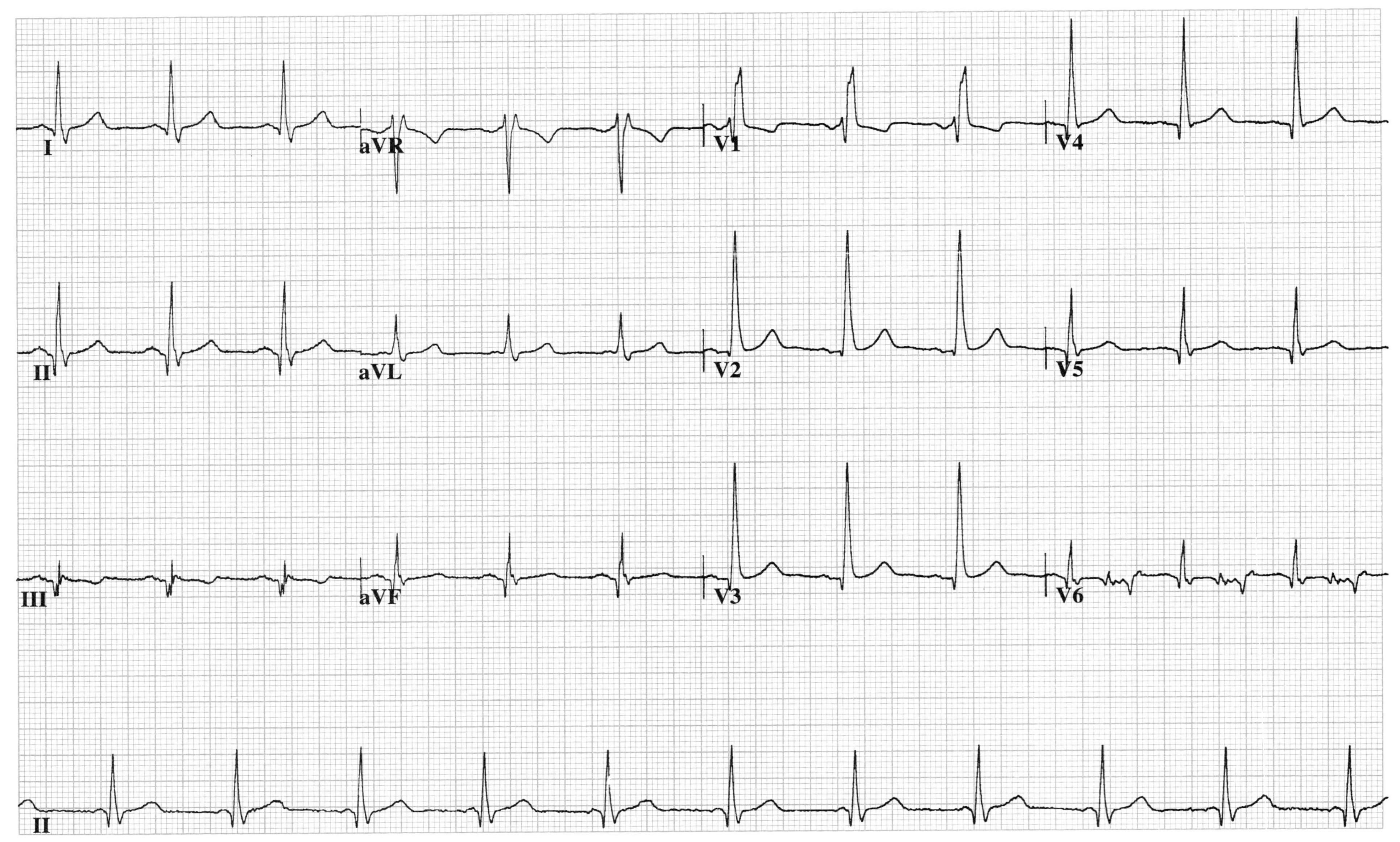

1. GENERAL FEATURES

☐ a. Normal ECG
☐ b. Borderline normal ECG or normal variant
☐ c. Incorrect electrode placement
☐ d. Artifact due to tremor

2. ATRIAL RHYTHMS

☐ a. Sinus rhythm
☐ b. Sinus arrhythmia
☐ c. Sinus bradycardia (< 60)
☐ d. Sinus tachycardia (> 100)
☐ e. Sinus pause or arrest
☐ f. Sinoatrial exit block
☐ g. Ecoptic atrial rhythm
☐ h. Wandering atrial pacemaker
☐ i. Atrial premature complexes, normally conducted
☐ j. Atrial premature complexes, nonconducted
☐ k. Atrial premature complexes with aberrant intraventricular conduction
☐ l. Atrial tachycardia (regular, sustained, 1:1 conduction)
☐ m. Atrial tachycardia, repetitive (short paroxysms)
☐ n. Atrial tachycardia, multifocal
☐ o. Atrial tachycardia with AV block
☐ p. Supraventricular tachycardia, unspecific
☐ q. Supraventricular tachycardia, paroxysmal
☐ r. Atrial flutter
☐ s. Atrial fibrillation
☐ t. Retrograde atrial activation

3. AV JUNCTIONAL RHYTHMS

☐ a. AV junctional premature complexes
☐ b. AV junctional escape complexes
☐ c. AV junctional rhythm, accelerated
☐ d. AV junctional rhythm

4. VENTRICULAR RHYTHMS

☐ a. Ventricular premature complex(es), uniform, fixed coupling
☐ b. Ventricular premature complex(es), uniform, nonfixed coupling
☐ c. Ventricular premature complexes(es), multiform
☐ d. Ventricular premature complexes, in pairs
☐ e. Ventricular parasystole
☐ f. Ventricular tachycardia (≥ 3 consecutive complexes)
☐ g. Accelerated idioventricular rhythm
☐ h. Ventricular escape complexes or rhythm
☐ i. Ventricular fibrillation

5. ATRIAL-VENTRICULAR INTERACTIONS IN ARRHYTHMIAS

☐ a. Fusion complexes
☐ b. Reciprocal (echo) complexes
☐ c. Ventricular capture complexes
☐ d. AV dissociation
☐ e. Ventriculophasic sinus arrhythmia

6. AV CONDUCTION ABNORMALITIES

☐ a. AV block, 1°
☐ b. AV block, 2° - Mobitz type I (Wenckebach)
☐ c. AV block, 2° - Mobitz type II
☐ d. AV block, 2:1
☐ e. AV block, 3°
☐ f. AV block, variable
☐ g. Short PR interval (with sinus rhythm and normal QRS duration)
☐ h. Wolff-Parkinson-White pattern

7. INTRAVENTRICULAR CONDUCTION DISTURBANCES

☐ a. RBBB, incomplete
☐ b. RBBB, complete
☐ c. Left anterior fascicular block
☐ d. Left posterior fascicular block
☐ e. LBBB, with ST-T wave suggestive of acute myocardial injury or infarction
☐ f. LBBB, complete
☐ g. LBBB, intermittent
☐ h. Intraventricular conduction disturbance, nonspecific
☐ i. Aberrant intraventricular conduction with supraventricular arrhythmia

8. P WAVE ABNORMALITIES

☐ a. Right atrial abnormality
☐ b. Left atrial abnormalities
☐ c. Nonspecific atrial abnormality

9. ABNORMALITIES OF QRS VOLTAGE OR AXIS

☐ a. Low voltage, limb leads only
☐ b. Low voltage, limb and precordial leads
☐ c. Left axis deviation (> - 30%)
☐ d. Right axis deviation (> + 100)
☐ e. Electrical alternans

10. VENTRICULAR HYPERTROPHY

☐ a. LVH by voltage only
☐ b. LVH by voltage and ST-T segment abnormalities
☐ c. RVH
☐ d. Combined ventricular hypertrophy

11. Q WAVE MYOCARDIAL INFARCTION

	Probably Acute or Recent	Probably Old or Age Indeterminate
Anterolateral	☐ a.	☐ g.
Anterior	☐ b.	☐ h.
Anteroseptal	☐ c.	☐ i.
Lateral/High lateral	☐ d.	☐ j.
Inferior	☐ e.	☐ k.
Posterior	☐ f.	☐ l.

☐ m. Probably ventricular aneurysm

12. ST, T, U, WAVE ABNORMALITIES

☐ a. Normal variant, early repolarization
☐ b. Normal variant, juvenile T waves
☐ c. Nonspecific ST and/or T wave abnormalities
☐ d. ST and/or T wave abnormalities suggesting myocardial ischemia
☐ e. ST and/or T wave abnormalities suggesting myocardial injury
☐ f. ST and/or T wave abnormalities suggesting acute pericarditis
☐ g. ST-T segment abnormalities secondary to intraventricular conduction disturbance or hypertrophy
☐ h. Post-extrasystolic T wave abnormality
☐ i. Isolated J point depression
☐ j. Peaked T waves
☐ k. Prolonged QT interval
☐ l. Prominent U waves

13. PACEMAKER FUNCTION AND RHYTHM

☐ a. Atrial or coronary sinus pacing
☐ b. Ventricular demand pacing
☐ c. AV sequential pacing
☐ d. Ventricular pacing, complete control
☐ e. Dual chamber, atrial sensing pacemaker
☐ f. Pacemaker malfunction, not constantly capturing (atrium or ventricle)
☐ g. Pacemaker malfunction, not constantly sensing (atrium or ventricle)
☐ h. Pacemaker malfunction, not firing
☐ i. Pacemaker malfunction, slowing

14. SUGGESTED OR PROBABLE CLINICAL DISORDERS

☐ a. Digitalis effect
☐ b. Digitalis toxicity
☐ c. Antiarrhythmic drug effect
☐ d. Antiarrhythmic drug toxicity
☐ e. Hyperkalemia
☐ f. Hypokalemia
☐ g. Hypercalcemia
☐ h. Hypocalcemia
☐ i. Atrial septal defect, secundum
☐ j. Atrial septal defect, primum
☐ k. Dextrocardia, mirror image
☐ l. Mitral valve disease
☐ m. Chronic lung disease
☐ n. Acute cor pulmonale, including pulmonary embolus
☐ o. Pericardial effusion
☐ p. Acute pericarditis
☐ q. Hypertrophic cardiomyopathy
☐ r. Coronary artery disease
☐ s. Central nervous system disorder
☐ t. Myxedema
☐ u. Hypothermia
☐ v. Sick sinus syndrome

ECG 44 was obtained in a 52-year-old male with a history of heart disease. The tracing shows sinus rhythm, RBBB (arrow), and age indeterminate myocardial infarction involving the inferior and anterolateral walls; posterior MI is difficult to diagnose due to the presence of RBBB. The unusual undulation of the baseline in lead V_6 (asterisk) is artifactual, and is most likely due to a bad electrode (or contact). This ECG is consistent with coronary artery disease.

Codes:

2a	Sinus rhythm
7b	RBBB, complete
11g	Anterolateral Q wave MI, probably old or age indeterminate
11k	Inferior Q wave MI, probably old or age indeterminate
14r	Coronary artery disease

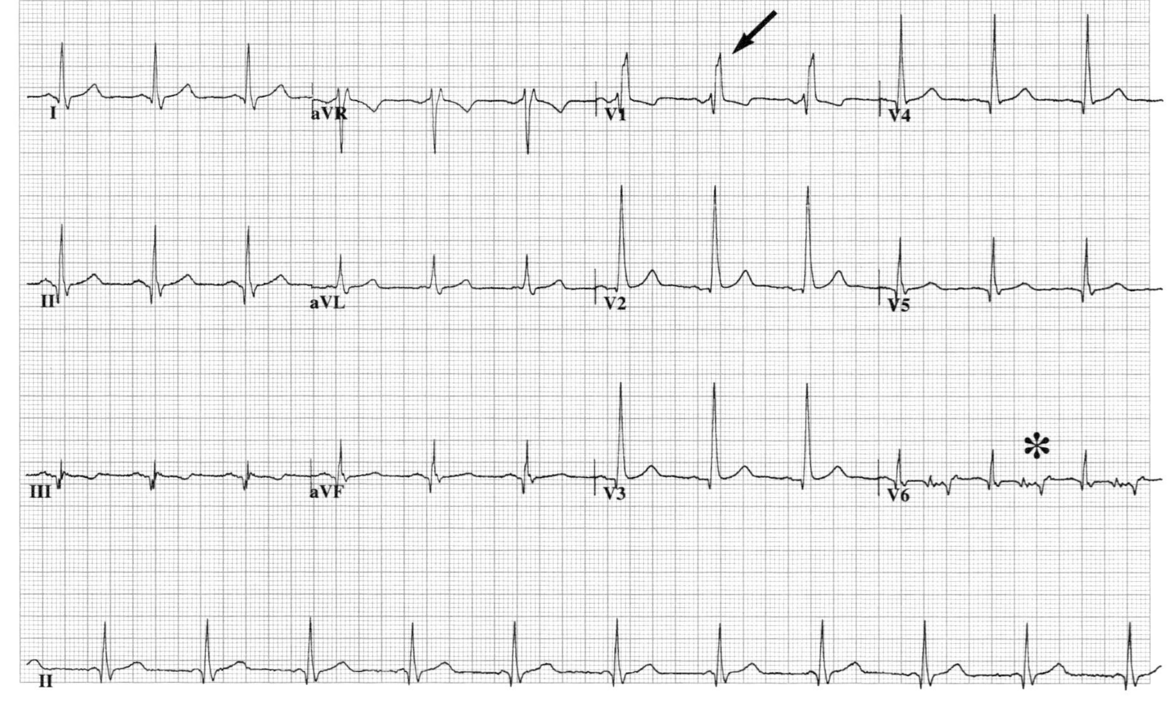

Questions: ECG 44

1. Findings in this ECG that can also be found in pulmonary embolism include:

   a. S_1Q_3
   b. Q-waves in leads II, III, and aVF
   c. Right bundle branch block
   d. Inverted T waves in the right precordial leads

2. The presence of right bundle branch block affects the ECG diagnosis of acute myocardial infarction:

   a. True
   b. False

3. Which of the following statements about Q waves are true?

   a. Small Q waves may be present in one or more inferior leads in > 50% of normal adults
   b. Q wave duration of 0.04 seconds is virtually always pathological
   c. When present, "normal" Q wave amplitude in the limb leads is usually < 4 mm and < 25% the height of the R wave

4. Clinical conditions associated with abnormal Q waves include:

   a. Hypertrophic obstructive cardiomyopathy
   b. Muscular dystrophy
   c. Scleroderma of the heart
   d. Amyloid heart
   e. Primary and metastatic tumors of the heart
   f. Myocardial contusion
   g. Mitral valve prolapse

Answers: ECG 44

1. ECG changes often accompany large pulmonary emboli associated with elevated pulmonary artery pressures, right ventricular dilation and strain, and clockwise rotation of the heart: ***S_1Q_3 or $S_1Q_3T_3$*** occurs in up to 30% of cases and lasts for 1-2 weeks; ***right bundle branch block (RBBB)*** (incomplete or complete) may be seen in up to 25% of cases and usually lasts less than 1 week; and ***inverted T waves*** secondary to right ventricular strain may be seen in the right precordial leads and can last for months. Other ECG findings include right axis deviation, nonspecific ST and T wave changes, and P pulmonale. Arrhythmias and conduction disturbances include sinus tachycardia (most common), atrial fibrillation, atrial flutter, atrial tachycardia, and first-degree AV block. The clinical

presentation and ECG of acute pulmonary embolism may sometimes be confused with acute inferior MI. While Q waves and T wave inversions may be seen in leads III and aVF in both conditions, a Q wave in lead II is uncommon in pulmonary embolism and suggests MI. (Answer: a, c)

2. Right bundle branch block does not interfere with the diagnosis of acute Q-wave myocardial infarction. In contrast, left bundle branch block often masks the presence of acute MI. (Answer: b)

3. Ventricular activation begins at the mid-portion of the left interventricular system and spreads across the septum in a left-to-right direction. Small (< 0.04 sec in duration) "septal" Q waves are inscribed in the leads opposite these initial electrical forces; when the heart is vertical, they appear in the inferior leads, and when the heart is horizontal, they appear in leads I and aVL. Septal Q waves are common in normal patients, and may be up to 0.04 seconds in duration in lead III. (Answer: All)

4. Patients with hypertrophic cardiomyopathy often demonstrate abnormal (> 0.04 sec in duration) Q waves in leads I, aVL, and V_4 - V_6, reflecting exaggerated septal Q waves from marked septal hypertrophy. Q waves also occur in conditions where electrically active tissue is replaced by fibrous tissue or electrically inert substances, as in muscular dystrophy, scleroderma, amyloid, and primary and metastatic tumors of the heart. Q waves can also be seen in areas of intramyocardial hemorrhage and edema following myocardial contusion, in conjunction with nonspecific ST and T wave changes and various degrees of heart block (if the conduction system is involved). Mitral valve prolapse has rarely been associated with Q waves in leads III and aVF. Other cardiac conditions associated with abnormal Q waves include left bundle branch block, left anterior fascicular block, left and right ventricular hypertrophy, and dilated cardiomyopathy. In the WPW syndrome, the Q waves are actually negative delta waves. (Answer: All)

— Quick Review 44 —

Artifact	
Commonly due to tremor	
• Parkinson's tremor simulates atrial ____ with a rate of ____ per second	flutter 4-6
• Physiologic tremor rate is ____ per second	7-9
• Tremor is most prominent in (limb/precordial) leads	limb
Anterolateral MI, age indeterminate or probably old	
• Abnormal Q waves (with/without) ST segment elevation in leads ____	without V_4-V_6

Common Dilemmas in ECG Interpretation

Problem

Atrial fibrillation is present with intermittent episodes of atrial flutter. Should atrial fibrillation or atrial flutter be coded?

Recommendation

Atrial fibrillation. Atrial fibrillation often manifests as "fib/flutter;" however, on formal testing, you must choose one or the other. The best strategy in this setting is to code atrial fibrillation; atrial flutter should be reserved for tracings that show continuous atrial flutter without interspersed episodes of fibrillation.

ECG 45. 31-year-old male with palpitations:

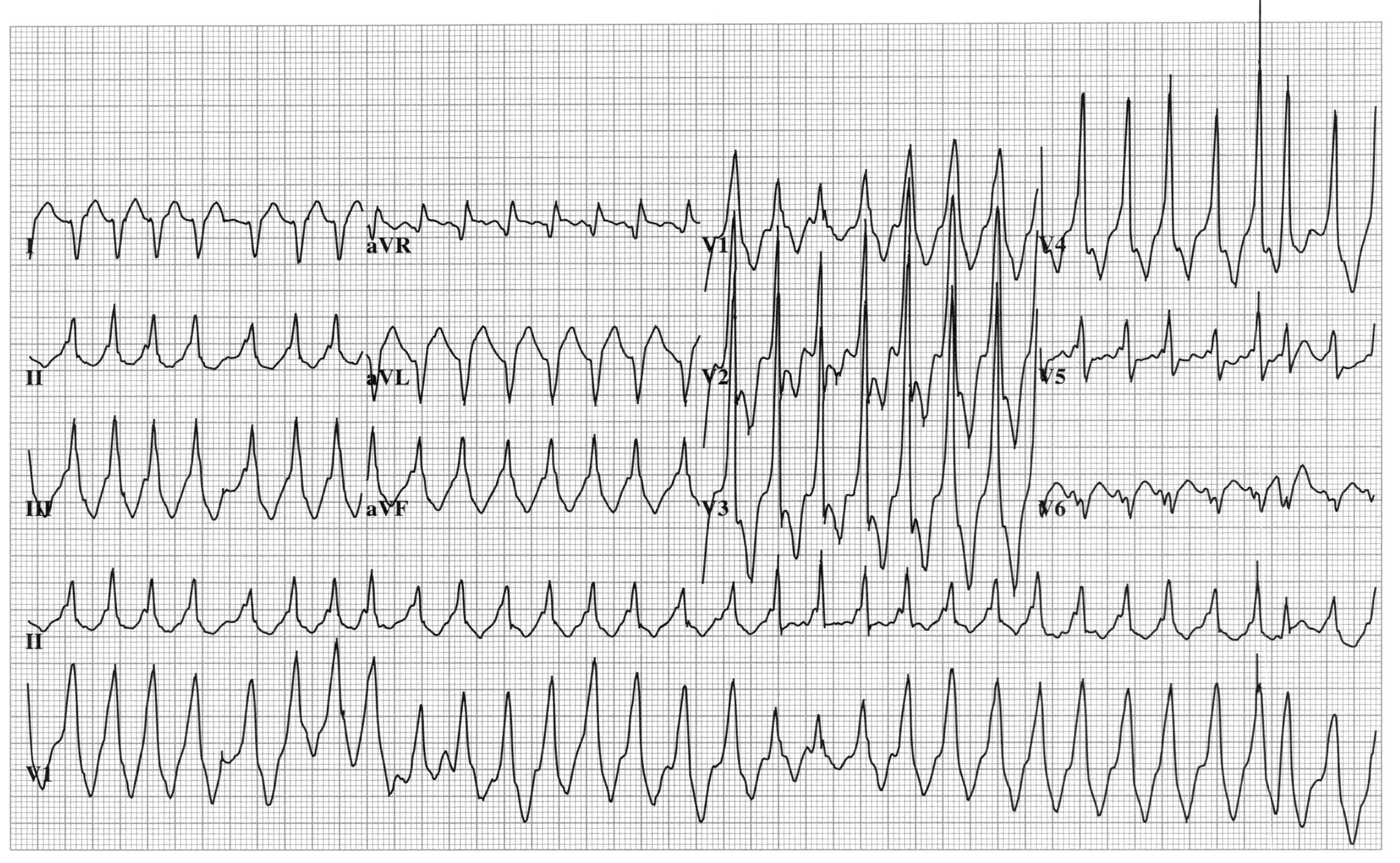

1. GENERAL FEATURES

☐ a. Normal ECG
☐ b. Borderline normal ECG or normal variant
☐ c. Incorrect electrode placement
☐ d. Artifact due to tremor

2. ATRIAL RHYTHMS

☐ a. Sinus rhythm
☐ b. Sinus arrhythmia
☐ c. Sinus bradycardia (< 60)
☐ d. Sinus tachycardia (> 100)
☐ e. Sinus pause or arrest
☐ f. Sinoatrial exit block
☐ g. Ecoptic atrial rhythm
☐ h. Wandering atrial pacemaker
☐ i. Atrial premature complexes, normally conducted
☐ j. Atrial premature complexes, nonconducted
☐ k. Atrial premature complexes with aberrant intraventricular conduction
☐ l. Atrial tachycardia (regular, sustained, 1:1 conduction)
☐ m. Atrial tachycardia, repetitive (short paroxysms)
☐ n. Atrial tachycardia, multifocal
☐ o. Atrial tachycardia with AV block
☐ p. Supraventricular tachycardia, unspecific
☐ q. Supraventricular tachycardia, paroxysmal
☐ r. Atrial flutter
☐ s. Atrial fibrillation
☐ t. Retrograde atrial activation

3. AV JUNCTIONAL RHYTHMS

☐ a. AV junctional premature complexes
☐ b. AV junctional escape complexes
☐ c. AV junctional rhythm, accelerated
☐ d. AV junctional rhythm

4. VENTRICULAR RHYTHMS

☐ a. Ventricular premature complex(es), uniform, fixed coupling
☐ b. Ventricular premature complex(es), uniform, nonfixed coupling
☐ c. Ventricular premature complexes(es), multiform
☐ d. Ventricular premature complexes, in pairs
☐ e. Ventricular parasystole
☐ f. Ventricular tachycardia (≥ 3 consecutive complexes)
☐ g. Accelerated idioventricular rhythm
☐ h. Ventricular escape complexes or rhythm
☐ i. Ventricular fibrillation

5. ATRIAL-VENTRICULAR INTERACTIONS IN ARRHYTHMIAS

☐ a. Fusion complexes
☐ b. Reciprocal (echo) complexes
☐ c. Ventricular capture complexes
☐ d. AV dissociation
☐ e. Ventriculophasic sinus arrhythmia

6. AV CONDUCTION ABNORMALITIES

☐ a. AV block, 1°
☐ b. AV block, 2° - Mobitz type I (Wenckebach)
☐ c. AV block, 2° - Mobitz type II
☐ d. AV block, 2:1
☐ e. AV block, 3°
☐ f. AV block, variable
☐ g. Short PR interval (with sinus rhythm and normal QRS duration)
☐ h. Wolff-Parkinson-White pattern

7. INTRAVENTRICULAR CONDUCTION DISTURBANCES

☐ a. RBBB, incomplete
☐ b. RBBB, complete
☐ c. Left anterior fascicular block
☐ d. Left posterior fascicular block
☐ e. LBBB, with ST-T wave suggestive of acute myocardial injury or infarction
☐ f. LBBB, complete
☐ g. LBBB, intermittent
☐ h. Intraventricular conduction disturbance, nonspecific
☐ i. Aberrant intraventricular conduction with supraventricular arrhythmia

8. P WAVE ABNORMALITIES

☐ a. Right atrial abnormality
☐ b. Left atrial abnormalities
☐ c. Nonspecific atrial abnormality

9. ABNORMALITIES OF QRS VOLTAGE OR AXIS

☐ a. Low voltage, limb leads only
☐ b. Low voltage, limb and precordial leads
☐ c. Left axis deviation (> - 30%)
☐ d. Right axis deviation (> + 100)
☐ e. Electrical alternans

10. VENTRICULAR HYPERTROPHY

☐ a. LVH by voltage only
☐ b. LVH by voltage and ST-T segment abnormalities
☐ c. RVH
☐ d. Combined ventricular hypertrophy

11. Q WAVE MYOCARDIAL INFARCTION

	Probably Acute or Recent	Probably Old or Age Indeterminate
Anterolateral	☐ a.	☐ g.
Anterior	☐ b.	☐ h.
Anteroseptal	☐ c.	☐ i.
Lateral/High lateral	☐ d.	☐ j.
Inferior	☐ e.	☐ k.
Posterior	☐ f.	☐ l.

☐ m. Probably ventricular aneurysm

12. ST, T, U, WAVE ABNORMALITIES

☐ a. Normal variant, early repolarization
☐ b. Normal variant, juvenile T waves
☐ c. Nonspecific ST and/or T wave abnormalities
☐ d. ST and/or T wave abnormalities suggesting myocardial ischemia
☐ e. ST and/or T wave abnormalities suggesting myocardial injury
☐ f. ST and/or T wave abnormalities suggesting acute pericarditis
☐ g. ST-T segment abnormalities secondary to intraventricular conduction disturbance or hypertrophy
☐ h. Post-extrasystolic T wave abnormality
☐ i. Isolated J point depression
☐ j. Peaked T waves
☐ k. Prolonged QT interval
☐ l. Prominent U waves

13. PACEMAKER FUNCTION AND RHYTHM

☐ a. Atrial or coronary sinus pacing
☐ b. Ventricular demand pacing
☐ c. AV sequential pacing
☐ d. Ventricular pacing, complete control
☐ e. Dual chamber, atrial sensing pacemaker
☐ f. Pacemaker malfunction, not constantly capturing (atrium or ventricle)
☐ g. Pacemaker malfunction, not constantly sensing (atrium or ventricle)
☐ h. Pacemaker malfunction, not firing
☐ i. Pacemaker malfunction, slowing

14. SUGGESTED OR PROBABLE CLINICAL DISORDERS

☐ a. Digitalis effect
☐ b. Digitalis toxicity
☐ c. Antiarrhythmic drug effect
☐ d. Antiarrhythmic drug toxicity
☐ e. Hyperkalemia
☐ f. Hypokalemia
☐ g. Hypercalcemia
☐ h. Hypocalcemia
☐ i. Atrial septal defect, secundum
☐ j. Atrial septal defect, primum
☐ k. Dextrocardia, mirror image
☐ l. Mitral valve disease
☐ m. Chronic lung disease
☐ n. Acute cor pulmonale, including pulmonary embolus
☐ o. Pericardial effusion
☐ p. Acute pericarditis
☐ q. Hypertrophic cardiomyopathy
☐ r. Coronary artery disease
☐ s. Central nervous system disorder
☐ t. Myxedema
☐ u. Hypothermia
☐ v. Sick sinus syndrome

ECG 45 was obtained in a 31-year-old male with palpitations. The ECG shows an irregular wide complex tachycardia, consistent with atrial fibrillation in a patient with Wolff-Parkinson-White syndrome. Fusion complexes are present as well as ST-T changes secondary to the intraventricular conduction abnormality.

Codes:

2s	Atrial fibrillation
5a	Fusion complexes
6h	Wolff-Parkinson-White pattern
9d	Right axis deviation (> +100°)
12g	ST-T segment abnormalities secondary to IVCD or hypertrophy

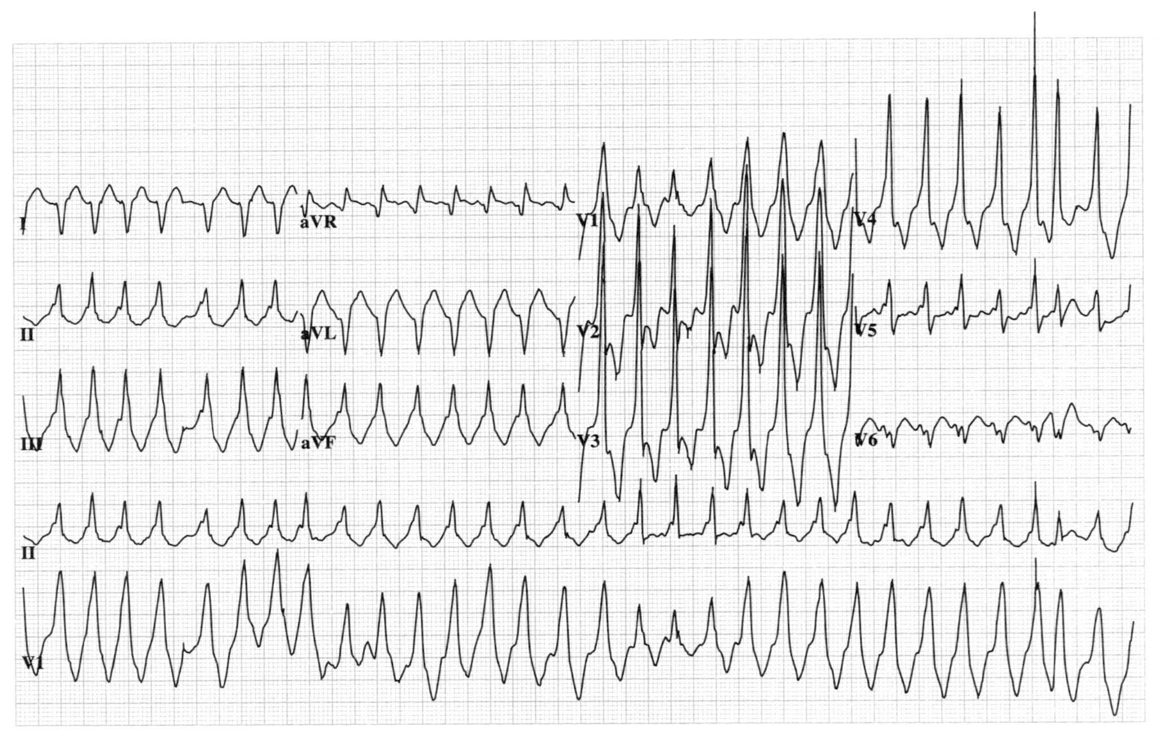

Questions: ECG 45

1. The PR interval in Wolff-Parkinson-White pattern is characteristically less than ___ seconds:

   a. 0.08
   b. 0.10
   c. 0.12
   d. 0.14

2. The QRS duration in Wolff-Parkinson-White pattern should be ___ seconds:

   a. < 0.08
   b. 0.08-0.10
   c. 0.10-0.14
   d. > 0.14

3. In the setting of WPW, the PJ interval (beginning of the P wave to the end of the QRS) remains constant despite varying degrees of pre-excitation:

   a. True
   b. False

Answers: ECG 45

1. The PR interval is the time from the onset of atrial depolarization to the onset of ventricular depolarization. In Wolff-Parkinson-White, AV conduction over the accessory pathway (Bundle of Kent) bypasses the AV node (and AV nodal conduction delay), resulting in pre-excitation of the ventricles and a short PR interval (typically less than 0.12 seconds). Up to 10% of patients with WPW may have PR intervals ≥ 0.12 seconds. (Answer: c)

2. The QRS duration in WPW pattern is typically 0.10-0.14 seconds. The widened QRS complexes represent fusion between electrical wavefronts conducted down the accessory pathway (delta wave) and the AV node. Differing degrees of pre-excitation (fusion) may be present, resulting in variability in the delta wave and QRS duration. (Answer: c)

3. Despite varying degrees of pre-excitation, the PJ interval remains constant. This is due to an inverse relationship between the PR interval and QRS duration — if the PR interval shortens, the QRS widens; if the PR interval lengthens, the QRS narrows. (Answer: a)

— Quick Review 45 —

Atrial fibrillation	
• ____ waves are absent	P
• Atrial activity is totally ____ and represented by fibrillatory (f) waves of varying amplitudes, duration and morphology	irregular
• Atrial activity is best seen in the ____ and ____ leads	right precordial, inferior
• Ventricular rhythm is (regularly/irregularly) irregular	irregularly
• ____ toxicity may result in regularization of the RR interval due to complete heart block with junctional tachycardia	Digitalis
• Ventricular rate is usually ____ per minute in the absence of drugs	100-180
▸ Think ____ if the ventricular rate is > 200 per minute and the QRS is > 0.12 seconds	Wolff-Parkinson-White
Fusion complexes	
• Due to simultaneous activation of the ventricle from ____ sources, resulting in a QRS complex that is ____ in morphology between each source	2 intermediate
Wolff-Parkinson-White pattern	
• (Sinus/nonsinus) P wave	sinus
• PR interval < ____ seconds	0.12
• Initial slurring of QRS (____ wave) resulting in QRS duration > ____ seconds	delta 0.10
• Secondary ST-T wave changes occur (true/false)	true
• PJ interval (beginning of P wave to end of QRS) (is constant/varies)	is constant

Differential Diagnosis

Right Axis Deviation and/or a Dominant R Wave possibly mimicking RVH

- Posterior or inferoposterolateral wall MI (item 11f)
- Right bundle branch block (item 7b)
- Wolff-Parkinson-White syndrome (item 6h)
- Dextrocardia
- Left posterior fascicular block (item 7d)
- Normal variant (especially in children)

ECG 46. 58-year-old female with chronic tobacco use. asthma, and exertional dyspnea:

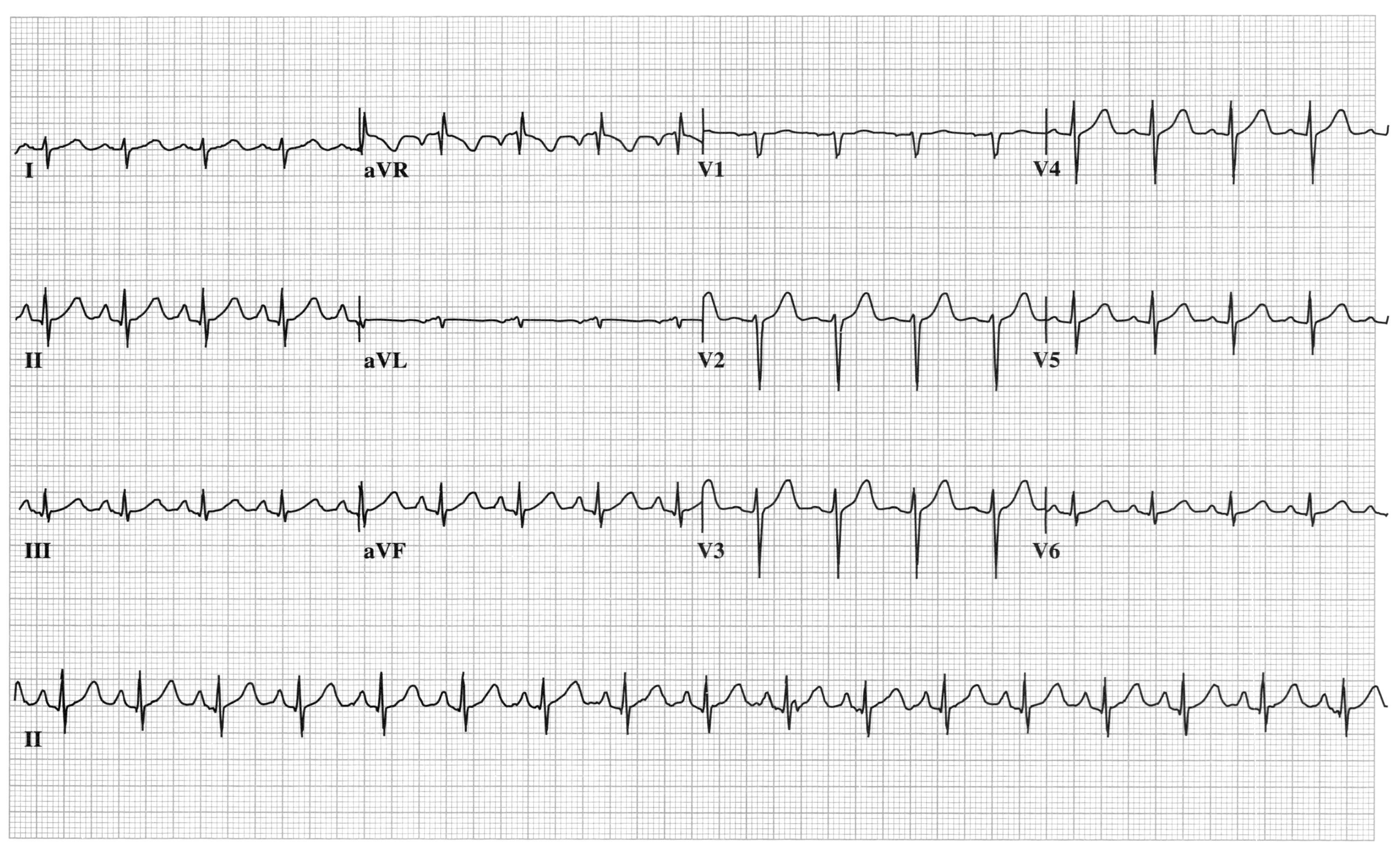

1. GENERAL FEATURES

- ☐ a. Normal ECG
- ☐ b. Borderline normal ECG or normal variant
- ☐ c. Incorrect electrode placement
- ☐ d. Artifact due to tremor

2. ATRIAL RHYTHMS

- ☐ a. Sinus rhythm
- ☐ b. Sinus arrhythmia
- ☐ c. Sinus bradycardia (< 60)
- ☐ d. Sinus tachycardia (> 100)
- ☐ e. Sinus pause or arrest
- ☐ f. Sinoatrial exit block
- ☐ g. Ecoptic atrial rhythm
- ☐ h. Wandering atrial pacemaker
- ☐ i. Atrial premature complexes, normally conducted
- ☐ j. Atrial premature complexes, nonconducted
- ☐ k. Atrial premature complexes with aberrant intraventricular conduction
- ☐ l. Atrial tachycardia (regular, sustained, 1:1 conduction)
- ☐ m. Atrial tachycardia, repetitive (short paroxysms)
- ☐ n. Atrial tachycardia, multifocal
- ☐ o. Atrial tachycardia with AV block
- ☐ p. Supraventricular tachycardia, unspecific
- ☐ q. Supraventricular tachycardia, paroxysmal
- ☐ r. Atrial flutter
- ☐ s. Atrial fibrillation
- ☐ t. Retrograde atrial activation

3. AV JUNCTIONAL RHYTHMS

- ☐ a. AV junctional premature complexes
- ☐ b. AV junctional escape complexes
- ☐ c. AV junctional rhythm, accelerated
- ☐ d. AV junctional rhythm

4. VENTRICULAR RHYTHMS

- ☐ a. Ventricular premature complex(es), uniform, fixed coupling
- ☐ b. Ventricular premature complex(es), uniform, nonfixed coupling
- ☐ c. Ventricular premature complexes(es), multiform
- ☐ d. Ventricular premature complexes, in pairs
- ☐ e. Ventricular parasystole
- ☐ f. Ventricular tachycardia (≥ 3 consecutive complexes)
- ☐ g. Accelerated idioventricular rhythm
- ☐ h. Ventricular escape complexes or rhythm
- ☐ i. Ventricular fibrillation

5. ATRIAL-VENTRICULAR INTERACTIONS IN ARRHYTHMIAS

- ☐ a. Fusion complexes
- ☐ b. Reciprocal (echo) complexes
- ☐ c. Ventricular capture complexes
- ☐ d. AV dissociation
- ☐ e. Ventriculophasic sinus arrhythmia

6. AV CONDUCTION ABNORMALITIES

- ☐ a. AV block, 1°
- ☐ b. AV block, 2° - Mobitz type I (Wenckebach)
- ☐ c. AV block, 2° - Mobitz type II
- ☐ d. AV block, 2:1
- ☐ e. AV block, 3°
- ☐ f. AV block, variable
- ☐ g. Short PR interval (with sinus rhythm and normal QRS duration)
- ☐ h. Wolff-Parkinson-White pattern

7. INTRAVENTRICULAR CONDUCTION DISTURBANCES

- ☐ a. RBBB, incomplete
- ☐ b. RBBB, complete
- ☐ c. Left anterior fascicular block
- ☐ d. Left posterior fascicular block
- ☐ e. LBBB, with ST-T wave suggestive of acute myocardial injury or infarction
- ☐ f. LBBB, complete
- ☐ g. LBBB, intermittent
- ☐ h. Intraventricular conduction disturbance, nonspecific
- ☐ i. Aberrant intraventricular conduction with supraventricular arrhythmia

8. P WAVE ABNORMALITIES

- ☐ a. Right atrial abnormality
- ☐ b. Left atrial abnormalities
- ☐ c. Nonspecific atrial abnormality

9. ABNORMALITIES OF QRS VOLTAGE OR AXIS

- ☐ a. Low voltage, limb leads only
- ☐ b. Low voltage, limb and precordial leads
- ☐ c. Left axis deviation (> - 30%)
- ☐ d. Right axis deviation (> + 100)
- ☐ e. Electrical alternans

10. VENTRICULAR HYPERTROPHY

- ☐ a. LVH by voltage only
- ☐ b. LVH by voltage and ST-T segment abnormalities
- ☐ c. RVH
- ☐ d. Combined ventricular hypertrophy

11. Q WAVE MYOCARDIAL INFARCTION

	Probably Acute or Recent	Probably Old or Age Indeterminate
Anterolateral	☐ a.	☐ g.
Anterior	☐ b.	☐ h.
Anteroseptal	☐ c.	☐ i.
Lateral/High lateral	☐ d.	☐ j.
Inferior	☐ e.	☐ k.
Posterior	☐ f.	☐ l.

- ☐ m. Probably ventricular aneurysm

12. ST, T, U, WAVE ABNORMALITIES

- ☐ a. Normal variant, early repolarization
- ☐ b. Normal variant, juvenile T waves
- ☐ c. Nonspecific ST and/or T wave abnormalities
- ☐ d. ST and/or T wave abnormalities suggesting myocardial ischemia
- ☐ e. ST and/or T wave abnormalities suggesting myocardial injury
- ☐ f. ST and/or T wave abnormalities suggesting acute pericarditis
- ☐ g. ST-T segment abnormalities secondary to intraventricular conduction disturbance or hypertrophy
- ☐ h. Post-extrasystolic T wave abnormality
- ☐ i. Isolated J point depression
- ☐ j. Peaked T waves
- ☐ k. Prolonged QT interval
- ☐ l. Prominent U waves

13. PACEMAKER FUNCTION AND RHYTHM

- ☐ a. Atrial or coronary sinus pacing
- ☐ b. Ventricular demand pacing
- ☐ c. AV sequential pacing
- ☐ d. Ventricular pacing, complete control
- ☐ e. Dual chamber, atrial sensing pacemaker
- ☐ f. Pacemaker malfunction, not constantly capturing (atrium or ventricle)
- ☐ g. Pacemaker malfunction, not constantly sensing (atrium or ventricle)
- ☐ h. Pacemaker malfunction, not firing
- ☐ i. Pacemaker malfunction, slowing

14. SUGGESTED OR PROBABLE CLINICAL DISORDERS

- ☐ a. Digitalis effect
- ☐ b. Digitalis toxicity
- ☐ c. Antiarrhythmic drug effect
- ☐ d. Antiarrhythmic drug toxicity
- ☐ e. Hyperkalemia
- ☐ f. Hypokalemia
- ☐ g. Hypercalcemia
- ☐ h. Hypocalcemia
- ☐ i. Atrial septal defect, secundum
- ☐ j. Atrial septal defect, primum
- ☐ k. Dextrocardia, mirror image
- ☐ l. Mitral valve disease
- ☐ m. Chronic lung disease
- ☐ n. Acute cor pulmonale, including pulmonary embolus
- ☐ o. Pericardial effusion
- ☐ p. Acute pericarditis
- ☐ q. Hypertrophic cardiomyopathy
- ☐ r. Coronary artery disease
- ☐ s. Central nervous system disorder
- ☐ t. Myxedema
- ☐ u. Hypothermia
- ☐ v. Sick sinus syndrome

ECG 46 was obtained in a 58-year-old female with a history of chronic tobacco use and asthma, who was being evaluated for ex[illegible] The ECG show sinus tachycardia, right axis deviation, and right atrial abnormality (arrow). Slow R wave progression is precordial leads (often referred to as clockwise rotation of the transitional zone), with equiphasic QRS complexes (R=S) first V_5 (asterisk). This constellation of findings is typical for patients with chronic lung disease (COPD).

Codes:

2d	Sinus tachycardia
8a	Right atrial abnormality
9d	Right axis deviation (> + 100°)
14m	Chronic lung disease

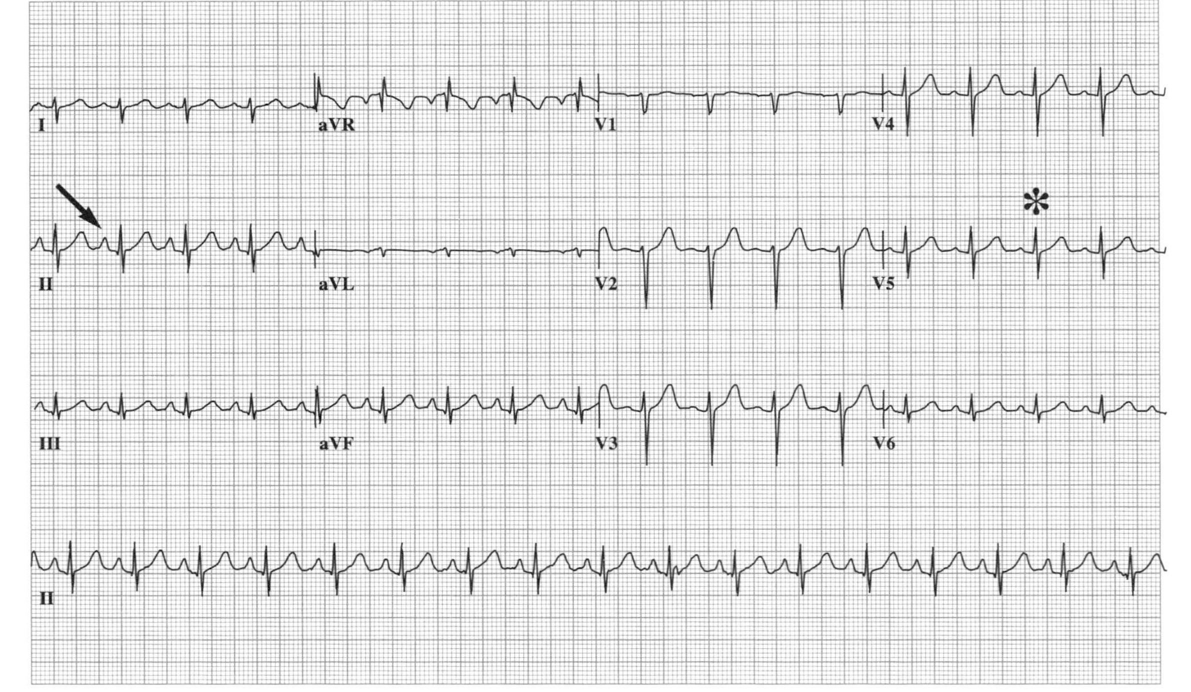

Questions: ECG 46

1. Causes of right axis deviation include:

    a. Right ventricular hypertrophy
    b. Right bundle branch block
    c. Lateral myocardial infarction
    d. Wolff-Parkinson-White syndrome
    e. Dextrocardia
    f. COPD

2. Is left posterior fascicular block present in this tracing?

    a. Yes
    b. No

3. ECG findings consistent with COPD include:

    a. Right ventricular hypertrophy
    b. Right atrial abnormality
    c. Right axis deviation
    d. Poor R wave progression
    e. Low voltage QRS
    f. Pseudo-infarct pattern in the anteroseptal leads
    g. Right bundle branch block

Answers: ECG 46

1. Right axis deviation can be seen as a normal variant, but is more often associated with COPD, cor pulmonale, right ventricular hypertrophy, lateral MI, left posterior fascicular block (LPFB), dextrocardia, lead reversal, and Wolff-Parkinson-White syndrome. Right bundle branch block does not cause right axis deviation unless complicated by LPFB. Right axis deviation (QRS axis 90° to 180°) must be distinguished from right *superior* axis (-90° to -180°), which can be caused by left anterior fascicular block with right ventricular hypertrophy, left anterior fascicular with lateral MI, right ventricular hypertrophy alone, and COPD. (Answer: All except b)

2. While many of the criteria associated with left posterior fascicular block (LPFB) are present in this tracing (right axis deviation; rS in lead I; qR in leads II, III, aVF), LPFB remains a diagnosis of exclusion, and should not be coded when other causes of right axis deviation are evident. In the present tracing, right axis deviation can be attributed to COPD. (Answer: b)

3. Chronic obstructive pulmonary disease (COPD) results in hyperinflation of the lungs, flattening of the diaphragms, and vertical and clockwise rotation of the heart (along its longitudinal axis). Since the hyperinflated lung is a poor electrical conductor, low voltage QRS may be present. Other ECG findings that can be seen in COPD include right ventricular hypertrophy, right

atrial abnormality, right axis deviation, poor R-wave progression (late transitional zone), and at times, a pseudo-infarct pattern in the anteroseptal leads. Right bundle branch block is not a typical feature of COPD, although incomplete right bundle branch block is commonly observed in conditions leading to acute right ventricular strain, such as pulmonary embolism. (Answer: All except g)

— Quick Review 46 —

Sinus tachycardia	
• Rate > ____ per minute	100
• P wave amplitude often (increases/decreases) and PR interval often (increases/decreases) with increasing heart rate	increases shortens
Right atrial abnormality	
• Upright P wave > ____ mm in leads II, III and aVF *or* > ____ mm in leads V_1 or V_2	2.5 1.5
• P wave axis ≥ ____ degrees	70
Chronic lung disease	
• (Right/left) ventricular hypertrophy	Right
• (Right/left) axis deviation	Right
• (Right/left) atrial abnormality	Right
• Shift of transitional zone (clockwise/counterclockwise)	Clockwise
• (High/low) voltage QRS	Low
• Pseudoinfarct pattern in the ____ leads	anteroseptal
• S waves in leads ____ (S_1 S_2 S_3 pattern)	I, II, and III
• May also see sinus tachycardia, junctional rhythm, various degrees of AV block, IVCD, and bundle branch block (true/false)	true

Don't Get Confused!

Atrial Tachycardia with AV Block

P wave axis or morphology different from sinus node; atrial rate of 150-240 per minute; isoelectric intervals between P waves in all leads; second- or third-degree AV block; rhythm is regular

May be confused with:

Atrial flutter

Atrial tachycardia with AV block has a distinct isoelectric baseline between P waves and an atrial rate of 150-240 per minute, whereas atrial flutter lacks an isoelectric baseline (except in lead V_1) and has an atrial rate of 240-340 per minute.

ECG 47. 80-year-old female with history of CHF being treated with a diuretic & digitalis presents with 1 week of profound generalized weakness:

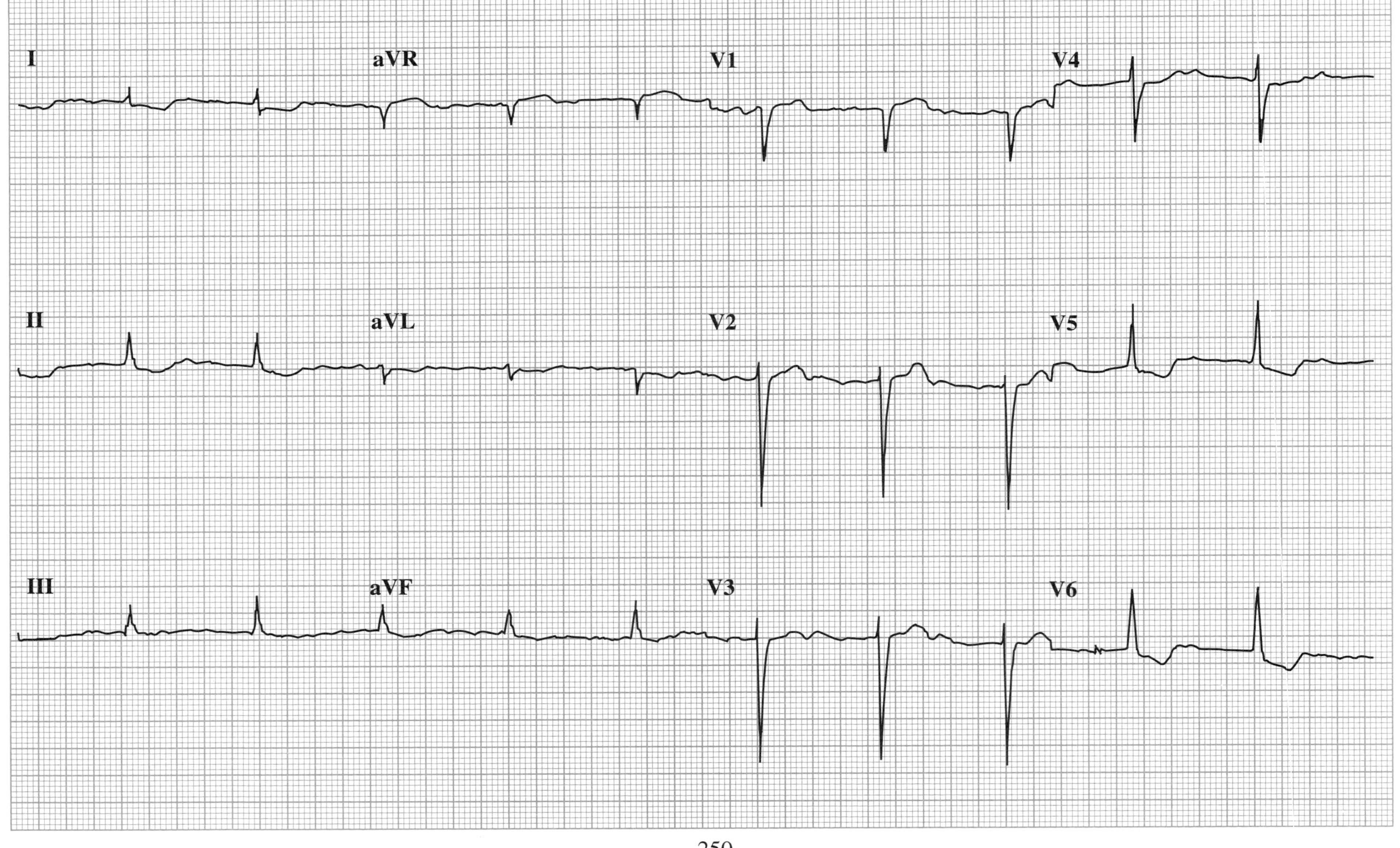

1. GENERAL FEATURES

☐ a. Normal ECG
☐ b. Borderline normal ECG or normal variant
☐ c. Incorrect electrode placement
☐ d. Artifact due to tremor

2. ATRIAL RHYTHMS

☐ a. Sinus rhythm
☐ b. Sinus arrhythmia
☐ c. Sinus bradycardia (< 60)
☐ d. Sinus tachycardia (> 100)
☐ e. Sinus pause or arrest
☐ f. Sinoatrial exit block
☐ g. Ecoptic atrial rhythm
☐ h. Wandering atrial pacemaker
☐ i. Atrial premature complexes, normally conducted
☐ j. Atrial premature complexes, nonconducted
☐ k. Atrial premature complexes with aberrant intraventricular conduction
☐ l. Atrial tachycardia (regular, sustained, 1:1 conduction)
☐ m. Atrial tachycardia, repetitive (short paroxysms)
☐ n. Atrial tachycardia, multifocal
☐ o. Atrial tachycardia with AV block
☐ p. Supraventricular tachycardia, unspecific
☐ q. Supraventricular tachycardia, paroxysmal
☐ r. Atrial flutter
☐ s. Atrial fibrillation
☐ t. Retrograde atrial activation

3. AV JUNCTIONAL RHYTHMS

☐ a. AV junctional premature complexes
☐ b. AV junctional escape complexes
☐ c. AV junctional rhythm, accelerated
☐ d. AV junctional rhythm

4. VENTRICULAR RHYTHMS

☐ a. Ventricular premature complex(es), uniform, fixed coupling
☐ b. Ventricular premature complex(es), uniform, nonfixed coupling
☐ c. Ventricular premature complexes(es), multiform
☐ d. Ventricular premature complexes, in pairs
☐ e. Ventricular parasystole
☐ f. Ventricular tachycardia (≥ 3 consecutive complexes)
☐ g. Accelerated idioventricular rhythm
☐ h. Ventricular escape complexes or rhythm
☐ i. Ventricular fibrillation

5. ATRIAL-VENTRICULAR INTERACTIONS IN ARRHYTHMIAS

☐ a. Fusion complexes
☐ b. Reciprocal (echo) complexes
☐ c. Ventricular capture complexes
☐ d. AV dissociation
☐ e. Ventriculophasic sinus arrhythmia

6. AV CONDUCTION ABNORMALITIES

☐ a. AV block, 1°
☐ b. AV block, 2° - Mobitz type I (Wenckebach)
☐ c. AV block, 2° - Mobitz type II
☐ d. AV block, 2:1
☐ e. AV block, 3°
☐ f. AV block, variable
☐ g. Short PR interval (with sinus rhythm and normal QRS duration)
☐ h. Wolff-Parkinson-White pattern

7. INTRAVENTRICULAR CONDUCTION DISTURBANCES

☐ a. RBBB, incomplete
☐ b. RBBB, complete
☐ c. Left anterior fascicular block
☐ d. Left posterior fascicular block
☐ e. LBBB, with ST-T wave suggestive of acute myocardial injury or infarction
☐ f. LBBB, complete
☐ g. LBBB, intermittent
☐ h. Intraventricular conduction disturbance, nonspecific
☐ i. Aberrant intraventricular conduction with supraventricular arrhythmia

8. P WAVE ABNORMALITIES

☐ a. Right atrial abnormality
☐ b. Left atrial abnormalities
☐ c. Nonspecific atrial abnormality

9. ABNORMALITIES OF QRS VOLTAGE OR AXIS

☐ a. Low voltage, limb leads only
☐ b. Low voltage, limb and precordial leads
☐ c. Left axis deviation (> - 30%)
☐ d. Right axis deviation (> + 100)
☐ e. Electrical alternans

10. VENTRICULAR HYPERTROPHY

☐ a. LVH by voltage only
☐ b. LVH by voltage and ST-T segment abnormalities
☐ c. RVH
☐ d. Combined ventricular hypertrophy

11. Q WAVE MYOCARDIAL INFARCTION

	Probably Acute or Recent	Probably Old or Age Indeterminate
Anterolateral	☐ a.	☐ g.
Anterior	☐ b.	☐ h.
Anteroseptal	☐ c.	☐ i.
Lateral/High lateral	☐ d.	☐ j.
Inferior	☐ e.	☐ k.
Posterior	☐ f.	☐ l.

☐ m. Probably ventricular aneurysm

12. ST, T, U, WAVE ABNORMALITIES

☐ a. Normal variant, early repolarization
☐ b. Normal variant, juvenile T waves
☐ c. Nonspecific ST and/or T wave abnormalities
☐ d. ST and/or T wave abnormalities suggesting myocardial ischemia
☐ e. ST and/or T wave abnormalities suggesting myocardial injury
☐ f. ST and/or T wave abnormalities suggesting acute pericarditis
☐ g. ST-T segment abnormalities secondary to intraventricular conduction disturbance or hypertrophy
☐ h. Post-extrasystolic T wave abnormality
☐ i. Isolated J point depression
☐ j. Peaked T waves
☐ k. Prolonged QT interval
☐ l. Prominent U waves

13. PACEMAKER FUNCTION AND RHYTHM

☐ a. Atrial or coronary sinus pacing
☐ b. Ventricular demand pacing
☐ c. AV sequential pacing
☐ d. Ventricular pacing, complete control
☐ e. Dual chamber, atrial sensing pacemaker
☐ f. Pacemaker malfunction, not constantly capturing (atrium or ventricle)
☐ g. Pacemaker malfunction, not constantly sensing (atrium or ventricle)
☐ h. Pacemaker malfunction, not firing
☐ i. Pacemaker malfunction, slowing

14. SUGGESTED OR PROBABLE CLINICAL DISORDERS

☐ a. Digitalis effect
☐ b. Digitalis toxicity
☐ c. Antiarrhythmic drug effect
☐ d. Antiarrhythmic drug toxicity
☐ e. Hyperkalemia
☐ f. Hypokalemia
☐ g. Hypercalcemia
☐ h. Hypocalcemia
☐ i. Atrial septal defect, secundum
☐ j. Atrial septal defect, primum
☐ k. Dextrocardia, mirror image
☐ l. Mitral valve disease
☐ m. Chronic lung disease
☐ n. Acute cor pulmonale, including pulmonary embolus
☐ o. Pericardial effusion
☐ p. Acute pericarditis
☐ q. Hypertrophic cardiomyopathy
☐ r. Coronary artery disease
☐ s. Central nervous system disorder
☐ t. Myxedema
☐ u. Hypothermia
☐ v. Sick sinus syndrome

ECG 47 was obtained in an 80-year-old female with a history of congestive heart failure being treated with a diuretic and digitalis, who presented with several days of profound generalized weakness. The ECG shows underlying atrial fibrillation with a regular rhythm, which is consistent with complete heart block with an accelerated junctional rhythm (junctional rate = 70/minute). Prominent U waves (arrow) and a nonspecific intraventricular conduction defect (QRS in $V_4 = 0.11$ sec) with secondary ST-T changes are also present. These findings are suggestive of digitalis toxicity and hypokalemia (which can predispose to digitalis toxicity). This patient's diuretic dose had recently been increased; at the time the ECG was taken, her potassium level was 2.0 mEq/L and digitalis level was 2.5 ng/mL.

Codes:

2s	Atrial fibrillation
3c	AV junctional rhythm, accelerated
7h	IVCD, nonspecific type
12g	ST-T segment abnormalities secondary to IVCD or hypertrophy
12l	Prominent U waves
14b	Digitalis toxicity
14f	Hypokalemia

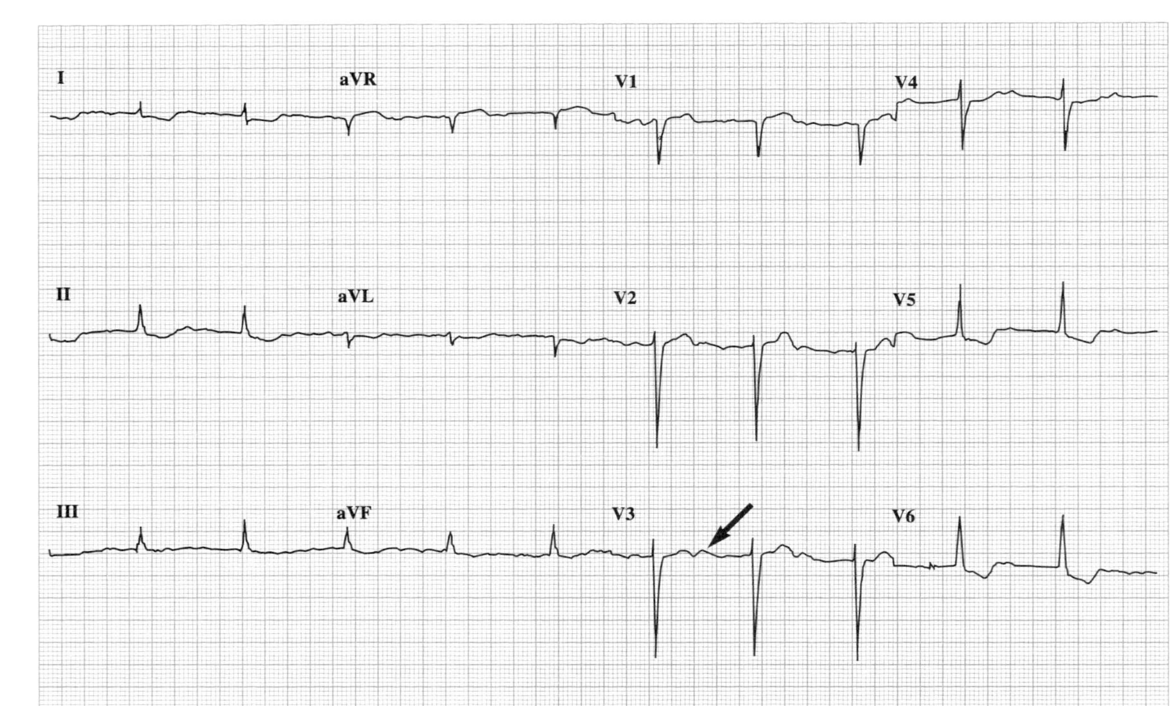

Questions: ECG 47

1. In the setting of atrial fibrillation, digitalis toxicity often manifests as:

   a. Accelerated conduction through the AV node with increased ventricular rates
   b. Complete heart block with an accelerated junctional rhythm
   c. Complete heart block with an idioventricular rhythm
   d. Protracted asystole after electrocardioversion

2. Hypokalemia is associated with:

   a. Prominent U waves
   b. Decreased T wave amplitude
   c. Shortening of the corrected QT
   d. Cardiac arrhythmias including ventricular tachycardia

3. ECG manifestations of hypokalemia are predictably seen when the serum potassium level is below:

   a. 2.7 mEq/L
   b. 3.0 mEq/L
   c. 3.3 mEq/L
   d. 3.6 mEq/L

Answers: ECG 47

1. In the setting of atrial fibrillation, digitalis toxicity most commonly manifests as regularization of the RR interval due to high-grade or complete AV block with an accelerated junctional or idioventricular rhythm. Digitalis toxicity can also cause protracted asystole after cardioversion for atrial fibrillation. Digitalis results in decreased (not increased) AV nodal conduction and slowing (not acceleration) of the ventricular response. (Answer: b, c, d)

2. ECG features of hypokalemia include ST segment depression, decreased T wave amplitude, and prominent U waves. Arrhythmias associated with hypokalemia include frequent VPCs, ventricular tachycardia and fibrillation, first-degree and second-degree AV block, and AV dissociation. Hypokalemia can predispose to digitalis toxicity. (Answer: a, b, d)

3. The ST-T and U wave changes of hypokalemia are seen in approximately 80% of patients with potassium levels of patients below 2.7 mEq/L, compared to 35% of patients with levels of 2.7-3.0 mEq/L and 10% with levels above 3.0 mEq/L. (Answer: a)

— Quick Review 47 —

AV junctional rhythm, accelerated	
• Regular QRS rhythm at rate > ____ per minute	60
• P wave may proceed, be buried in, or follow the QRS complex (true/false)	true
• QRS is usually narrow but may be wide if _____	aberrant or IVCD
• If retrograde block is present, the atria remain in sinus rhythm with ____	AV dissociation
• If retrograde atrial activation occurs, a (constant/variable) QRS-P interval will be present	constant
Prominent U waves	
• Amplitude ≥ ____ mm	1.5
• The U wave is normally ____% the height of the T wave, and is largest in leads ____	5-25 V_2, V_3
Digitalis effect	
• ____ ST segment depression with upward (concavity/convexity)	Sagging concavity
• T wave flat, inverted, or ____	biphasic
• QT interval (shortened/prolonged)	shortened
• U wave amplitude (increased/decreased)	increased
• PR interval (shortened/prolonged)	prolonged

— Quick Review 47 —

Digitalis toxicity	
• Digitalis toxicity can cause almost any type of cardiac dysrhythmia or conduction disturbance except _____	bundle branch block
• Typical abnormalities include:	
▸ Paroxysmal ____ tachycardia with block	atrial
▸ Atrial fibrillation with ____ heart block	complete
▸ Second or third-degree ____ block	AV
▸ Complete heart block with accelerated ____ or ____ rhythm	junctional idioventricular
▸ Supraventricular tachycardia with ____ bundle branch block	alternating
Hypokalemia	
• Prominent ____ waves	U
• ST segment (depression/elevation)	depression
• Flattened ____ waves	T
• Prolonged ____ interval	QT
• Arrhythmias and conduction disturbances, including paroxysmal atrial tachycardia with block, first-degree AV block, Type I second-degree AV block, AV dissociation, VPCs, ventricular tachycardia, and ventricular fibrillation (true/false)	true

Don't Forget!

- When a VPC originates on the same side as a bundle branch block, the resulting fusion complex can be narrow
- Think of parasystole when you see ventricular complexes with nonfixed coupling and fusion beats
- Look for ventricular capture complexes (item 5c) and fusion beats (item 5a) as markers for VT in the setting of a wide QRS tachycardia
- Classical Wenckebach periodicity may not always be evident, especially when sinus arrhythmia is present or an abrupt change in autonomic tone occurs
- 2:1 AV block can be Mobitz Type I or Type II
- In WPW, the PJ interval (beginning of P wave to end of QRS complex) is constant and $\leq$ 0.26 seconds
- Think WPW when atrial fibrillation or flutter is associated with a QRS that varies in width (generally wide) and has a rate >200 per minute

ECG 48. 78-year-old female with a history of syncope:

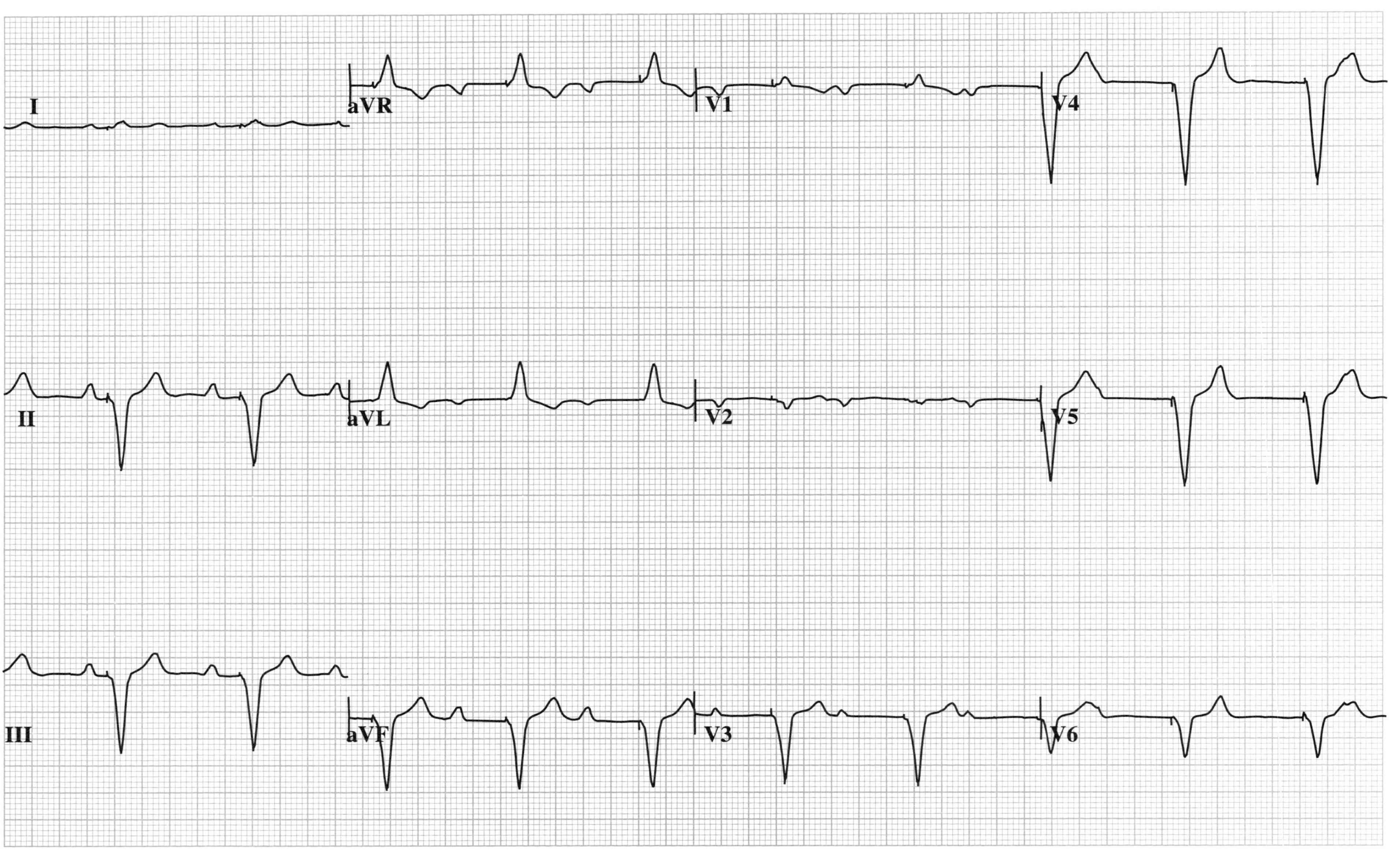

1. GENERAL FEATURES

☐ a. Normal ECG
☐ b. Borderline normal ECG or normal variant
☐ c. Incorrect electrode placement
☐ d. Artifact due to tremor

2. ATRIAL RHYTHMS

☐ a. Sinus rhythm
☐ b. Sinus arrhythmia
☐ c. Sinus bradycardia (< 60)
☐ d. Sinus tachycardia (> 100)
☐ e. Sinus pause or arrest
☐ f. Sinoatrial exit block
☐ g. Ecoptic atrial rhythm
☐ h. Wandering atrial pacemaker
☐ i. Atrial premature complexes, normally conducted
☐ j. Atrial premature complexes, nonconducted
☐ k. Atrial premature complexes with aberrant intraventricular conduction
☐ l. Atrial tachycardia (regular, sustained, 1:1 conduction)
☐ m. Atrial tachycardia, repetitive (short paroxysms)
☐ n. Atrial tachycardia, multifocal
☐ o. Atrial tachycardia with AV block
☐ p. Supraventricular tachycardia, unspecific
☐ q. Supraventricular tachycardia, paroxysmal
☐ r. Atrial flutter
☐ s. Atrial fibrillation
☐ t. Retrograde atrial activation

3. AV JUNCTIONAL RHYTHMS

☐ a. AV junctional premature complexes
☐ b. AV junctional escape complexes
☐ c. AV junctional rhythm, accelerated
☐ d. AV junctional rhythm

4. VENTRICULAR RHYTHMS

☐ a. Ventricular premature complex(es), uniform, fixed coupling
☐ b. Ventricular premature complex(es), uniform, nonfixed coupling
☐ c. Ventricular premature complexes(es), multiform
☐ d. Ventricular premature complexes, in pairs
☐ e. Ventricular parasystole
☐ f. Ventricular tachycardia (≥ 3 consecutive complexes)
☐ g. Accelerated idioventricular rhythm
☐ h. Ventricular escape complexes or rhythm
☐ i. Ventricular fibrillation

5. ATRIAL-VENTRICULAR INTERACTIONS IN ARRHYTHMIAS

☐ a. Fusion complexes
☐ b. Reciprocal (echo) complexes
☐ c. Ventricular capture complexes
☐ d. AV dissociation

☐ e. Ventriculophasic sinus arrhythmia

6. AV CONDUCTION ABNORMALITIES

☐ a. AV block, 1°
☐ b. AV block, 2° - Mobitz type I (Wenckebach)
☐ c. AV block, 2° - Mobitz type II
☐ d. AV block, 2:1
☐ e. AV block, 3°
☐ f. AV block, variable
☐ g. Short PR interval (with sinus rhythm and normal QRS duration)
☐ h. Wolff-Parkinson-White pattern

7. INTRAVENTRICULAR CONDUCTION DISTURBANCES

☐ a. RBBB, incomplete
☐ b. RBBB, complete
☐ c. Left anterior fascicular block
☐ d. Left posterior fascicular block
☐ e. LBBB, with ST-T wave suggestive of acute myocardial injury or infarction
☐ f. LBBB, complete
☐ g. LBBB, intermittent
☐ h. Intraventricular conduction disturbance, nonspecific
☐ i. Aberrant intraventricular conduction with supraventricular arrhythmia

8. P WAVE ABNORMALITIES

☐ a. Right atrial abnormality
☐ b. Left atrial abnormalities
☐ c. Nonspecific atrial abnormality

9. ABNORMALITIES OF QRS VOLTAGE OR AXIS

☐ a. Low voltage, limb leads only
☐ b. Low voltage, limb and precordial leads
☐ c. Left axis deviation (> - 30%)
☐ d. Right axis deviation (> + 100)
☐ e. Electrical alternans

10. VENTRICULAR HYPERTROPHY

☐ a. LVH by voltage only
☐ b. LVH by voltage and ST-T segment abnormalities
☐ c. RVH
☐ d. Combined ventricular hypertrophy

11. Q WAVE MYOCARDIAL INFARCTION

	Probably Acute or Recent	Probably Old or Age Indeterminate
Anterolateral	☐ a.	☐ g.
Anterior	☐ b.	☐ h.
Anteroseptal	☐ c.	☐ i.
Lateral/High lateral	☐ d.	☐ j.
Inferior	☐ e.	☐ k.
Posterior	☐ f.	☐ l.

☐ m. Probably ventricular aneurysm

12. ST, T, U, WAVE ABNORMALITIES

☐ a. Normal variant, early repolarization
☐ b. Normal variant, juvenile T waves
☐ c. Nonspecific ST and/or T wave abnormalities
☐ d. ST and/or T wave abnormalities suggesting myocardial ischemia
☐ e. ST and/or T wave abnormalities suggesting myocardial injury
☐ f. ST and/or T wave abnormalities suggesting acute pericarditis
☐ g. ST-T segment abnormalities secondary to intraventricular conduction disturbance or hypertrophy
☐ h. Post-extrasystolic T wave abnormality
☐ i. Isolated J point depression
☐ j. Peaked T waves
☐ k. Prolonged QT interval
☐ l. Prominent U waves

13. PACEMAKER FUNCTION AND RHYTHM

☐ a. Atrial or coronary sinus pacing
☐ b. Ventricular demand pacing
☐ c. AV sequential pacing
☐ d. Ventricular pacing, complete control
☐ e. Dual chamber, atrial sensing pacemaker
☐ f. Pacemaker malfunction, not constantly capturing (atrium or ventricle)
☐ g. Pacemaker malfunction, not constantly sensing (atrium or ventricle)
☐ h. Pacemaker malfunction, not firing
☐ i. Pacemaker malfunction, slowing

14. SUGGESTED OR PROBABLE CLINICAL DISORDERS

☐ a. Digitalis effect
☐ b. Digitalis toxicity
☐ c. Antiarrhythmic drug effect
☐ d. Antiarrhythmic drug toxicity
☐ e. Hyperkalemia
☐ f. Hypokalemia
☐ g. Hypercalcemia
☐ h. Hypocalcemia
☐ i. Atrial septal defect, secundum
☐ j. Atrial septal defect, primum
☐ k. Dextrocardia, mirror image
☐ l. Mitral valve disease
☐ m. Chronic lung disease
☐ n. Acute cor pulmonale, including pulmonary embolus
☐ o. Pericardial effusion
☐ p. Acute pericarditis
☐ q. Hypertrophic cardiomyopathy
☐ r. Coronary artery disease
☐ s. Central nervous system disorder
☐ t. Myxedema
☐ u. Hypothermia
☐ v. Sick sinus syndrome

ECG 48 was obtained from a 78-year-old female with a history of syncope. Ventricular pacing at 64 beats/minute is noted throughout the tracing (asterisks). It is impossible to tell whether this is VVI or VOO pacing; however, since no demonstrable output inhibition is noted, it is best to code this as fixed rate ventricular pacing (VOO). The underlying rhythm is sinus with complete heart block. Criteria are met for right atrial abnormality (arrowhead) and left atrial abnormality (arrow).

Codes:

2a	Sinus rhythm
6e	AV block, 3°
8a	Right atrial abnormality
8b	Left atrial abnormality
13d	Ventricular pacing, complete control

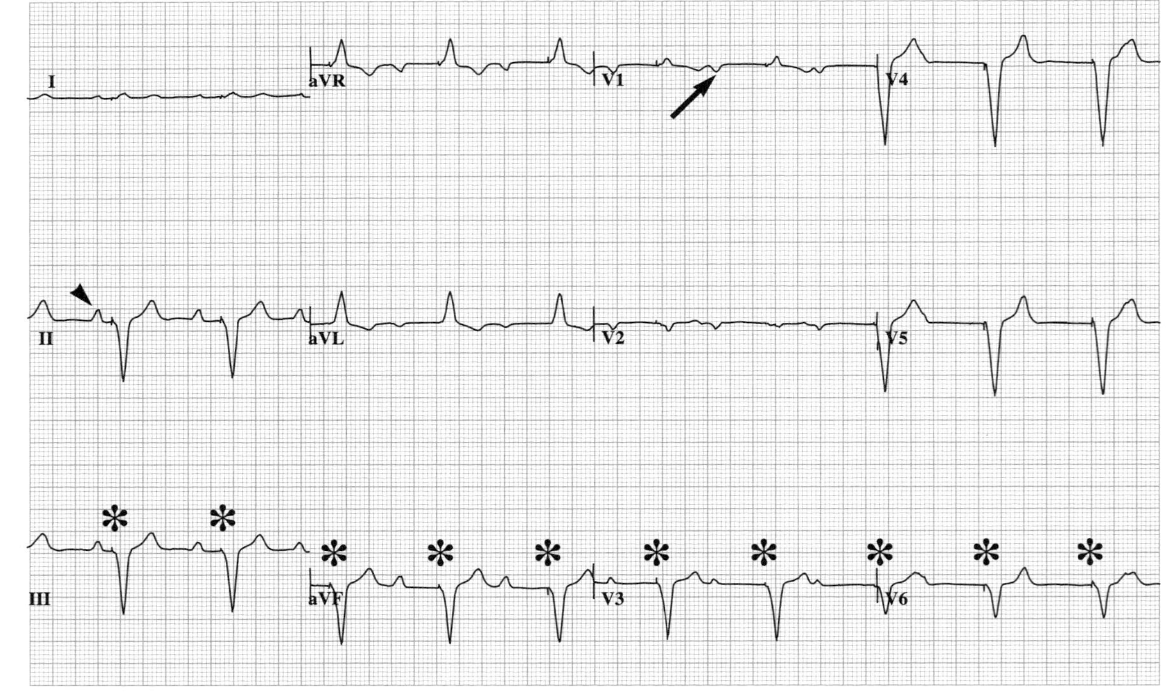

Questions: ECG 48

1. In the setting of VVI pacing, the native P waves are usually independent of the paced ventricular activity:

   a. True
   b. False

2. Ventricular pacing does not interfere with the diagnosis of acute myocardial infarction or ischemia:

   a. True
   b. False

Answers: ECG 48

1. By definition, VVI pacemakers do not sense the atrium. If underlying atrial activity is present (native P waves) but the native ventricular rate is slower than the rate setting on the pacemaker, the ventricle will be paced irrespective of the atrial rate. (Answer: a)

2. Ventricular pacing should be considered the equivalent of LBBB when it comes to identifying acute myocardial infarction. Ventricular pacing results in an abnormal ventricular activation pattern, resulting in wide QRS complexes with secondary ST-T abnormalities; this makes the diagnosis of acute myocardial ischemia and/or infarction extremely difficult unless portions of the ECG show unpaced QRS complexes. The ST-T changes secondary to ventricular pacing should be coded as 12g (ST and T abnormalities secondary to intraventricular conduction disturbance or hypertrophy). (Answer: b)

— Quick Review 48 —

AV block, 3°	
• Atrial and ventricular rhythms are ____ of each other	independent
• Atrial rate is generally (faster/slower) than the ventricular rate	faster
Left atrial abnormality	
• Notched P wave with a duration ≥ ____ seconds in leads II, III or aVF, *or*	0.12
• Terminal negative portion of the P wave in lead V_1 ≥ 1 mm deep and ≥ ____ seconds in duration	0.04
Ventricular pacing, fixed rate (asynchronous)	
• Ventricular pacing (with/without) demonstrable output inhibition by intrinsic QRS complexes	without

ECG 49. 76-year-old female with chest pain and syncope:

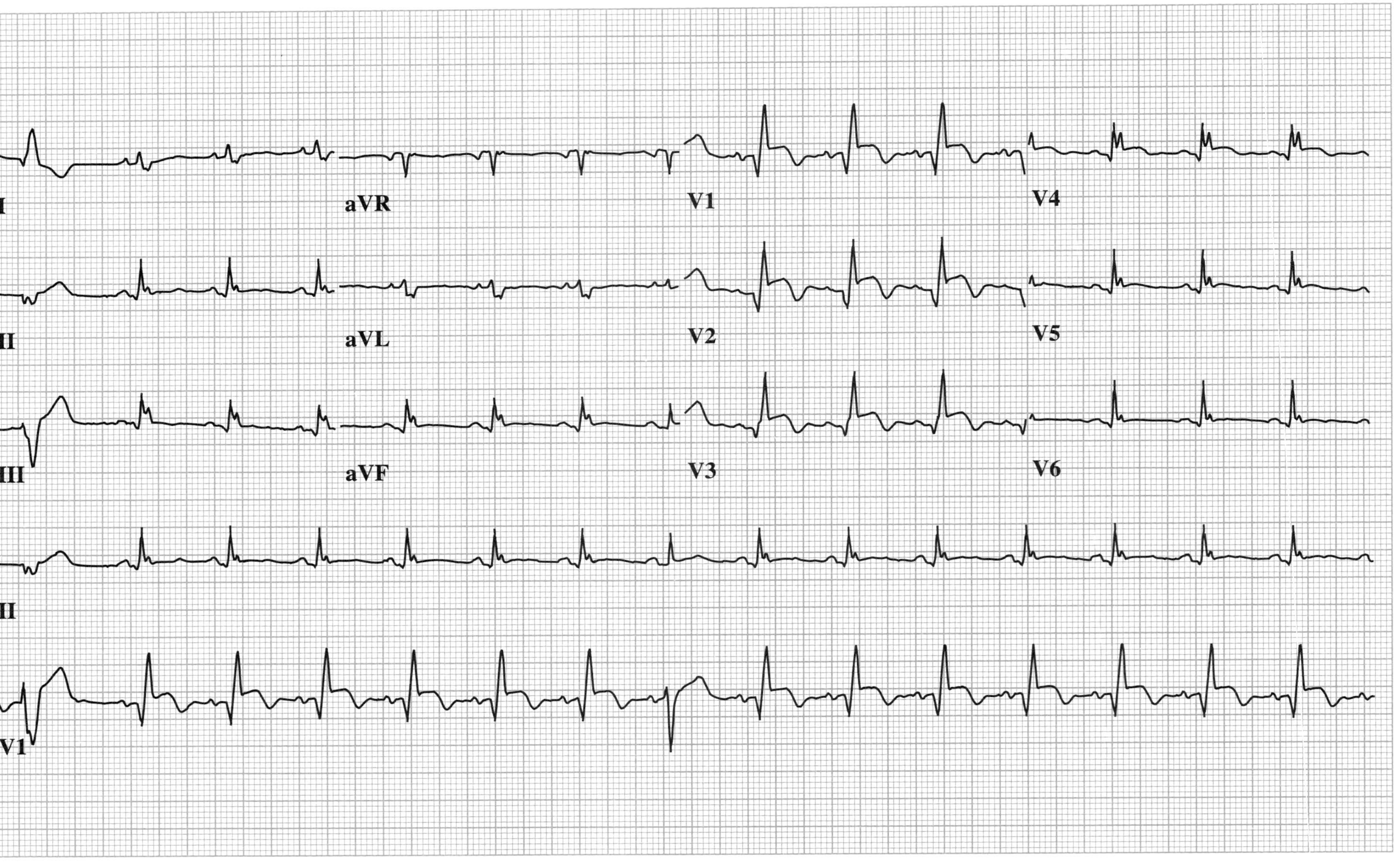

1. GENERAL FEATURES

☐ a. Normal ECG
☐ b. Borderline normal ECG or normal variant
☐ c. Incorrect electrode placement
☐ d. Artifact due to tremor

2. ATRIAL RHYTHMS

☐ a. Sinus rhythm
☐ b. Sinus arrhythmia
☐ c. Sinus bradycardia (< 60)
☐ d. Sinus tachycardia (> 100)
☐ e. Sinus pause or arrest
☐ f. Sinoatrial exit block
☐ g. Ecoptic atrial rhythm
☐ h. Wandering atrial pacemaker
☐ i. Atrial premature complexes, normally conducted
☐ j. Atrial premature complexes, nonconducted
☐ k. Atrial premature complexes with aberrant intraventricular conduction
☐ l. Atrial tachycardia (regular, sustained, 1:1 conduction)
☐ m. Atrial tachycardia, repetitive (short paroxysms)
☐ n. Atrial tachycardia, multifocal
☐ o. Atrial tachycardia with AV block
☐ p. Supraventricular tachycardia, unspecific
☐ q. Supraventricular tachycardia, paroxysmal
☐ r. Atrial flutter
☐ s. Atrial fibrillation
☐ t. Retrograde atrial activation

3. AV JUNCTIONAL RHYTHMS

☐ a. AV junctional premature complexes
☐ b. AV junctional escape complexes
☐ c. AV junctional rhythm, accelerated
☐ d. AV junctional rhythm

4. VENTRICULAR RHYTHMS

☐ a. Ventricular premature complex(es), uniform, fixed coupling
☐ b. Ventricular premature complex(es), uniform, nonfixed coupling
☐ c. Ventricular premature complexes(es), multiform
☐ d. Ventricular premature complexes, in pairs
☐ e. Ventricular parasystole
☐ f. Ventricular tachycardia (≥ 3 consecutive complexes)
☐ g. Accelerated idioventricular rhythm
☐ h. Ventricular escape complexes or rhythm
☐ i. Ventricular fibrillation

5. ATRIAL-VENTRICULAR INTERACTIONS IN ARRHYTHMIAS

☐ a. Fusion complexes
☐ b. Reciprocal (echo) complexes
☐ c. Ventricular capture complexes
☐ d. AV dissociation
☐ e. Ventriculophasic sinus arrhythmia

6. AV CONDUCTION ABNORMALITIES

☐ a. AV block, 1°
☐ b. AV block, 2° - Mobitz type I (Wenckebach)
☐ c. AV block, 2° - Mobitz type II
☐ d. AV block, 2:1
☐ e. AV block, 3°
☐ f. AV block, variable
☐ g. Short PR interval (with sinus rhythm and normal QRS duration)
☐ h. Wolff-Parkinson-White pattern

7. INTRAVENTRICULAR CONDUCTION DISTURBANCES

☐ a. RBBB, incomplete
☐ b. RBBB, complete
☐ c. Left anterior fascicular block
☐ d. Left posterior fascicular block
☐ e. LBBB, with ST-T wave suggestive of acute myocardial injury or infarction
☐ f. LBBB, complete
☐ g. LBBB, intermittent
☐ h. Intraventricular conduction disturbance, nonspecific
☐ i. Aberrant intraventricular conduction with supraventricular arrhythmia

8. P WAVE ABNORMALITIES

☐ a. Right atrial abnormality
☐ b. Left atrial abnormalities
☐ c. Nonspecific atrial abnormality

9. ABNORMALITIES OF QRS VOLTAGE OR AXIS

☐ a. Low voltage, limb leads only
☐ b. Low voltage, limb and precordial leads
☐ c. Left axis deviation (> - 30%)
☐ d. Right axis deviation (> + 100)
☐ e. Electrical alternans

10. VENTRICULAR HYPERTROPHY

☐ a. LVH by voltage only
☐ b. LVH by voltage and ST-T segment abnormalities
☐ c. RVH
☐ d. Combined ventricular hypertrophy

11. Q WAVE MYOCARDIAL INFARCTION

	Probably Acute or Recent	Probably Old or Age Indeterminate
Anterolateral	☐ a.	☐ g.
Anterior	☐ b.	☐ h.
Anteroseptal	☐ c.	☐ i.
Lateral/High lateral	☐ d.	☐ j.
Inferior	☐ e.	☐ k.
Posterior	☐ f.	☐ l.

☐ m. Probably ventricular aneurysm

12. ST, T, U, WAVE ABNORMALITIES

☐ a. Normal variant, early repolarization
☐ b. Normal variant, juvenile T waves
☐ c. Nonspecific ST and/or T wave abnormalities
☐ d. ST and/or T wave abnormalities suggesting myocardial ischemia
☐ e. ST and/or T wave abnormalities suggesting myocardial injury
☐ f. ST and/or T wave abnormalities suggesting acute pericarditis
☐ g. ST-T segment abnormalities secondary to intraventricular conduction disturbance or hypertrophy
☐ h. Post-extrasystolic T wave abnormality
☐ i. Isolated J point depression
☐ j. Peaked T waves
☐ k. Prolonged QT interval
☐ l. Prominent U waves

13. PACEMAKER FUNCTION AND RHYTHM

☐ a. Atrial or coronary sinus pacing
☐ b. Ventricular demand pacing
☐ c. AV sequential pacing
☐ d. Ventricular pacing, complete control
☐ e. Dual chamber, atrial sensing pacemaker
☐ f. Pacemaker malfunction, not constantly capturing (atrium or ventricle)
☐ g. Pacemaker malfunction, not constantly sensing (atrium or ventricle)
☐ h. Pacemaker malfunction, not firing
☐ i. Pacemaker malfunction, slowing

14. SUGGESTED OR PROBABLE CLINICAL DISORDERS

☐ a. Digitalis effect
☐ b. Digitalis toxicity
☐ c. Antiarrhythmic drug effect
☐ d. Antiarrhythmic drug toxicity
☐ e. Hyperkalemia
☐ f. Hypokalemia
☐ g. Hypercalcemia
☐ h. Hypocalcemia
☐ i. Atrial septal defect, secundum
☐ j. Atrial septal defect, primum
☐ k. Dextrocardia, mirror image
☐ l. Mitral valve disease
☐ m. Chronic lung disease
☐ n. Acute cor pulmonale, including pulmonary embolus
☐ o. Pericardial effusion
☐ p. Acute pericarditis
☐ q. Hypertrophic cardiomyopathy
☐ r. Coronary artery disease
☐ s. Central nervous system disorder
☐ t. Myxedema
☐ u. Hypothermia
☐ v. Sick sinus syndrome

ECG 49 was obtained in a 76-year-old female with chest pain and syncope. The ECG shows normal sinus rhythm with ventricular premature complexes (arrowhead). The second VPC (arrow) is a fusion complex, which is intermediate in morphology between a regular sinus beat and a VPC. Also present are RBBB and acute anteroseptal myocardial infarction, with Q waves and ST segment elevation most notable in leads V_1-V_3 (asterisks). ST-T changes suggesting myocardial injury and coronary artery disease should also be coded.

Codes:

2a	Sinus rhythm
4a	Ventricular premature complex(es), uniform, fixed coupling
5a	Fusion complexes
7b	RBBB, complete
11c	Anteroseptal Q wave MI, probably acute or recent
12e	ST and/or T wave abnormalities suggesting myocardial injury
14r	Coronary artery disease

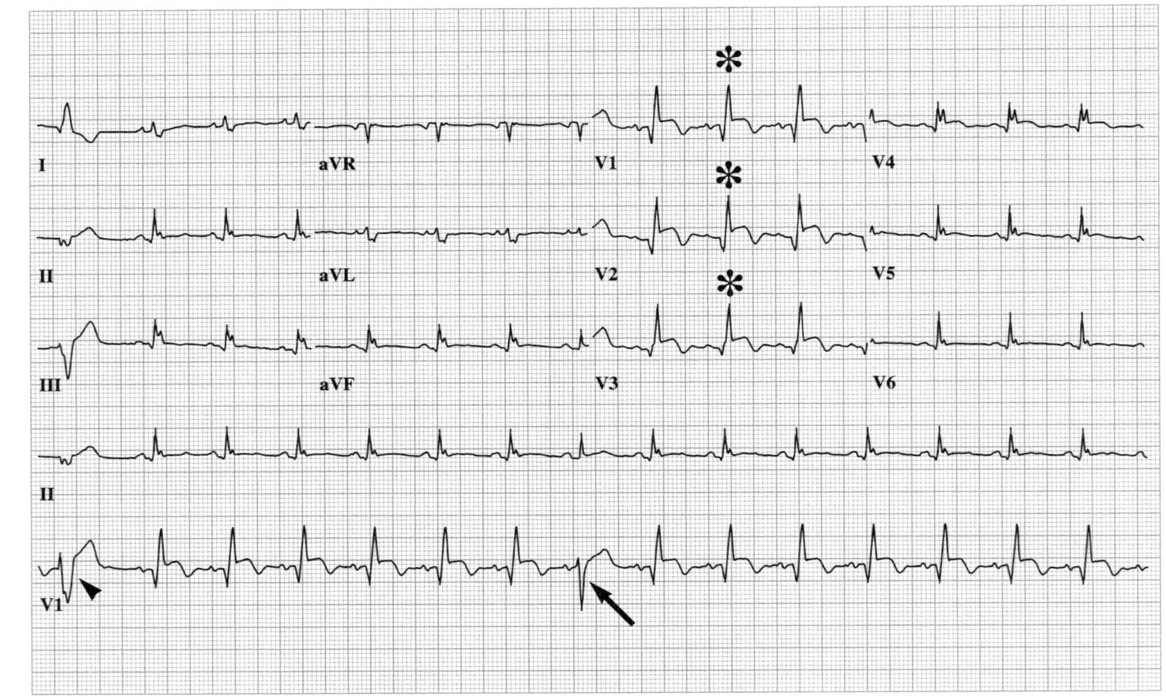

Questions: ECG 49

1. The presence of RBBB invalidates the usual criteria for diagnosing acute anteroseptal myocardial infarction:

   a. True
   b. False

Answers: ECG 49

1. Right bundle branch block is occasionally found in normal adults (incidence ~ 2/1000) without underlying structural heart disease (unlike LBBB). These patients have essentially the same prognosis as the general population. However, among patients with coronary artery disease, RBBB is associated with a 2-fold increase in mortality, and LBBB with a 5-fold increase in mortality (compared to patients with coronary disease but without bundle branch block). RBBB is not usually associated with extensive baseline ST segment repolarization abnormalities (unlike LBBB), and the initial QRS complex is formed by the intact left bundle; therefore, RBBB does not interfere with identification of the Q waves or ST segment elevation of acute myocardial infarction. (Answer: b)

— Quick Review 49 —

Ventricular premature complex(es), uniform, fixed coupling	
• A wide, notched or slurred ____ complex that is premature relative to the normal RR interval and is not preceded by a ____ wave	QRS P
• QRS duration is almost always > ____ seconds	0.12
• Initial direction of the QRS is often (similar to/different from) the QRS during sinus rhythm	different from
• Secondary ST & T wave changes in the (same/opposite) direction as the major deflection of the QRS (i.e., ST depression & T wave inversion in leads with a dominant ____wave; ST elevation and upright T wave in leads with a dominant ____ wave or ____ complex)	opposite R S QS
• Coupling interval is constant or varies by < ____ seconds	0.08
• Morphology of VPCs in any given lead is (the same/different)	the same
• Retrograde capture of atria may occur (true/false)	true
• A full ____ pause (PP interval containing the VPC is twice the normal PP interval) is usually evident	compensatory
Anteroseptal MI, recent or probably acute	
• Abnormal Q or QS deflection and ST elevation in leads ____ (and sometimes V_4)	V_1-V_3
• The presence of a Q wave in lead ____ distinguishes anteroseptal from anterior infarction	V_1

— Quick Review 49 —	
ST and/or T wave changes suggesting myocardial injury	
• Acute ST segment (elevation/depression) with upward (convexity/concavity) in the leads representing the area of infarction	elevation convexity
• T waves invert (before/after) ST segments return to baseline	before
• Associated ST (elevation/depression) in the noninfarct leads is common	depression
• Acute ____ wall injury often has horizontal or downsloping ST segment depression with upright T waves in V_1-V_3, with or without a prominent R wave in these same leads	posterior

— POP QUIZ —

Make The Diagnosis

Instructions: Determine the ECG diagnosis that best corresponds to the ECG features listed below (see score sheet for options)

ECG Features	Diagnosis
• Abnormal Q waves (duration ≥ 0.03 seconds) and ST segment elevation in leads V_4-V_6	Anterolateral MI, acute or recent
• rS in lead V_1, *followed by* QS or QR complexes (Q wave duration ≥ 0.03 seconds) and ST elevation in two of leads V_2-V_4, *or* decreasing R wave amplitude from V_2-V_5	Anterior MI, acute or recent
• Abnormal Q or QS deflection and ST elevation in V_1-V_3 (and sometimes V_4)	Anteroseptal MI, acute or recent
• Abnormal Q waves and ST elevation in leads I and aVL	Lateral MI, acute or recent
• Abnormal Q waves and ST elevation in at least two of leads II, III, and aVF • Associated ST depression usually evident in leads I, aVL, V_1-V_3	Inferior MI, probably acute or recent
• Initial R wave ≥ 0.04 seconds in leads V_1 and V_2 with R wave amplitude > S wave amplitude, *and* ST segment depression with upright T waves • Usually seen in the setting of acute inferior MI	Posterior MI, probably acute or recent
• ST segment elevation ≥ 1 mm persisting 4 or more weeks after acute MI in leads with abnormal Q waves	Probable ventricular aneurysm

ECG 50. 13-year-old male with a family history of sudden cardiac death:

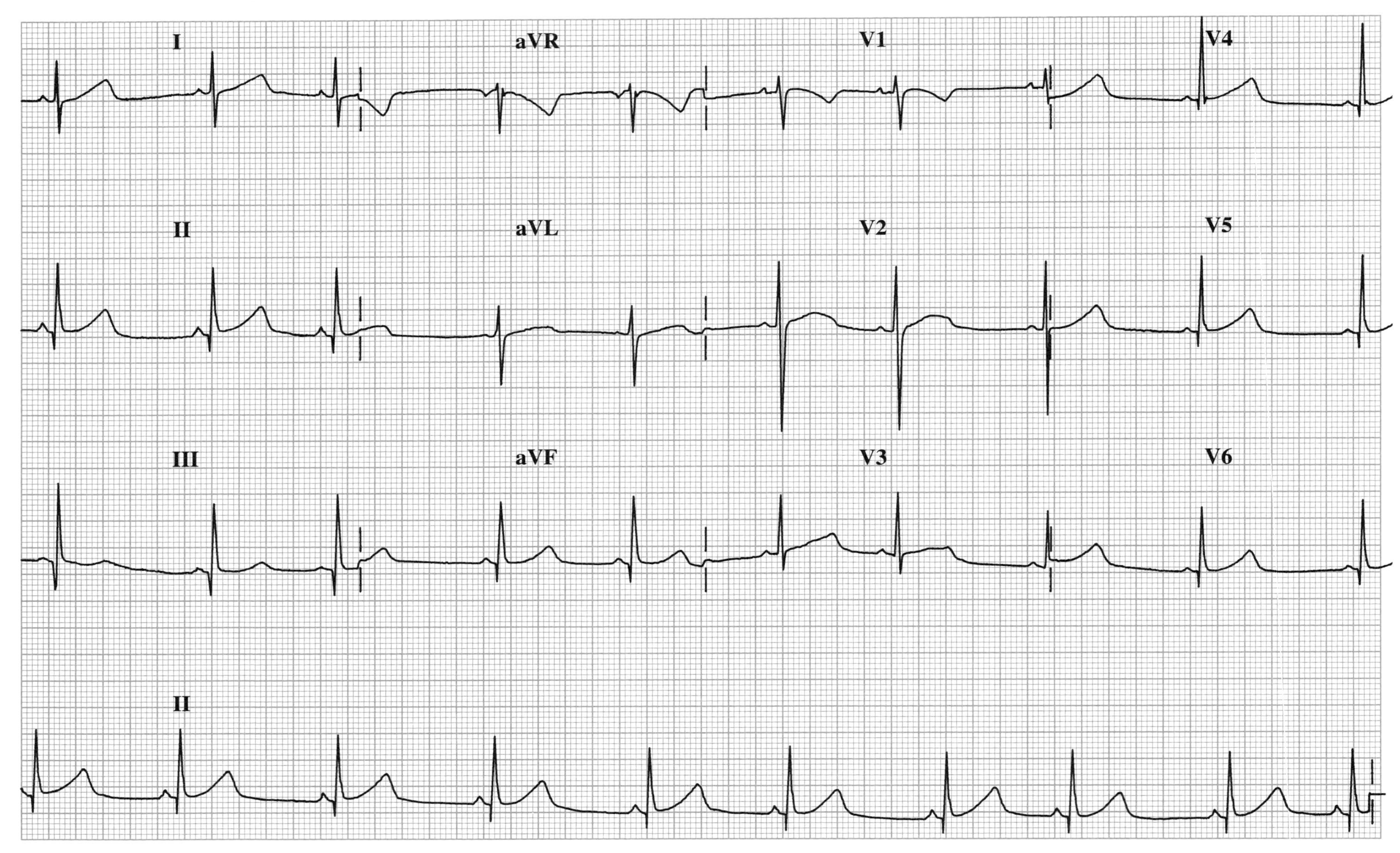

1. GENERAL FEATURES

☐ a. Normal ECG
☐ b. Borderline normal ECG or normal variant
☐ c. Incorrect electrode placement
☐ d. Artifact due to tremor

2. ATRIAL RHYTHMS

☐ a. Sinus rhythm
☐ b. Sinus arrhythmia
☐ c. Sinus bradycardia (< 60)
☐ d. Sinus tachycardia (> 100)
☐ e. Sinus pause or arrest
☐ f. Sinoatrial exit block
☐ g. Ecoptic atrial rhythm
☐ h. Wandering atrial pacemaker
☐ i. Atrial premature complexes, normally conducted
☐ j. Atrial premature complexes, nonconducted
☐ k. Atrial premature complexes with aberrant intraventricular conduction
☐ l. Atrial tachycardia (regular, sustained, 1:1 conduction)
☐ m. Atrial tachycardia, repetitive (short paroxysms)
☐ n. Atrial tachycardia, multifocal
☐ o. Atrial tachycardia with AV block
☐ p. Supraventricular tachycardia, unspecific
☐ q. Supraventricular tachycardia, paroxysmal
☐ r. Atrial flutter
☐ s. Atrial fibrillation
☐ t. Retrograde atrial activation

3. AV JUNCTIONAL RHYTHMS

☐ a. AV junctional premature complexes
☐ b. AV junctional escape complexes
☐ c. AV junctional rhythm, accelerated
☐ d. AV junctional rhythm

4. VENTRICULAR RHYTHMS

☐ a. Ventricular premature complex(es), uniform, fixed coupling
☐ b. Ventricular premature complex(es), uniform, nonfixed coupling
☐ c. Ventricular premature complexes(es), multiform
☐ d. Ventricular premature complexes, in pairs
☐ e. Ventricular parasystole
☐ f. Ventricular tachycardia (≥ 3 consecutive complexes)
☐ g. Accelerated idioventricular rhythm
☐ h. Ventricular escape complexes or rhythm
☐ i. Ventricular fibrillation

5. ATRIAL-VENTRICULAR INTERACTIONS IN ARRHYTHMIAS

☐ a. Fusion complexes
☐ b. Reciprocal (echo) complexes
☐ c. Ventricular capture complexes
☐ d. AV dissociation
☐ e. Ventriculophasic sinus arrhythmia

6. AV CONDUCTION ABNORMALITIES

☐ a. AV block, 1°
☐ b. AV block, 2° - Mobitz type I (Wenckebach)
☐ c. AV block, 2° - Mobitz type II
☐ d. AV block, 2:1
☐ e. AV block, 3°
☐ f. AV block, variable
☐ g. Short PR interval (with sinus rhythm and normal QRS duration)
☐ h. Wolff-Parkinson-White pattern

7. INTRAVENTRICULAR CONDUCTION DISTURBANCES

☐ a. RBBB, incomplete
☐ b. RBBB, complete
☐ c. Left anterior fascicular block
☐ d. Left posterior fascicular block
☐ e. LBBB, with ST-T wave suggestive of acute myocardial injury or infarction
☐ f. LBBB, complete
☐ g. LBBB, intermittent
☐ h. Intraventricular conduction disturbance, nonspecific
☐ i. Aberrant intraventricular conduction with supraventricular arrhythmia

8. P WAVE ABNORMALITIES

☐ a. Right atrial abnormality
☐ b. Left atrial abnormalities
☐ c. Nonspecific atrial abnormality

9. ABNORMALITIES OF QRS VOLTAGE OR AXIS

☐ a. Low voltage, limb leads only
☐ b. Low voltage, limb and precordial leads
☐ c. Left axis deviation (> - 30%)
☐ d. Right axis deviation (> + 100)
☐ e. Electrical alternans

10. VENTRICULAR HYPERTROPHY

☐ a. LVH by voltage only
☐ b. LVH by voltage and ST-T segment abnormalities
☐ c. RVH
☐ d. Combined ventricular hypertrophy

11. Q WAVE MYOCARDIAL INFARCTION

	Probably Acute or Recent	Probably Old or Age Indeterminate
Anterolateral	☐ a.	☐ g.
Anterior	☐ b.	☐ h.
Anteroseptal	☐ c.	☐ i.
Lateral/High lateral	☐ d.	☐ j.
Inferior	☐ e.	☐ k.
Posterior	☐ f.	☐ l.

☐ m. Probably ventricular aneurysm

12. ST, T, U, WAVE ABNORMALITIES

☐ a. Normal variant, early repolarization
☐ b. Normal variant, juvenile T waves
☐ c. Nonspecific ST and/or T wave abnormalities
☐ d. ST and/or T wave abnormalities suggesting myocardial ischemia
☐ e. ST and/or T wave abnormalities suggesting myocardial injury
☐ f. ST and/or T wave abnormalities suggesting acute pericarditis
☐ g. ST-T segment abnormalities secondary to intraventricular conduction disturbance or hypertrophy
☐ h. Post-extrasystolic T wave abnormality
☐ i. Isolated J point depression
☐ j. Peaked T waves
☐ k. Prolonged QT interval
☐ l. Prominent U waves

13. PACEMAKER FUNCTION AND RHYTHM

☐ a. Atrial or coronary sinus pacing
☐ b. Ventricular demand pacing
☐ c. AV sequential pacing
☐ d. Ventricular pacing, complete control
☐ e. Dual chamber, atrial sensing pacemaker
☐ f. Pacemaker malfunction, not constantly capturing (atrium or ventricle)
☐ g. Pacemaker malfunction, not constantly sensing (atrium or ventricle)
☐ h. Pacemaker malfunction, not firing
☐ i. Pacemaker malfunction, slowing

14. SUGGESTED OR PROBABLE CLINICAL DISORDERS

☐ a. Digitalis effect
☐ b. Digitalis toxicity
☐ c. Antiarrhythmic drug effect
☐ d. Antiarrhythmic drug toxicity
☐ e. Hyperkalemia
☐ f. Hypokalemia
☐ g. Hypercalcemia
☐ h. Hypocalcemia
☐ i. Atrial septal defect, secundum
☐ j. Atrial septal defect, primum
☐ k. Dextrocardia, mirror image
☐ l. Mitral valve disease
☐ m. Chronic lung disease
☐ n. Acute cor pulmonale, including pulmonary embolus
☐ o. Pericardial effusion
☐ p. Acute pericarditis
☐ q. Hypertrophic cardiomyopathy
☐ r. Coronary artery disease
☐ s. Central nervous system disorder
☐ t. Myxedema
☐ u. Hypothermia
☐ v. Sick sinus syndrome

ECG 50 was obtained in a 13-year-old male with a family history of sudden cardiac death. This tracing shows a sinus rhythm at 60 BPM with sinus arrhythmia and a prolonged QT interval (the corrected QT interval measures 560 msec in leads V_2 and V_3). The axis is vertical but does not meet criteria for right axis deviation. Q waves are present in leads II, III and aVF (arrows); however, they are < 0.03 seconds in duration and thus are not pathological. This patient, one of his siblings, and his mother were all diagnosed with "long-QT syndrome."

Codes:

2a	Sinus rhythm
2b	Sinus arrhythmia
12k	Prolonged QT interval

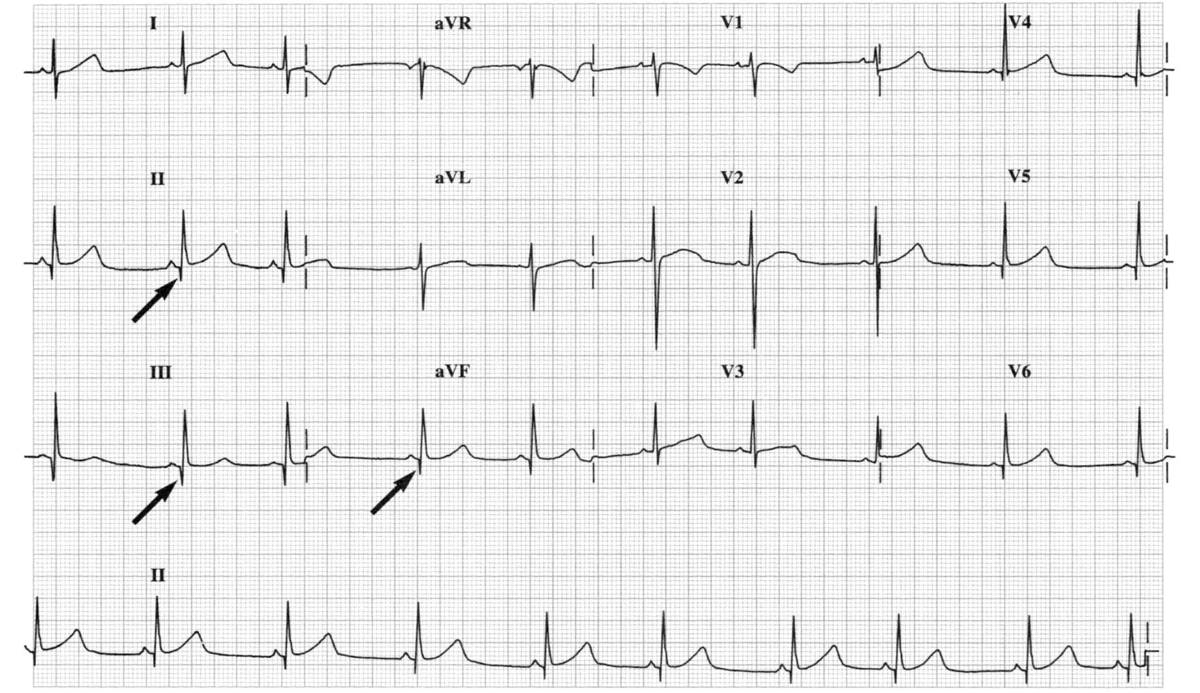

Questions: ECG 50

1. Which of the following statements about the QT interval are true:

   a. Represents the period of ventricular depolarization
   b. Normally lengthens as heart rate falls
   c. Is longer while awake than while asleep

2. What is responsible for the early appearance of the 6th, 8th, and 10th beats in the rhythm strip:

   a. Premature atrial contractions
   b. Junctional premature contractions with retrograde atrial activation
   c. Wenkebach phenomenon
   d. Sinus arrhythmia

Answers: ECG 50

1. The QT interval represents the period of ventricular electrical systole (i.e., the time required for ventricular depolarization and repolarization to occur), varies inversely with heart rate, and is longer while asleep than while awake (presumably due to vagal hypertonia). (Answer: b)

2. The early appearance of the 6th and 10th beats in the rhythm strip is due to sinus arrhythmia, which is diagnosed when the sinus PP interval varies by > 0.16 seconds. Since the P wave morphology of beats 6 and 10 is identical to that of the normal sinus beats, the diagnosis of premature atrial or junctional contractions is excluded. Wenckebach phenomenon is associated with a regular PP interval and does not cause premature beats. (Answer: d)

— Quick Review 50 —

Sinus arrhythmia	
• (Sinus/nonsinus) P wave	Sinus
• Longest and shortest PP intervals vary by > ____ seconds or 10%	0.16
• Sinus arrhythmia differs from "ventriculophasic" sinus arrhythmia, the latter of which occurs in the setting of ____	heart block
Prolonged QT interval	
• Corrected QT interval (QTc) ≥ ____ seconds, where QTc = QT interval divided by the square root of the preceding ____ interval	0.42-0.46 RR
• QT interval varies (directly/inversely) with heart rate	inversely
• The normal QT interval should be (less than/greater than) 50% of the RR interval	less than

ECG 51. Asymptomatic 77-year-old female:

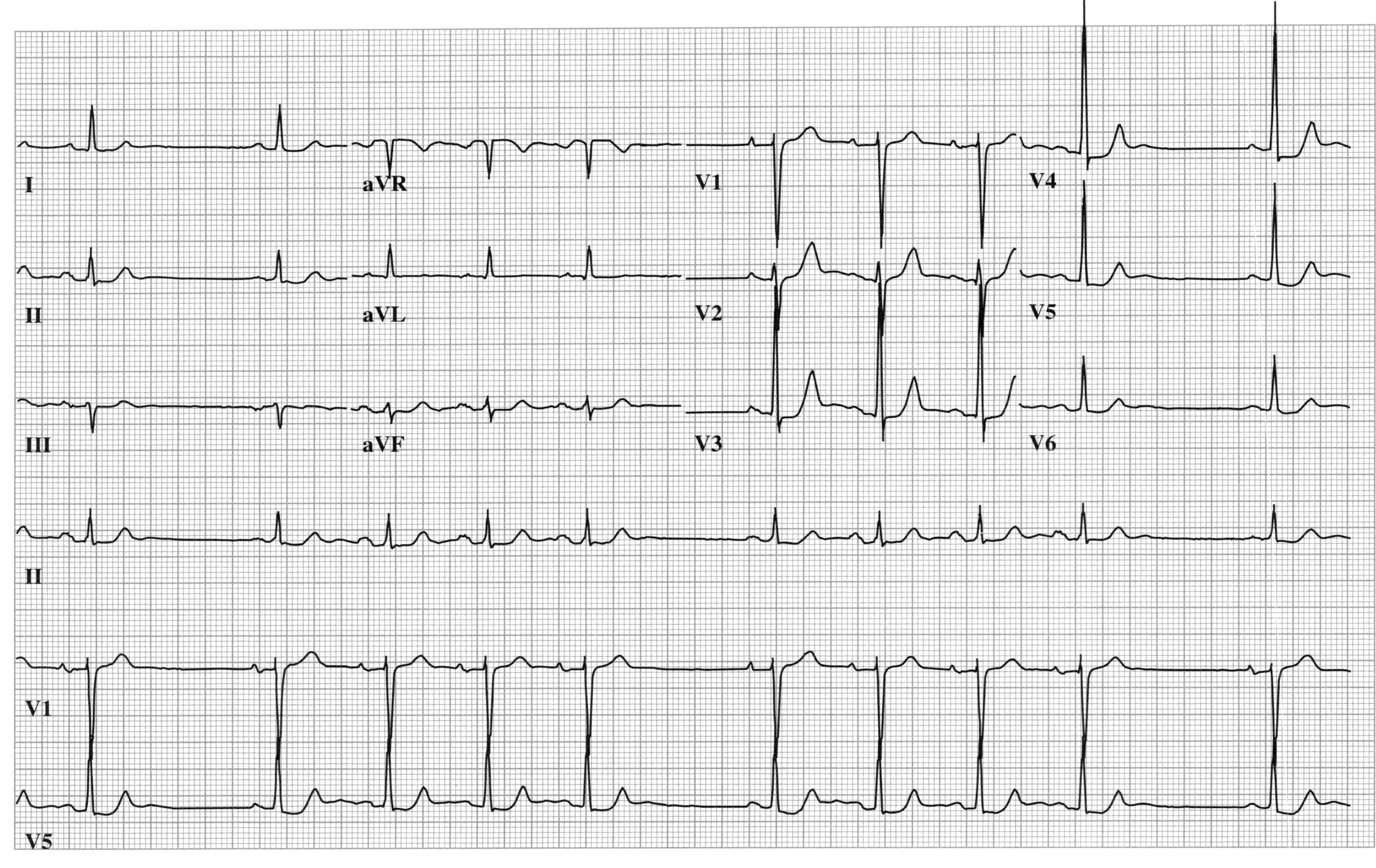

1. GENERAL FEATURES

☐ a. Normal ECG
☐ b. Borderline normal ECG or normal variant
☐ c. Incorrect electrode placement
☐ d. Artifact due to tremor

2. ATRIAL RHYTHMS

☐ a. Sinus rhythm
☐ b. Sinus arrhythmia
☐ c. Sinus bradycardia (< 60)
☐ d. Sinus tachycardia (> 100)
☐ e. Sinus pause or arrest
☐ f. Sinoatrial exit block
☐ g. Ecoptic atrial rhythm
☐ h. Wandering atrial pacemaker
☐ i. Atrial premature complexes, normally conducted
☐ j. Atrial premature complexes, nonconducted
☐ k. Atrial premature complexes with aberrant intraventricular conduction
☐ l. Atrial tachycardia (regular, sustained, 1:1 conduction)
☐ m. Atrial tachycardia, repetitive (short paroxysms)
☐ n. Atrial tachycardia, multifocal
☐ o. Atrial tachycardia with AV block
☐ p. Supraventricular tachycardia, unspecific
☐ q. Supraventricular tachycardia, paroxysmal
☐ r. Atrial flutter
☐ s. Atrial fibrillation
☐ t. Retrograde atrial activation

3. AV JUNCTIONAL RHYTHMS

☐ a. AV junctional premature complexes
☐ b. AV junctional escape complexes
☐ c. AV junctional rhythm, accelerated
☐ d. AV junctional rhythm

4. VENTRICULAR RHYTHMS

☐ a. Ventricular premature complex(es), uniform, fixed coupling
☐ b. Ventricular premature complex(es), uniform, nonfixed coupling
☐ c. Ventricular premature complexes(es), multiform
☐ d. Ventricular premature complexes, in pairs
☐ e. Ventricular parasystole
☐ f. Ventricular tachycardia (≥ 3 consecutive complexes)
☐ g. Accelerated idioventricular rhythm
☐ h. Ventricular escape complexes or rhythm
☐ i. Ventricular fibrillation

5. ATRIAL-VENTRICULAR INTERACTIONS IN ARRHYTHMIAS

☐ a. Fusion complexes
☐ b. Reciprocal (echo) complexes
☐ c. Ventricular capture complexes
☐ d. AV dissociation
☐ e. Ventriculophasic sinus arrhythmia

6. AV CONDUCTION ABNORMALITIES

☐ a. AV block, 1°
☐ b. AV block, 2° - Mobitz type I (Wenckebach)
☐ c. AV block, 2° - Mobitz type II
☐ d. AV block, 2:1
☐ e. AV block, 3°
☐ f. AV block, variable
☐ g. Short PR interval (with sinus rhythm and normal QRS duration)
☐ h. Wolff-Parkinson-White pattern

7. INTRAVENTRICULAR CONDUCTION DISTURBANCES

☐ a. RBBB, incomplete
☐ b. RBBB, complete
☐ c. Left anterior fascicular block
☐ d. Left posterior fascicular block
☐ e. LBBB, with ST-T wave suggestive of acute myocardial injury or infarction
☐ f. LBBB, complete
☐ g. LBBB, intermittent
☐ h. Intraventricular conduction disturbance, nonspecific
☐ i. Aberrant intraventricular conduction with supraventricular arrhythmia

8. P WAVE ABNORMALITIES

☐ a. Right atrial abnormality
☐ b. Left atrial abnormalities
☐ c. Nonspecific atrial abnormality

9. ABNORMALITIES OF QRS VOLTAGE OR AXIS

☐ a. Low voltage, limb leads only
☐ b. Low voltage, limb and precordial leads
☐ c. Left axis deviation (> - 30%)
☐ d. Right axis deviation (> + 100)
☐ e. Electrical alternans

10. VENTRICULAR HYPERTROPHY

☐ a. LVH by voltage only
☐ b. LVH by voltage and ST-T segment abnormalities
☐ c. RVH
☐ d. Combined ventricular hypertrophy

11. Q WAVE MYOCARDIAL INFARCTION

	Probably Acute or Recent	Probably Old or Age Indeterminate
Anterolateral	☐ a.	☐ g.
Anterior	☐ b.	☐ h.
Anteroseptal	☐ c.	☐ i.
Lateral/High lateral	☐ d.	☐ j.
Inferior	☐ e.	☐ k.
Posterior	☐ f.	☐ l.

☐ m. Probably ventricular aneurysm

12. ST, T, U, WAVE ABNORMALITIES

☐ a. Normal variant, early repolarization
☐ b. Normal variant, juvenile T waves
☐ c. Nonspecific ST and/or T wave abnormalities
☐ d. ST and/or T wave abnormalities suggesting myocardial ischemia
☐ e. ST and/or T wave abnormalities suggesting myocardial injury
☐ f. ST and/or T wave abnormalities suggesting acute pericarditis
☐ g. ST-T segment abnormalities secondary to intraventricular conduction disturbance or hypertrophy
☐ h. Post-extrasystolic T wave abnormality
☐ i. Isolated J point depression
☐ j. Peaked T waves
☐ k. Prolonged QT interval
☐ l. Prominent U waves

13. PACEMAKER FUNCTION AND RHYTHM

☐ a. Atrial or coronary sinus pacing
☐ b. Ventricular demand pacing
☐ c. AV sequential pacing
☐ d. Ventricular pacing, complete control
☐ e. Dual chamber, atrial sensing pacemaker
☐ f. Pacemaker malfunction, not constantly capturing (atrium or ventricle)
☐ g. Pacemaker malfunction, not constantly sensing (atrium or ventricle)
☐ h. Pacemaker malfunction, not firing
☐ i. Pacemaker malfunction, slowing

14. SUGGESTED OR PROBABLE CLINICAL DISORDERS

☐ a. Digitalis effect
☐ b. Digitalis toxicity
☐ c. Antiarrhythmic drug effect
☐ d. Antiarrhythmic drug toxicity
☐ e. Hyperkalemia
☐ f. Hypokalemia
☐ g. Hypercalcemia
☐ h. Hypocalcemia
☐ i. Atrial septal defect, secundum
☐ j. Atrial septal defect, primum
☐ k. Dextrocardia, mirror image
☐ l. Mitral valve disease
☐ m. Chronic lung disease
☐ n. Acute cor pulmonale, including pulmonary embolus
☐ o. Pericardial effusion
☐ p. Acute pericarditis
☐ q. Hypertrophic cardiomyopathy
☐ r. Coronary artery disease
☐ s. Central nervous system disorder
☐ t. Myxedema
☐ u. Hypothermia
☐ v. Sick sinus syndrome

ECG 51 was obtained in an asymptomatic 77-year-old female. The ECG shows a sinus rhythm at approximately 70 BPM with intermittent Mobitz II SA exit block, manifesting as PP pauses approximately twice the normal PP interval (asterisks). Left ventricular hypertrophy (S wave in V_1 + R wave in V_5 > 35 mm) with secondary ST-T abnormalities are also noted. This tracing is compatible with sick sinus syndrome.

Codes:

2a	Sinus rhythm
2f	Sinoatrial exit block
10b	LVH by both voltage and ST-T segment abnormalities
12g	ST-T segment abnormalities secondary to IVCD or hypertrophy
14v	Sick sinus syndrome

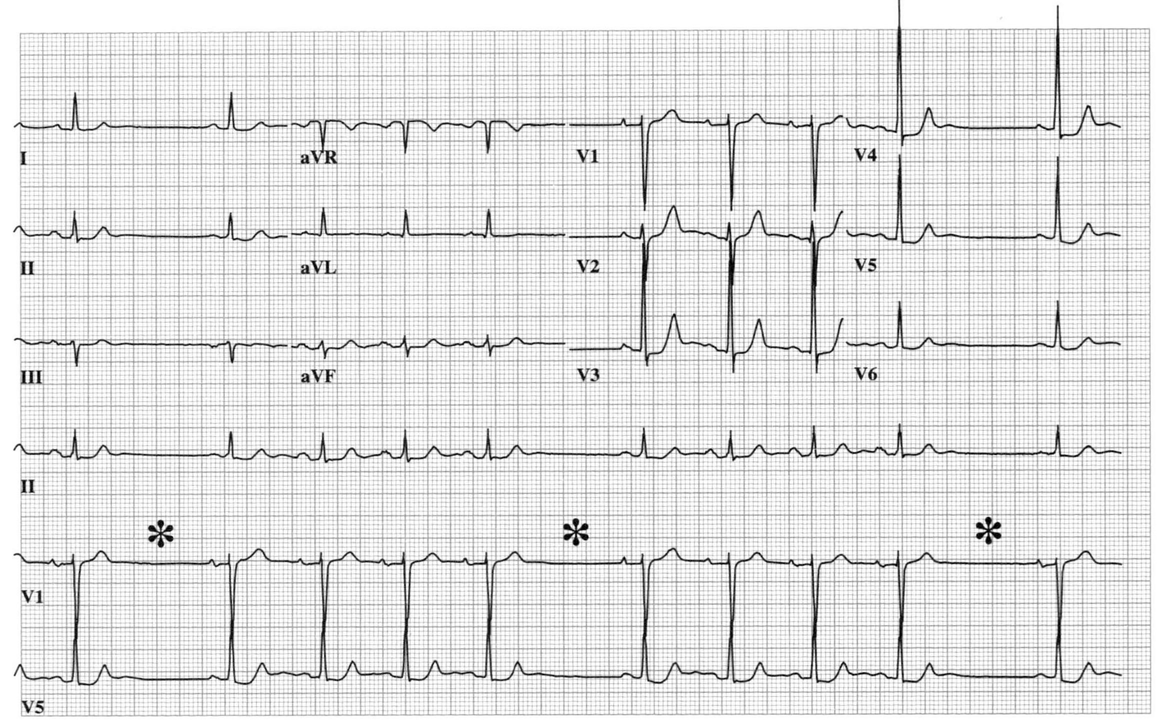

Questions: ECG 51

1. ECG manifestations of Mobitz II SA exit block include:

   a. Sinus pauses that are a multiple of normal PP interval
   b. Lengthening of the PR interval
   c. Narrowing of the QRS complex
   d. Shortening of the PP interval

2. At a heart rate of 70 beats/minute, the normal QT interval should be _____ ± 0.07 seconds:

   a. 0.38
   b. 0.44
   c. 0.42
   d. 0.40

Answers: ECG 51

1. In ***Mobitz II*** SA exit block, sinus impulses occur at a constant rate but occasionally fail to capture the atria, resulting in intermittent absence of a P wave. The typical ECG finding is a PP pause that is a multiple (2x, 3x, etc.) of the basic PP interval. ***Mobitz I*** SA exit block is suggested by the presence of recurring pauses ("group beating") with PP intervals less than two times the basic PP interval. SA exit block is often a component of sick sinus syndrome, and is an important consideration when evaluating the etiology of a PP pause. (Answer: a)

2. The easiest method to assess the corrected QT interval is to assume that the normal QT interval for a heart rate of 70 BPM is 0.40 ± 0.07 sec. Then, for every 10 BPM change in heart rate from 70 BPM, the QT interval is adjusted by 0.02 seconds up or down (inversely with the heart rate). Thus, at a heart rate of 50 BPM, the corrected QT interval should be (0.40) + (2 x 0.02) = 0.44 ± .07 sec. At heart rates of 60 BPM and 80 BPM, the corrected QT intervals should be 0.42 ± .07 seconds and 0.38 ± .07 seconds, respectively. (Answer: d)

— Quick Review 51 —

Sinoatrial (SA) exit block	
First-degree: Conduction of sinus impulses to the atrium is (normal/delayed), but ____:1 response is maintained	delayed, 1
• First-degree SA exit block (is/is not) detectable on the surface ECG	is not
Second-degree: Some sinus impulses fail to ____the atria	capture
• Type I (Mobitz I):	
▸ Sinus P wave (true/false)	true
▸ "____ beating" with:	Group
(1) (Shortening/lengthening) of the PP interval prior to absent P wave	Shortening
(2) (Constant/variable) PR interval	Constant
(3) PP pause less than ____ times the normal PP interval	2
• Type II (Mobitz II): Constant PP interval followed by a pause that (is/is not) a multiple (2x, 3x, etc.) of the normal PP interval	is
Third-degree:	
• Complete failure of ____ conduction	sinoatrial
• Cannot be differentiated from ____	complete sinus arrest

— Quick Review 51 —

Sick sinus syndrome	
• Marked sinus ____	bradycardia
• ____ arrest or ____ exit block	Sinus, sinoatrial
• Bradycardia alternating with ____	tachycardia
• Atrial fibrillation with ____ ventricular response preceded or followed by sinus bradycardia, sinus arrest, or sinoatrial exit block	slow
• Prolonged sinus node ____ time after atrial premature complex or atrial tachyarrhythmias	recovery
• AV junctional ____ rhythm	escape
• Additional conduction system disease is often present, including AV block, IVCD, and/or bundle branch block (true/false)	true

— Comic Relief —

Do you get the feeling that the good doctor will be running a little behind schedule today?

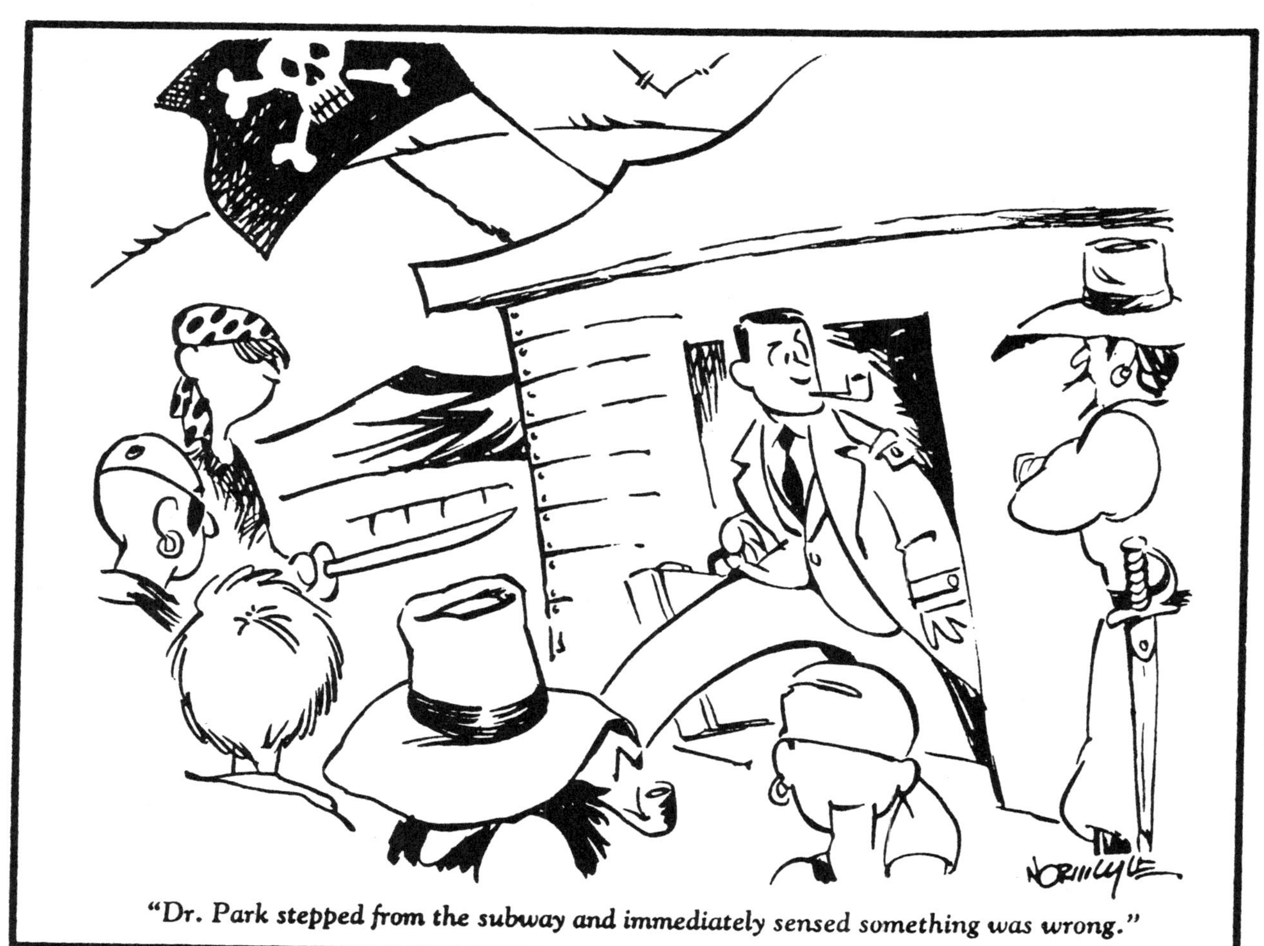

"Dr. Park stepped from the subway and immediately sensed something was wrong."

ECG 52. Healthy 32-year-old male being screened for an insurance physical exam:

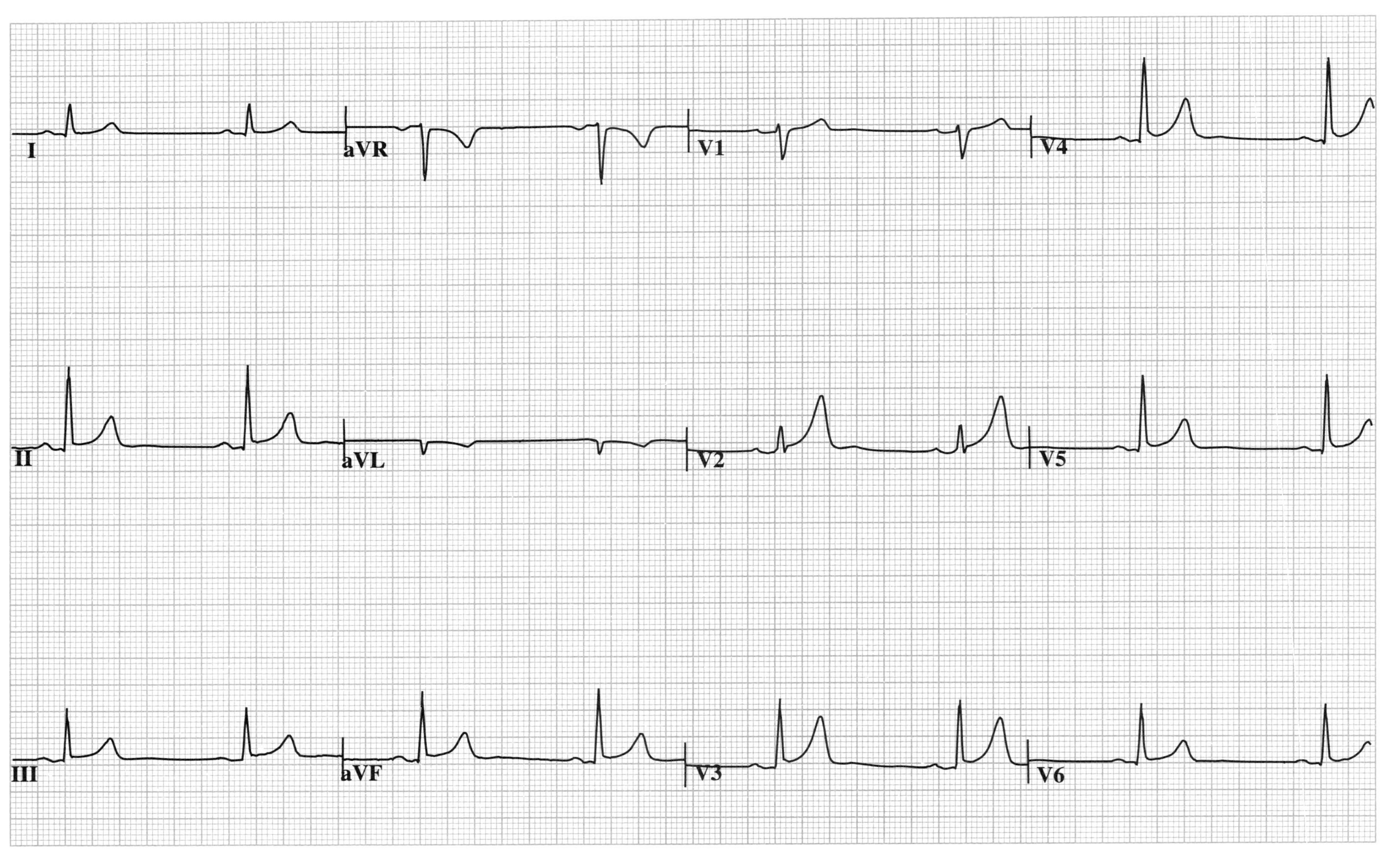

1. GENERAL FEATURES
- ☐ a. Normal ECG
- ☐ b. Borderline normal ECG or normal variant
- ☐ c. Incorrect electrode placement
- ☐ d. Artifact due to tremor

2. ATRIAL RHYTHMS
- ☐ a. Sinus rhythm
- ☐ b. Sinus arrhythmia
- ☐ c. Sinus bradycardia (< 60)
- ☐ d. Sinus tachycardia (> 100)
- ☐ e. Sinus pause or arrest
- ☐ f. Sinoatrial exit block
- ☐ g. Ecoptic atrial rhythm
- ☐ h. Wandering atrial pacemaker
- ☐ i. Atrial premature complexes, normally conducted
- ☐ j. Atrial premature complexes, nonconducted
- ☐ k. Atrial premature complexes with aberrant intraventricular conduction
- ☐ l. Atrial tachycardia (regular, sustained, 1:1 conduction)
- ☐ m. Atrial tachycardia, repetitive (short paroxysms)
- ☐ n. Atrial tachycardia, multifocal
- ☐ o. Atrial tachycardia with AV block
- ☐ p. Supraventricular tachycardia, unspecific
- ☐ q. Supraventricular tachycardia, paroxysmal
- ☐ r. Atrial flutter
- ☐ s. Atrial fibrillation
- ☐ t. Retrograde atrial activation

3. AV JUNCTIONAL RHYTHMS
- ☐ a. AV junctional premature complexes
- ☐ b. AV junctional escape complexes
- ☐ c. AV junctional rhythm, accelerated
- ☐ d. AV junctional rhythm

4. VENTRICULAR RHYTHMS
- ☐ a. Ventricular premature complex(es), uniform, fixed coupling
- ☐ b. Ventricular premature complex(es), uniform, nonfixed coupling
- ☐ c. Ventricular premature complexes(es), multiform
- ☐ d. Ventricular premature complexes, in pairs
- ☐ e. Ventricular parasystole
- ☐ f. Ventricular tachycardia (≥ 3 consecutive complexes)
- ☐ g. Accelerated idioventricular rhythm
- ☐ h. Ventricular escape complexes or rhythm
- ☐ i. Ventricular fibrillation

5. ATRIAL-VENTRICULAR INTERACTIONS IN ARRHYTHMIAS
- ☐ a. Fusion complexes
- ☐ b. Reciprocal (echo) complexes
- ☐ c. Ventricular capture complexes
- ☐ d. AV dissociation
- ☐ e. Ventriculophasic sinus arrhythmia

6. AV CONDUCTION ABNORMALITIES
- ☐ a. AV block, 1°
- ☐ b. AV block, 2° - Mobitz type I (Wenckebach)
- ☐ c. AV block, 2° - Mobitz type II
- ☐ d. AV block, 2:1
- ☐ e. AV block, 3°
- ☐ f. AV block, variable
- ☐ g. Short PR interval (with sinus rhythm and normal QRS duration)
- ☐ h. Wolff-Parkinson-White pattern

7. INTRAVENTRICULAR CONDUCTION DISTURBANCES
- ☐ a. RBBB, incomplete
- ☐ b. RBBB, complete
- ☐ c. Left anterior fascicular block
- ☐ d. Left posterior fascicular block
- ☐ e. LBBB, with ST-T wave suggestive of acute myocardial injury or infarction
- ☐ f. LBBB, complete
- ☐ g. LBBB, intermittent
- ☐ h. Intraventricular conduction disturbance, nonspecific
- ☐ i. Aberrant intraventricular conduction with supraventricular arrhythmia

8. P WAVE ABNORMALITIES
- ☐ a. Right atrial abnormality
- ☐ b. Left atrial abnormalities
- ☐ c. Nonspecific atrial abnormality

9. ABNORMALITIES OF QRS VOLTAGE OR AXIS
- ☐ a. Low voltage, limb leads only
- ☐ b. Low voltage, limb and precordial leads
- ☐ c. Left axis deviation (> - 30%)
- ☐ d. Right axis deviation (> + 100)
- ☐ e. Electrical alternans

10. VENTRICULAR HYPERTROPHY
- ☐ a. LVH by voltage only
- ☐ b. LVH by voltage and ST-T segment abnormalities
- ☐ c. RVH
- ☐ d. Combined ventricular hypertrophy

11. Q WAVE MYOCARDIAL INFARCTION

	Probably Acute or Recent	Probably Old or Age Indeterminate
Anterolateral	☐ a.	☐ g.
Anterior	☐ b.	☐ h.
Anteroseptal	☐ c.	☐ i.
Lateral/High lateral	☐ d.	☐ j.
Inferior	☐ e.	☐ k.
Posterior	☐ f.	☐ l.

☐ m. Probably ventricular aneurysm

12. ST, T, U, WAVE ABNORMALITIES
- ☐ a. Normal variant, early repolarization
- ☐ b. Normal variant, juvenile T waves
- ☐ c. Nonspecific ST and/or T wave abnormalities
- ☐ d. ST and/or T wave abnormalities suggesting myocardial ischemia
- ☐ e. ST and/or T wave abnormalities suggesting myocardial injury
- ☐ f. ST and/or T wave abnormalities suggesting acute pericarditis
- ☐ g. ST-T segment abnormalities secondary to intraventricular conduction disturbance or hypertrophy
- ☐ h. Post-extrasystolic T wave abnormality
- ☐ i. Isolated J point depression
- ☐ j. Peaked T waves
- ☐ k. Prolonged QT interval
- ☐ l. Prominent U waves

13. PACEMAKER FUNCTION AND RHYTHM
- ☐ a. Atrial or coronary sinus pacing
- ☐ b. Ventricular demand pacing
- ☐ c. AV sequential pacing
- ☐ d. Ventricular pacing, complete control
- ☐ e. Dual chamber, atrial sensing pacemaker
- ☐ f. Pacemaker malfunction, not constantly capturing (atrium or ventricle)
- ☐ g. Pacemaker malfunction, not constantly sensing (atrium or ventricle)
- ☐ h. Pacemaker malfunction, not firing
- ☐ i. Pacemaker malfunction, slowing

14. SUGGESTED OR PROBABLE CLINICAL DISORDERS
- ☐ a. Digitalis effect
- ☐ b. Digitalis toxicity
- ☐ c. Antiarrhythmic drug effect
- ☐ d. Antiarrhythmic drug toxicity
- ☐ e. Hyperkalemia
- ☐ f. Hypokalemia
- ☐ g. Hypercalcemia
- ☐ h. Hypocalcemia
- ☐ i. Atrial septal defect, secundum
- ☐ j. Atrial septal defect, primum
- ☐ k. Dextrocardia, mirror image
- ☐ l. Mitral valve disease
- ☐ m. Chronic lung disease
- ☐ n. Acute cor pulmonale, including pulmonary embolus
- ☐ o. Pericardial effusion
- ☐ p. Acute pericarditis
- ☐ q. Hypertrophic cardiomyopathy
- ☐ r. Coronary artery disease
- ☐ s. Central nervous system disorder
- ☐ t. Myxedema
- ☐ u. Hypothermia
- ☐ v. Sick sinus syndrome

ECG 52 was obtained from a healthy 32-year-old male being screened for an insurance physical exam. Sinus bradycardia and normal variant early repolarization abnormalities (most apparent in leads II, III, aVF, V_2-V_6; arrows) are present. Criteria are also met for peaked T waves (asterisks), both in the limb leads (6 mm) and in the precordial leads (10 mm). Subtle notching of the J point is present (most apparent in V_3) and is characteristic of normal variant early repolarization abnormalities. All the findings in this tracing are consistent with a normal variant ECG.

Codes:

1b	Borderline normal ECG or normal variant
2c	Sinus bradycardia (< 60)
12a	Normal variant, early repolarization
12j	Peaked T waves

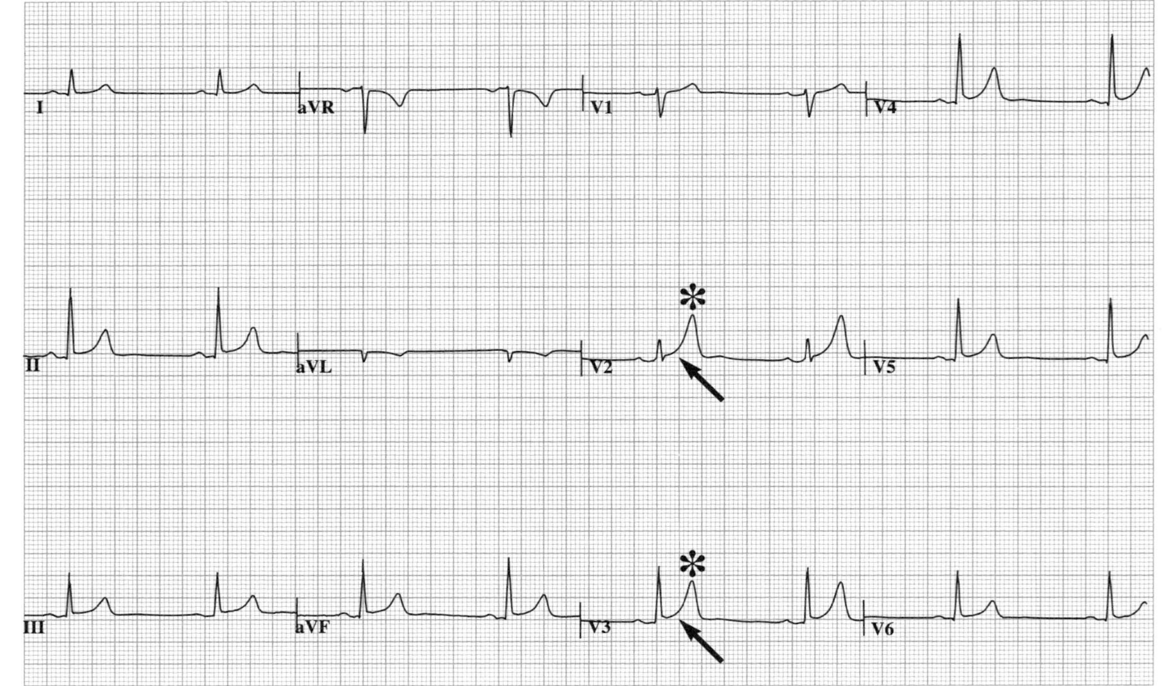

Questions: ECG 52

1. Causes of diffuse ST elevation include:

   a. Acute MI
   b. Pericarditis
   c. Left ventricular hypertrophy
   d. Hyperkalemia
   e. LV aneurysm
   f. Variant (Printzmetal's) angina
   g. Early repolarization

2. Which of the following statements about ST elevation are true?

   Ventricular aneurysm:
   a. Q wave or QS is usually present in the same leads with ST elevation
   b. ST and T wave changes remain stable over time

   Pericarditis:
   a. Reciprocal ST depression is common
   b. Q waves are often evident
   c. ST and T wave changes remain stable over time
   d. T waves become inverted after ST segments return to baseline

3. Normal variant findings on the ECG include:

   a. Small negative T waves in V_1 - V_3
   b. S waves in leads I - III
   c. Amplitude of R wave equal to depth of S wave in V_1
   d. Amplitude of R wave equal to depth of S wave in V_2
   e. ST elevation of 1-2 mm in V_2 and V_3
   f. Q wave duration ≥ 0.04 seconds
   g. ST depression in precordial leads
   h. U wave
   i. RSR' or rSR' in V_1 with a QRS duration < 0.12 seconds

Answers: ECG 52

1. Causes of diffuse ST elevation include pericarditis, severe hyperkalemia ("dialyzable current of injury"), and early repolarization (although ST elevation is usually most apparent in leads V_2 - V_5 and II, III, aVF). Localized ST elevation may occur in acute myocardial infarction, LV aneurysm, and variant angina, and is usually confined to the distribution of the culprit vessel. (Answer: b, d, g)

2. The ST elevation of ventricular aneurysm differs from pericarditis in several ways: In ventricular aneurysm, ST

levation is localized, Q waves are usually present in the same leads with ST elevation, and ST and T wave changes remain stable over time. In pericarditis, ST elevation is diffuse, Q waves are not evident (unless pericarditis follows acute MI), and ST and T wave changes evolve and are transient. The ST elevation of pericarditis differs from acute MI in that reciprocal ST depression does not occur, and T waves become inverted *after* the ST segment has returned to baseline. (Answers: Ventricular aneurysm: a, b; Pericarditis: d)

3. A tall R wave in lead V_1, Q waves > 0.04 seconds, and ST depression in the precordial leads are abnormal findings. The transition zone, defined as the lead where the amplitude of the positive and negative QRS deflections are equal (R/S = 1), typically occurs at V_2 - V_4. When the R wave is taller than the S wave in V_1, *counterclockwise rotation* is said to be present, which is abnormal in adults; conditions associated with this finding include posterior MI, right ventricular hypertrophy, WPW syndrome, and COPD. Q wave duration > 0.03 seconds is abnormal for most leads. A Q wave ≥ 0.04 seconds is required for infarcts involving leads III, aVL, aVF and V_1. Conditions associated with abnormal Q waves include myocardial infarction, cardiomyopathy, pulmonary embolism, infiltrative myocardial disorders (e.g., amyloid, sarcoid, muscular dystrophy), CNS disorders and others. Finally, ST depression in the precordial leads is abnormal, although ST depression or elevation of 1 mm in the limb leads and ST elevation of 1-2 mm in the precordial leads (especially V_2, V_3) may be found in normals. (Answer: All but c, f, g)

— Quick Review 52 —

Normal variant, early repolarization	
• Elevated ____ of the ST segment at the J junction	take-off
• (Concave/convex) upward ST elevation ending with a symmetrical upright T wave, which is often of large amplitude	Concave
• Distinct notch or slur on downstroke of ____ wave	R
• Most commonly involves leads ____	V_2-V_5
• Reciprocal ST segment depression is present (true/false)	false
• Some degree of ST elevation is present in the majority of young healthy individuals, especially in the precordial leads (true/false)	true
Peaked T waves	
• T wave > ____ mm in the limb leads or > ____ mm in the precordial leads	6, 10

Differential Diagnosis

Electrical Alternans

(Alternation in the amplitude and/or direction of P, QRS, and/or T waves)

- Pericardial effusion (item 14o). (If electrical alternans involves the P, QRS, and T ["total alternans"], effusion with tamponade is often present. Yet, only 12% of patients with pericardial effusions have electrical alternans.)
- Severe left ventricular failure
- Hypertension
- Coronary artery disease
- Rheumatic heart disease
- Supraventricular or ventricular tachycardia
- Deep respirations

ECG 53. 62-year-old male with a history of MI three months ago now with dyspnea on exertion:

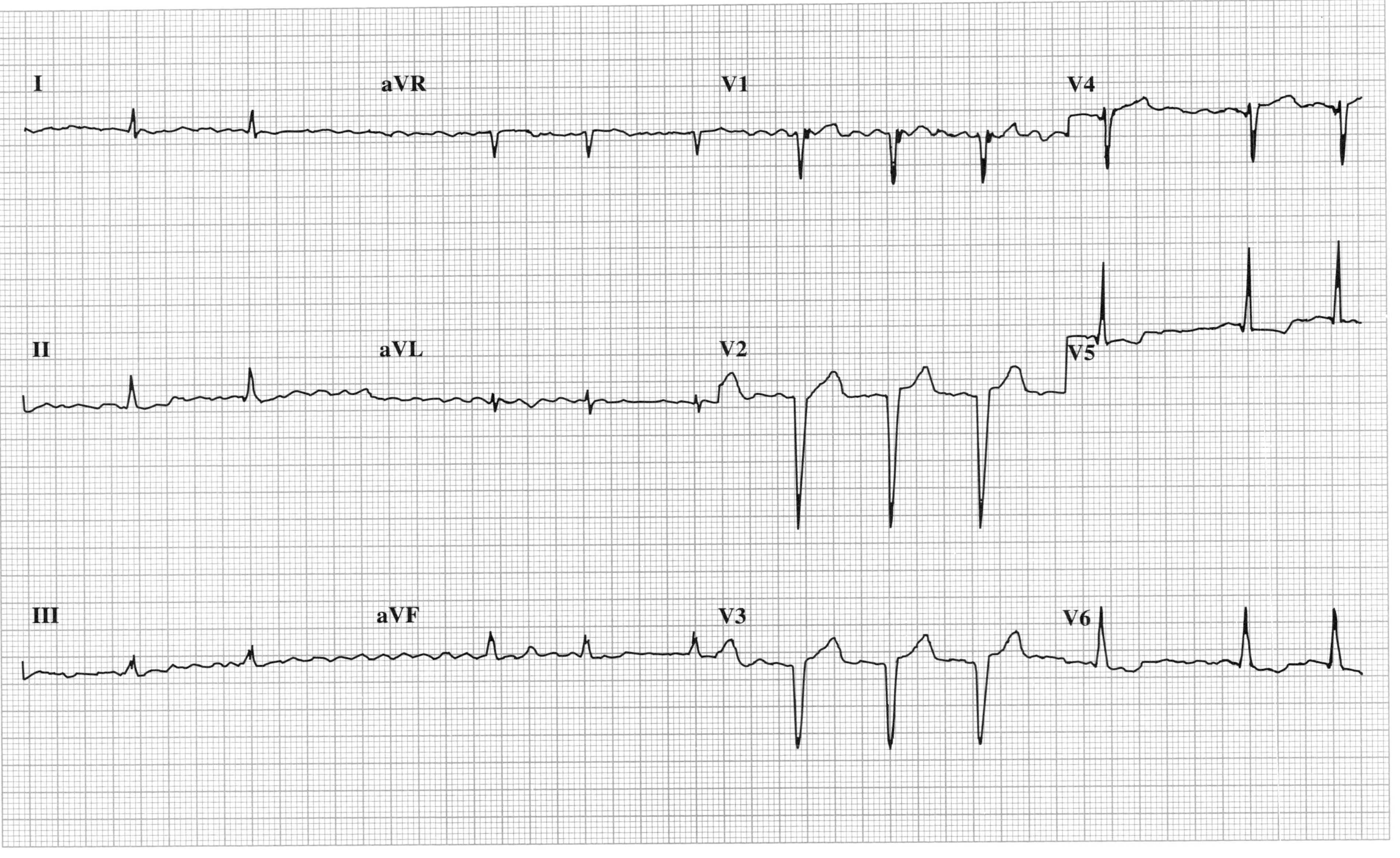

1. GENERAL FEATURES
- ☐ a. Normal ECG
- ☐ b. Borderline normal ECG or normal variant
- ☐ c. Incorrect electrode placement
- ☐ d. Artifact due to tremor

2. ATRIAL RHYTHMS
- ☐ a. Sinus rhythm
- ☐ b. Sinus arrhythmia
- ☐ c. Sinus bradycardia (< 60)
- ☐ d. Sinus tachycardia (> 100)
- ☐ e. Sinus pause or arrest
- ☐ f. Sinoatrial exit block
- ☐ g. Ecoptic atrial rhythm
- ☐ h. Wandering atrial pacemaker
- ☐ i. Atrial premature complexes, normally conducted
- ☐ j. Atrial premature complexes, nonconducted
- ☐ k. Atrial premature complexes with aberrant intraventricular conduction
- ☐ l. Atrial tachycardia (regular, sustained, 1:1 conduction)
- ☐ m. Atrial tachycardia, repetitive (short paroxysms)
- ☐ n. Atrial tachycardia, multifocal
- ☐ o. Atrial tachycardia with AV block
- ☐ p. Supraventricular tachycardia, unspecific
- ☐ q. Supraventricular tachycardia, paroxysmal
- ☐ r. Atrial flutter
- ☐ s. Atrial fibrillation
- ☐ t. Retrograde atrial activation

3. AV JUNCTIONAL RHYTHMS
- ☐ a. AV junctional premature complexes
- ☐ b. AV junctional escape complexes
- ☐ c. AV junctional rhythm, accelerated
- ☐ d. AV junctional rhythm

4. VENTRICULAR RHYTHMS
- ☐ a. Ventricular premature complex(es), uniform, fixed coupling
- ☐ b. Ventricular premature complex(es), uniform, nonfixed coupling
- ☐ c. Ventricular premature complexes(es), multiform
- ☐ d. Ventricular premature complexes, in pairs
- ☐ e. Ventricular parasystole
- ☐ f. Ventricular tachycardia (≥ 3 consecutive complexes)
- ☐ g. Accelerated idioventricular rhythm
- ☐ h. Ventricular escape complexes or rhythm
- ☐ i. Ventricular fibrillation

5. ATRIAL-VENTRICULAR INTERACTIONS IN ARRHYTHMIAS
- ☐ a. Fusion complexes
- ☐ b. Reciprocal (echo) complexes
- ☐ c. Ventricular capture complexes
- ☐ d. AV dissociation
- ☐ e. Ventriculophasic sinus arrhythmia

6. AV CONDUCTION ABNORMALITIES
- ☐ a. AV block, 1°
- ☐ b. AV block, 2° - Mobitz type I (Wenckebach)
- ☐ c. AV block, 2° - Mobitz type II
- ☐ d. AV block, 2:1
- ☐ e. AV block, 3°
- ☐ f. AV block, variable
- ☐ g. Short PR interval (with sinus rhythm and normal QRS duration)
- ☐ h. Wolff-Parkinson-White pattern

7. INTRAVENTRICULAR CONDUCTION DISTURBANCES
- ☐ a. RBBB, incomplete
- ☐ b. RBBB, complete
- ☐ c. Left anterior fascicular block
- ☐ d. Left posterior fascicular block
- ☐ e. LBBB, with ST-T wave suggestive of acute myocardial injury or infarction
- ☐ f. LBBB, complete
- ☐ g. LBBB, intermittent
- ☐ h. Intraventricular conduction disturbance, nonspecific
- ☐ i. Aberrant intraventricular conduction with supraventricular arrhythmia

8. P WAVE ABNORMALITIES
- ☐ a. Right atrial abnormality
- ☐ b. Left atrial abnormalities
- ☐ c. Nonspecific atrial abnormality

9. ABNORMALITIES OF QRS VOLTAGE OR AXIS
- ☐ a. Low voltage, limb leads only
- ☐ b. Low voltage, limb and precordial leads
- ☐ c. Left axis deviation (> - 30%)
- ☐ d. Right axis deviation (> + 100)
- ☐ e. Electrical alternans

10. VENTRICULAR HYPERTROPHY
- ☐ a. LVH by voltage only
- ☐ b. LVH by voltage and ST-T segment abnormalities
- ☐ c. RVH
- ☐ d. Combined ventricular hypertrophy

11. Q WAVE MYOCARDIAL INFARCTION

	Probably Acute or Recent	Probably Old or Age Indeterminate
Anterolateral	☐ a.	☐ g.
Anterior	☐ b.	☐ h.
Anteroseptal	☐ c.	☐ i.
Lateral/High lateral	☐ d.	☐ j.
Inferior	☐ e.	☐ k.
Posterior	☐ f.	☐ l.

- ☐ m. Probably ventricular aneurysm

12. ST, T, U, WAVE ABNORMALITIES
- ☐ a. Normal variant, early repolarization
- ☐ b. Normal variant, juvenile T waves
- ☐ c. Nonspecific ST and/or T wave abnormalities
- ☐ d. ST and/or T wave abnormalities suggesting myocardial ischemia
- ☐ e. ST and/or T wave abnormalities suggesting myocardial injury
- ☐ f. ST and/or T wave abnormalities suggesting acute pericarditis
- ☐ g. ST-T segment abnormalities secondary to intraventricular conduction disturbance or hypertrophy
- ☐ h. Post-extrasystolic T wave abnormality
- ☐ i. Isolated J point depression
- ☐ j. Peaked T waves
- ☐ k. Prolonged QT interval
- ☐ l. Prominent U waves

13. PACEMAKER FUNCTION AND RHYTHM
- ☐ a. Atrial or coronary sinus pacing
- ☐ b. Ventricular demand pacing
- ☐ c. AV sequential pacing
- ☐ d. Ventricular pacing, complete control
- ☐ e. Dual chamber, atrial sensing pacemaker
- ☐ f. Pacemaker malfunction, not constantly capturing (atrium or ventricle)
- ☐ g. Pacemaker malfunction, not constantly sensing (atrium or ventricle)
- ☐ h. Pacemaker malfunction, not firing
- ☐ i. Pacemaker malfunction, slowing

14. SUGGESTED OR PROBABLE CLINICAL DISORDERS
- ☐ a. Digitalis effect
- ☐ b. Digitalis toxicity
- ☐ c. Antiarrhythmic drug effect
- ☐ d. Antiarrhythmic drug toxicity
- ☐ e. Hyperkalemia
- ☐ f. Hypokalemia
- ☐ g. Hypercalcemia
- ☐ h. Hypocalcemia
- ☐ i. Atrial septal defect, secundum
- ☐ j. Atrial septal defect, primum
- ☐ k. Dextrocardia, mirror image
- ☐ l. Mitral valve disease
- ☐ m. Chronic lung disease
- ☐ n. Acute cor pulmonale, including pulmonary embolus
- ☐ o. Pericardial effusion
- ☐ p. Acute pericarditis
- ☐ q. Hypertrophic cardiomyopathy
- ☐ r. Coronary artery disease
- ☐ s. Central nervous system disorder
- ☐ t. Myxedema
- ☐ u. Hypothermia
- ☐ v. Sick sinus syndrome

ECG 53 was obtained in a 62-year-old male with a history of myocardial infarction 3 months ago, who now has dyspnea on exertion. The ECG demonstrates coarse atrial fibrillation with evidence for an old anteroseptal myocardial infarction. Persisting ST segment elevation is noted in leads V_2-V_4 (arrowheads), consistent with probable ventricular aneurysm. Also present are nonspecific ST-T abnormalities (arrows), which could be due to digoxin, as well as evidence for coronary artery disease.

Codes:

2s	Atrial fibrillation
11i	Anteroseptal Q wave MI, probably old or age indeterminate
11m	Probable ventricular aneurysm
12c	Nonspecific ST and/or T wave abnormalities
14a	Digitalis effect
14r	Coronary artery disease

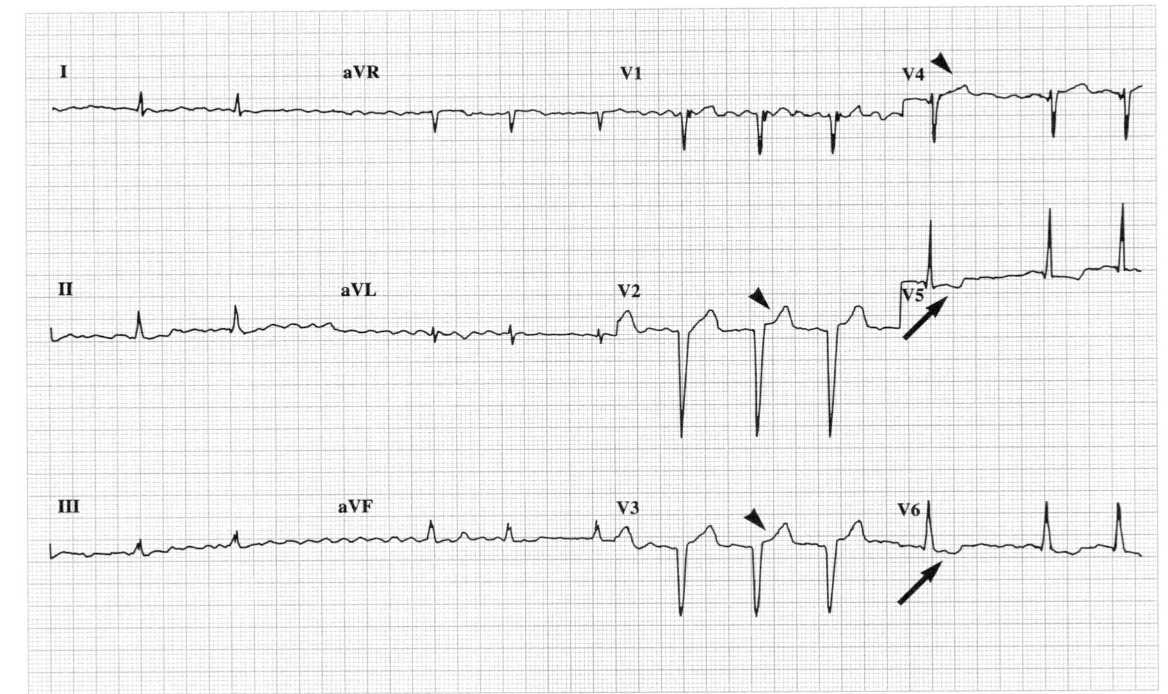

Questions: ECG 53

1. Leads containing Q waves and persistent ST elevation after acute myocardial infarction can be used to predict the location of a ventricular aneurysm:

   a. True
   b. False

2. The most common site for aneurysm formation after myocardial infarction is:

   a. Anteroseptal
   b. Anterolateral
   c. Posterior
   d. Inferior

Answers: ECG 53

1. ST segment elevation persisting 4 or more weeks after acute Q wave myocardial infarction should raise the suspicion of left ventricular aneurysm, which forms at the site of extensive transmural myocardial necrosis. The size of the aneurysm is not necessarily related to the magnitude of ST segment elevation. (Answer: a)

2. Anteroseptal infarctions account for approximately 80% of the aneurysms noted after myocardial infarction, and posterior aneurysms account for the other 20%. Rupture of a ventricular aneurysm generally occurs within the first 10 days after acute transmural myocardial infarction and is almost uniformly a fatal event. In contrast, chronic aneurysms (≥ 4 weeks) almost never rupture. They are, however, associated with systemic thromboembolization (especially during the first 3 months after acute MI). For this reason, chronic anticoagulation is recommended when the aneurysm is large. (Answer: a)

— Quick Review 53 —	
Anteroseptal MI, age indeterminate or probably old	
• Abnormal Q or QS deflection (with/without) ST elevation in leads ____ (and sometimes V_4)	without V_1-V_3
• The presence of a Q wave in lead ____ distinguishes anteroseptal from anterior infarction	V_1
Probable ventricular aneurysm	
• ST segment elevation ≥ ____ mm persisting ____ or more weeks after acute MI in leads with abnormal Q waves	1, 4

ECG 54. 66-year-old female complaining of intermittent irregularity of her heart:

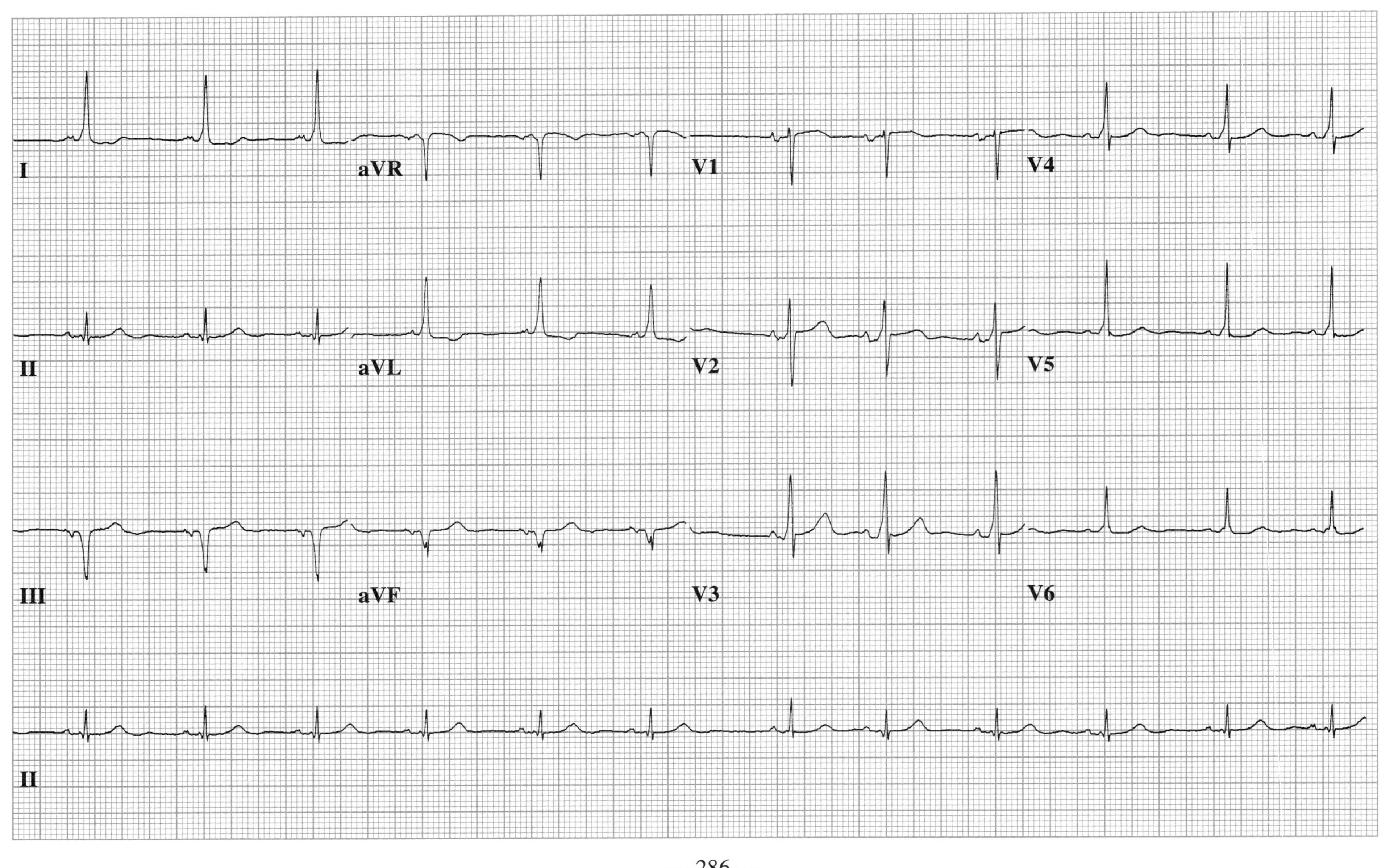

1. GENERAL FEATURES

☐ a. Normal ECG
☐ b. Borderline normal ECG or normal variant
☐ c. Incorrect electrode placement
☐ d. Artifact due to tremor

2. ATRIAL RHYTHMS

☐ a. Sinus rhythm
☐ b. Sinus arrhythmia
☐ c. Sinus bradycardia (< 60)
☐ d. Sinus tachycardia (> 100)
☐ e. Sinus pause or arrest
☐ f. Sinoatrial exit block
☐ g. Ecoptic atrial rhythm
☐ h. Wandering atrial pacemaker
☐ i. Atrial premature complexes, normally conducted
☐ j. Atrial premature complexes, nonconducted
☐ k. Atrial premature complexes with aberrant intraventricular conduction
☐ l. Atrial tachycardia (regular, sustained, 1:1 conduction)
☐ m. Atrial tachycardia, repetitive (short paroxysms)
☐ n. Atrial tachycardia, multifocal
☐ o. Atrial tachycardia with AV block
☐ p. Supraventricular tachycardia, unspecific
☐ q. Supraventricular tachycardia, paroxysmal
☐ r. Atrial flutter
☐ s. Atrial fibrillation
☐ t. Retrograde atrial activation

3. AV JUNCTIONAL RHYTHMS

☐ a. AV junctional premature complexes
☐ b. AV junctional escape complexes
☐ c. AV junctional rhythm, accelerated
☐ d. AV junctional rhythm

4. VENTRICULAR RHYTHMS

☐ a. Ventricular premature complex(es), uniform, fixed coupling
☐ b. Ventricular premature complex(es), uniform, nonfixed coupling
☐ c. Ventricular premature complexes(es), multiform
☐ d. Ventricular premature complexes, in pairs
☐ e. Ventricular parasystole
☐ f. Ventricular tachycardia (≥ 3 consecutive complexes)
☐ g. Accelerated idioventricular rhythm
☐ h. Ventricular escape complexes or rhythm
☐ i. Ventricular fibrillation

5. ATRIAL-VENTRICULAR INTERACTIONS IN ARRHYTHMIAS

☐ a. Fusion complexes
☐ b. Reciprocal (echo) complexes
☐ c. Ventricular capture complexes
☐ d. AV dissociation
☐ e. Ventriculophasic sinus arrhythmia

6. AV CONDUCTION ABNORMALITIES

☐ a. AV block, 1°
☐ b. AV block, 2° - Mobitz type I (Wenckebach)
☐ c. AV block, 2° - Mobitz type II
☐ d. AV block, 2:1
☐ e. AV block, 3°
☐ f. AV block, variable
☐ g. Short PR interval (with sinus rhythm and normal QRS duration)
☐ h. Wolff-Parkinson-White pattern

7. INTRAVENTRICULAR CONDUCTION DISTURBANCES

☐ a. RBBB, incomplete
☐ b. RBBB, complete
☐ c. Left anterior fascicular block
☐ d. Left posterior fascicular block
☐ e. LBBB, with ST-T wave suggestive of acute myocardial injury or infarction
☐ f. LBBB, complete
☐ g. LBBB, intermittent
☐ h. Intraventricular conduction disturbance, nonspecific
☐ i. Aberrant intraventricular conduction with supraventricular arrhythmia

8. P WAVE ABNORMALITIES

☐ a. Right atrial abnormality
☐ b. Left atrial abnormalities
☐ c. Nonspecific atrial abnormality

9. ABNORMALITIES OF QRS VOLTAGE OR AXIS

☐ a. Low voltage, limb leads only
☐ b. Low voltage, limb and precordial leads
☐ c. Left axis deviation (> - 30%)
☐ d. Right axis deviation (> + 100)
☐ e. Electrical alternans

10. VENTRICULAR HYPERTROPHY

☐ a. LVH by voltage only
☐ b. LVH by voltage and ST-T segment abnormalities
☐ c. RVH
☐ d. Combined ventricular hypertrophy

11. Q WAVE MYOCARDIAL INFARCTION

	Probably Acute or Recent	Probably Old or Age Indeterminate
Anterolateral	☐ a.	☐ g.
Anterior	☐ b.	☐ h.
Anteroseptal	☐ c.	☐ i.
Lateral/High lateral	☐ d.	☐ j.
Inferior	☐ e.	☐ k.
Posterior	☐ f.	☐ l.

☐ m. Probably ventricular aneurysm

12. ST, T, U, WAVE ABNORMALITIES

☐ a. Normal variant, early repolarization
☐ b. Normal variant, juvenile T waves
☐ c. Nonspecific ST and/or T wave abnormalities
☐ d. ST and/or T wave abnormalities suggesting myocardial ischemia
☐ e. ST and/or T wave abnormalities suggesting myocardial injury
☐ f. ST and/or T wave abnormalities suggesting acute pericarditis
☐ g. ST-T segment abnormalities secondary to intraventricular conduction disturbance or hypertrophy
☐ h. Post-extrasystolic T wave abnormality
☐ i. Isolated J point depression
☐ j. Peaked T waves
☐ k. Prolonged QT interval
☐ l. Prominent U waves

13. PACEMAKER FUNCTION AND RHYTHM

☐ a. Atrial or coronary sinus pacing
☐ b. Ventricular demand pacing
☐ c. AV sequential pacing
☐ d. Ventricular pacing, complete control
☐ e. Dual chamber, atrial sensing pacemaker
☐ f. Pacemaker malfunction, not constantly capturing (atrium or ventricle)
☐ g. Pacemaker malfunction, not constantly sensing (atrium or ventricle)
☐ h. Pacemaker malfunction, not firing
☐ i. Pacemaker malfunction, slowing

14. SUGGESTED OR PROBABLE CLINICAL DISORDERS

☐ a. Digitalis effect
☐ b. Digitalis toxicity
☐ c. Antiarrhythmic drug effect
☐ d. Antiarrhythmic drug toxicity
☐ e. Hyperkalemia
☐ f. Hypokalemia
☐ g. Hypercalcemia
☐ h. Hypocalcemia
☐ i. Atrial septal defect, secundum
☐ j. Atrial septal defect, primum
☐ k. Dextrocardia, mirror image
☐ l. Mitral valve disease
☐ m. Chronic lung disease
☐ n. Acute cor pulmonale, including pulmonary embolus
☐ o. Pericardial effusion
☐ p. Acute pericarditis
☐ q. Hypertrophic cardiomyopathy
☐ r. Coronary artery disease
☐ s. Central nervous system disorder
☐ t. Myxedema
☐ u. Hypothermia
☐ v. Sick sinus syndrome

ECG 54 was obtained in a 66-year-old female complaining of intermittent irregularity of her heart. The tracing shows sinus arrhythmia. Delta waves are present (arrows) suggesting Wolff-Parkinson-White pattern. The QRS complexes represent fusion between electrical wavefronts progressing through the AV node and the accessory pathway. The seventh beat on the rhythm strip (asterisk; also see full-size ECG on previous page for closer inspection) shows a normal QRS complex with a smaller delta wave, which represents variation in the degree of fusion and is a common finding in WPW.

Codes:

2b	Sinus arrhythmia
5a	Fusion complexes
6h	Wolff-Parkinson-White pattern

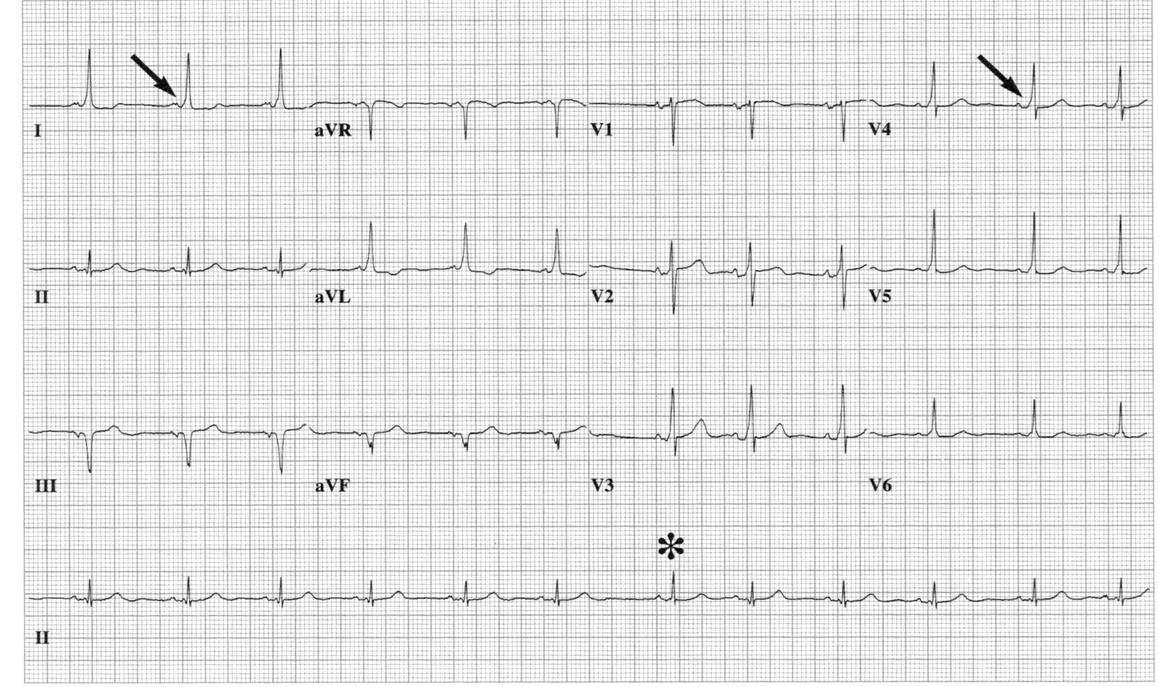

Questions: ECG 54

1. Which of the following statements about Wolff-Parkinson-White syndrome are true?

   a. WPW may interfere with ECG recognition of left and right ventricular hypertrophy
   b. WPW may interfere with ECG recognition of bundle branch block
   c. WPW may interfere with ECG recognition of acute myocardial infarction
   d. The polarity of the delta waves can be used to accurately predict the location of the bypass tract
   e. A short QT interval is commonly seen in WPW

Answers: ECG 54

1. Wolff-Parkinson-White syndrome (WPW) is characterized by the presence of an abnormal muscular network of specialized conduction tissue that connects the atrium to the ventricle and bypasses conduction through the AV node. It is found in 0.2-0.4% of the overall population and is more common in males and younger patients. Most patients with WPW do not have structural heart disease, although there is an increased prevalence of this disorder among patients with Epstein's anomaly (downward displacement of the tricuspid valve into the right ventricle due to anomalous attachment of the tricuspid leaflets), hypertrophic cardiomyopathy, mitral valve prolapse, and dilated cardiomyopathy. ECG manifestations include a short PR interval (< 0.12 seconds) and a widened QRS complex (> 0.10 seconds) with slurring of the initial 30-50 milliseconds (delta wave). Two types of accessory pathways (AP) exist: In ***manifest*** AP, antegrade conduction occurs over the AP and results in preexcitation on baseline ECG (which may be intermittent). In ***concealed*** AP, antegrade conduction occurs via the AV node and retrograde conduction occurs over the AP, so preexcitation is not evident on the baseline ECG. Approximately 50% of patients with WPW manifest tachyarrhythmias, of which 80% is AV reentry tachycardia, 15% is atrial fibrillation, and 5% is atrial flutter. Asymptomatic individuals have an excellent prognosis. For patients with recurrent tachycardias, the overall prognosis is good but sudden death may occur. The presence of

delta waves and secondary repolarization abnormalities can lead to a false positive or false negative diagnosis of ventricular hypertrophy, bundle branch block, or acute myocardial infarction. The polarity of the delta waves can be used to predict the location of the bypass tract. (Answer: All except e)

— Quick Review 54 —

Sinus arrhythmia	
• (Sinus/nonsinus) P wave	Sinus
• Longest and shortest PP intervals vary by > ____ seconds or 10%	0.16
• Sinus arrhythmia differs from "ventriculophasic" sinus arrhythmia, the latter of which occurs in the setting of ____	heart block
Fusion complexes	
• Due to simultaneous activation of the ventricle from ____ sources, resulting in a QRS complex that is ____ in morphology between each source	2 intermediate
Wolff-Parkinson-White pattern	
• (Sinus/nonsinus) P wave	sinus
• PR interval < ____ seconds	0.12
• Initial slurring of QRS (____ wave) resulting in QRS duration > ____ seconds	delta 0.10
• Secondary ST-T wave changes occur (true/false)	true
• PJ interval (beginning of P wave to end of QRS) (is constant/varies)	is constant

— POP QUIZ —

2:1 AV Block: Mobitz Type I or II

Instructions: Decide if the ECG features listed below favor Mobitz Type I (Wenkebach) or Mobitz Type II second-degree AV block

ECG Feature	Mobitz Type I or II
Narrow QRS complex	I
AV block worsens in response to maneuvers that increase heart rate & AV conduction (e.g., atropine, exercise)	II
AV block worsens in response to maneuvers that reduce heart rate & AV conduction (e.g., carotid sinus massage)	I
2:1 block develops during inferior MI	I
Type I on another part of ECG	I
History of syncope	II

ECG 55. 76-year-old male with a history of coronary artery disease:

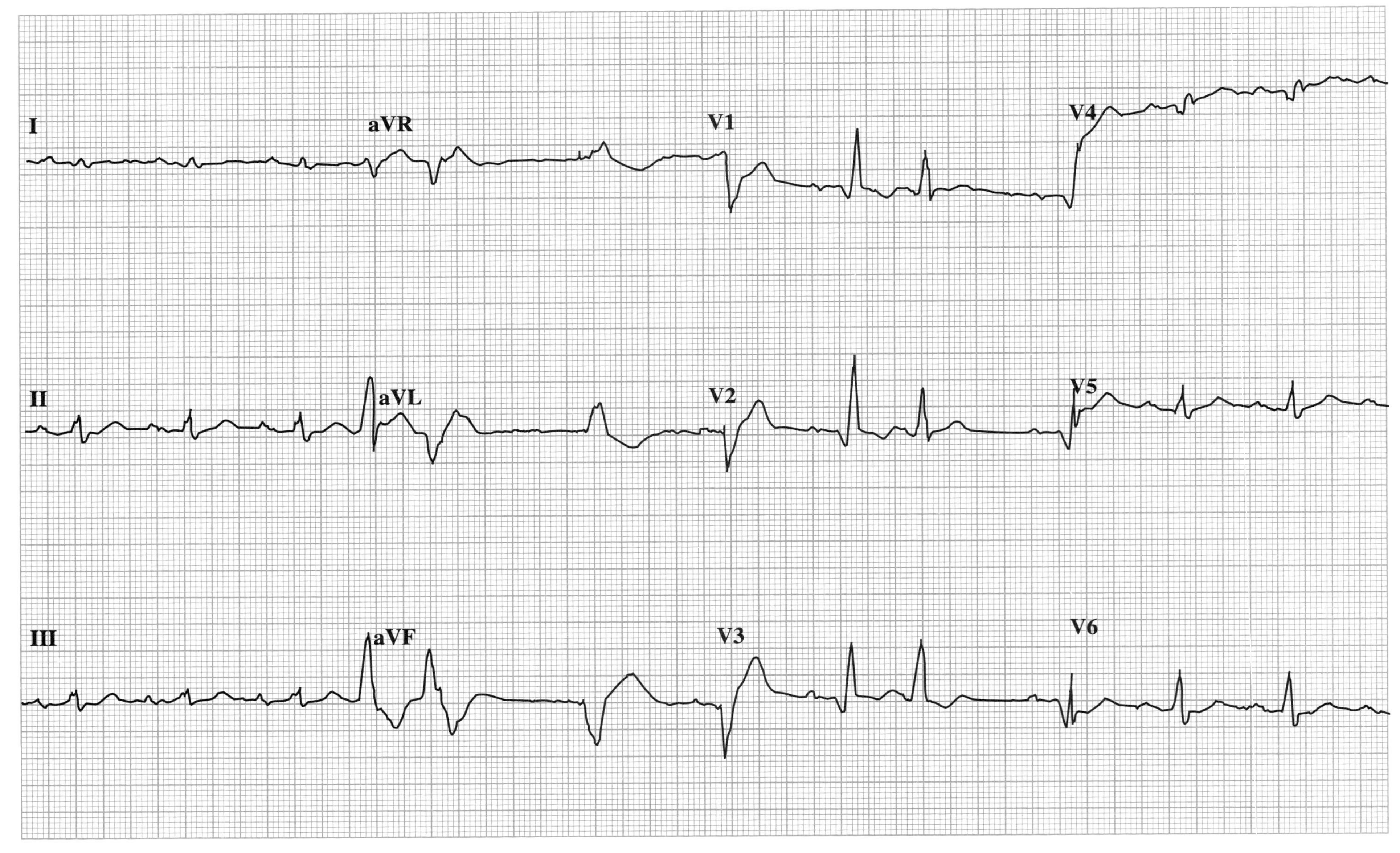

1. GENERAL FEATURES

☐ a. Normal ECG
☐ b. Borderline normal ECG or normal variant
☐ c. Incorrect electrode placement
☐ d. Artifact due to tremor

2. ATRIAL RHYTHMS

☐ a. Sinus rhythm
☐ b. Sinus arrhythmia
☐ c. Sinus bradycardia (< 60)
☐ d. Sinus tachycardia (> 100)
☐ e. Sinus pause or arrest
☐ f. Sinoatrial exit block
☐ g. Ecoptic atrial rhythm
☐ h. Wandering atrial pacemaker
☐ i. Atrial premature complexes, normally conducted
☐ j. Atrial premature complexes, nonconducted
☐ k. Atrial premature complexes with aberrant intraventricular conduction
☐ l. Atrial tachycardia (regular, sustained, 1:1 conduction)
☐ m. Atrial tachycardia, repetitive (short paroxysms)
☐ n. Atrial tachycardia, multifocal
☐ o. Atrial tachycardia with AV block
☐ p. Supraventricular tachycardia, unspecific
☐ q. Supraventricular tachycardia, paroxysmal
☐ r. Atrial flutter
☐ s. Atrial fibrillation
☐ t. Retrograde atrial activation

3. AV JUNCTIONAL RHYTHMS

☐ a. AV junctional premature complexes
☐ b. AV junctional escape complexes
☐ c. AV junctional rhythm, accelerated
☐ d. AV junctional rhythm

4. VENTRICULAR RHYTHMS

☐ a. Ventricular premature complex(es), uniform, fixed coupling
☐ b. Ventricular premature complex(es), uniform, nonfixed coupling
☐ c. Ventricular premature complexes(es), multiform
☐ d. Ventricular premature complexes, in pairs
☐ e. Ventricular parasystole
☐ f. Ventricular tachycardia (≥ 3 consecutive complexes)
☐ g. Accelerated idioventricular rhythm
☐ h. Ventricular escape complexes or rhythm
☐ i. Ventricular fibrillation

5. ATRIAL-VENTRICULAR INTERACTIONS IN ARRHYTHMIAS

☐ a. Fusion complexes
☐ b. Reciprocal (echo) complexes
☐ c. Ventricular capture complexes
☐ d. AV dissociation

☐ e. Ventriculophasic sinus arrhythmia

6. AV CONDUCTION ABNORMALITIES

☐ a. AV block, 1°
☐ b. AV block, 2° - Mobitz type I (Wenckebach)
☐ c. AV block, 2° - Mobitz type II
☐ d. AV block, 2:1
☐ e. AV block, 3°
☐ f. AV block, variable
☐ g. Short PR interval (with sinus rhythm and normal QRS duration)
☐ h. Wolff-Parkinson-White pattern

7. INTRAVENTRICULAR CONDUCTION DISTURBANCES

☐ a. RBBB, incomplete
☐ b. RBBB, complete
☐ c. Left anterior fascicular block
☐ d. Left posterior fascicular block
☐ e. LBBB, with ST-T wave suggestive of acute myocardial injury or infarction
☐ f. LBBB, complete
☐ g. LBBB, intermittent
☐ h. Intraventricular conduction disturbance, nonspecific
☐ i. Aberrant intraventricular conduction with supraventricular arrhythmia

8. P WAVE ABNORMALITIES

☐ a. Right atrial abnormality
☐ b. Left atrial abnormalities
☐ c. Nonspecific atrial abnormality

9. ABNORMALITIES OF QRS VOLTAGE OR AXIS

☐ a. Low voltage, limb leads only
☐ b. Low voltage, limb and precordial leads
☐ c. Left axis deviation (> - 30%)
☐ d. Right axis deviation (> + 100)
☐ e. Electrical alternans

10. VENTRICULAR HYPERTROPHY

☐ a. LVH by voltage only
☐ b. LVH by voltage and ST-T segment abnormalities
☐ c. RVH
☐ d. Combined ventricular hypertrophy

11. Q WAVE MYOCARDIAL INFARCTION

	Probably Acute or Recent	Probably Old or Age Indeterminate
Anterolateral	☐ a.	☐ g.
Anterior	☐ b.	☐ h.
Anteroseptal	☐ c.	☐ i.
Lateral/High lateral	☐ d.	☐ j.
Inferior	☐ e.	☐ k.
Posterior	☐ f.	☐ l.

☐ m. Probably ventricular aneurysm

12. ST, T, U, WAVE ABNORMALITIES

☐ a. Normal variant, early repolarization
☐ b. Normal variant, juvenile T waves
☐ c. Nonspecific ST and/or T wave abnormalities
☐ d. ST and/or T wave abnormalities suggesting myocardial ischemia
☐ e. ST and/or T wave abnormalities suggesting myocardial injury
☐ f. ST and/or T wave abnormalities suggesting acute pericarditis
☐ g. ST-T segment abnormalities secondary to intraventricular conduction disturbance or hypertrophy
☐ h. Post-extrasystolic T wave abnormality
☐ i. Isolated J point depression
☐ j. Peaked T waves
☐ k. Prolonged QT interval
☐ l. Prominent U waves

13. PACEMAKER FUNCTION AND RHYTHM

☐ a. Atrial or coronary sinus pacing
☐ b. Ventricular demand pacing
☐ c. AV sequential pacing
☐ d. Ventricular pacing, complete control
☐ e. Dual chamber, atrial sensing pacemaker
☐ f. Pacemaker malfunction, not constantly capturing (atrium or ventricle)
☐ g. Pacemaker malfunction, not constantly sensing (atrium or ventricle)
☐ h. Pacemaker malfunction, not firing
☐ i. Pacemaker malfunction, slowing

14. SUGGESTED OR PROBABLE CLINICAL DISORDERS

☐ a. Digitalis effect
☐ b. Digitalis toxicity
☐ c. Antiarrhythmic drug effect
☐ d. Antiarrhythmic drug toxicity
☐ e. Hyperkalemia
☐ f. Hypokalemia
☐ g. Hypercalcemia
☐ h. Hypocalcemia
☐ i. Atrial septal defect, secundum
☐ j. Atrial septal defect, primum
☐ k. Dextrocardia, mirror image
☐ l. Mitral valve disease
☐ m. Chronic lung disease
☐ n. Acute cor pulmonale, including pulmonary embolus
☐ o. Pericardial effusion
☐ p. Acute pericarditis
☐ q. Hypertrophic cardiomyopathy
☐ r. Coronary artery disease
☐ s. Central nervous system disorder
☐ t. Myxedema
☐ u. Hypothermia
☐ v. Sick sinus syndrome

ECG 55 was obtained in a 76-year-old male with a long history of coronary artery disease. The ECG demonstrates sinus rhythm, first-degree AV block, and left atrial abnormality (notched P wave in lead II $\geq$ 0.12 seconds). Ventricular premature complexes (VPC) are present, including one couplet (asterisk). After the pair, a compensatory pause triggers a demand ventricular pacemaker (pacer spiker best seen in aVR; arrowhead), which fires for two beats at approximately 60 beats/minute. The QRS complex in the second of the paced beats is a fusion complex (intermediate between a normal sinus beat and a ventricular paced beat). Also present are previous anteroseptal MI (arrows) and RBBB with secondary ST-T changes. The first complex in leads V_4-V_6 demonstrates a subtle aberration in the normal T wave configuration that is probably the result of the preceding VPC (although it can be argued that this clinically insignificant finding may not be present). Remember to code for ventricular demand pacing and coronary artery disease.

Codes:

2a	Sinus rhythm	11i	Anteroseptal Q wave MI, probably old or age indeterminate
4d	VPCs, in pairs (2 consecutive)	12g	ST-T segment abnormalities secondary to IVCD or hypertrophy
5a	Fusion complexes	12h	Post-extrasystolic T wave abnormality
6a	AV block, 1°	13b	Ventricular pacing, complete control (or ventricular demand pacing)
7b	RBBB, complete	14r	Coronary artery disease
8b	Left atrial abnormality		

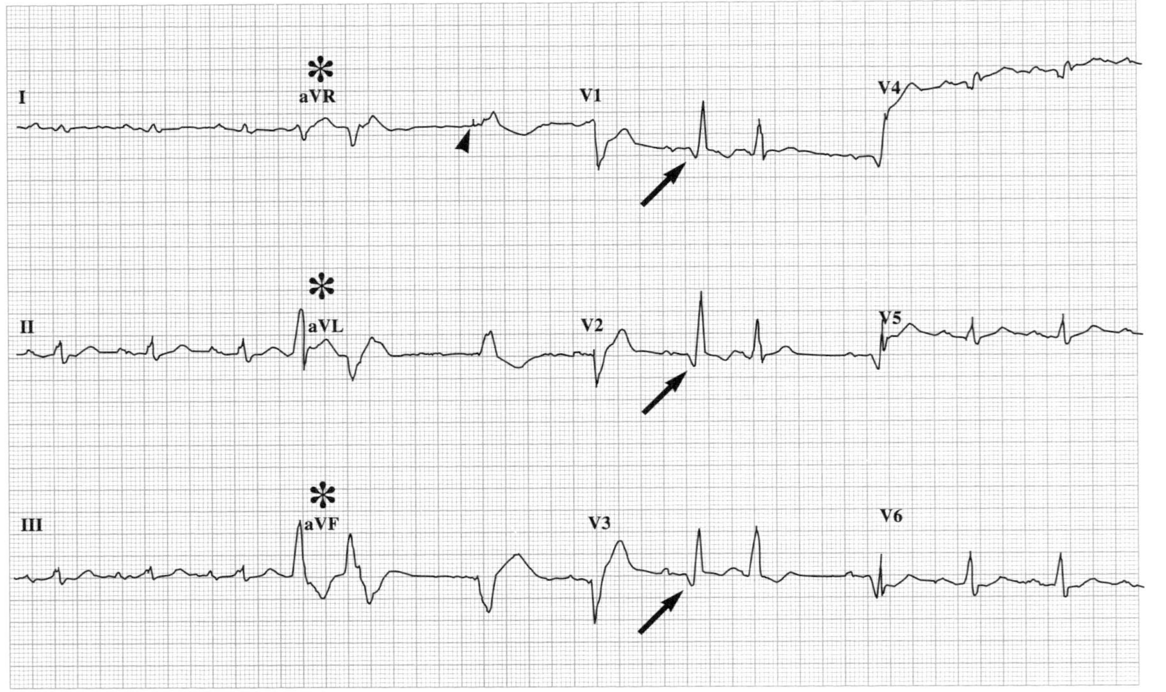

Questions: ECG 55

1. Which of the following statements about post-extrasystolic T wave abnormality are true:

   a. Involves any alteration in the contour, amplitude, and/or direction of the T wave in the sinus beat following the ectopic beat
   b. Can occur after single ventricular premature complexes or ventricular tachycardia

2. The presence of RBBB usually distorts the Q waves of previous myocardial infarction:

   a. True
   b. False

Answers: ECG 55

1. Post-extrasystolic T wave abnormality is characterized by any alteration in the contour, amplitude and/or direction of the T wave in the sinus beats following an ectopic beat or repetitive ectopic beats (e.g., ventricular tachycardia). It is often a relatively subtle finding, as it is on this tracing. (Answer: All)

2. RBBB results in delay of the terminal forces of the QRS complex. Since the Q wave involves the initial or unblocked portion of the QRS, RBBB usually does not interfere with the diagnosis of Q-wave myocardial infarction. (Answer: b)

— Quick Review 55 —

AV block, 1°	
• PR interval ≥ ____ seconds	0.20
Left atrial abnormality	
• Notched P wave with a duration ≥ ____ seconds in leads II, III or aVF, *or*	0.12
• Terminal negative portion of the P wave in lead V_1 ≥ 1 mm deep and ≥ ____ seconds in duration	0.04
Ventricular demand pacing	
• Pacemaker stimulus followed by a QRS complex that has (the same/different) morphology compared to the intrinsic QRS	different
• Must demonstrate ____ of pacemaker output in response to intrinsic QRS	inhibition

ECG 56. 59-year-old male with a history of high blood pressure:

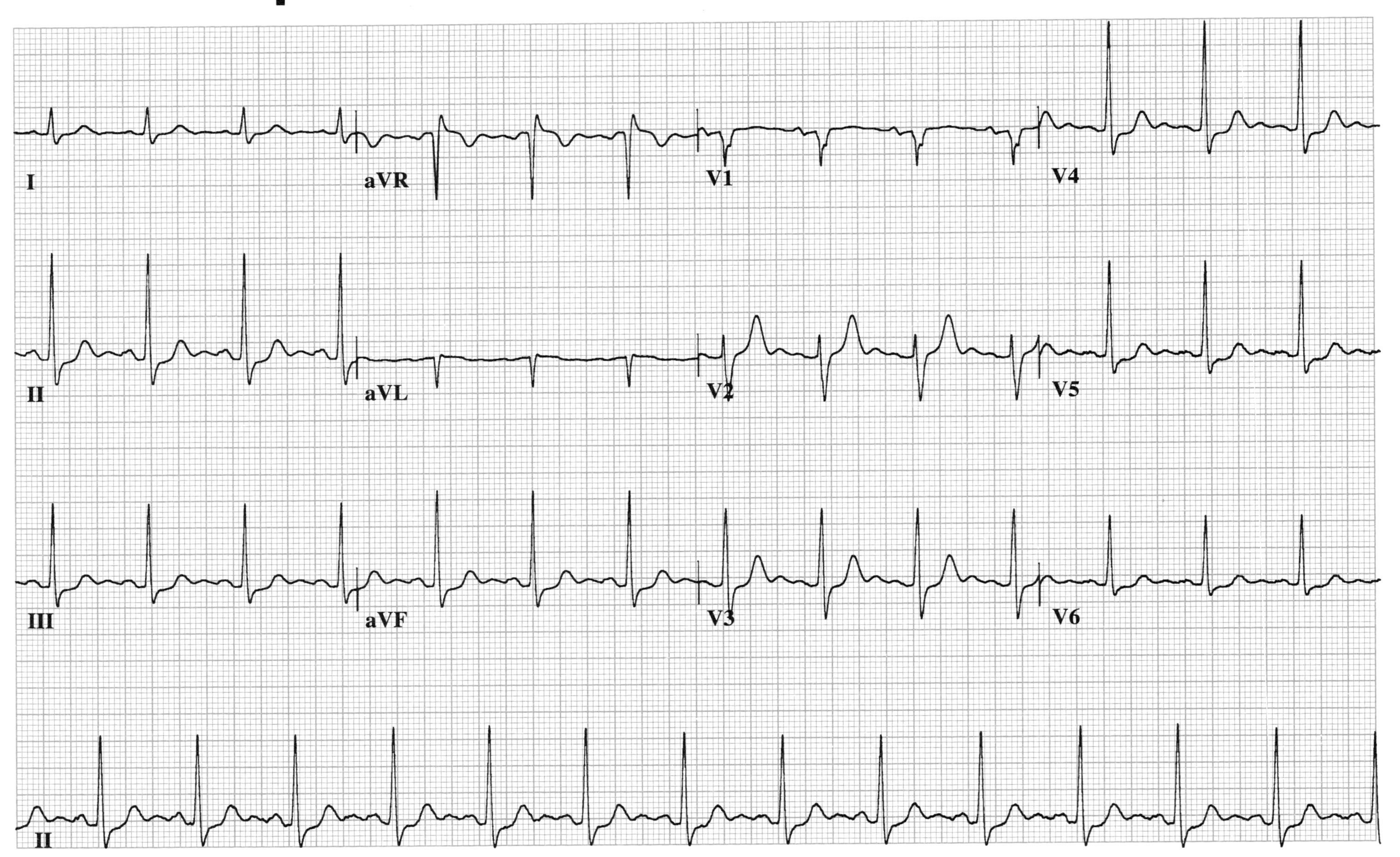

1. GENERAL FEATURES

- ☐ a. Normal ECG
- ☐ b. Borderline normal ECG or normal variant
- ☐ c. Incorrect electrode placement
- ☐ d. Artifact due to tremor

2. ATRIAL RHYTHMS

- ☐ a. Sinus rhythm
- ☐ b. Sinus arrhythmia
- ☐ c. Sinus bradycardia (< 60)
- ☐ d. Sinus tachycardia (> 100)
- ☐ e. Sinus pause or arrest
- ☐ f. Sinoatrial exit block
- ☐ g. Ecoptic atrial rhythm
- ☐ h. Wandering atrial pacemaker
- ☐ i. Atrial premature complexes, normally conducted
- ☐ j. Atrial premature complexes, nonconducted
- ☐ k. Atrial premature complexes with aberrant intraventricular conduction
- ☐ l. Atrial tachycardia (regular, sustained, 1:1 conduction)
- ☐ m. Atrial tachycardia, repetitive (short paroxysms)
- ☐ n. Atrial tachycardia, multifocal
- ☐ o. Atrial tachycardia with AV block
- ☐ p. Supraventricular tachycardia, unspecific
- ☐ q. Supraventricular tachycardia, paroxysmal
- ☐ r. Atrial flutter
- ☐ s. Atrial fibrillation
- ☐ t. Retrograde atrial activation

3. AV JUNCTIONAL RHYTHMS

- ☐ a. AV junctional premature complexes
- ☐ b. AV junctional escape complexes
- ☐ c. AV junctional rhythm, accelerated
- ☐ d. AV junctional rhythm

4. VENTRICULAR RHYTHMS

- ☐ a. Ventricular premature complex(es), uniform, fixed coupling
- ☐ b. Ventricular premature complex(es), uniform, nonfixed coupling
- ☐ c. Ventricular premature complexes(es), multiform
- ☐ d. Ventricular premature complexes, in pairs
- ☐ e. Ventricular parasystole
- ☐ f. Ventricular tachycardia (≥ 3 consecutive complexes)
- ☐ g. Accelerated idioventricular rhythm
- ☐ h. Ventricular escape complexes or rhythm
- ☐ i. Ventricular fibrillation

5. ATRIAL-VENTRICULAR INTERACTIONS IN ARRHYTHMIAS

- ☐ a. Fusion complexes
- ☐ b. Reciprocal (echo) complexes
- ☐ c. Ventricular capture complexes
- ☐ d. AV dissociation
- ☐ e. Ventriculophasic sinus arrhythmia

6. AV CONDUCTION ABNORMALITIES

- ☐ a. AV block, 1°
- ☐ b. AV block, 2° - Mobitz type I (Wenckebach)
- ☐ c. AV block, 2° - Mobitz type II
- ☐ d. AV block, 2:1
- ☐ e. AV block, 3°
- ☐ f. AV block, variable
- ☐ g. Short PR interval (with sinus rhythm and normal QRS duration)
- ☐ h. Wolff-Parkinson-White pattern

7. INTRAVENTRICULAR CONDUCTION DISTURBANCES

- ☐ a. RBBB, incomplete
- ☐ b. RBBB, complete
- ☐ c. Left anterior fascicular block
- ☐ d. Left posterior fascicular block
- ☐ e. LBBB, with ST-T wave suggestive of acute myocardial injury or infarction
- ☐ f. LBBB, complete
- ☐ g. LBBB, intermittent
- ☐ h. Intraventricular conduction disturbance, nonspecific
- ☐ i. Aberrant intraventricular conduction with supraventricular arrhythmia

8. P WAVE ABNORMALITIES

- ☐ a. Right atrial abnormality
- ☐ b. Left atrial abnormalities
- ☐ c. Nonspecific atrial abnormality

9. ABNORMALITIES OF QRS VOLTAGE OR AXIS

- ☐ a. Low voltage, limb leads only
- ☐ b. Low voltage, limb and precordial leads
- ☐ c. Left axis deviation (> - 30%)
- ☐ d. Right axis deviation (> + 100)
- ☐ e. Electrical alternans

10. VENTRICULAR HYPERTROPHY

- ☐ a. LVH by voltage only
- ☐ b. LVH by voltage and ST-T segment abnormalities
- ☐ c. RVH
- ☐ d. Combined ventricular hypertrophy

11. Q WAVE MYOCARDIAL INFARCTION

	Probably Acute or Recent	Probably Old or Age Indeterminate
Anterolateral	☐ a.	☐ g.
Anterior	☐ b.	☐ h.
Anteroseptal	☐ c.	☐ i.
Lateral/High lateral	☐ d.	☐ j.
Inferior	☐ e.	☐ k.
Posterior	☐ f.	☐ l.

- ☐ m. Probably ventricular aneurysm

12. ST, T, U, WAVE ABNORMALITIES

- ☐ a. Normal variant, early repolarization
- ☐ b. Normal variant, juvenile T waves
- ☐ c. Nonspecific ST and/or T wave abnormalities
- ☐ d. ST and/or T wave abnormalities suggesting myocardial ischemia
- ☐ e. ST and/or T wave abnormalities suggesting myocardial injury
- ☐ f. ST and/or T wave abnormalities suggesting acute pericarditis
- ☐ g. ST-T segment abnormalities secondary to intraventricular conduction disturbance or hypertrophy
- ☐ h. Post-extrasystolic T wave abnormality
- ☐ i. Isolated J point depression
- ☐ j. Peaked T waves
- ☐ k. Prolonged QT interval
- ☐ l. Prominent U waves

13. PACEMAKER FUNCTION AND RHYTHM

- ☐ a. Atrial or coronary sinus pacing
- ☐ b. Ventricular demand pacing
- ☐ c. AV sequential pacing
- ☐ d. Ventricular pacing, complete control
- ☐ e. Dual chamber, atrial sensing pacemaker
- ☐ f. Pacemaker malfunction, not constantly capturing (atrium or ventricle)
- ☐ g. Pacemaker malfunction, not constantly sensing (atrium or ventricle)
- ☐ h. Pacemaker malfunction, not firing
- ☐ i. Pacemaker malfunction, slowing

14. SUGGESTED OR PROBABLE CLINICAL DISORDERS

- ☐ a. Digitalis effect
- ☐ b. Digitalis toxicity
- ☐ c. Antiarrhythmic drug effect
- ☐ d. Antiarrhythmic drug toxicity
- ☐ e. Hyperkalemia
- ☐ f. Hypokalemia
- ☐ g. Hypercalcemia
- ☐ h. Hypocalcemia
- ☐ i. Atrial septal defect, secundum
- ☐ j. Atrial septal defect, primum
- ☐ k. Dextrocardia, mirror image
- ☐ l. Mitral valve disease
- ☐ m. Chronic lung disease
- ☐ n. Acute cor pulmonale, including pulmonary embolus
- ☐ o. Pericardial effusion
- ☐ p. Acute pericarditis
- ☐ q. Hypertrophic cardiomyopathy
- ☐ r. Coronary artery disease
- ☐ s. Central nervous system disorder
- ☐ t. Myxedema
- ☐ u. Hypothermia
- ☐ v. Sick sinus syndrome

ECG 56 was obtained from a 59-year-old male with a history of high blood pressure. The tracing shows sinus rhythm, a nonspecific IVCD (asterisk), and a nonspecific atrial abnormality (the P wave is abnormally wide and notched but does not quite meet criteria for either left or right atrial abnormality) (arrowhead). Prominent U waves (arrow) and nonspecific ST-T changes are also present.

Codes:

2a	Sinus rhythm
7h	IVCD, nonspecific type
8c	Nonspecific atrial abnormality
12c	Nonspecific ST and/or T wave abnormalities
12l	Prominent U waves

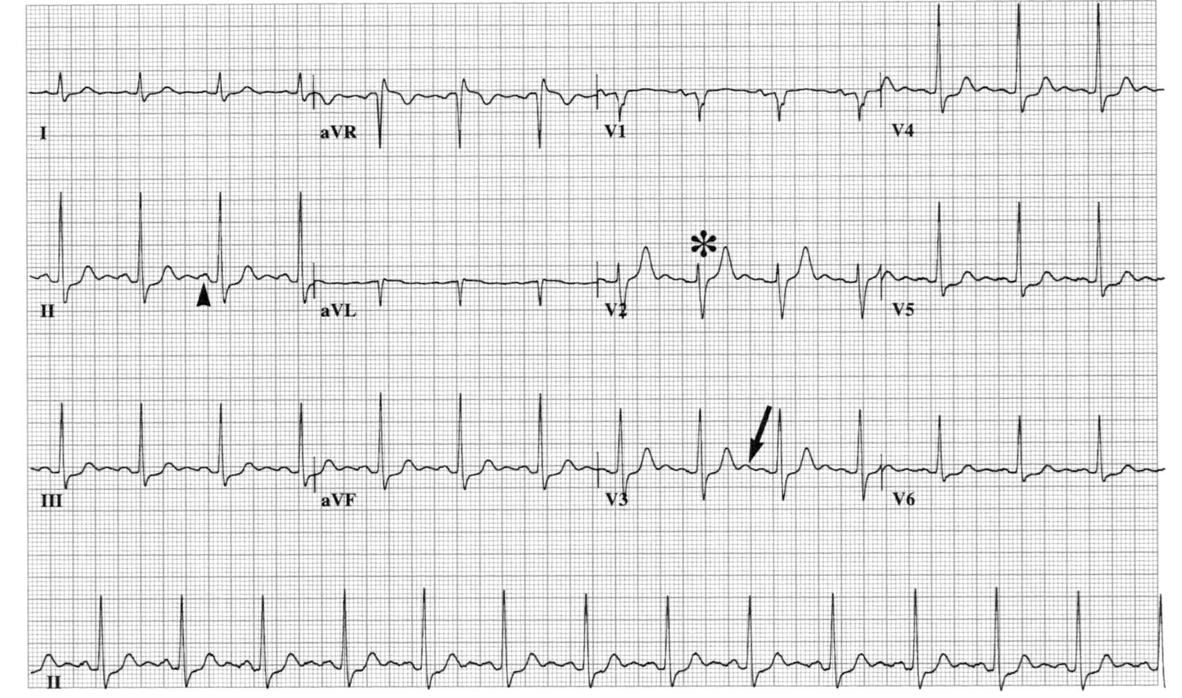

Questions: ECG 56

1. Conditions associated with intraventricular conduction disturbance (IVCD) includes:

   a. Antiarrhythmic drug toxicity
   b. Hyperkalemia
   c. Hypothermia
   d. Hypercalcemia

2. Match of the clinical disorders in question 1 to the following ECG findings:

   a. IVCD, atrial fibrillation, prolonged PR interval, prolonged QT interval, J wave (Osborne wave) in terminal QRS
   b. IVCD, wide QRS complex, tall and peaked T waves, sinoventricular conduction
   c. IVCD, wide QRS complex, prolonged QT interval, U wave

3. Which of the following statements about U waves are true?

   a. Large U waves (> 2 mm) are considered a normal variant
   b. U waves are usually upright in all leads except aVR
   c. U waves are more pronounced at slower heart rates
   d. The U wave may overlap the T wave to result in pseudo-prolongation of the QT interval
   e. Inverted U waves can be seen in LVH and ischemic heart disease, but is rarely seen in normal hearts

Answers: ECG 56

1. Intraventricular conduction delay (IVCD), defined as a wide QRS complex (> 0.12 seconds) not fitting the criteria for left or right bundle branch block, is seen with Type IA and IC antiarrhythmics, hyperkalemia, and hypothermia. Hypercalcemia does not cause IVCD. (Answer: a - c)

2. Answer: a: hypothermia
   b: hyperkalemia
   c: antiarrhythmic drug toxicity

3. The U wave is a small deflection following the T wave. It is usually upright, more pronounced at slower heart rates, and may be superimposed on the preceding T wave. U wave amplitude may reach 2-3 mm in leads V_2 and V_3, but is usually $\leq$ 2 mm in most leads. (Answer: b - e)

— Quick Review 56 —

Intraventricular conduction disturbance, nonspecific type	
• QRS ≥ ____ seconds in duration but morphology does not meet criteria for LBBB or RBBB, *or*	0.11
abnormal ____ without widening of the QRS complex	notching
Nonspecific ST and/or T wave abnormalities	
• Slight ____ segment depression or elevation	ST
• Slightly inverted or flat ____ wave	T

— POP QUIZ —

Make The Diagnosis

Instructions: Determine the ECG diagnosis that best corresponds to the ECG features listed below (see score sheet for options)

ECG Features	Diagnosis
• Ventricular rate of 40-60 per minute • QRS morphology similar to sinus/supraventricular impulse • QRS complex occurs in response to decreased sinus impulse formation or conduction, or high-degree AV block; the atrial mechanism may be sinus rhythm, paroxysmal atrial tachycardia, atrial flutter, or atrial fibrillation	AV junctional escape complex
• Ventricular ectopic beats occur at a rate of 30-50 per minute (can range from 20-400 per minute) • VPCs show nonfixed coupling • Fusion complexes may be present • All interectopic intervals are a multiple of the shortest interectopic interval	Ventricular parasystole
• Regular ventricular rhythm at a rate of 60-110 bpm • QRS morphology is similar to VPCs • Ventricular capture complexes, fusion beats, and AV dissociation are common	Accelerated idioventricular rhythm
• Ventricular rate of 30-40 per minute • QRS morphology is similar to VPCs • QRS complex occurs as a secondary phenomenon in response to decreased sinus impulse formation or conduction, or high-degree AV block	Ventricular escape beats or rhythm
• Due to simultaneous activation of the ventricle from 2 sources, resulting in a QRS complex that is intermediate in morphology between each source	Fusion complexes

ECG 57. 76-year-old female with severe substernal chest pressure:

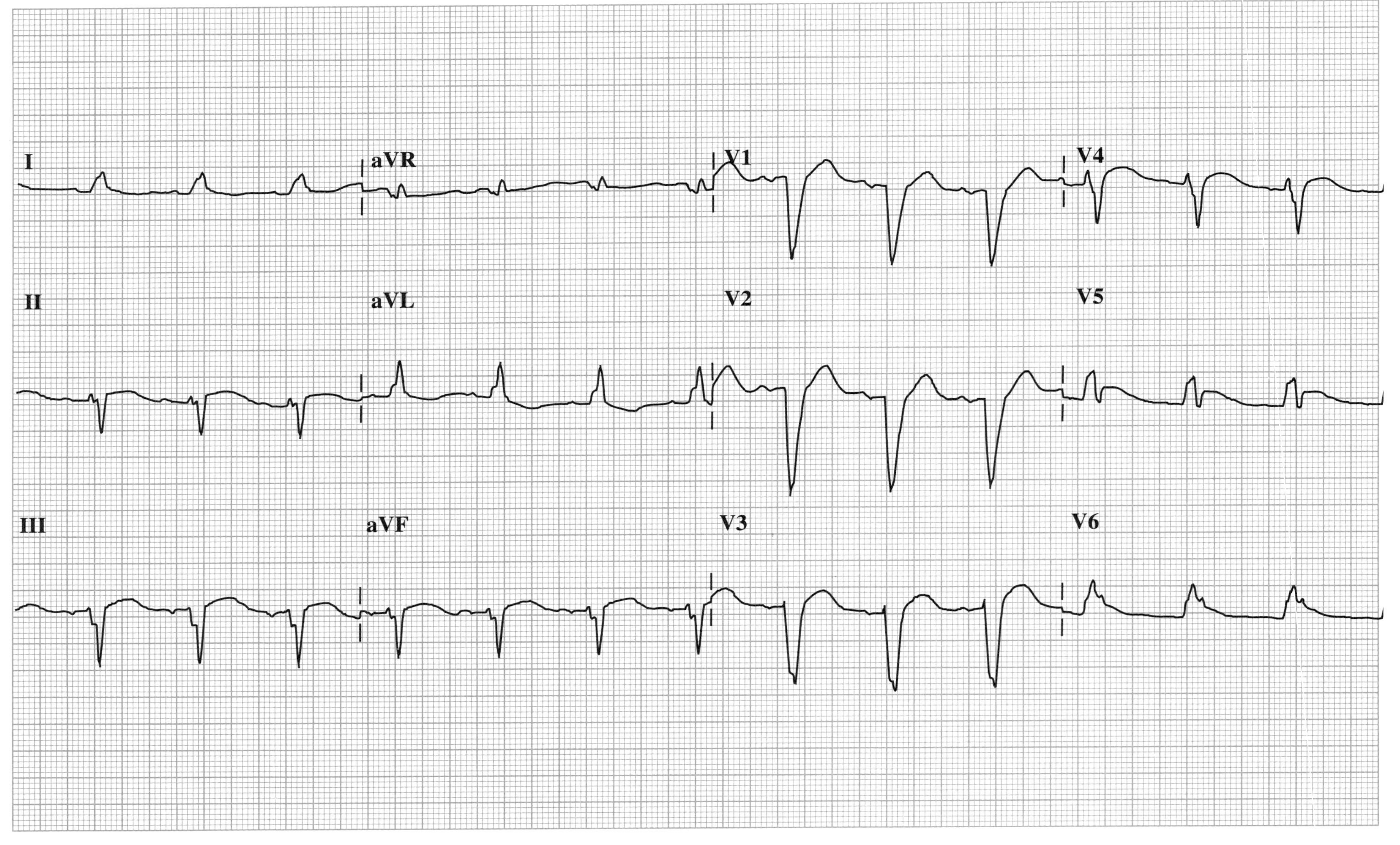

1. GENERAL FEATURES

- ☐ a. Normal ECG
- ☐ b. Borderline normal ECG or normal variant
- ☐ c. Incorrect electrode placement
- ☐ d. Artifact due to tremor

2. ATRIAL RHYTHMS

- ☐ a. Sinus rhythm
- ☐ b. Sinus arrhythmia
- ☐ c. Sinus bradycardia (< 60)
- ☐ d. Sinus tachycardia (> 100)
- ☐ e. Sinus pause or arrest
- ☐ f. Sinoatrial exit block
- ☐ g. Ecoptic atrial rhythm
- ☐ h. Wandering atrial pacemaker
- ☐ i. Atrial premature complexes, normally conducted
- ☐ j. Atrial premature complexes, nonconducted
- ☐ k. Atrial premature complexes with aberrant intraventricular conduction
- ☐ l. Atrial tachycardia (regular, sustained, 1:1 conduction)
- ☐ m. Atrial tachycardia, repetitive (short paroxysms)
- ☐ n. Atrial tachycardia, multifocal
- ☐ o. Atrial tachycardia with AV block
- ☐ p. Supraventricular tachycardia, unspecific
- ☐ q. Supraventricular tachycardia, paroxysmal
- ☐ r. Atrial flutter
- ☐ s. Atrial fibrillation
- ☐ t. Retrograde atrial activation

3. AV JUNCTIONAL RHYTHMS

- ☐ a. AV junctional premature complexes
- ☐ b. AV junctional escape complexes
- ☐ c. AV junctional rhythm, accelerated
- ☐ d. AV junctional rhythm

4. VENTRICULAR RHYTHMS

- ☐ a. Ventricular premature complex(es), uniform, fixed coupling
- ☐ b. Ventricular premature complex(es), uniform, nonfixed coupling
- ☐ c. Ventricular premature complexes(es), multiform
- ☐ d. Ventricular premature complexes, in pairs
- ☐ e. Ventricular parasystole
- ☐ f. Ventricular tachycardia (≥ 3 consecutive complexes)
- ☐ g. Accelerated idioventricular rhythm
- ☐ h. Ventricular escape complexes or rhythm
- ☐ i. Ventricular fibrillation

5. ATRIAL-VENTRICULAR INTERACTIONS IN ARRHYTHMIAS

- ☐ a. Fusion complexes
- ☐ b. Reciprocal (echo) complexes
- ☐ c. Ventricular capture complexes
- ☐ d. AV dissociation
- ☐ e. Ventriculophasic sinus arrhythmia

6. AV CONDUCTION ABNORMALITIES

- ☐ a. AV block, 1°
- ☐ b. AV block, 2° - Mobitz type I (Wenckebach)
- ☐ c. AV block, 2° - Mobitz type II
- ☐ d. AV block, 2:1
- ☐ e. AV block, 3°
- ☐ f. AV block, variable
- ☐ g. Short PR interval (with sinus rhythm and normal QRS duration)
- ☐ h. Wolff-Parkinson-White pattern

7. INTRAVENTRICULAR CONDUCTION DISTURBANCES

- ☐ a. RBBB, incomplete
- ☐ b. RBBB, complete
- ☐ c. Left anterior fascicular block
- ☐ d. Left posterior fascicular block
- ☐ e. LBBB, with ST-T wave suggestive of acute myocardial injury or infarction
- ☐ f. LBBB, complete
- ☐ g. LBBB, intermittent
- ☐ h. Intraventricular conduction disturbance, nonspecific
- ☐ i. Aberrant intraventricular conduction with supraventricular arrhythmia

8. P WAVE ABNORMALITIES

- ☐ a. Right atrial abnormality
- ☐ b. Left atrial abnormalities
- ☐ c. Nonspecific atrial abnormality

9. ABNORMALITIES OF QRS VOLTAGE OR AXIS

- ☐ a. Low voltage, limb leads only
- ☐ b. Low voltage, limb and precordial leads
- ☐ c. Left axis deviation (> - 30%)
- ☐ d. Right axis deviation (> + 100)
- ☐ e. Electrical alternans

10. VENTRICULAR HYPERTROPHY

- ☐ a. LVH by voltage only
- ☐ b. LVH by voltage and ST-T segment abnormalities
- ☐ c. RVH
- ☐ d. Combined ventricular hypertrophy

11. Q WAVE MYOCARDIAL INFARCTION

	Probably Acute or Recent	Probably Old or Age Indeterminate
Anterolateral	☐ a.	☐ g.
Anterior	☐ b.	☐ h.
Anteroseptal	☐ c.	☐ i.
Lateral/High lateral	☐ d.	☐ j.
Inferior	☐ e.	☐ k.
Posterior	☐ f.	☐ l.

- ☐ m. Probably ventricular aneurysm

12. ST, T, U, WAVE ABNORMALITIES

- ☐ a. Normal variant, early repolarization
- ☐ b. Normal variant, juvenile T waves
- ☐ c. Nonspecific ST and/or T wave abnormalities
- ☐ d. ST and/or T wave abnormalities suggesting myocardial ischemia
- ☐ e. ST and/or T wave abnormalities suggesting myocardial injury
- ☐ f. ST and/or T wave abnormalities suggesting acute pericarditis
- ☐ g. ST-T segment abnormalities secondary to intraventricular conduction disturbance or hypertrophy
- ☐ h. Post-extrasystolic T wave abnormality
- ☐ i. Isolated J point depression
- ☐ j. Peaked T waves
- ☐ k. Prolonged QT interval
- ☐ l. Prominent U waves

13. PACEMAKER FUNCTION AND RHYTHM

- ☐ a. Atrial or coronary sinus pacing
- ☐ b. Ventricular demand pacing
- ☐ c. AV sequential pacing
- ☐ d. Ventricular pacing, complete control
- ☐ e. Dual chamber, atrial sensing pacemaker
- ☐ f. Pacemaker malfunction, not constantly capturing (atrium or ventricle)
- ☐ g. Pacemaker malfunction, not constantly sensing (atrium or ventricle)
- ☐ h. Pacemaker malfunction, not firing
- ☐ i. Pacemaker malfunction, slowing

14. SUGGESTED OR PROBABLE CLINICAL DISORDERS

- ☐ a. Digitalis effect
- ☐ b. Digitalis toxicity
- ☐ c. Antiarrhythmic drug effect
- ☐ d. Antiarrhythmic drug toxicity
- ☐ e. Hyperkalemia
- ☐ f. Hypokalemia
- ☐ g. Hypercalcemia
- ☐ h. Hypocalcemia
- ☐ i. Atrial septal defect, secundum
- ☐ j. Atrial septal defect, primum
- ☐ k. Dextrocardia, mirror image
- ☐ l. Mitral valve disease
- ☐ m. Chronic lung disease
- ☐ n. Acute cor pulmonale, including pulmonary embolus
- ☐ o. Pericardial effusion
- ☐ p. Acute pericarditis
- ☐ q. Hypertrophic cardiomyopathy
- ☐ r. Coronary artery disease
- ☐ s. Central nervous system disorder
- ☐ t. Myxedema
- ☐ u. Hypothermia
- ☐ v. Sick sinus syndrome

ECG 57 was obtained in a 76-year-old female with severe substernal chest pressure associated with diaphoresis and pallor. The ECG shows sinus rhythm, LBBB, left atrial abnormality, and left axis deviation. Concordant ST segment elevation is apparent in leads V_5 and V_6 (arrows) consistent with an acute injury pattern. However, since pathological Q waves are not present, Q wave myocardial infarction should not be coded. This ECG is consistent with coronary artery disease.

Codes:

2a	Sinus rhythm
7e	LBBB, complete with ST-T wave suggestive of acute myocardial injury or infarction
8b	Left atrial abnormality
9c	Left axis deviation (> -30°)
12e	ST and/or T wave abnormalities suggesting myocardial injury
14r	Coronary artery disease

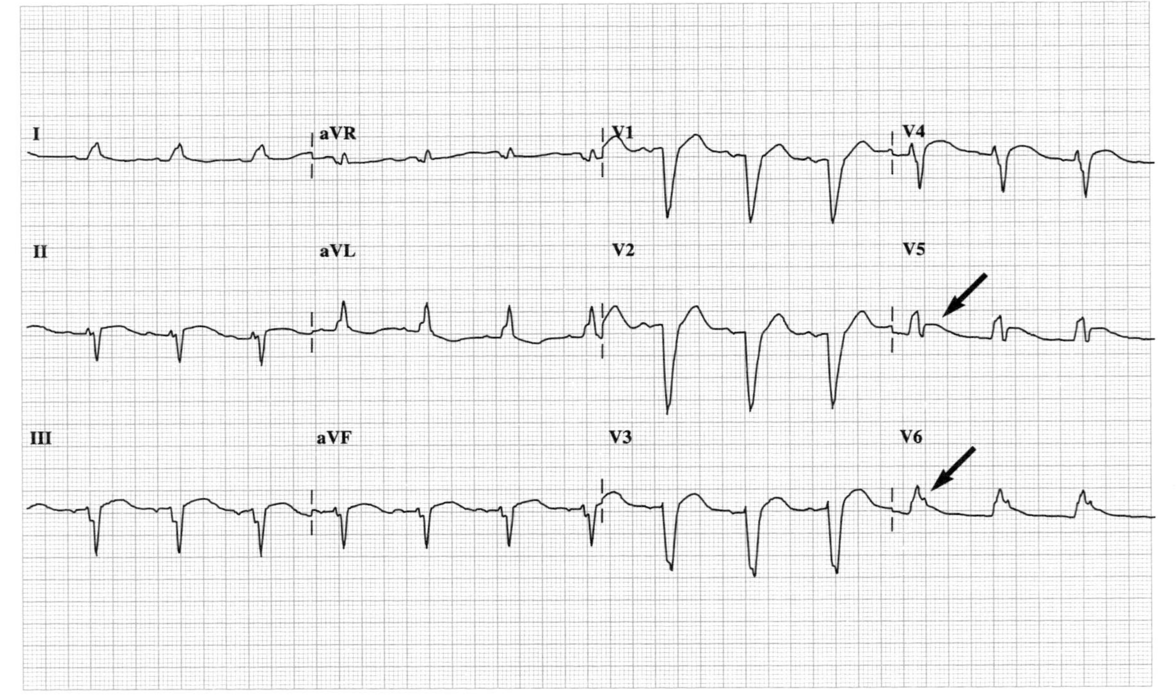

Questions: ECG 57

1. The most specific finding for an acute injury pattern in the setting of LBBB is:

   a. Discordant ST segment elevation >1 mm
   b. Q waves in leads V_1-V_3
   c. Concordant ST segment elevation
   d. Concordant ST segment depression

2. Concordant ST segment depression in leads V_1-V_3 in the setting of LBBB of more than ___ mm is consistent with acute ischemia:

   a. 1
   b. 2
   c. 3
   d. 4

Answers: ECG 57

1. In the setting of LBBB, acute myocardial infarction is very difficult to diagnosis and the usual criteria do not apply. Q waves are often normally present in the anteroseptal leads and cannot be considered pathologic. In addition, ST depression and T wave inversion is commonly seen with LBBB in the absence of acute ischemia. On the other hand, concordant ST segment elevation > 1 mm is an unusual finding in LBBB and is generally considered to be a sign of myocardial injury. (Answer: c)

2. In the setting of LBBB, concordant ST segment depression >1 mm or discordant ST segment elevation in leads V_1-V_3 suggests acute myocardial injury. (Answer: a)

— Quick Review 57 —

LBBB, complete with ST-T waves suggestive of acute myocardial injury or infarction	
• ST elevation ≥ ____ mm concordant to (same direction as) the major deflection of the QRS	1
• ST depression ≥ ____ mm in V_1, V_2, or V_3	1
• ST elevation ≥ ____ mm discordant with (opposite direction to) the major deflection of the QRS	5
ST and/or T wave changes suggesting myocardial injury	
• Acute ST segment (elevation/depression) with upward (convexity/concavity) in the leads representing the area of infarction	elevation convexity
• T waves invert (before/after) ST segments return to baseline	before
• Associated ST (elevation/depression) in the noninfarct leads is common	depression
• Acute ____ wall injury often has horizontal or downsloping ST segment depression with upright T waves in V_1-V_3, with or without a prominent R wave in these same leads	posterior

— POP QUIZ —

Make The Diagnosis

Instructions: Determine the ECG diagnosis that best corresponds to the ECG features listed below (see score sheet for options)

ECG Features	Diagnosis
• Elevated take-off of the ST segment at the J junction • Concave upward ST elevation ending with a symmetrical upright T wave, which is often of large amplitude • Distinct notch or slur on downstroke of R wave • Most commonly involves leads V_2-V_5	Normal variant, early repolarization
• Persistently negative T waves, which are usually not symmetrical or deep, in leads V_1-V_3 in normal adults • Upright T waves in leads I, II, V_5, V_6 • Most frequently seen in young healthy females	Normal variant, juvenile T waves
• Abnormally tall, symmetrical, inverted T waves • Horizontal or downsloping ST segments with or without T wave inversion	ST-T changes of myocardial ischemia
• Acute ST segment elevation with upward convexity in the leads representing the area of infarction • T waves invert before ST segments return to baseline	ST-T changes of myocardial injury

ECG 58. 42-year-old female with scleroderma:

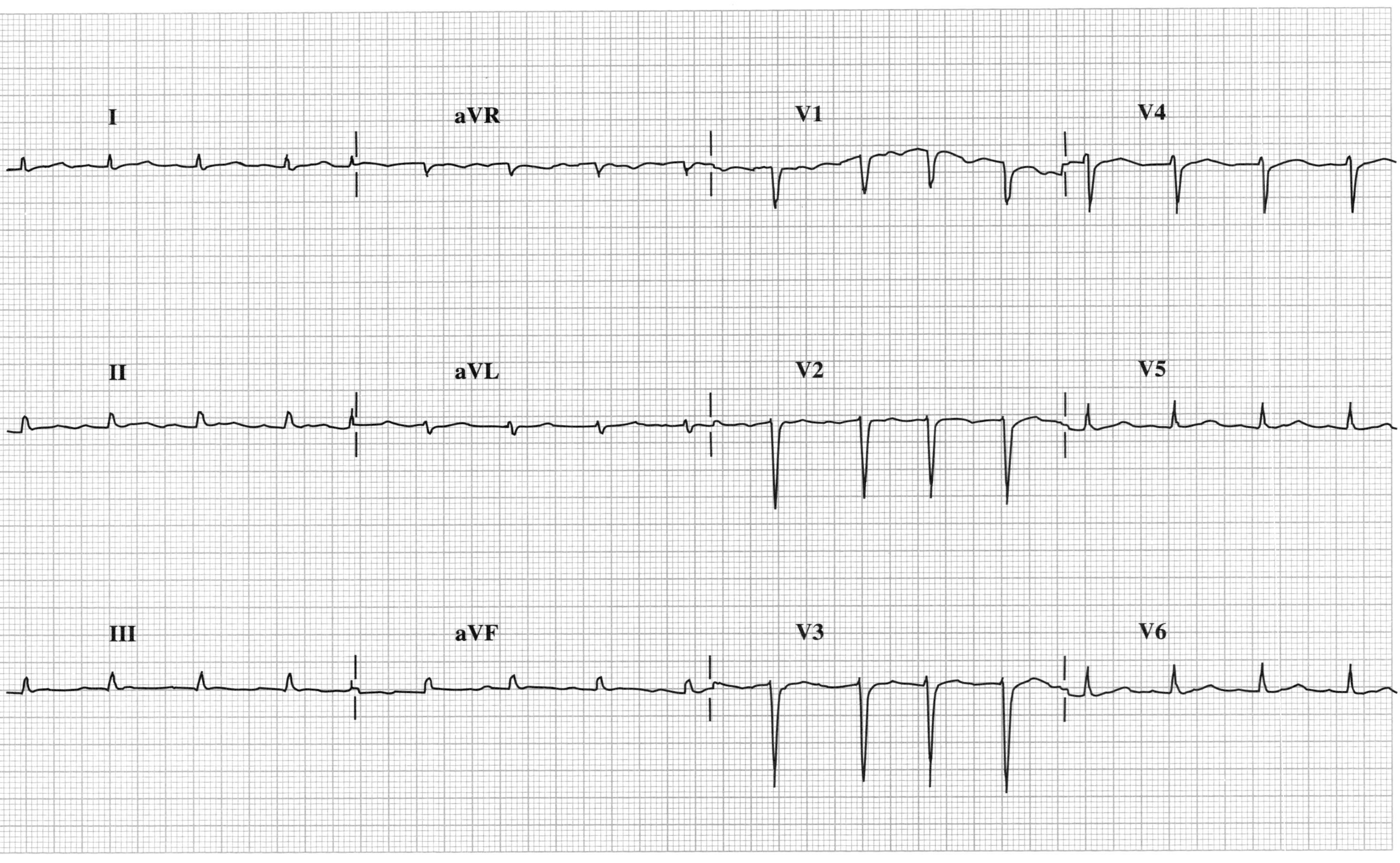

1. GENERAL FEATURES

- ☐ a. Normal ECG
- ☐ b. Borderline normal ECG or normal variant
- ☐ c. Incorrect electrode placement
- ☐ d. Artifact due to tremor

2. ATRIAL RHYTHMS

- ☐ a. Sinus rhythm
- ☐ b. Sinus arrhythmia
- ☐ c. Sinus bradycardia (< 60)
- ☐ d. Sinus tachycardia (> 100)
- ☐ e. Sinus pause or arrest
- ☐ f. Sinoatrial exit block
- ☐ g. Ecoptic atrial rhythm
- ☐ h. Wandering atrial pacemaker
- ☐ i. Atrial premature complexes, normally conducted
- ☐ j. Atrial premature complexes, nonconducted
- ☐ k. Atrial premature complexes with aberrant intraventricular conduction
- ☐ l. Atrial tachycardia (regular, sustained, 1:1 conduction)
- ☐ m. Atrial tachycardia, repetitive (short paroxysms)
- ☐ n. Atrial tachycardia, multifocal
- ☐ o. Atrial tachycardia with AV block
- ☐ p. Supraventricular tachycardia, unspecific
- ☐ q. Supraventricular tachycardia, paroxysmal
- ☐ r. Atrial flutter
- ☐ s. Atrial fibrillation
- ☐ t. Retrograde atrial activation

3. AV JUNCTIONAL RHYTHMS

- ☐ a. AV junctional premature complexes
- ☐ b. AV junctional escape complexes
- ☐ c. AV junctional rhythm, accelerated
- ☐ d. AV junctional rhythm

4. VENTRICULAR RHYTHMS

- ☐ a. Ventricular premature complex(es), uniform, fixed coupling
- ☐ b. Ventricular premature complex(es), uniform, nonfixed coupling
- ☐ c. Ventricular premature complexes(es), multiform
- ☐ d. Ventricular premature complexes, in pairs
- ☐ e. Ventricular parasystole
- ☐ f. Ventricular tachycardia (≥ 3 consecutive complexes)
- ☐ g. Accelerated idioventricular rhythm
- ☐ h. Ventricular escape complexes or rhythm
- ☐ i. Ventricular fibrillation

5. ATRIAL-VENTRICULAR INTERACTIONS IN ARRHYTHMIAS

- ☐ a. Fusion complexes
- ☐ b. Reciprocal (echo) complexes
- ☐ c. Ventricular capture complexes
- ☐ d. AV dissociation
- ☐ e. Ventriculophasic sinus arrhythmia

6. AV CONDUCTION ABNORMALITIES

- ☐ a. AV block, 1°
- ☐ b. AV block, 2° - Mobitz type I (Wenckebach)
- ☐ c. AV block, 2° - Mobitz type II
- ☐ d. AV block, 2:1
- ☐ e. AV block, 3°
- ☐ f. AV block, variable
- ☐ g. Short PR interval (with sinus rhythm and normal QRS duration)
- ☐ h. Wolff-Parkinson-White pattern

7. INTRAVENTRICULAR CONDUCTION DISTURBANCES

- ☐ a. RBBB, incomplete
- ☐ b. RBBB, complete
- ☐ c. Left anterior fascicular block
- ☐ d. Left posterior fascicular block
- ☐ e. LBBB, with ST-T wave suggestive of acute myocardial injury or infarction
- ☐ f. LBBB, complete
- ☐ g. LBBB, intermittent
- ☐ h. Intraventricular conduction disturbance, nonspecific
- ☐ i. Aberrant intraventricular conduction with supraventricular arrhythmia

8. P WAVE ABNORMALITIES

- ☐ a. Right atrial abnormality
- ☐ b. Left atrial abnormalities
- ☐ c. Nonspecific atrial abnormality

9. ABNORMALITIES OF QRS VOLTAGE OR AXIS

- ☐ a. Low voltage, limb leads only
- ☐ b. Low voltage, limb and precordial leads
- ☐ c. Left axis deviation (> - 30%)
- ☐ d. Right axis deviation (> + 100)
- ☐ e. Electrical alternans

10. VENTRICULAR HYPERTROPHY

- ☐ a. LVH by voltage only
- ☐ b. LVH by voltage and ST-T segment abnormalities
- ☐ c. RVH
- ☐ d. Combined ventricular hypertrophy

11. Q WAVE MYOCARDIAL INFARCTION

	Probably Acute or Recent	Probably Old or Age Indeterminate
Anterolateral	☐ a.	☐ g.
Anterior	☐ b.	☐ h.
Anteroseptal	☐ c.	☐ i.
Lateral/High lateral	☐ d.	☐ j.
Inferior	☐ e.	☐ k.
Posterior	☐ f.	☐ l.

- ☐ m. Probably ventricular aneurysm

12. ST, T, U, WAVE ABNORMALITIES

- ☐ a. Normal variant, early repolarization
- ☐ b. Normal variant, juvenile T waves
- ☐ c. Nonspecific ST and/or T wave abnormalities
- ☐ d. ST and/or T wave abnormalities suggesting myocardial ischemia
- ☐ e. ST and/or T wave abnormalities suggesting myocardial injury
- ☐ f. ST and/or T wave abnormalities suggesting acute pericarditis
- ☐ g. ST-T segment abnormalities secondary to intraventricular conduction disturbance or hypertrophy
- ☐ h. Post-extrasystolic T wave abnormality
- ☐ i. Isolated J point depression
- ☐ j. Peaked T waves
- ☐ k. Prolonged QT interval
- ☐ l. Prominent U waves

13. PACEMAKER FUNCTION AND RHYTHM

- ☐ a. Atrial or coronary sinus pacing
- ☐ b. Ventricular demand pacing
- ☐ c. AV sequential pacing
- ☐ d. Ventricular pacing, complete control
- ☐ e. Dual chamber, atrial sensing pacemaker
- ☐ f. Pacemaker malfunction, not constantly capturing (atrium or ventricle)
- ☐ g. Pacemaker malfunction, not constantly sensing (atrium or ventricle)
- ☐ h. Pacemaker malfunction, not firing
- ☐ i. Pacemaker malfunction, slowing

14. SUGGESTED OR PROBABLE CLINICAL DISORDERS

- ☐ a. Digitalis effect
- ☐ b. Digitalis toxicity
- ☐ c. Antiarrhythmic drug effect
- ☐ d. Antiarrhythmic drug toxicity
- ☐ e. Hyperkalemia
- ☐ f. Hypokalemia
- ☐ g. Hypercalcemia
- ☐ h. Hypocalcemia
- ☐ i. Atrial septal defect, secundum
- ☐ j. Atrial septal defect, primum
- ☐ k. Dextrocardia, mirror image
- ☐ l. Mitral valve disease
- ☐ m. Chronic lung disease
- ☐ n. Acute cor pulmonale, including pulmonary embolus
- ☐ o. Pericardial effusion
- ☐ p. Acute pericarditis
- ☐ q. Hypertrophic cardiomyopathy
- ☐ r. Coronary artery disease
- ☐ s. Central nervous system disorder
- ☐ t. Myxedema
- ☐ u. Hypothermia
- ☐ v. Sick sinus syndrome

ECG 58 was obtained from a 42-year-old female with a diagnosis of scleroderma. The ECG shows a sinus tachycardia at approximately 102 beats/minute. Also noted is an APC in the anterior precordial leads (asterisks), low voltage in the limb leads, and subtle electrical alternans in the anterior precordial leads (double asterisk). These findings are consistent with pericardial effusion. This patient was documented to have a moderate sized pericardial effusion felt to be related to her collagen vascular disease.

Codes:

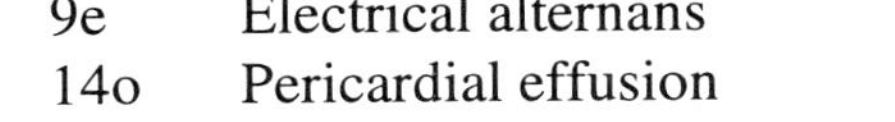

2d	Sinus tachycardia
2i	Atrial premature complexes, normally conducted
9a	Low voltage, limb leads only
9e	Electrical alternans
14o	Pericardial effusion

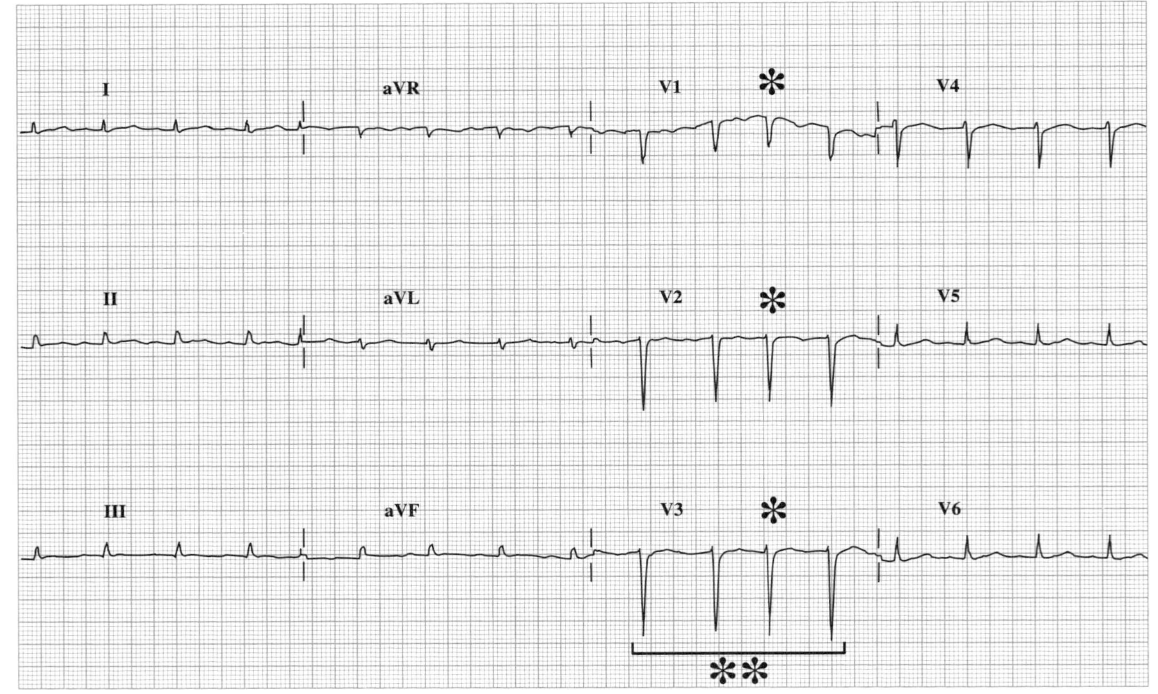

Questions: ECG 58

1. Electrical alternans may be seen with:

   a. Pericardial effusion
   b. Left ventricular hypertrophy
   c. Complete heart block
   d. Ventricular tachycardia

2. Pericardial effusion with threatened tamponade is suggested by:

   a. Electrical alternans
   b. Low QRS voltage
   c. Sinus tachycardia

Answers: ECG 58

1. Electrical alternans (alternation in the amplitude and/or direction of the P, QRS, and/or T waves) is most commonly associated with pericardial effusion, but may be seen in congestive heart failure, hypertensive heart disease, coronary artery disease, rheumatic heart disease, deep respirations, supraventricular tachycardia, and ventricular tachycardia. Electrical alternans is not typically associated with complete heart block. (Answer: a, b, d)

2. Sizeable pericardial effusions electrically "insulate" the heart and result in low QRS voltage on the surface ECG. Electrical alternans, commonly associated with pericardial effusion, is due to swinging of the heart in the pericardial fluid during the cardiac cycle. If the pericardial effusion progresses to cardiac tamponade with overt or pending hemodynamic collapse, sinus tachycardia is almost always present. (Answer: All)

— Quick Review 58 —

Sinus tachycardia (>100)	
• Rate > ____ per minute	100
• P wave amplitude often (increases/decreases) and PR interval often (increases/decreases) with increasing heart rate	increases shortens
Low voltage, limb leads only	
• Amplitude of the entire QRS complex (R+S) < ____ mm in all limb leads	5
Pericardial effusion	
• (High/low) voltage QRS	Low
• Electrical ____, especially if complicated by cardiac ____	alternans tamponade
• Other features of acute ____ may also be present	pericarditis

ECG 59. 82-year-old male with hypertension:

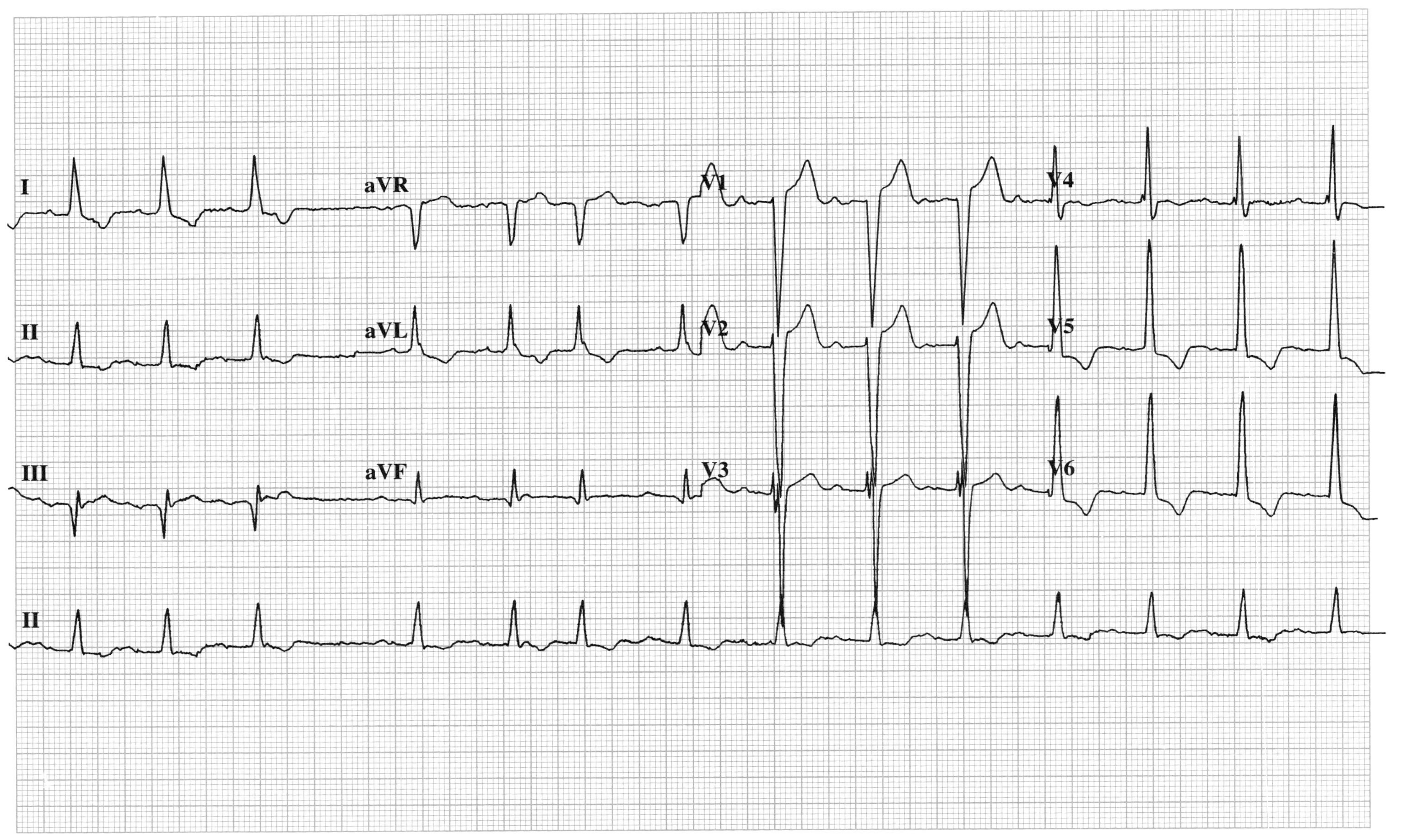

1. GENERAL FEATURES
- ☐ a. Normal ECG
- ☐ b. Borderline normal ECG or normal variant
- ☐ c. Incorrect electrode placement
- ☐ d. Artifact due to tremor

2. ATRIAL RHYTHMS
- ☐ a. Sinus rhythm
- ☐ b. Sinus arrhythmia
- ☐ c. Sinus bradycardia (< 60)
- ☐ d. Sinus tachycardia (> 100)
- ☐ e. Sinus pause or arrest
- ☐ f. Sinoatrial exit block
- ☐ g. Ecoptic atrial rhythm
- ☐ h. Wandering atrial pacemaker
- ☐ i. Atrial premature complexes, normally conducted
- ☐ j. Atrial premature complexes, nonconducted
- ☐ k. Atrial premature complexes with aberrant intraventricular conduction
- ☐ l. Atrial tachycardia (regular, sustained, 1:1 conduction)
- ☐ m. Atrial tachycardia, repetitive (short paroxysms)
- ☐ n. Atrial tachycardia, multifocal
- ☐ o. Atrial tachycardia with AV block
- ☐ p. Supraventricular tachycardia, unspecific
- ☐ q. Supraventricular tachycardia, paroxysmal
- ☐ r. Atrial flutter
- ☐ s. Atrial fibrillation
- ☐ t. Retrograde atrial activation

3. AV JUNCTIONAL RHYTHMS
- ☐ a. AV junctional premature complexes
- ☐ b. AV junctional escape complexes
- ☐ c. AV junctional rhythm, accelerated
- ☐ d. AV junctional rhythm

4. VENTRICULAR RHYTHMS
- ☐ a. Ventricular premature complex(es), uniform, fixed coupling
- ☐ b. Ventricular premature complex(es), uniform, nonfixed coupling
- ☐ c. Ventricular premature complexes(es), multiform
- ☐ d. Ventricular premature complexes, in pairs
- ☐ e. Ventricular parasystole
- ☐ f. Ventricular tachycardia (≥ 3 consecutive complexes)
- ☐ g. Accelerated idioventricular rhythm
- ☐ h. Ventricular escape complexes or rhythm
- ☐ i. Ventricular fibrillation

5. ATRIAL-VENTRICULAR INTERACTIONS IN ARRHYTHMIAS
- ☐ a. Fusion complexes
- ☐ b. Reciprocal (echo) complexes
- ☐ c. Ventricular capture complexes
- ☐ d. AV dissociation
- ☐ e. Ventriculophasic sinus arrhythmia

6. AV CONDUCTION ABNORMALITIES
- ☐ a. AV block, 1°
- ☐ b. AV block, 2° - Mobitz type I (Wenckebach)
- ☐ c. AV block, 2° - Mobitz type II
- ☐ d. AV block, 2:1
- ☐ e. AV block, 3°
- ☐ f. AV block, variable
- ☐ g. Short PR interval (with sinus rhythm and normal QRS duration)
- ☐ h. Wolff-Parkinson-White pattern

7. INTRAVENTRICULAR CONDUCTION DISTURBANCES
- ☐ a. RBBB, incomplete
- ☐ b. RBBB, complete
- ☐ c. Left anterior fascicular block
- ☐ d. Left posterior fascicular block
- ☐ e. LBBB, with ST-T wave suggestive of acute myocardial injury or infarction
- ☐ f. LBBB, complete
- ☐ g. LBBB, intermittent
- ☐ h. Intraventricular conduction disturbance, nonspecific
- ☐ i. Aberrant intraventricular conduction with supraventricular arrhythmia

8. P WAVE ABNORMALITIES
- ☐ a. Right atrial abnormality
- ☐ b. Left atrial abnormalities
- ☐ c. Nonspecific atrial abnormality

9. ABNORMALITIES OF QRS VOLTAGE OR AXIS
- ☐ a. Low voltage, limb leads only
- ☐ b. Low voltage, limb and precordial leads
- ☐ c. Left axis deviation (> - 30%)
- ☐ d. Right axis deviation (> + 100)
- ☐ e. Electrical alternans

10. VENTRICULAR HYPERTROPHY
- ☐ a. LVH by voltage only
- ☐ b. LVH by voltage and ST-T segment abnormalities
- ☐ c. RVH
- ☐ d. Combined ventricular hypertrophy

11. Q WAVE MYOCARDIAL INFARCTION

	Probably Acute or Recent	Probably Old or Age Indeterminate
Anterolateral	☐ a.	☐ g.
Anterior	☐ b.	☐ h.
Anteroseptal	☐ c.	☐ i.
Lateral/High lateral	☐ d.	☐ j.
Inferior	☐ e.	☐ k.
Posterior	☐ f.	☐ l.

☐ m. Probably ventricular aneurysm

12. ST, T, U, WAVE ABNORMALITIES
- ☐ a. Normal variant, early repolarization
- ☐ b. Normal variant, juvenile T waves
- ☐ c. Nonspecific ST and/or T wave abnormalities
- ☐ d. ST and/or T wave abnormalities suggesting myocardial ischemia
- ☐ e. ST and/or T wave abnormalities suggesting myocardial injury
- ☐ f. ST and/or T wave abnormalities suggesting acute pericarditis
- ☐ g. ST-T segment abnormalities secondary to intraventricular conduction disturbance or hypertrophy
- ☐ h. Post-extrasystolic T wave abnormality
- ☐ i. Isolated J point depression
- ☐ j. Peaked T waves
- ☐ k. Prolonged QT interval
- ☐ l. Prominent U waves

13. PACEMAKER FUNCTION AND RHYTHM
- ☐ a. Atrial or coronary sinus pacing
- ☐ b. Ventricular demand pacing
- ☐ c. AV sequential pacing
- ☐ d. Ventricular pacing, complete control
- ☐ e. Dual chamber, atrial sensing pacemaker
- ☐ f. Pacemaker malfunction, not constantly capturing (atrium or ventricle)
- ☐ g. Pacemaker malfunction, not constantly sensing (atrium or ventricle)
- ☐ h. Pacemaker malfunction, not firing
- ☐ i. Pacemaker malfunction, slowing

14. SUGGESTED OR PROBABLE CLINICAL DISORDERS
- ☐ a. Digitalis effect
- ☐ b. Digitalis toxicity
- ☐ c. Antiarrhythmic drug effect
- ☐ d. Antiarrhythmic drug toxicity
- ☐ e. Hyperkalemia
- ☐ f. Hypokalemia
- ☐ g. Hypercalcemia
- ☐ h. Hypocalcemia
- ☐ i. Atrial septal defect, secundum
- ☐ j. Atrial septal defect, primum
- ☐ k. Dextrocardia, mirror image
- ☐ l. Mitral valve disease
- ☐ m. Chronic lung disease
- ☐ n. Acute cor pulmonale, including pulmonary embolus
- ☐ o. Pericardial effusion
- ☐ p. Acute pericarditis
- ☐ q. Hypertrophic cardiomyopathy
- ☐ r. Coronary artery disease
- ☐ s. Central nervous system disorder
- ☐ t. Myxedema
- ☐ u. Hypothermia
- ☐ v. Sick sinus syndrome

ECG 59 was obtained in an 82-year-old male with hypertension. The ECG shows sinus rhythm with a conducted APC (arrow) and a nonconducted APC (arrowhead). First-degree AV block, nonspecific intraventricular conduct defect, and LVH with ST-T abnormalities are also present. Voltage-based criteria for LVH on this tracing include: an R wave in aVL + S wave in $V_3 > 24$ mm; and an S wave in V_1 + R wave in V_5 or $V_6 > 35$ mm.

Codes:

2a	Sinus rhythm
2i	Atrial premature complexes, normally conducted
2j	Atrial premature complexes, nonconducted
6a	AV block, 1°
7h	IVCD, nonspecific type
10b	LVH by both voltage and ST-T segment abnormalities
12g	ST-T segment abnormalities secondary to IVCD or hypertrophy

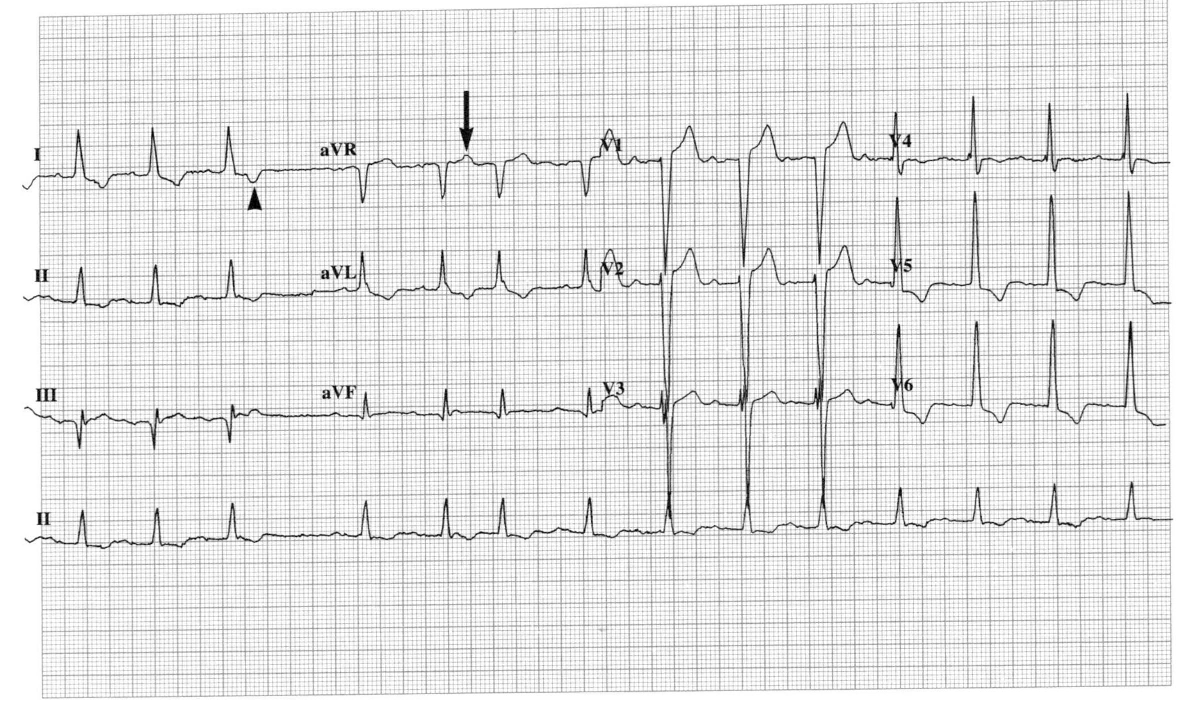

Questions: ECG 59

1. The pause following an atrial premature complex (APC) is typically fully compensatory:

   a. True
   b. False

2. Aberrantly conducted APCs are characterized by:

   a. Initial QRS vector opposite to initial QRS vector of normally conducted beats
   b. Late QRS vector in same direction or opposite to late QRS vector of normally conducted beats
   c. RBBB configuration

Answers: ECG 59

1. The post-APC pause is typically noncompensatory (i.e., the PP interval containing the APC is less than twice the basic PP interval). In contrast, the post-VPC pause is typically fully compensatory (i.e., the PP interval containing the VPC is twice the basic PP interval). (Answer: b)

2. Aberrant conduction of atrial premature complexes typically manifests as variable widening or distortion of the normal QRS. The initial QRS vector is in the same direction as the normally-conducted beats, while the more terminal portion of the QRS may be in a different vector. Aberrantly conducted APCs often display an RBBB configuration; the longer refractory period of the right bundle (compared to the left bundle) increases the likelihood that an APC will conduct down the left bundle while the right bundle is still refractory. (Answer: b, c)

— Quick Review 59 —

LVH by voltage only	
Cornell Criteria (most accurate): R wave in aVL + S wave in V_3 > ____ mm in males or > ____ mm in females	24, 20
• **Other commonly used voltage-based criteria**	
▸ Precordial leads (one or more)	
(1) R wave in V_5 or V_6 + S wave in V_1	
▸ > ____ mm if age > 30 years	35
▸ > ____ mm if age 20-30 years	40
▸ > ____ mm if age 16-19 years	60
(2) Maximum R wave + S wave in precordial leads > ____ mm	45
(3) R wave in V_5 > ____ mm	26
(4) R wave in V_6 > ____ mm	20
▸ Limb leads (one or more)	
(1) R wave in lead I + S wave in lead II ≥ ____ mm	26
(2) R wave in lead I ≥ ____ mm	14
(3) S wave in aVR ≥ ____ mm	15
(4) R wave in aVL ≥ ____ mm	12
(5) R wave in aVF ≥ ____ mm	21
• **Non-voltage related criteria for LVH**	
▸ (Left/right) atrial abnormality	left
▸ (Left/right) axis deviation	left
▸ Onset of intrinsicoid deflection > ____ seconds	0.05
▸ Small or absent R waves in leads ____	V_1-V_3
▸ Absent ____ waves in leads I, V_5, V_6	Q
▸ Abnormal ____ waves in leads II, III, aVF	Q
▸ Prominent ____ waves, especially in leads with large R and T waves	U
▸ R wave amplitude in V_6 (greater than/less than) V_5, provided there are dominant R waves in these leads	greater than

— Quick Review 59 —

ST and/or T wave changes secondary to IVCD or hypertrophy	
• ***LVH:*** ST (elevation/depression) & T wave inversion when QRS is mainly positive (leads ___); subtle ST (elevation/depression) & upright T waves when the QRS is mainly negative (leads V_1, V_2)	depression I, V_5, V_6 elevation
• ***RVH:*** ST segment depression & T wave inversion in leads ____ and sometimes in leads II, III, aVF	V_1-V_3
• ***LBBB:*** ST segment & T wave displacement (opposite to/ in same direction as) the major QRS deflection	opposite to
• ***RBBB:*** Uncomplicated RBBB has little ST displacement (true/false). T wave vector is (opposite to/in same direction as) the terminal slurred portion of the QRS	true opposite to

Don't Get Confused!

Multifocal Atrial Tachycardia

Atrial rate >100 per minute; P waves with ≥ 3 morphologies; varying PR, RR and RP intervals

***May be confused with*:**

Sinus tachycardia with multifocal APCs

Demonstrates one dominant atrial pacemaker (i.e., the sinus node). In contrast, in multifocal atrial tachycardia, *no* dominant atrial pacemaker (i.e., no dominant P wave morphology) is present.

Atrial fibrillation/flutter

Atrial fibrillation/flutter lacks an isoelectric baseline. In contrast, multifocal atrial tachycardia demonstrates a distinct isoelectric baseline and P waves.

ECG 60. 64-year-old female with recurrent syncope:

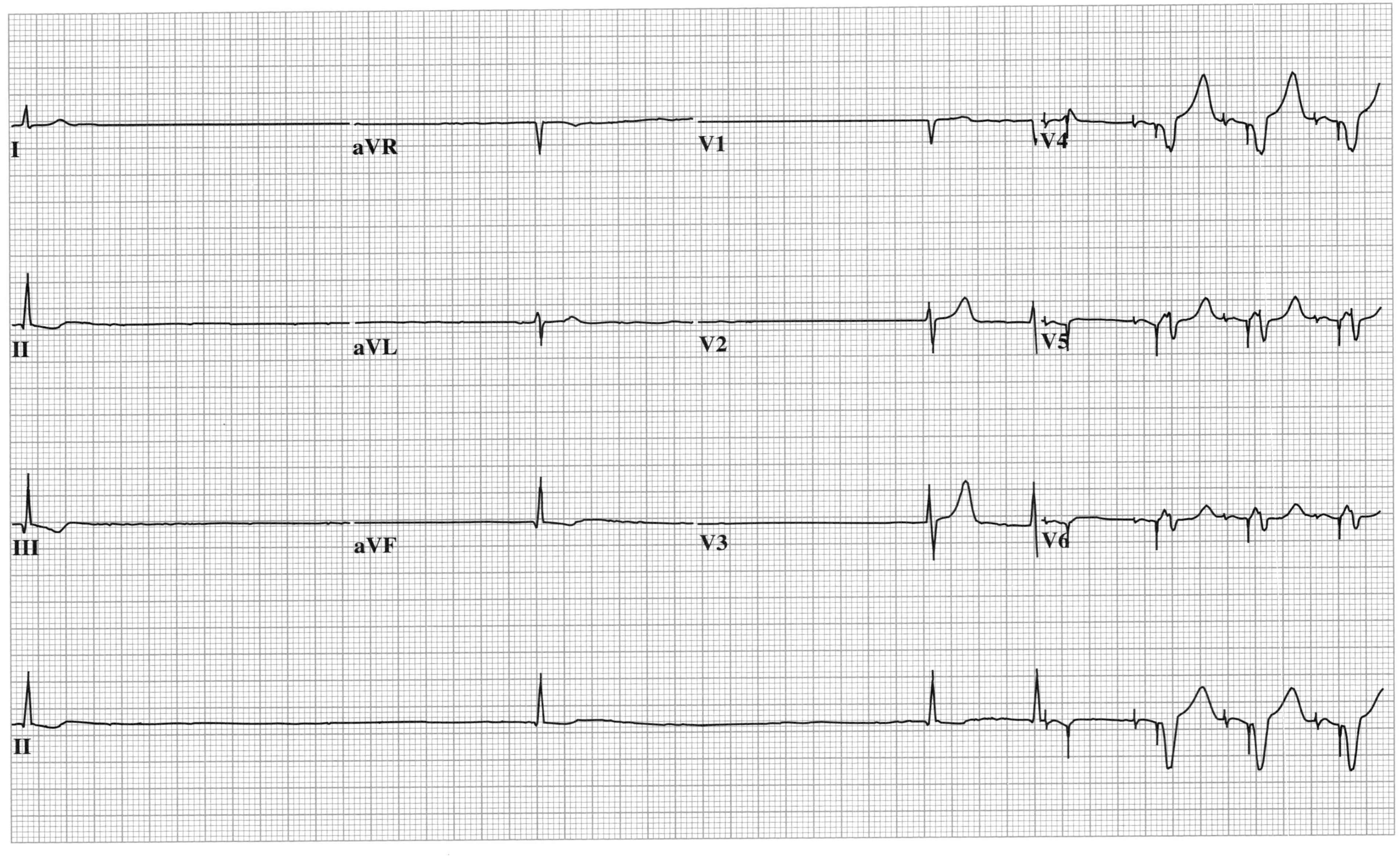

1. GENERAL FEATURES
- ☐ a. Normal ECG
- ☐ b. Borderline normal ECG or normal variant
- ☐ c. Incorrect electrode placement
- ☐ d. Artifact due to tremor

2. ATRIAL RHYTHMS
- ☐ a. Sinus rhythm
- ☐ b. Sinus arrhythmia
- ☐ c. Sinus bradycardia (< 60)
- ☐ d. Sinus tachycardia (> 100)
- ☐ e. Sinus pause or arrest
- ☐ f. Sinoatrial exit block
- ☐ g. Ecoptic atrial rhythm
- ☐ h. Wandering atrial pacemaker
- ☐ i. Atrial premature complexes, normally conducted
- ☐ j. Atrial premature complexes, nonconducted
- ☐ k. Atrial premature complexes with aberrant intraventricular conduction
- ☐ l. Atrial tachycardia (regular, sustained, 1:1 conduction)
- ☐ m. Atrial tachycardia, repetitive (short paroxysms)
- ☐ n. Atrial tachycardia, multifocal
- ☐ o. Atrial tachycardia with AV block
- ☐ p. Supraventricular tachycardia, unspecific
- ☐ q. Supraventricular tachycardia, paroxysmal
- ☐ r. Atrial flutter
- ☐ s. Atrial fibrillation
- ☐ t. Retrograde atrial activation

3. AV JUNCTIONAL RHYTHMS
- ☐ a. AV junctional premature complexes
- ☐ b. AV junctional escape complexes
- ☐ c. AV junctional rhythm, accelerated
- ☐ d. AV junctional rhythm

4. VENTRICULAR RHYTHMS
- ☐ a. Ventricular premature complex(es), uniform, fixed coupling
- ☐ b. Ventricular premature complex(es), uniform, nonfixed coupling
- ☐ c. Ventricular premature complexes(es), multiform
- ☐ d. Ventricular premature complexes, in pairs
- ☐ e. Ventricular parasystole
- ☐ f. Ventricular tachycardia (≥ 3 consecutive complexes)
- ☐ g. Accelerated idioventricular rhythm
- ☐ h. Ventricular escape complexes or rhythm
- ☐ i. Ventricular fibrillation

5. ATRIAL-VENTRICULAR INTERACTIONS IN ARRHYTHMIAS
- ☐ a. Fusion complexes
- ☐ b. Reciprocal (echo) complexes
- ☐ c. Ventricular capture complexes
- ☐ d. AV dissociation
- ☐ e. Ventriculophasic sinus arrhythmia

6. AV CONDUCTION ABNORMALITIES
- ☐ a. AV block, 1°
- ☐ b. AV block, 2° - Mobitz type I (Wenckebach)
- ☐ c. AV block, 2° - Mobitz type II
- ☐ d. AV block, 2:1
- ☐ e. AV block, 3°
- ☐ f. AV block, variable
- ☐ g. Short PR interval (with sinus rhythm and normal QRS duration)
- ☐ h. Wolff-Parkinson-White pattern

7. INTRAVENTRICULAR CONDUCTION DISTURBANCES
- ☐ a. RBBB, incomplete
- ☐ b. RBBB, complete
- ☐ c. Left anterior fascicular block
- ☐ d. Left posterior fascicular block
- ☐ e. LBBB, with ST-T wave suggestive of acute myocardial injury or infarction
- ☐ f. LBBB, complete
- ☐ g. LBBB, intermittent
- ☐ h. Intraventricular conduction disturbance, nonspecific
- ☐ i. Aberrant intraventricular conduction with supraventricular arrhythmia

8. P WAVE ABNORMALITIES
- ☐ a. Right atrial abnormality
- ☐ b. Left atrial abnormalities
- ☐ c. Nonspecific atrial abnormality

9. ABNORMALITIES OF QRS VOLTAGE OR AXIS
- ☐ a. Low voltage, limb leads only
- ☐ b. Low voltage, limb and precordial leads
- ☐ c. Left axis deviation (> - 30%)
- ☐ d. Right axis deviation (> + 100)
- ☐ e. Electrical alternans

10. VENTRICULAR HYPERTROPHY
- ☐ a. LVH by voltage only
- ☐ b. LVH by voltage and ST-T segment abnormalities
- ☐ c. RVH
- ☐ d. Combined ventricular hypertrophy

11. Q WAVE MYOCARDIAL INFARCTION

	Probably Acute or Recent	Probably Old or Age Indeterminate
Anterolateral	☐ a.	☐ g.
Anterior	☐ b.	☐ h.
Anteroseptal	☐ c.	☐ i.
Lateral/High lateral	☐ d.	☐ j.
Inferior	☐ e.	☐ k.
Posterior	☐ f.	☐ l.

☐ m. Probably ventricular aneurysm

12. ST, T, U, WAVE ABNORMALITIES
- ☐ a. Normal variant, early repolarization
- ☐ b. Normal variant, juvenile T waves
- ☐ c. Nonspecific ST and/or T wave abnormalities
- ☐ d. ST and/or T wave abnormalities suggesting myocardial ischemia
- ☐ e. ST and/or T wave abnormalities suggesting myocardial injury
- ☐ f. ST and/or T wave abnormalities suggesting acute pericarditis
- ☐ g. ST-T segment abnormalities secondary to intraventricular conduction disturbance or hypertrophy
- ☐ h. Post-extrasystolic T wave abnormality
- ☐ i. Isolated J point depression
- ☐ j. Peaked T waves
- ☐ k. Prolonged QT interval
- ☐ l. Prominent U waves

13. PACEMAKER FUNCTION AND RHYTHM
- ☐ a. Atrial or coronary sinus pacing
- ☐ b. Ventricular demand pacing
- ☐ c. AV sequential pacing
- ☐ d. Ventricular pacing, complete control
- ☐ e. Dual chamber, atrial sensing pacemaker
- ☐ f. Pacemaker malfunction, not constantly capturing (atrium or ventricle)
- ☐ g. Pacemaker malfunction, not constantly sensing (atrium or ventricle)
- ☐ h. Pacemaker malfunction, not firing
- ☐ i. Pacemaker malfunction, slowing

14. SUGGESTED OR PROBABLE CLINICAL DISORDERS
- ☐ a. Digitalis effect
- ☐ b. Digitalis toxicity
- ☐ c. Antiarrhythmic drug effect
- ☐ d. Antiarrhythmic drug toxicity
- ☐ e. Hyperkalemia
- ☐ f. Hypokalemia
- ☐ g. Hypercalcemia
- ☐ h. Hypocalcemia
- ☐ i. Atrial septal defect, secundum
- ☐ j. Atrial septal defect, primum
- ☐ k. Dextrocardia, mirror image
- ☐ l. Mitral valve disease
- ☐ m. Chronic lung disease
- ☐ n. Acute cor pulmonale, including pulmonary embolus
- ☐ o. Pericardial effusion
- ☐ p. Acute pericarditis
- ☐ q. Hypertrophic cardiomyopathy
- ☐ r. Coronary artery disease
- ☐ s. Central nervous system disorder
- ☐ t. Myxedema
- ☐ u. Hypothermia
- ☐ v. Sick sinus syndrome

ECG 60 was obtained in a 64-year-old female with recurrent syncope. The ECG shows sinus arrest (asterisk) with junctional escape complexes (arrows). Near the end of the tracing is a normally conducted junctional premature beat (arrowhead), which is followed immediately by output from an AV sequential pacemaker (double asterisk). The pacemaker fails to sense the premature beat, fails to capture the ventricle the first time it fires (since the myocardium has not yet repolarized), and fails to fire during the sinus arrest. Thus, pacemaker malfunction is noted, both with respect to undersensing and oversensing. The sinus arrest is suggestive of sick sinus syndrome.

Codes:

2e	Sinus pause or arrest
3a	AV junctional premature complexes
3b	AV junctional escape complexes
13c	AV sequential pacing
13g	Pacemaker malfunction, not constantly sensing (atrium or ventricle)
13h	Pacemaker malfunction, not firing
14v	Sick sinus syndrome

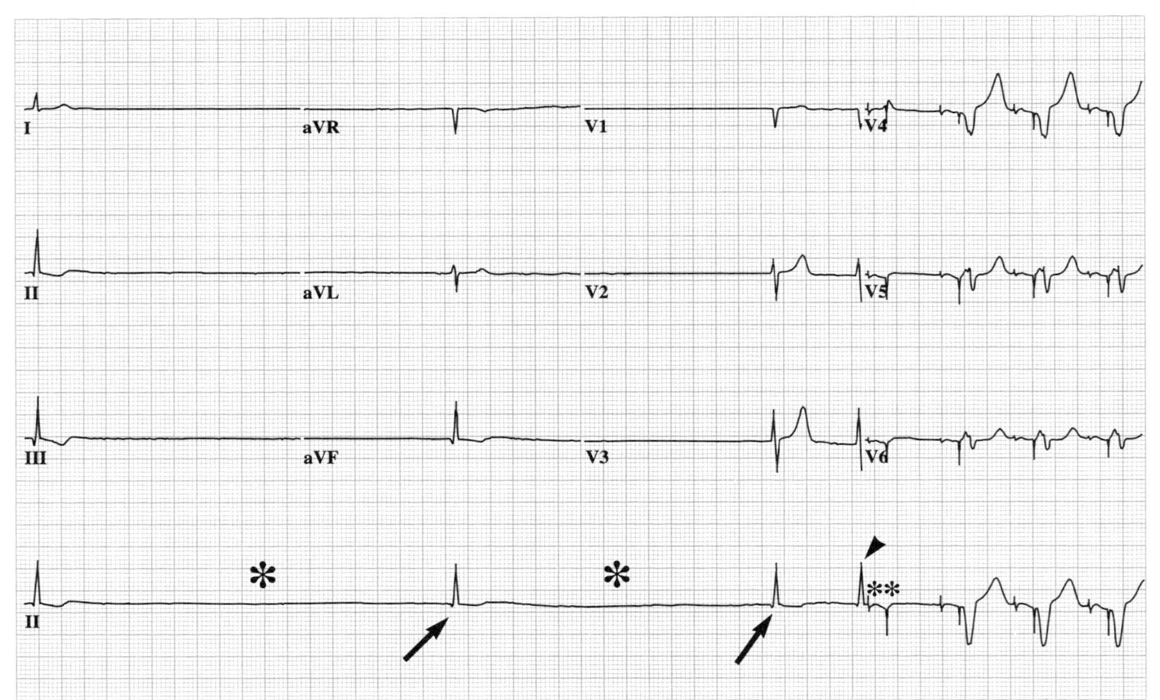

Questions: ECG 60

1. Abnormal sensing with a ventricular pacemaker can be diagnosed when:

   a. A ventricular premature complex falls within the programmed refractory period of the pacemaker
   b. A pacemaker stimulus occurs within the QRS complex
   c. A pacemaker stimulus does not result in appropriate capture
   d. The ventricular pacemaker fails to be inhibited by a QRS complex falling in an appropriate range

Answers: ECG 60

1. Pacemaker sensing malfunction can involve the atrium and/or the ventricle. For a pacemaker in the inhibited mode, failure to sense is manifest as inappropriate pacing after a complex that fell in a range that would normally inhibit pacemaker output. For a pacemaker in the triggered mode (e.g., DDD), failure to sense is manifest as failure to trigger appropriately following a native event (such as a P wave). If premature depolarizations fall within the programmed refractory period of the pacemaker they will not be sensed. Any pacemaker spike falling within the QRS complex generally does not represent sensing malfunction. A pacemaker stimulus that does not depolarize the chamber is defined as a capture malfunction rather than a sensing malfunction. Failure to sense occurs when pacemaker timing is not reset by an intrinsic or ectopic beat, resulting in asynchronous firing of the pacemaker (i.e., paced rhythm competes with the intrinsic rhythm); this occurs with low amplitude signals (especially VPCs), inappropriate programming of the sensitivity, and all causes of failure to capture. Failure to sense can often be corrected by reprogramming the sensitivity of the pacemaker. (Answer: d)

— Quick Review 60 —

Sinus pause or arrest	
• PP interval > _____ seconds	1.6-2.0
• Resumption of sinus rhythm at a PP interval that (is/is not) a multiple of the basic sinus PP interval	is not
• If sinus rhythm resumes at a multiple of the basic PP, consider _____	sinoatrial exit block
AV sequential pacing	
• Atrial followed by ____ pacing	ventricular
Pacemaker malfunction, not constantly sensing (atrium or ventricle)	
• Pacemakers in the inhibited mode: Pacemaker fails to be ____ by an appropriate intrinsic depolarization	inhibited
• Pacemakers in the triggered mode: Pacemaker fails to be ____ by an appropriate intrinsic depolarization	triggered
• Premature depolarizations may not be sensed if they fall within the programmed ____ period of the pacemaker, *or* have insufficient ____ at the sensing electrode site	refractory amplitude

Common Dilemmas in ECG Interpretation

Problem

Mobitz Type I second-degree AV block is present. Should first-degree AV block also be coded if the PR interval exceeds 0.20 seconds?

Recommendation

Not necessarily. Mobitz Type I second-degree AV block (Wenckebach) can occur with or without first-degree AV block. If the ***shortest*** PR interval — usually the first PR interval after a nonconducted P wave — exceeds 0.20 seconds, first-degree AV block (item 6a) should be coded..

ECG 61. 67-year-old female with hypertension:

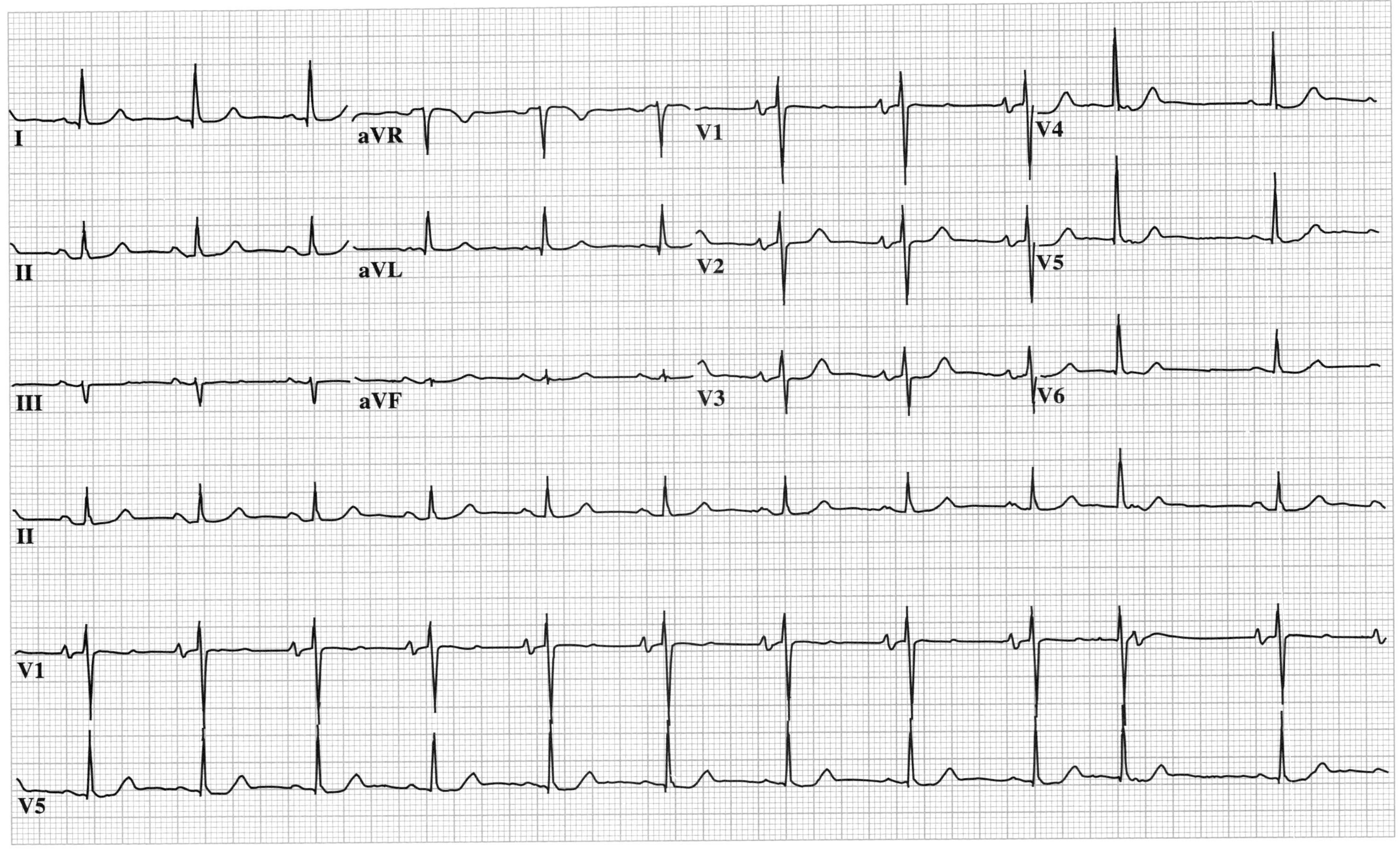

1. GENERAL FEATURES
- ☐ a. Normal ECG
- ☐ b. Borderline normal ECG or normal variant
- ☐ c. Incorrect electrode placement
- ☐ d. Artifact due to tremor

2. ATRIAL RHYTHMS
- ☐ a. Sinus rhythm
- ☐ b. Sinus arrhythmia
- ☐ c. Sinus bradycardia (< 60)
- ☐ d. Sinus tachycardia (> 100)
- ☐ e. Sinus pause or arrest
- ☐ f. Sinoatrial exit block
- ☐ g. Ecoptic atrial rhythm
- ☐ h. Wandering atrial pacemaker
- ☐ i. Atrial premature complexes, normally conducted
- ☐ j. Atrial premature complexes, nonconducted
- ☐ k. Atrial premature complexes with aberrant intraventricular conduction
- ☐ l. Atrial tachycardia (regular, sustained, 1:1 conduction)
- ☐ m. Atrial tachycardia, repetitive (short paroxysms)
- ☐ n. Atrial tachycardia, multifocal
- ☐ o. Atrial tachycardia with AV block
- ☐ p. Supraventricular tachycardia, unspecific
- ☐ q. Supraventricular tachycardia, paroxysmal
- ☐ r. Atrial flutter
- ☐ s. Atrial fibrillation
- ☐ t. Retrograde atrial activation

3. AV JUNCTIONAL RHYTHMS
- ☐ a. AV junctional premature complexes
- ☐ b. AV junctional escape complexes
- ☐ c. AV junctional rhythm, accelerated
- ☐ d. AV junctional rhythm

4. VENTRICULAR RHYTHMS
- ☐ a. Ventricular premature complex(es), uniform, fixed coupling
- ☐ b. Ventricular premature complex(es), uniform, nonfixed coupling
- ☐ c. Ventricular premature complexes(es), multiform
- ☐ d. Ventricular premature complexes, in pairs
- ☐ e. Ventricular parasystole
- ☐ f. Ventricular tachycardia (≥ 3 consecutive complexes)
- ☐ g. Accelerated idioventricular rhythm
- ☐ h. Ventricular escape complexes or rhythm
- ☐ i. Ventricular fibrillation

5. ATRIAL-VENTRICULAR INTERACTIONS IN ARRHYTHMIAS
- ☐ a. Fusion complexes
- ☐ b. Reciprocal (echo) complexes
- ☐ c. Ventricular capture complexes
- ☐ d. AV dissociation
- ☐ e. Ventriculophasic sinus arrhythmia

6. AV CONDUCTION ABNORMALITIES
- ☐ a. AV block, 1°
- ☐ b. AV block, 2° - Mobitz type I (Wenckebach)
- ☐ c. AV block, 2° - Mobitz type II
- ☐ d. AV block, 2:1
- ☐ e. AV block, 3°
- ☐ f. AV block, variable
- ☐ g. Short PR interval (with sinus rhythm and normal QRS duration)
- ☐ h. Wolff-Parkinson-White pattern

7. INTRAVENTRICULAR CONDUCTION DISTURBANCES
- ☐ a. RBBB, incomplete
- ☐ b. RBBB, complete
- ☐ c. Left anterior fascicular block
- ☐ d. Left posterior fascicular block
- ☐ e. LBBB, with ST-T wave suggestive of acute myocardial injury or infarction
- ☐ f. LBBB, complete
- ☐ g. LBBB, intermittent
- ☐ h. Intraventricular conduction disturbance, nonspecific
- ☐ i. Aberrant intraventricular conduction with supraventricular arrhythmia

8. P WAVE ABNORMALITIES
- ☐ a. Right atrial abnormality
- ☐ b. Left atrial abnormalities
- ☐ c. Nonspecific atrial abnormality

9. ABNORMALITIES OF QRS VOLTAGE OR AXIS
- ☐ a. Low voltage, limb leads only
- ☐ b. Low voltage, limb and precordial leads
- ☐ c. Left axis deviation (> - 30%)
- ☐ d. Right axis deviation (> + 100)
- ☐ e. Electrical alternans

10. VENTRICULAR HYPERTROPHY
- ☐ a. LVH by voltage only
- ☐ b. LVH by voltage and ST-T segment abnormalities
- ☐ c. RVH
- ☐ d. Combined ventricular hypertrophy

11. Q WAVE MYOCARDIAL INFARCTION

	Probably Acute or Recent	Probably Old or Age Indeterminate
Anterolateral	☐ a.	☐ g.
Anterior	☐ b.	☐ h.
Anteroseptal	☐ c.	☐ i.
Lateral/High lateral	☐ d.	☐ j.
Inferior	☐ e.	☐ k.
Posterior	☐ f.	☐ l.

☐ m. Probably ventricular aneurysm

12. ST, T, U, WAVE ABNORMALITIES
- ☐ a. Normal variant, early repolarization
- ☐ b. Normal variant, juvenile T waves
- ☐ c. Nonspecific ST and/or T wave abnormalities
- ☐ d. ST and/or T wave abnormalities suggesting myocardial ischemia
- ☐ e. ST and/or T wave abnormalities suggesting myocardial injury
- ☐ f. ST and/or T wave abnormalities suggesting acute pericarditis
- ☐ g. ST-T segment abnormalities secondary to intraventricular conduction disturbance or hypertrophy
- ☐ h. Post-extrasystolic T wave abnormality
- ☐ i. Isolated J point depression
- ☐ j. Peaked T waves
- ☐ k. Prolonged QT interval
- ☐ l. Prominent U waves

13. PACEMAKER FUNCTION AND RHYTHM
- ☐ a. Atrial or coronary sinus pacing
- ☐ b. Ventricular demand pacing
- ☐ c. AV sequential pacing
- ☐ d. Ventricular pacing, complete control
- ☐ e. Dual chamber, atrial sensing pacemaker
- ☐ f. Pacemaker malfunction, not constantly capturing (atrium or ventricle)
- ☐ g. Pacemaker malfunction, not constantly sensing (atrium or ventricle)
- ☐ h. Pacemaker malfunction, not firing
- ☐ i. Pacemaker malfunction, slowing

14. SUGGESTED OR PROBABLE CLINICAL DISORDERS
- ☐ a. Digitalis effect
- ☐ b. Digitalis toxicity
- ☐ c. Antiarrhythmic drug effect
- ☐ d. Antiarrhythmic drug toxicity
- ☐ e. Hyperkalemia
- ☐ f. Hypokalemia
- ☐ g. Hypercalcemia
- ☐ h. Hypocalcemia
- ☐ i. Atrial septal defect, secundum
- ☐ j. Atrial septal defect, primum
- ☐ k. Dextrocardia, mirror image
- ☐ l. Mitral valve disease
- ☐ m. Chronic lung disease
- ☐ n. Acute cor pulmonale, including pulmonary embolus
- ☐ o. Pericardial effusion
- ☐ p. Acute pericarditis
- ☐ q. Hypertrophic cardiomyopathy
- ☐ r. Coronary artery disease
- ☐ s. Central nervous system disorder
- ☐ t. Myxedema
- ☐ u. Hypothermia
- ☐ v. Sick sinus syndrome

ECG 61 was obtained in this 67-year-old female with hypertension. The ECG shows sinus rhythm with right atrial abnormality (arrowhead marks positive deflection of P wave > 1.5 mm in V_1), left atrial abnormality (arrow marks prominent negative deflection of P wave in V_1), and nonspecific ST-T wave changes. The 10th QRS complex (asterisk) is a junctional premature complex — it appears early, is not preceded by a P wave, has normal morphology, and does not disrupt the sinus rhythm (so the PP interval remains constant). The atrium was activated by the sinus node and not retrogradely by the junction, suggesting retrograde conduction block between the junctional focus and the atrium.

Codes:

2a	Sinus rhythm
3a	AV junctional premature complexes
8a	Right atrial abnormality
8b	Left atrial abnormality
12c	Nonspecific ST and/or T wave abnormalities

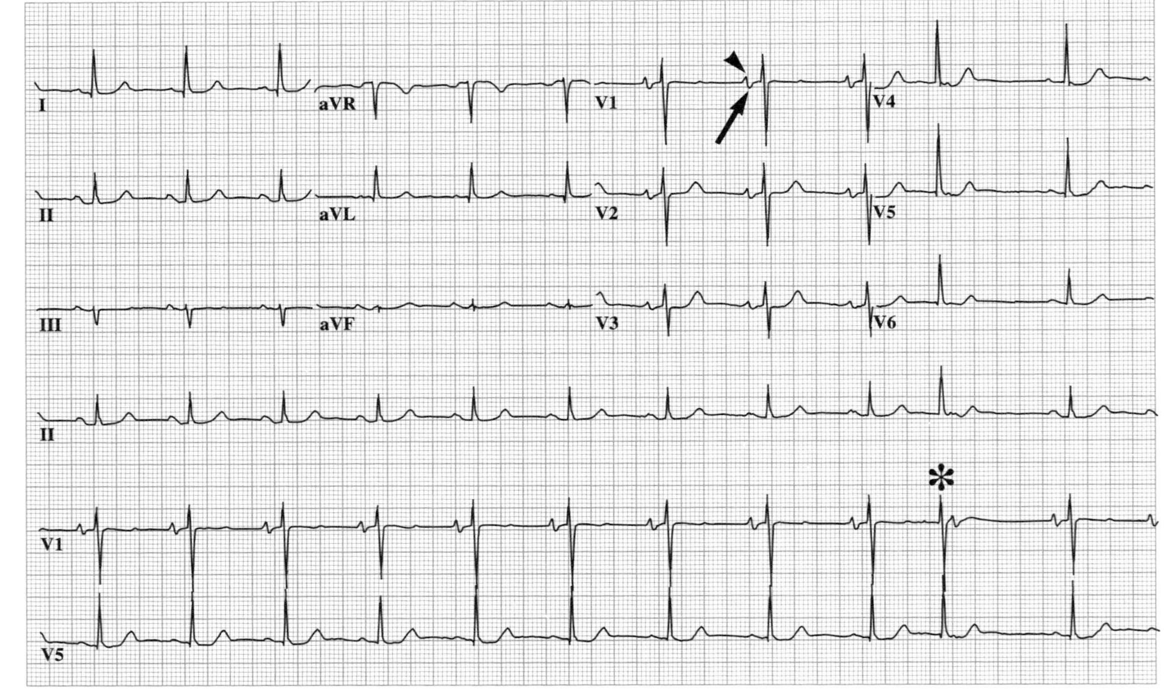

Questions: ECG 61

1. Which of the following statements about the P wave of an AV junctional premature complex are true:

    a. Can precede the QRS by 0.11 seconds or less
    b. Can follow the QRS complex
    c. Can be superimposed on the QRS complex
    d. Is inverted in leads II, III, and aVF
    e. Is upright in leads I and aVL
    f. Has normal morphology if retrograde ventriculo-atrial block is present

2. Junctional premature complexes are distinguished from junctional escape complexes by:

    a. The presence of retrograde atrial activation with junctional premature but not escape complexes
    b. Junctional premature complexes occur early in the cycle

Answers: ECG 61

1. A premature junctional complex occurs in the region of the AV node and His bundle, then spreads retrograde to the atrium and antegrade to the ventricle. The retrograde activation of the atrium results in a P wave that can precede the QRS by 0.11 seconds or less, follow the QRS, or be superimposed on the QRS. Since the P wave originates in the region of the AV node (rather than the sinus node), the spread of atrial activation is away from (rather than towards) leads II, III, and aVF, resulting in inverted (rather than upright) P waves in these leads. Since atrial activation also spreads toward the left side of the heart, upright P waves in the lateral leads (I and aVL) are also evident. The P wave morphology will resemble that of sinus rhythm if the AV junctional impulse cannot activate the atrium due to retrograde block (as in the present case), or the sinus node activates the atrium before the AV junctional impulse. (Answer: All)

2. Junctional premature complexes occur early in the cycle whereas escape complexes do not (hence the term "premature"). Both junctional premature complexes and junctional escape complexes can activate the atrium in a retrograde fashion to result in P waves that are inverted in leads II, III and aVF, and upright in leads I and aVL. (Answer: b)

— Quick Review 61 —

AV junctional premature complexes	
• Premature ____ complex (relative to the basic RR interval), which may be narrow or aberrant	QRS
• Inverted P waves in leads ____ and upright P waves in leads ____ are common	II, III, aVF I, aVL
• The P wave may precede, be buried in, or follow the QRS complex (true/false)	true
• A (fixed/nonfixed) coupling interval and (compensatory/noncompensatory) pause are common	fixed non-compensatory
Right atrial abnormality	
• Upright P wave > ____ mm in leads II, III and aVF *or* > ____ mm in leads V_1 or V_2	2.5 1.5
• P wave axis ≥ ____ degrees	70
Left atrial abnormality	
• Notched P wave with a duration ≥ ____ seconds in leads II, III or aVF, *or*	0.12
• Terminal negative portion of the P wave in lead V_1 ≥ 1 mm deep and ≥ ____ seconds in duration	0.04

— POP QUIZ —

Make The Diagnosis

Instructions: Determine the ECG diagnosis that best corresponds to the ECG features listed below (see score sheet for options)

ECG Features	Diagnosis
• Pacemaker stimulus followed by an atrial depolarization	Atrial pacing
• Pacemaker stimulus followed by a QRS complex that has different morphology compared to the intrinsic QRS • Must demonstrate inhibition of pacemaker output in response to intrinsic QRS	Ventricular demand pacing
• Atrial followed by ventricular pacing	AV sequential pacing
• Ventricular pacing without demonstrable output inhibition by intrinsic QRS complexes	Ventricular pacing, fixed rate, asynchronous
• Increase in stimulus intervals over the programmed intervals • Usually an indicator of battery end of life • Often noted first during magnet application	Pacemaker malfunction, slowing

ECG 62. 76-year-old male with a history of coronary artery bypass graft surgery:

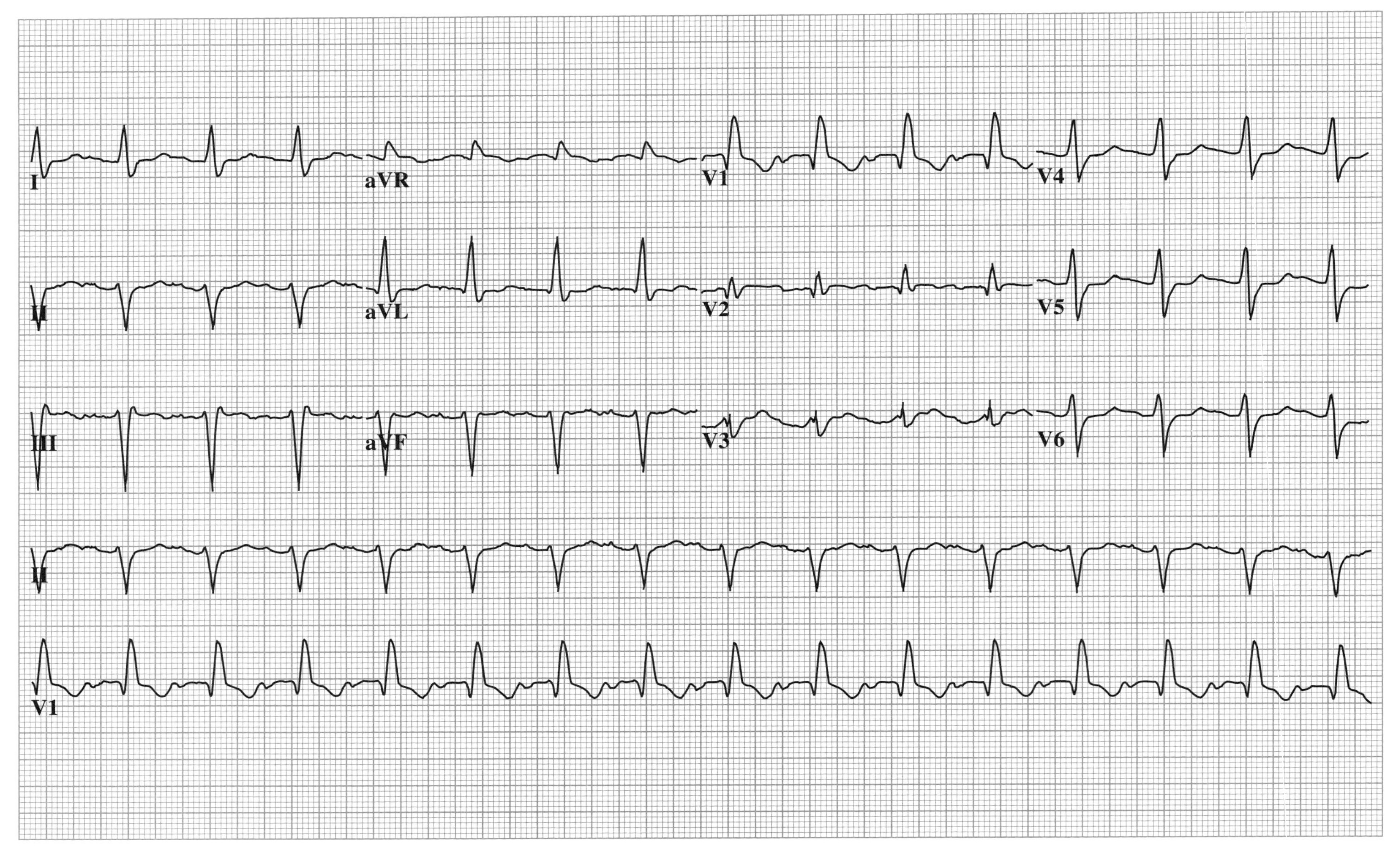

1. GENERAL FEATURES

- ☐ a. Normal ECG
- ☐ b. Borderline normal ECG or normal variant
- ☐ c. Incorrect electrode placement
- ☐ d. Artifact due to tremor

2. ATRIAL RHYTHMS

- ☐ a. Sinus rhythm
- ☐ b. Sinus arrhythmia
- ☐ c. Sinus bradycardia (< 60)
- ☐ d. Sinus tachycardia (> 100)
- ☐ e. Sinus pause or arrest
- ☐ f. Sinoatrial exit block
- ☐ g. Ecoptic atrial rhythm
- ☐ h. Wandering atrial pacemaker
- ☐ i. Atrial premature complexes, normally conducted
- ☐ j. Atrial premature complexes, nonconducted
- ☐ k. Atrial premature complexes with aberrant intraventricular conduction
- ☐ l. Atrial tachycardia (regular, sustained, 1:1 conduction)
- ☐ m. Atrial tachycardia, repetitive (short paroxysms)
- ☐ n. Atrial tachycardia, multifocal
- ☐ o. Atrial tachycardia with AV block
- ☐ p. Supraventricular tachycardia, unspecific
- ☐ q. Supraventricular tachycardia, paroxysmal
- ☐ r. Atrial flutter
- ☐ s. Atrial fibrillation
- ☐ t. Retrograde atrial activation

3. AV JUNCTIONAL RHYTHMS

- ☐ a. AV junctional premature complexes
- ☐ b. AV junctional escape complexes
- ☐ c. AV junctional rhythm, accelerated
- ☐ d. AV junctional rhythm

4. VENTRICULAR RHYTHMS

- ☐ a. Ventricular premature complex(es), uniform, fixed coupling
- ☐ b. Ventricular premature complex(es), uniform, nonfixed coupling
- ☐ c. Ventricular premature complexes(es), multiform
- ☐ d. Ventricular premature complexes, in pairs
- ☐ e. Ventricular parasystole
- ☐ f. Ventricular tachycardia (≥ 3 consecutive complexes)
- ☐ g. Accelerated idioventricular rhythm
- ☐ h. Ventricular escape complexes or rhythm
- ☐ i. Ventricular fibrillation

5. ATRIAL-VENTRICULAR INTERACTIONS IN ARRHYTHMIAS

- ☐ a. Fusion complexes
- ☐ b. Reciprocal (echo) complexes
- ☐ c. Ventricular capture complexes
- ☐ d. AV dissociation
- ☐ e. Ventriculophasic sinus arrhythmia

6. AV CONDUCTION ABNORMALITIES

- ☐ a. AV block, 1°
- ☐ b. AV block, 2° - Mobitz type I (Wenckebach)
- ☐ c. AV block, 2° - Mobitz type II
- ☐ d. AV block, 2:1
- ☐ e. AV block, 3°
- ☐ f. AV block, variable
- ☐ g. Short PR interval (with sinus rhythm and normal QRS duration)
- ☐ h. Wolff-Parkinson-White pattern

7. INTRAVENTRICULAR CONDUCTION DISTURBANCES

- ☐ a. RBBB, incomplete
- ☐ b. RBBB, complete
- ☐ c. Left anterior fascicular block
- ☐ d. Left posterior fascicular block
- ☐ e. LBBB, with ST-T wave suggestive of acute myocardial injury or infarction
- ☐ f. LBBB, complete
- ☐ g. LBBB, intermittent
- ☐ h. Intraventricular conduction disturbance, nonspecific
- ☐ i. Aberrant intraventricular conduction with supraventricular arrhythmia

8. P WAVE ABNORMALITIES

- ☐ a. Right atrial abnormality
- ☐ b. Left atrial abnormalities
- ☐ c. Nonspecific atrial abnormality

9. ABNORMALITIES OF QRS VOLTAGE OR AXIS

- ☐ a. Low voltage, limb leads only
- ☐ b. Low voltage, limb and precordial leads
- ☐ c. Left axis deviation (> - 30%)
- ☐ d. Right axis deviation (> + 100)
- ☐ e. Electrical alternans

10. VENTRICULAR HYPERTROPHY

- ☐ a. LVH by voltage only
- ☐ b. LVH by voltage and ST-T segment abnormalities
- ☐ c. RVH
- ☐ d. Combined ventricular hypertrophy

11. Q WAVE MYOCARDIAL INFARCTION

	Probably Acute or Recent	Probably Old or Age Indeterminate
Anterolateral	☐ a.	☐ g.
Anterior	☐ b.	☐ h.
Anteroseptal	☐ c.	☐ i.
Lateral/High lateral	☐ d.	☐ j.
Inferior	☐ e.	☐ k.
Posterior	☐ f.	☐ l.

- ☐ m. Probably ventricular aneurysm

12. ST, T, U, WAVE ABNORMALITIES

- ☐ a. Normal variant, early repolarization
- ☐ b. Normal variant, juvenile T waves
- ☐ c. Nonspecific ST and/or T wave abnormalities
- ☐ d. ST and/or T wave abnormalities suggesting myocardial ischemia
- ☐ e. ST and/or T wave abnormalities suggesting myocardial injury
- ☐ f. ST and/or T wave abnormalities suggesting acute pericarditis
- ☐ g. ST-T segment abnormalities secondary to intraventricular conduction disturbance or hypertrophy
- ☐ h. Post-extrasystolic T wave abnormality
- ☐ i. Isolated J point depression
- ☐ j. Peaked T waves
- ☐ k. Prolonged QT interval
- ☐ l. Prominent U waves

13. PACEMAKER FUNCTION AND RHYTHM

- ☐ a. Atrial or coronary sinus pacing
- ☐ b. Ventricular demand pacing
- ☐ c. AV sequential pacing
- ☐ d. Ventricular pacing, complete control
- ☐ e. Dual chamber, atrial sensing pacemaker
- ☐ f. Pacemaker malfunction, not constantly capturing (atrium or ventricle)
- ☐ g. Pacemaker malfunction, not constantly sensing (atrium or ventricle)
- ☐ h. Pacemaker malfunction, not firing
- ☐ i. Pacemaker malfunction, slowing

14. SUGGESTED OR PROBABLE CLINICAL DISORDERS

- ☐ a. Digitalis effect
- ☐ b. Digitalis toxicity
- ☐ c. Antiarrhythmic drug effect
- ☐ d. Antiarrhythmic drug toxicity
- ☐ e. Hyperkalemia
- ☐ f. Hypokalemia
- ☐ g. Hypercalcemia
- ☐ h. Hypocalcemia
- ☐ i. Atrial septal defect, secundum
- ☐ j. Atrial septal defect, primum
- ☐ k. Dextrocardia, mirror image
- ☐ l. Mitral valve disease
- ☐ m. Chronic lung disease
- ☐ n. Acute cor pulmonale, including pulmonary embolus
- ☐ o. Pericardial effusion
- ☐ p. Acute pericarditis
- ☐ q. Hypertrophic cardiomyopathy
- ☐ r. Coronary artery disease
- ☐ s. Central nervous system disorder
- ☐ t. Myxedema
- ☐ u. Hypothermia
- ☐ v. Sick sinus syndrome

ECG 62 was obtained in a 76-year-old male with a remote history of coronary artery bypass graft surgery. The ECG shows a sinus rhythm at 93 beats/minute with first-degree AV block, left atrial abnormality (arrow), RBBB with secondary ST-T repolarization abnormality (asterisk), left anterior fascicular block, and left axis deviation. Q waves are evident in leads V_1 and V_2, but not in V_3, so anteroseptal myocardial infarction should not be coded.

Codes:

2a	Sinus rhythm
6a	AV block, 1°
7b	RBBB, complete
7c	Left anterior fascicular block
8b	Left atrial abnormality
9c	Left axis deviation (>-30°)
12g	ST-T segment abnormalities secondary to IVCD or hypertrophy

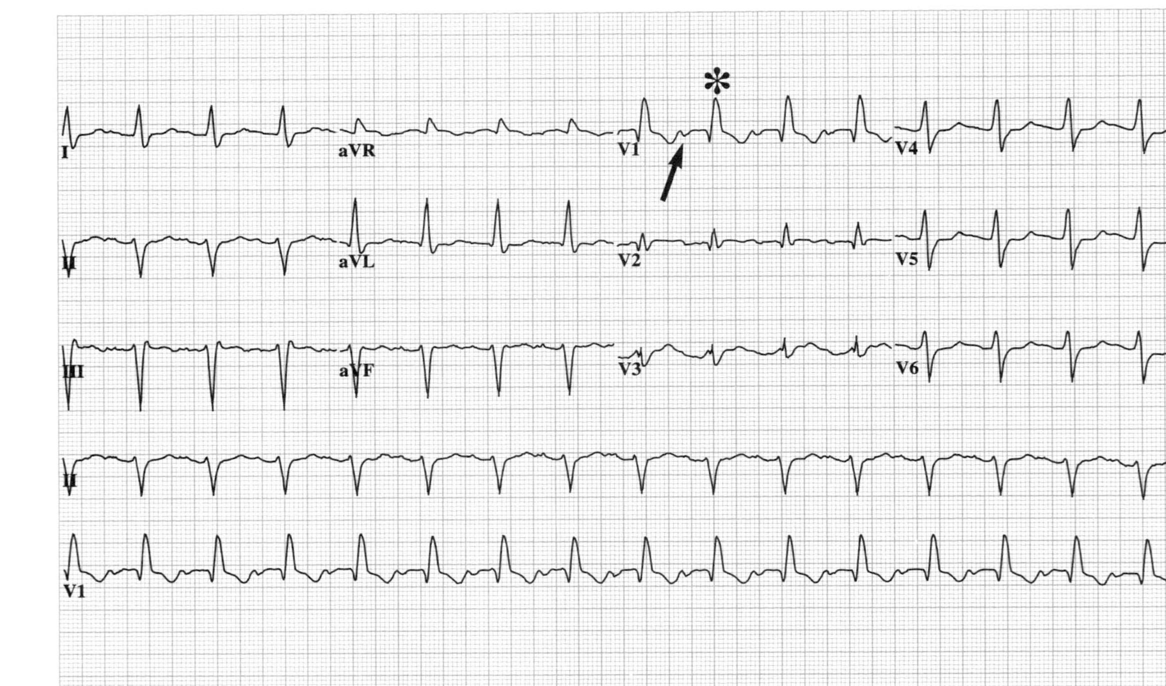

Questions: ECG 62

1. Which of the following statements are about right bundle branch block are true?

   a. RBBB obscures the diagnosis of MI
   b. RBBB obscures the diagnosis of LVH
   c. RBBB obscures the ability to determine QRS axis
   d. Most patients with RBBB have structural heart disease

2. Which of the following statements about left anterior fascicular block (LAFB) are true:

   a. LAFB always signifies the presence of structural heart disease
   b. LAFB reduces the specificity for the diagnosis of LVH by voltage criteria
   c. The most common cause of LAFB is coronary artery disease
   d. In the presence of inferior MI, the specificity of ECG criteria for the diagnosis of LAFB is reduced

3 Which of the following statements about first-degree AV block are true?

   a. Prolongation of the PR interval may be due to conduction delay at the level of the sinoatrial node, AV node, or His bundle
   b. Conduction delay is most often within the AV node when the QRS complex is narrow
   c. Conduction delay is most often within the His bundle when the QRS complex is wide

Answers: ECG 62

1. Most patients with right bundle branch block (RBBB) have organic heart disease, including coronary artery disease (most common cause), hypertensive heart disease, myocarditis, cardiomyopathy, rheumatic heart disease, cor pulmonale (acute or chronic), degenerative disease of the conduction system (Lenegre's disease), and sclerosis of the cardiac skeleton (Lev's disease). RBBB may obscure the ECG diagnosis of LVH; patients with RBBB and anatomical LVH may not manifest increased QRS voltage. The first 0.04 - 0.06 seconds of the QRS is unaffected by RBBB and can be used to determine QRS axis and identify abnormal Q waves of myocardial infarction. (Answer: b, d)

2. The left bundle branch supplies the Purkinje fibers to the left ventricle via an anterior fascicle (anterior and lateral ventricle)

in the left anterior fascicle results in late activation of the anterior and lateral ventricular walls, shifting the mean QRS axis to the left. The most common cause of left anterior fascicular block (LAFB) is coronary artery disease, but this conduction abnormality can be seen in patients without structural heart disease. LAFB reduces the specificity for the diagnosis of LVH based on voltage criteria in leads I and aVL. Inferior myocardial infarction (MI), which can shift the mean QRS axis superior and leftward (from unopposed anterior and lateral forces), can cause left axis deviation despite normal conduction down the left anterior fascicle. When QS complexes are present in the inferior leads, inferior MI and LAFB may both be present. (Answer: b, c)

3. The PR interval represents the interval from the onset of atrial depolarization to the onset of ventricular depolarization; it does not, however, represent conduction from the sinoatrial node to the atrium. Prolongation of the PR interval, therefore, may be caused by conduction delay within the atrium, AV node, His bundle or bundle branches, but not the sinoatrial node. When the QRS complex is narrow, conduction delay usually occurs at the level of the AV node. When the QRS complex is wide, conduction delay usually occurs within the bundle branches. (Answer: b,c)

— Quick Review 62 —

AV block, 1°	
• PR interval ≥ ____ seconds	0.20
Left anterior fascicular block	
• ____ axis deviation with a mean QRS axis between ____ and ____ degrees	left -45, -90
• (qR/rS) complex in leads I and aVL	qR
• (qR/rS) complex in lead III	rS
• Normal or slightly prolonged QRS duration (true/false)	true
• No other cause for left axis deviation should be present (true/false)	true
• Poor R wave progression is (common/uncommon)	common
Left axis deviation	
• Mean QRS axis between ____ and ____ degrees	-30, -60

Differential Diagnosis

RIGHT AXIS DEVIATION (>+100°)

- RVH (item 10c)
- Vertical heart
- Chronic obstructive pulmonary disease (item 14m)
- Pulmonary embolus (item 14n)
- Left posterior fascicular block (item 7d)
- Lateral wall myocardial infarction (items 11d, j)
- Dextrocardia (item 14k)
- Lead reversal (item 1c)
- Ostium secundum ASD (item 14i)

ECG 63. 53-year-old male with dyspnea on exertion:

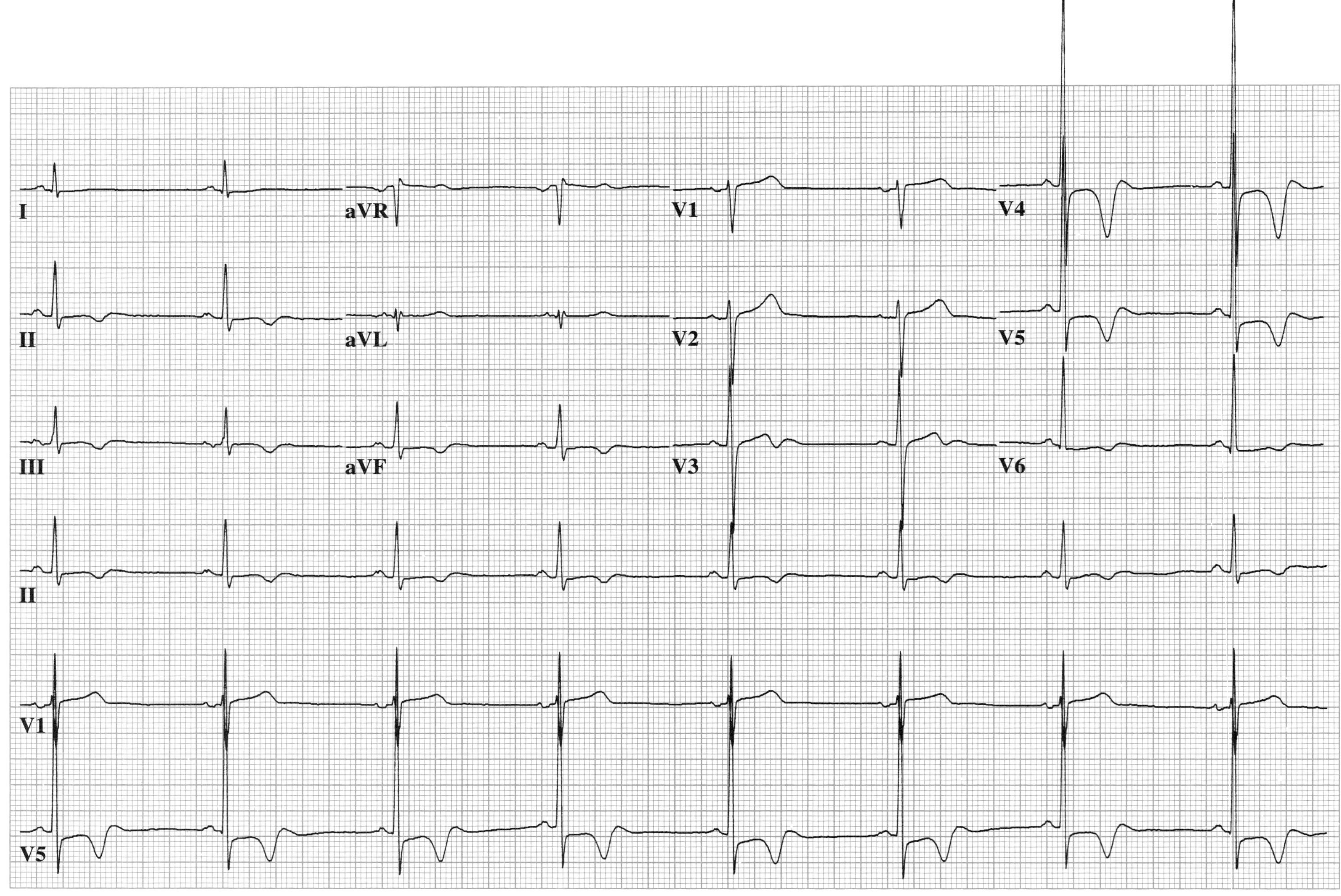

1. GENERAL FEATURES

- ☐ a. Normal ECG
- ☐ b. Borderline normal ECG or normal variant
- ☐ c. Incorrect electrode placement
- ☐ d. Artifact due to tremor

2. ATRIAL RHYTHMS

- ☐ a. Sinus rhythm
- ☐ b. Sinus arrhythmia
- ☐ c. Sinus bradycardia (< 60)
- ☐ d. Sinus tachycardia (> 100)
- ☐ e. Sinus pause or arrest
- ☐ f. Sinoatrial exit block
- ☐ g. Ecoptic atrial rhythm
- ☐ h. Wandering atrial pacemaker
- ☐ i. Atrial premature complexes, normally conducted
- ☐ j. Atrial premature complexes, nonconducted
- ☐ k. Atrial premature complexes with aberrant intraventricular conduction
- ☐ l. Atrial tachycardia (regular, sustained, 1:1 conduction)
- ☐ m. Atrial tachycardia, repetitive (short paroxysms)
- ☐ n. Atrial tachycardia, multifocal
- ☐ o. Atrial tachycardia with AV block
- ☐ p. Supraventricular tachycardia, unspecific
- ☐ q. Supraventricular tachycardia, paroxysmal
- ☐ r. Atrial flutter
- ☐ s. Atrial fibrillation
- ☐ t. Retrograde atrial activation

3. AV JUNCTIONAL RHYTHMS

- ☐ a. AV junctional premature complexes
- ☐ b. AV junctional escape complexes
- ☐ c. AV junctional rhythm, accelerated
- ☐ d. AV junctional rhythm

4. VENTRICULAR RHYTHMS

- ☐ a. Ventricular premature complex(es), uniform, fixed coupling
- ☐ b. Ventricular premature complex(es), uniform, nonfixed coupling
- ☐ c. Ventricular premature complexes(es), multiform
- ☐ d. Ventricular premature complexes, in pairs
- ☐ e. Ventricular parasystole
- ☐ f. Ventricular tachycardia (≥ 3 consecutive complexes)
- ☐ g. Accelerated idioventricular rhythm
- ☐ h. Ventricular escape complexes or rhythm
- ☐ i. Ventricular fibrillation

5. ATRIAL-VENTRICULAR INTERACTIONS IN ARRHYTHMIAS

- ☐ a. Fusion complexes
- ☐ b. Reciprocal (echo) complexes
- ☐ c. Ventricular capture complexes
- ☐ d. AV dissociation
- ☐ e. Ventriculophasic sinus arrhythmia

6. AV CONDUCTION ABNORMALITIES

- ☐ a. AV block, 1°
- ☐ b. AV block, 2° - Mobitz type I (Wenckebach)
- ☐ c. AV block, 2° - Mobitz type II
- ☐ d. AV block, 2:1
- ☐ e. AV block, 3°
- ☐ f. AV block, variable
- ☐ g. Short PR interval (with sinus rhythm and normal QRS duration)
- ☐ h. Wolff-Parkinson-White pattern

7. INTRAVENTRICULAR CONDUCTION DISTURBANCES

- ☐ a. RBBB, incomplete
- ☐ b. RBBB, complete
- ☐ c. Left anterior fascicular block
- ☐ d. Left posterior fascicular block
- ☐ e. LBBB, with ST-T wave suggestive of acute myocardial injury or infarction
- ☐ f. LBBB, complete
- ☐ g. LBBB, intermittent
- ☐ h. Intraventricular conduction disturbance, nonspecific
- ☐ i. Aberrant intraventricular conduction with supraventricular arrhythmia

8. P WAVE ABNORMALITIES

- ☐ a. Right atrial abnormality
- ☐ b. Left atrial abnormalities
- ☐ c. Nonspecific atrial abnormality

9. ABNORMALITIES OF QRS VOLTAGE OR AXIS

- ☐ a. Low voltage, limb leads only
- ☐ b. Low voltage, limb and precordial leads
- ☐ c. Left axis deviation (> - 30%)
- ☐ d. Right axis deviation (> + 100)
- ☐ e. Electrical alternans

10. VENTRICULAR HYPERTROPHY

- ☐ a. LVH by voltage only
- ☐ b. LVH by voltage and ST-T segment abnormalities
- ☐ c. RVH
- ☐ d. Combined ventricular hypertrophy

11. Q WAVE MYOCARDIAL INFARCTION

	Probably Acute or Recent	Probably Old or Age Indeterminate
Anterolateral	☐ a.	☐ g.
Anterior	☐ b.	☐ h.
Anteroseptal	☐ c.	☐ i.
Lateral/High lateral	☐ d.	☐ j.
Inferior	☐ e.	☐ k.
Posterior	☐ f.	☐ l.

☐ m. Probably ventricular aneurysm

12. ST, T, U, WAVE ABNORMALITIES

- ☐ a. Normal variant, early repolarization
- ☐ b. Normal variant, juvenile T waves
- ☐ c. Nonspecific ST and/or T wave abnormalities
- ☐ d. ST and/or T wave abnormalities suggesting myocardial ischemia
- ☐ e. ST and/or T wave abnormalities suggesting myocardial injury
- ☐ f. ST and/or T wave abnormalities suggesting acute pericarditis
- ☐ g. ST-T segment abnormalities secondary to intraventricular conduction disturbance or hypertrophy
- ☐ h. Post-extrasystolic T wave abnormality
- ☐ i. Isolated J point depression
- ☐ j. Peaked T waves
- ☐ k. Prolonged QT interval
- ☐ l. Prominent U waves

13. PACEMAKER FUNCTION AND RHYTHM

- ☐ a. Atrial or coronary sinus pacing
- ☐ b. Ventricular demand pacing
- ☐ c. AV sequential pacing
- ☐ d. Ventricular pacing, complete control
- ☐ e. Dual chamber, atrial sensing pacemaker
- ☐ f. Pacemaker malfunction, not constantly capturing (atrium or ventricle)
- ☐ g. Pacemaker malfunction, not constantly sensing (atrium or ventricle)
- ☐ h. Pacemaker malfunction, not firing
- ☐ i. Pacemaker malfunction, slowing

14. SUGGESTED OR PROBABLE CLINICAL DISORDERS

- ☐ a. Digitalis effect
- ☐ b. Digitalis toxicity
- ☐ c. Antiarrhythmic drug effect
- ☐ d. Antiarrhythmic drug toxicity
- ☐ e. Hyperkalemia
- ☐ f. Hypokalemia
- ☐ g. Hypercalcemia
- ☐ h. Hypocalcemia
- ☐ i. Atrial septal defect, secundum
- ☐ j. Atrial septal defect, primum
- ☐ k. Dextrocardia, mirror image
- ☐ l. Mitral valve disease
- ☐ m. Chronic lung disease
- ☐ n. Acute cor pulmonale, including pulmonary embolus
- ☐ o. Pericardial effusion
- ☐ p. Acute pericarditis
- ☐ q. Hypertrophic cardiomyopathy
- ☐ r. Coronary artery disease
- ☐ s. Central nervous system disorder
- ☐ t. Myxedema
- ☐ u. Hypothermia
- ☐ v. Sick sinus syndrome

ECG 63 was obtained in a 53-year-old male with dyspnea on exertion. The ECG shows sinus bradycardia at 46 beats/minute and marked LVH with secondary ST-T changes (arrowheads). Voltage-based criteria for LVH on this tracing include: an S wave in V_1 + R wave in $V_5 > 35$ mm; an R wave in $V_5 > 26$ mm; and the tallest precordial R wave + S wave > 45 mm. Prominent U waves, commonly seen in LVH and bradycardia, are also present (arrow). The magnitude of the voltage and repolarization abnormalities suggests a diagnosis of hypertrophic cardiomyopathy, which was later confirmed by echocardiography.

Codes:

2c	Sinus bradycardia < 60
10b	LVH by both voltage and ST-T segment abnormalities
12g	ST-T segment abnormalities secondary to IVCD or hypertrophy
12l	Prominent U waves
14q	Hypertrophic cardiomyopathy

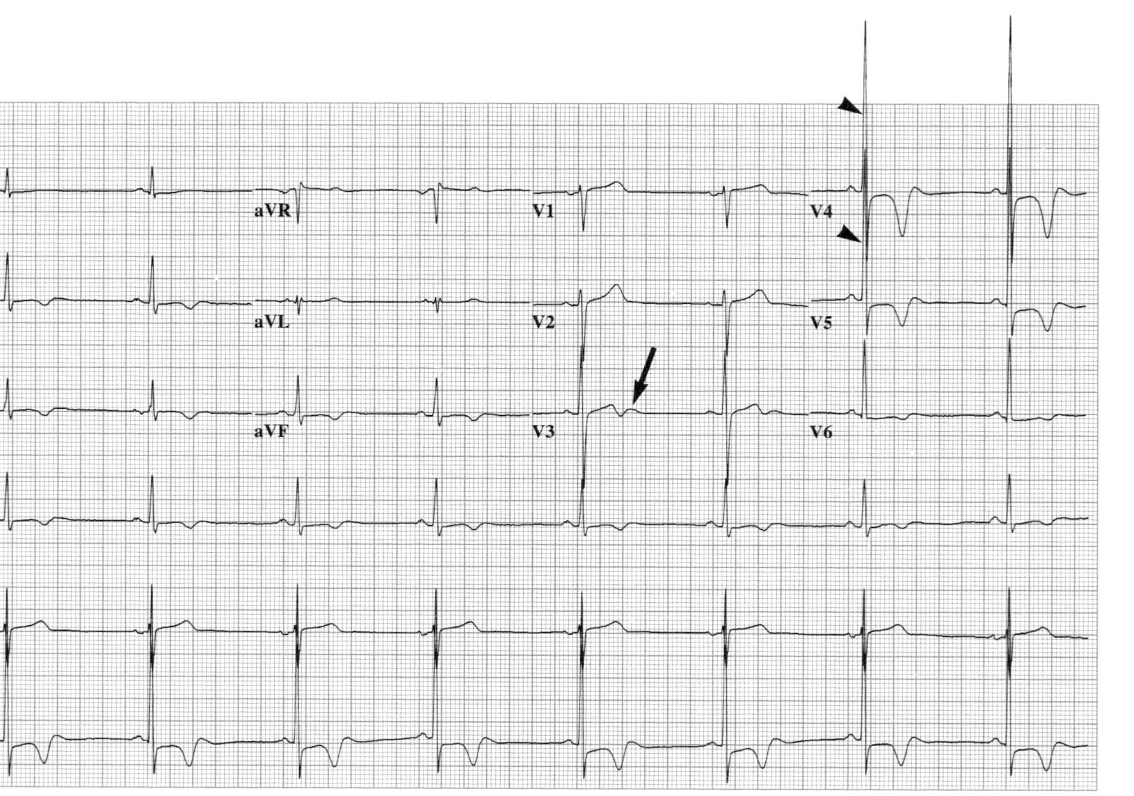

Questions: ECG 63

1. Apical hypertrophic cardiomyopathy typically results in deep T wave inversion in the ___ leads:

   a. Limb
   b. Precordial
   c. Limb and precordial

2. Common ECG findings of hypertrophic cardiomyopathy include:

   a. LVH with secondary ST-T wave changes
   b. Prominent U waves
   c. First-degree AV block
   d. Left atrial abnormality

3. Conditions associated with prominent U waves include all of the following except:

   a. LVH
   b. Hyperkalemia
   c. Hypokalemia
   d. Antiarrhythmic drug effect

Answers: ECG 63

1. Apical hypertrophic cardiomyopathy typically results in severe LVH with deep T wave inversions in the precordial leads. (Answer: b)

2. Common ECG findings in hypertrophic cardiomyopathy include LVH with secondary ST-T changes, prominent U waves, and left atrial abnormality. Other ECG findings may include a nonspecific intraventricular conduction defect, abnormal Q waves (causing a pseudo-infarction pattern), and ventricular dysrhythmias. First-degree AV block is not a typical ECG feature of hypertrophic cardiomyopathy. (Answer: a, b, d)

3. Prominent U waves (≥ 1.5 mm tall) can be seen in left ventricular hypertrophy, digitalis, electrolyte abnormalities (hypomagnesemia, hypocalcemia, hypokalemia), antiarrhythmic drug therapy, CNS disease, hyperthyroidism, mitral valve prolapse, bradycardia, prolonged QT syndrome, and myocardial ischemia. Hyperkalemia typically manifests peaked T waves, first-degree AV block, flattening of the P waves, QRS widening, and ST segment depression. Prominent U waves, however, are not typically seen in hyperkalemia. (Answer: b)

— Quick Review 63 —

Prominent U waves	
• Amplitude ≥ ____ mm	1.5
• The U wave is normally ____% the height of the T wave, and is largest in leads ____	5-25 V_2, V_3
Hypertrophic cardiomyopathy	
• (Right/left) atrial abnormality is common; (right/left) atrial abnormality on occasion	left right
• Majority have abnormal QRS complexes (true/false):	true
▸ (Small/large) amplitude QRS	large
▸ Large abnormal ____ waves (can give pseudoinfarct pattern in inferior, lateral, and anterior precordial leads)	Q
▸ Tall R wave with inverted T wave in V_1 simulating ____	RVH
▸ Nonspecific ST and/or T wave abnormalities are common (true/false)	false
▸ Apical variant of hypertrophic cardiomyopathy has deep T wave inversions in leads ____	V_4-V_6
▸ (Right/left) axis deviation in 20%	left

Common Dilemmas in ECG Interpretation

Problem

Should left axis deviation be coded when left anterior fascicular block is present? Similarly, should right axis deviation be coded when left posterior fascicular block is present?

Recommendation

Yes. The QRS axis is merely a descriptor of the major QRS vector. If left anterior fascicular block or left posterior fascicular block is present, the axis should also be coded.

ECG 64. 72-year-old female with presyncope:

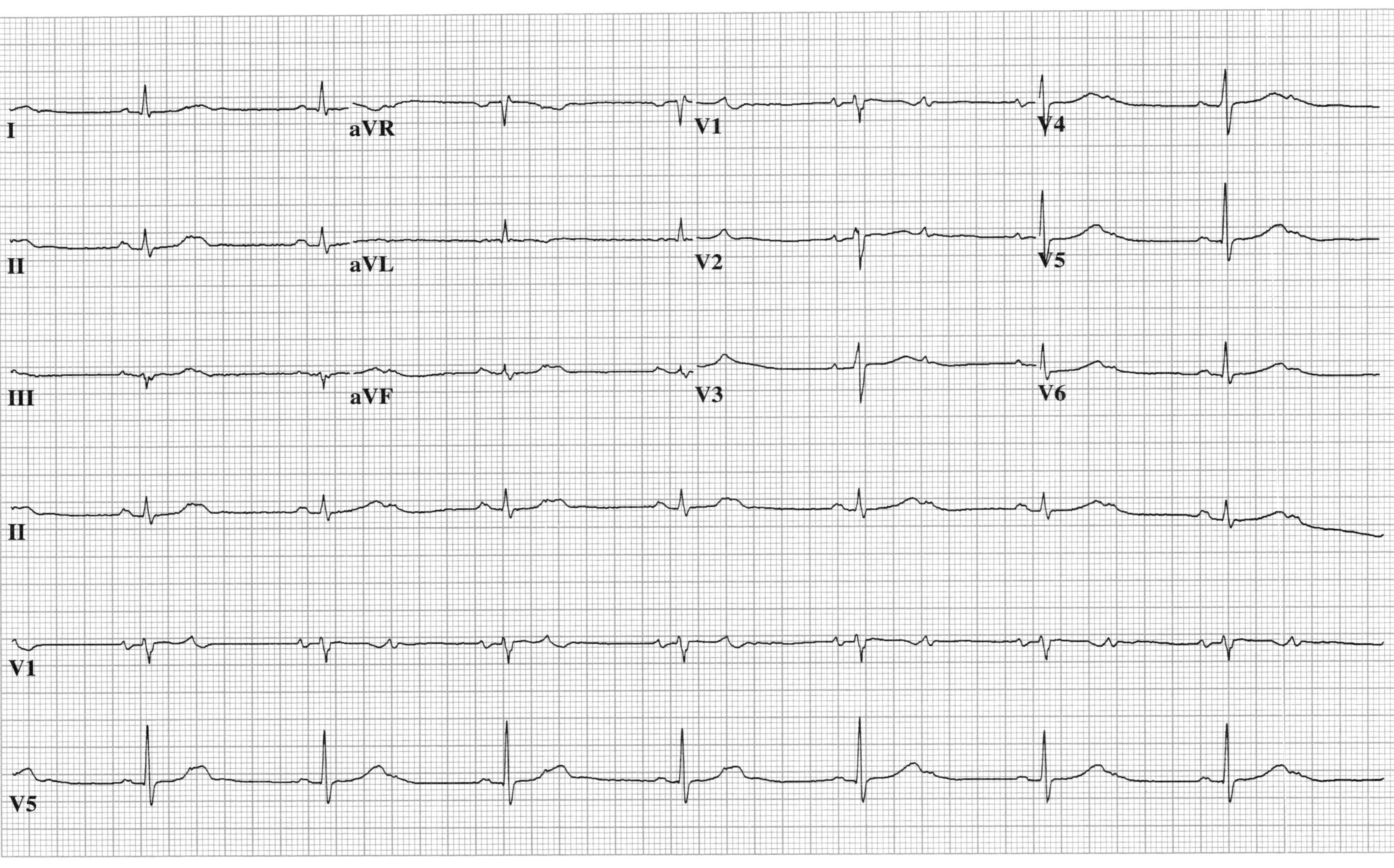

1. GENERAL FEATURES

☐ a. Normal ECG
☐ b. Borderline normal ECG or normal variant
☐ c. Incorrect electrode placement
☐ d. Artifact due to tremor

2. ATRIAL RHYTHMS

☐ a. Sinus rhythm
☐ b. Sinus arrhythmia
☐ c. Sinus bradycardia (< 60)
☐ d. Sinus tachycardia (> 100)
☐ e. Sinus pause or arrest
☐ f. Sinoatrial exit block
☐ g. Ecoptic atrial rhythm
☐ h. Wandering atrial pacemaker
☐ i. Atrial premature complexes, normally conducted
☐ j. Atrial premature complexes, nonconducted
☐ k. Atrial premature complexes with aberrant intraventricular conduction
☐ l. Atrial tachycardia (regular, sustained, 1:1 conduction)
☐ m. Atrial tachycardia, repetitive (short paroxysms)
☐ n. Atrial tachycardia, multifocal
☐ o. Atrial tachycardia with AV block
☐ p. Supraventricular tachycardia, unspecific
☐ q. Supraventricular tachycardia, paroxysmal
☐ r. Atrial flutter
☐ s. Atrial fibrillation
☐ t. Retrograde atrial activation

3. AV JUNCTIONAL RHYTHMS

☐ a. AV junctional premature complexes
☐ b. AV junctional escape complexes
☐ c. AV junctional rhythm, accelerated
☐ d. AV junctional rhythm

4. VENTRICULAR RHYTHMS

☐ a. Ventricular premature complex(es), uniform, fixed coupling
☐ b. Ventricular premature complex(es), uniform, nonfixed coupling
☐ c. Ventricular premature complexes(es), multiform
☐ d. Ventricular premature complexes, in pairs
☐ e. Ventricular parasystole
☐ f. Ventricular tachycardia (≥ 3 consecutive complexes)
☐ g. Accelerated idioventricular rhythm
☐ h. Ventricular escape complexes or rhythm
☐ i. Ventricular fibrillation

5. ATRIAL-VENTRICULAR INTERACTIONS IN ARRHYTHMIAS

☐ a. Fusion complexes
☐ b. Reciprocal (echo) complexes
☐ c. Ventricular capture complexes
☐ d. AV dissociation
☐ e. Ventriculophasic sinus arrhythmia

6. AV CONDUCTION ABNORMALITIES

☐ a. AV block, 1°
☐ b. AV block, 2° - Mobitz type I (Wenckebach)
☐ c. AV block, 2° - Mobitz type II
☐ d. AV block, 2:1
☐ e. AV block, 3°
☐ f. AV block, variable
☐ g. Short PR interval (with sinus rhythm and normal QRS duration)
☐ h. Wolff-Parkinson-White pattern

7. INTRAVENTRICULAR CONDUCTION DISTURBANCES

☐ a. RBBB, incomplete
☐ b. RBBB, complete
☐ c. Left anterior fascicular block
☐ d. Left posterior fascicular block
☐ e. LBBB, with ST-T wave suggestive of acute myocardial injury or infarction
☐ f. LBBB, complete
☐ g. LBBB, intermittent
☐ h. Intraventricular conduction disturbance, nonspecific
☐ i. Aberrant intraventricular conduction with supraventricular arrhythmia

8. P WAVE ABNORMALITIES

☐ a. Right atrial abnormality
☐ b. Left atrial abnormalities
☐ c. Nonspecific atrial abnormality

9. ABNORMALITIES OF QRS VOLTAGE OR AXIS

☐ a. Low voltage, limb leads only
☐ b. Low voltage, limb and precordial leads
☐ c. Left axis deviation (> - 30%)
☐ d. Right axis deviation (> + 100)
☐ e. Electrical alternans

10. VENTRICULAR HYPERTROPHY

☐ a. LVH by voltage only
☐ b. LVH by voltage and ST-T segment abnormalities
☐ c. RVH
☐ d. Combined ventricular hypertrophy

11. Q WAVE MYOCARDIAL INFARCTION

	Probably Acute or Recent	Probably Old or Age Indeterminate
Anterolateral	☐ a.	☐ g.
Anterior	☐ b.	☐ h.
Anteroseptal	☐ c.	☐ i.
Lateral/High lateral	☐ d.	☐ j.
Inferior	☐ e.	☐ k.
Posterior	☐ f.	☐ l.

☐ m. Probably ventricular aneurysm

12. ST, T, U, WAVE ABNORMALITIES

☐ a. Normal variant, early repolarization
☐ b. Normal variant, juvenile T waves
☐ c. Nonspecific ST and/or T wave abnormalities
☐ d. ST and/or T wave abnormalities suggesting myocardial ischemia
☐ e. ST and/or T wave abnormalities suggesting myocardial injury
☐ f. ST and/or T wave abnormalities suggesting acute pericarditis
☐ g. ST-T segment abnormalities secondary to intraventricular conduction disturbance or hypertrophy
☐ h. Post-extrasystolic T wave abnormality
☐ i. Isolated J point depression
☐ j. Peaked T waves
☐ k. Prolonged QT interval
☐ l. Prominent U waves

13. PACEMAKER FUNCTION AND RHYTHM

☐ a. Atrial or coronary sinus pacing
☐ b. Ventricular demand pacing
☐ c. AV sequential pacing
☐ d. Ventricular pacing, complete control
☐ e. Dual chamber, atrial sensing pacemaker
☐ f. Pacemaker malfunction, not constantly capturing (atrium or ventricle)
☐ g. Pacemaker malfunction, not constantly sensing (atrium or ventricle)
☐ h. Pacemaker malfunction, not firing
☐ i. Pacemaker malfunction, slowing

14. SUGGESTED OR PROBABLE CLINICAL DISORDERS

☐ a. Digitalis effect
☐ b. Digitalis toxicity
☐ c. Antiarrhythmic drug effect
☐ d. Antiarrhythmic drug toxicity
☐ e. Hyperkalemia
☐ f. Hypokalemia
☐ g. Hypercalcemia
☐ h. Hypocalcemia
☐ i. Atrial septal defect, secundum
☐ j. Atrial septal defect, primum
☐ k. Dextrocardia, mirror image
☐ l. Mitral valve disease
☐ m. Chronic lung disease
☐ n. Acute cor pulmonale, including pulmonary embolus
☐ o. Pericardial effusion
☐ p. Acute pericarditis
☐ q. Hypertrophic cardiomyopathy
☐ r. Coronary artery disease
☐ s. Central nervous system disorder
☐ t. Myxedema
☐ u. Hypothermia
☐ v. Sick sinus syndrome

ECG 64 was obtained from a 72-year-old female with presyncope. The ECG shows sinus rhythm with 2:1 AV block, ventriculophasic sinus arrhythmia (the sinus PP interval containing a QRS is shorter than the sinus PP interval without a QRS), and blocked atrial premature complexes (arrows).

Codes:

2a	Sinus rhythm
2j	Atrial premature complexes, nonconducted
5e	Ventriculophasic sinus arrhythmia
6d	AV block, 2:1

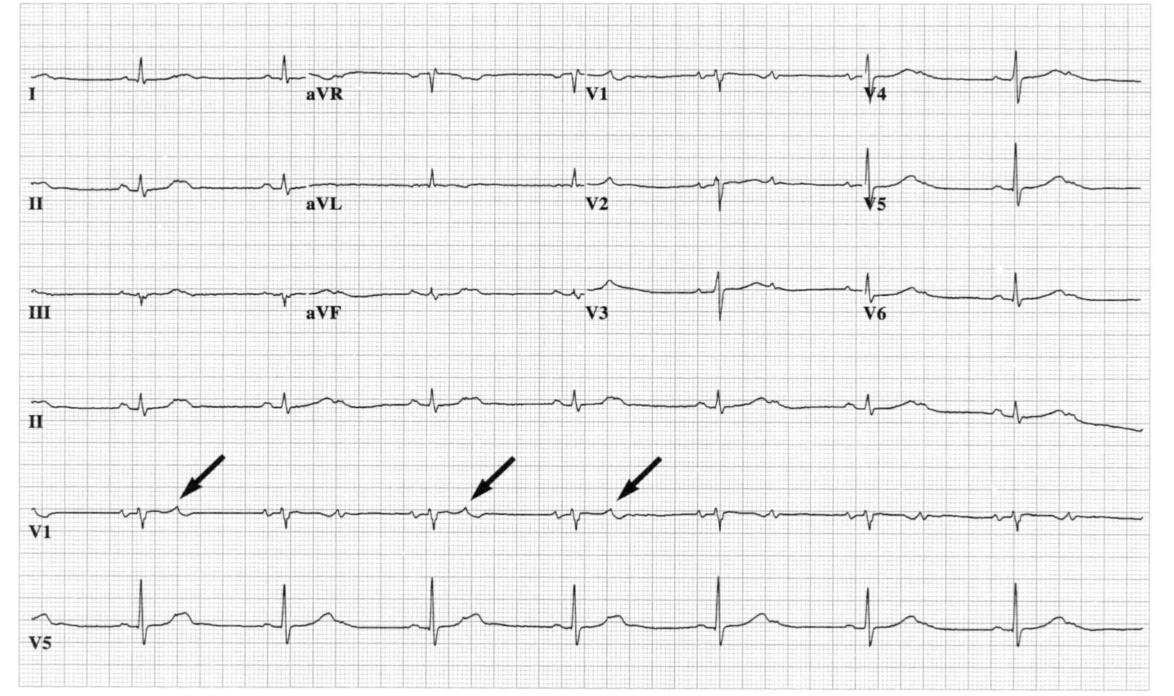

Questions: ECG 64

1. The irregularity in the PP interval in the present tracing is due to:

   a. Sinoatrial exit block
   b. Premature atrial contractions
   c. Ventriculophasic sinus arrhythmia

2. The dropped beats in the present tracing are due to:

   a. Blocked premature atrial contractions
   b. Second-degree AV block

3. The mechanism responsible for the 2:1 AV block in this tracing is:

   a. Mobitz Type I (Wenkebach)
   b. Mobitz Type II
   c. Unable to tell

4. The following features favor Mobitz Type I (Wenkebach) over Mobitz Type II when 2:1 AV block is present:

   a. Narrow QRS complex
   b. Presence of bundle branch block
   c. Atropine improves block
   d. Carotid sinus massage improves block
   e. History of syncope
   f. 2:1 AV block develops during acute inferior MI

5. Match each set of features to the condition below:

Features:

a. Congenital deafness; associated with syncope/ sudden death
b. Congenital; normal hearing associated with syncope and sudden death
c. Truncal obesity, moon facies, acne, hirsutism; ECG with prominent U wave
d. Dry skin, constipation, cold intolerance, memory difficulties; ECG with sinus bradycardia, low voltage, and prolonged PR
e. Adult respiratory distress syndrome, disseminated intravascular coagulation, severe liver dysfunction; ECG with atrial fibrillation and Osborne wave
f. Hemiparesis; ECG with deeply inverted T waves, ST elevation, and large U waves
g. Flu-like syndrome with abdominal pain, headache and dizziness progressing within 24 hours to psychosis, convulsions, and coma

Conditions:

1. Hypokalemia
2. Hypothermia
3. Organophosphorus poisoning
4. Intracranial hemorrhage
5. Hypothyroidism
6. Romano-Ward syndrome
7. Jervill and Lange-Nielsen syndrome

Answers: ECG 64

1. The irregularity in the PP interval is caused by ventriculophasic sinus arrhythmia, which should be coded in cases of partial or complete AV block when the sinus PP interval containing a QRS is shorter than the sinus PP interval without a QRS. Premature atrial contractions cause irregularity in the PP interval, but the morphology of the premature P wave is different from the sinus P wave, which is not the case in the present tracing. Sinoatrial exit block can also cause an irregular PP interval, but the diagnosis requires that the long PP intervals are exact multiples of the normal PP interval. (Answer: c)

2. Causes of dropped beats include blocked atrial premature complexes (APC) and second-degree AV block. These conditions can usually be distinguished from one another by the regularity of the PP interval and the morphology of the P wave. APCs are favored when there is irregularity in the PP interval and alteration in P wave morphology; second-degree AV block is favored when the PP interval and P wave morphology are constant, as seen in the present tracing. (Note: Second-degree AV block may show irregularity in the PP interval when ventriculophasic sinus arrhythmia coexists.) (Answer: b)

3. In the setting of 2:1 AV block, the surface ECG cannot be used to reliably distinguish Mobitz Type I (Wenckebach) from Mobitz Type II second-degree AV block. As discussed in question 4, below, the presence of certain features favor one mechanism over another. (Answer: c)

4. In the setting of 2:1 AV block, the presence of certain ECG and clinical features help to distinguish Mobitz Type I from Mobitz Type II second-degree AV block; exceptions, however, do exist. (Answer: Mobitz Type I: a, c, f; Mobitz Type II: b, d, e)

Features Suggesting the Mechanism of 2:1 AV Block

	Mobitz Type I	**Mobitz Type II**
Level of block	AV node	Intra- or infra-Hisian
QRS duration	Narrow	Wide (20% may be narrow)
Develops during MI	Inferior MI	Anterior MI
Response to atropine	Block improves	Block worsens
Response to carotid sinus massage	Block worsens	Block improves
Other	Mobitz I present in other portion of ECG	History of syncope

5. Answer: a: 7
b: 6
c: 1

d: 5
e: 2
f: 4
g: 3

— Quick Review 64 —	
Atrial premature complexes, nonconducted • Premature P wave with abnormal morphology not followed by a ____ complex	QRS-T
Ventriculophasic sinus arrhythmia • PP interval containing a QRS complex is (less than/equal to/greater than) the PP interval without a QRS complex	less than

ECG 65. 81-year-old female with sudden dyspnea and a normal ECG three weeks earlier:

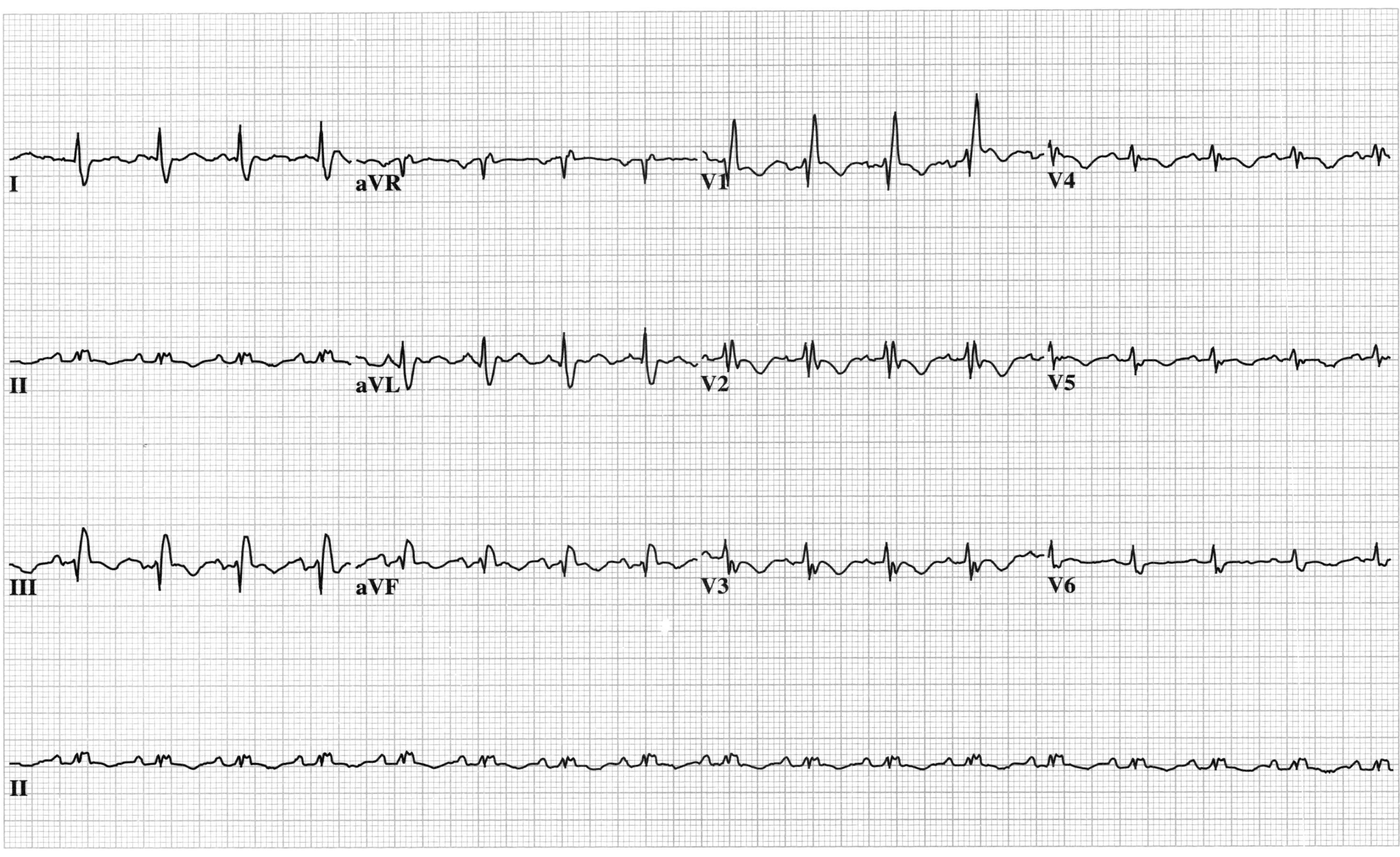

1. GENERAL FEATURES
- ☐ a. Normal ECG
- ☐ b. Borderline normal ECG or normal variant
- ☐ c. Incorrect electrode placement
- ☐ d. Artifact due to tremor

2. ATRIAL RHYTHMS
- ☐ a. Sinus rhythm
- ☐ b. Sinus arrhythmia
- ☐ c. Sinus bradycardia (< 60)
- ☐ d. Sinus tachycardia (> 100)
- ☐ e. Sinus pause or arrest
- ☐ f. Sinoatrial exit block
- ☐ g. Ecoptic atrial rhythm
- ☐ h. Wandering atrial pacemaker
- ☐ i. Atrial premature complexes, normally conducted
- ☐ j. Atrial premature complexes, nonconducted
- ☐ k. Atrial premature complexes with aberrant intraventricular conduction
- ☐ l. Atrial tachycardia (regular, sustained, 1:1 conduction)
- ☐ m. Atrial tachycardia, repetitive (short paroxysms)
- ☐ n. Atrial tachycardia, multifocal
- ☐ o. Atrial tachycardia with AV block
- ☐ p. Supraventricular tachycardia, unspecific
- ☐ q. Supraventricular tachycardia, paroxysmal
- ☐ r. Atrial flutter
- ☐ s. Atrial fibrillation
- ☐ t. Retrograde atrial activation

3. AV JUNCTIONAL RHYTHMS
- ☐ a. AV junctional premature complexes
- ☐ b. AV junctional escape complexes
- ☐ c. AV junctional rhythm, accelerated
- ☐ d. AV junctional rhythm

4. VENTRICULAR RHYTHMS
- ☐ a. Ventricular premature complex(es), uniform, fixed coupling
- ☐ b. Ventricular premature complex(es), uniform, nonfixed coupling
- ☐ c. Ventricular premature complexes(es), multiform
- ☐ d. Ventricular premature complexes, in pairs
- ☐ e. Ventricular parasystole
- ☐ f. Ventricular tachycardia (≥ 3 consecutive complexes)
- ☐ g. Accelerated idioventricular rhythm
- ☐ h. Ventricular escape complexes or rhythm
- ☐ i. Ventricular fibrillation

5. ATRIAL-VENTRICULAR INTERACTIONS IN ARRHYTHMIAS
- ☐ a. Fusion complexes
- ☐ b. Reciprocal (echo) complexes
- ☐ c. Ventricular capture complexes
- ☐ d. AV dissociation
- ☐ e. Ventriculophasic sinus arrhythmia

6. AV CONDUCTION ABNORMALITIES
- ☐ a. AV block, 1°
- ☐ b. AV block, 2° - Mobitz type I (Wenckebach)
- ☐ c. AV block, 2° - Mobitz type II
- ☐ d. AV block, 2:1
- ☐ e. AV block, 3°
- ☐ f. AV block, variable
- ☐ g. Short PR interval (with sinus rhythm and normal QRS duration)
- ☐ h. Wolff-Parkinson-White pattern

7. INTRAVENTRICULAR CONDUCTION DISTURBANCES
- ☐ a. RBBB, incomplete
- ☐ b. RBBB, complete
- ☐ c. Left anterior fascicular block
- ☐ d. Left posterior fascicular block
- ☐ e. LBBB, with ST-T wave suggestive of acute myocardial injury or infarction
- ☐ f. LBBB, complete
- ☐ g. LBBB, intermittent
- ☐ h. Intraventricular conduction disturbance, nonspecific
- ☐ i. Aberrant intraventricular conduction with supraventricular arrhythmia

8. P WAVE ABNORMALITIES
- ☐ a. Right atrial abnormality
- ☐ b. Left atrial abnormalities
- ☐ c. Nonspecific atrial abnormality

9. ABNORMALITIES OF QRS VOLTAGE OR AXIS
- ☐ a. Low voltage, limb leads only
- ☐ b. Low voltage, limb and precordial leads
- ☐ c. Left axis deviation (> - 30%)
- ☐ d. Right axis deviation (> + 100)
- ☐ e. Electrical alternans

10. VENTRICULAR HYPERTROPHY
- ☐ a. LVH by voltage only
- ☐ b. LVH by voltage and ST-T segment abnormalities
- ☐ c. RVH
- ☐ d. Combined ventricular hypertrophy

11. Q WAVE MYOCARDIAL INFARCTION

	Probably Acute or Recent	Probably Old or Age Indeterminate
Anterolateral	☐ a.	☐ g.
Anterior	☐ b.	☐ h.
Anteroseptal	☐ c.	☐ i.
Lateral/High lateral	☐ d.	☐ j.
Inferior	☐ e.	☐ k.
Posterior	☐ f.	☐ l.

☐ m. Probably ventricular aneurysm

12. ST, T, U, WAVE ABNORMALITIES
- ☐ a. Normal variant, early repolarization
- ☐ b. Normal variant, juvenile T waves
- ☐ c. Nonspecific ST and/or T wave abnormalities
- ☐ d. ST and/or T wave abnormalities suggesting myocardial ischemia
- ☐ e. ST and/or T wave abnormalities suggesting myocardial injury
- ☐ f. ST and/or T wave abnormalities suggesting acute pericarditis
- ☐ g. ST-T segment abnormalities secondary to intraventricular conduction disturbance or hypertrophy
- ☐ h. Post-extrasystolic T wave abnormality
- ☐ i. Isolated J point depression
- ☐ j. Peaked T waves
- ☐ k. Prolonged QT interval
- ☐ l. Prominent U waves

13. PACEMAKER FUNCTION AND RHYTHM
- ☐ a. Atrial or coronary sinus pacing
- ☐ b. Ventricular demand pacing
- ☐ c. AV sequential pacing
- ☐ d. Ventricular pacing, complete control
- ☐ e. Dual chamber, atrial sensing pacemaker
- ☐ f. Pacemaker malfunction, not constantly capturing (atrium or ventricle)
- ☐ g. Pacemaker malfunction, not constantly sensing (atrium or ventricle)
- ☐ h. Pacemaker malfunction, not firing
- ☐ i. Pacemaker malfunction, slowing

14. SUGGESTED OR PROBABLE CLINICAL DISORDERS
- ☐ a. Digitalis effect
- ☐ b. Digitalis toxicity
- ☐ c. Antiarrhythmic drug effect
- ☐ d. Antiarrhythmic drug toxicity
- ☐ e. Hyperkalemia
- ☐ f. Hypokalemia
- ☐ g. Hypercalcemia
- ☐ h. Hypocalcemia
- ☐ i. Atrial septal defect, secundum
- ☐ j. Atrial septal defect, primum
- ☐ k. Dextrocardia, mirror image
- ☐ l. Mitral valve disease
- ☐ m. Chronic lung disease
- ☐ n. Acute cor pulmonale, including pulmonary embolus
- ☐ o. Pericardial effusion
- ☐ p. Acute pericarditis
- ☐ q. Hypertrophic cardiomyopathy
- ☐ r. Coronary artery disease
- ☐ s. Central nervous system disorder
- ☐ t. Myxedema
- ☐ u. Hypothermia
- ☐ v. Sick sinus syndrome

ECG 65 was obtained in an 81-year-old female with sudden dyspnea and a normal ECG three weeks earlier. The ECG demonstrates sinus tachycardia with right bundle branch block (arrows mark wide rSR' complexes in leads V_1 and V_2 , and wide slurred S waves in leads I and V_6), and ST-T repolarization changes (asterisks) secondary to the RBBB. Given the patient's history, this ECG is most consistent with acute cor pulmonale due to a pulmonary embolus.

Codes:

2d	Sinus tachycardia
7b	RBBB, complete
12g	ST-T segment abnormality secondary to IVCD or hypertrophy
14n	Acute cor pulmonale, including pulmonary embolus

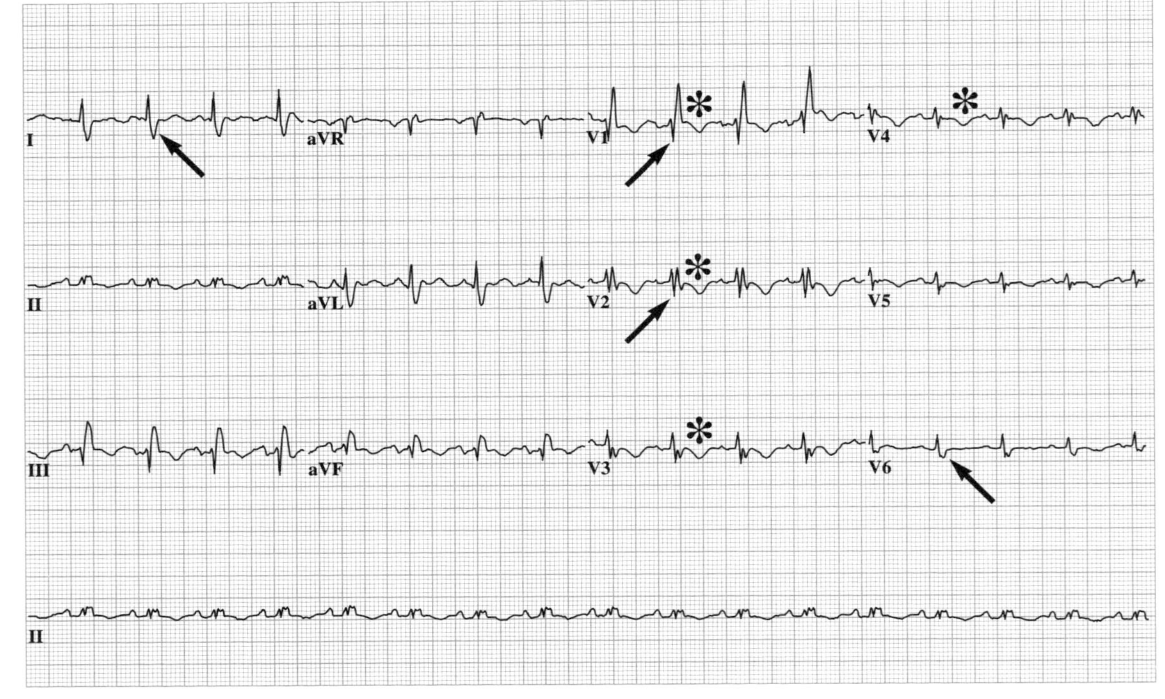

Questions: ECG 65

1. ECG findings consistent with acute cor pulmonale include:

   a. Sinus tachycardia
   b. Right atrial abnormality
   c. Inverted T wave in V_1-V_3
   d. Right axis deviation
   e. Pseudoinfarct pattern in the inferior leads
   f. New right bundle branch block

2. ECG abnormalities in patients with acute pulmonary embolus are often transient with a normal ECG recorded despite a persistent pulmonary embolus:

   a. True
   b. False

Answers: ECG 65

1. Acute cor pulmonale including pulmonary embolus can result in several ECG abnormalities. The most frequent abnormality is sinus tachycardia. Other supraventricular tachyarrhythmias can also be present. In addition, evidence of right ventricular pressure overload may be present, including right atrial abnormality, inverted T waves in V_1-V_3, and right axis deviation. Other findings consistent with acute cor pulmonale include an $S_1 Q_3 T_3$ pattern, transient RBBB, and a pseudoinfarct pattern in the inferior leads. (Answer: All)

2. Surprisingly, ECG abnormalities in patients with acute pulmonary embolus are often transient, and a normal ECG may be recorded despite persistence of the embolus. Sinus tachycardia, however, is usually present even when other ECG features of acute cor pulmonale are absent. (Answer: a)

— Quick Review 65 —

Acute cor pulmonale including pulmonary embolus	
• Sinus ____ (most common) and findings consistent	tachycardia
with (right/left) ventricular pressure overload:	right
▸ (Right/left) atrial abnormality	Right
▸ Inverted T waves in leads ____	V_1-V_3
▸ (Right/left) axis deviation	Right
▸ S_1Q_3 or S_1Q_3 ____ pattern	T_3
▸ Pseudoinfarct pattern in the ____ leads	inferior
▸ Incomplete or complete (RBBB/LBBB)	RBBB
▸ (Supraventricular/ventricular) tachyarrhythmias are common	Supraventricular
• ECG abnormalities are often (transient/persistent)	transient

ECG 66. 46-year-old female with a history of rheumatic fever now with dyspnea on exertion:

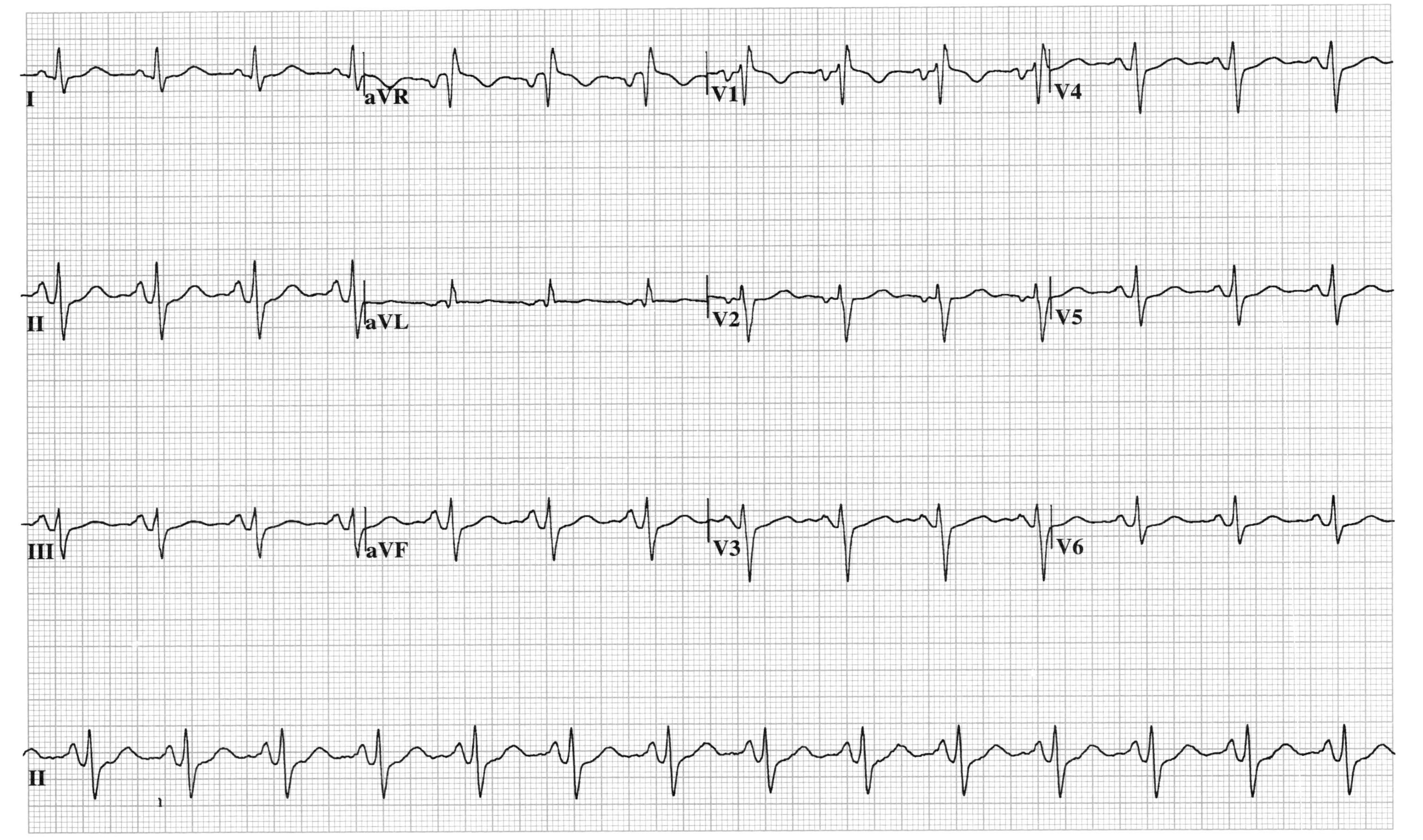

1. GENERAL FEATURES

- ☐ a. Normal ECG
- ☐ b. Borderline normal ECG or normal variant
- ☐ c. Incorrect electrode placement
- ☐ d. Artifact due to tremor

2. ATRIAL RHYTHMS

- ☐ a. Sinus rhythm
- ☐ b. Sinus arrhythmia
- ☐ c. Sinus bradycardia (< 60)
- ☐ d. Sinus tachycardia (> 100)
- ☐ e. Sinus pause or arrest
- ☐ f. Sinoatrial exit block
- ☐ g. Ecoptic atrial rhythm
- ☐ h. Wandering atrial pacemaker
- ☐ i. Atrial premature complexes, normally conducted
- ☐ j. Atrial premature complexes, nonconducted
- ☐ k. Atrial premature complexes with aberrant intraventricular conduction
- ☐ l. Atrial tachycardia (regular, sustained, 1:1 conduction)
- ☐ m. Atrial tachycardia, repetitive (short paroxysms)
- ☐ n. Atrial tachycardia, multifocal
- ☐ o. Atrial tachycardia with AV block
- ☐ p. Supraventricular tachycardia, unspecific
- ☐ q. Supraventricular tachycardia, paroxysmal
- ☐ r. Atrial flutter
- ☐ s. Atrial fibrillation
- ☐ t. Retrograde atrial activation

3. AV JUNCTIONAL RHYTHMS

- ☐ a. AV junctional premature complexes
- ☐ b. AV junctional escape complexes
- ☐ c. AV junctional rhythm, accelerated
- ☐ d. AV junctional rhythm

4. VENTRICULAR RHYTHMS

- ☐ a. Ventricular premature complex(es), uniform, fixed coupling
- ☐ b. Ventricular premature complex(es), uniform, nonfixed coupling
- ☐ c. Ventricular premature complexes(es), multiform
- ☐ d. Ventricular premature complexes, in pairs
- ☐ e. Ventricular parasystole
- ☐ f. Ventricular tachycardia (≥ 3 consecutive complexes)
- ☐ g. Accelerated idioventricular rhythm
- ☐ h. Ventricular escape complexes or rhythm
- ☐ i. Ventricular fibrillation

5. ATRIAL-VENTRICULAR INTERACTIONS IN ARRHYTHMIAS

- ☐ a. Fusion complexes
- ☐ b. Reciprocal (echo) complexes
- ☐ c. Ventricular capture complexes
- ☐ d. AV dissociation
- ☐ e. Ventriculophasic sinus arrhythmia

6. AV CONDUCTION ABNORMALITIES

- ☐ a. AV block, 1°
- ☐ b. AV block, 2° - Mobitz type I (Wenckebach)
- ☐ c. AV block, 2° - Mobitz type II
- ☐ d. AV block, 2:1
- ☐ e. AV block, 3°
- ☐ f. AV block, variable
- ☐ g. Short PR interval (with sinus rhythm and normal QRS duration)
- ☐ h. Wolff-Parkinson-White pattern

7. INTRAVENTRICULAR CONDUCTION DISTURBANCES

- ☐ a. RBBB, incomplete
- ☐ b. RBBB, complete
- ☐ c. Left anterior fascicular block
- ☐ d. Left posterior fascicular block
- ☐ e. LBBB, with ST-T wave suggestive of acute myocardial injury or infarction
- ☐ f. LBBB, complete
- ☐ g. LBBB, intermittent
- ☐ h. Intraventricular conduction disturbance, nonspecific
- ☐ i. Aberrant intraventricular conduction with supraventricular arrhythmia

8. P WAVE ABNORMALITIES

- ☐ a. Right atrial abnormality
- ☐ b. Left atrial abnormalities
- ☐ c. Nonspecific atrial abnormality

9. ABNORMALITIES OF QRS VOLTAGE OR AXIS

- ☐ a. Low voltage, limb leads only
- ☐ b. Low voltage, limb and precordial leads
- ☐ c. Left axis deviation (> - 30%)
- ☐ d. Right axis deviation (> + 100)
- ☐ e. Electrical alternans

10. VENTRICULAR HYPERTROPHY

- ☐ a. LVH by voltage only
- ☐ b. LVH by voltage and ST-T segment abnormalities
- ☐ c. RVH
- ☐ d. Combined ventricular hypertrophy

11. Q WAVE MYOCARDIAL INFARCTION

	Probably Acute or Recent	Probably Old or Age Indeterminate
Anterolateral	☐ a.	☐ g.
Anterior	☐ b.	☐ h.
Anteroseptal	☐ c.	☐ i.
Lateral/High lateral	☐ d.	☐ j.
Inferior	☐ e.	☐ k.
Posterior	☐ f.	☐ l.

☐ m. Probably ventricular aneurysm

12. ST, T, U, WAVE ABNORMALITIES

- ☐ a. Normal variant, early repolarization
- ☐ b. Normal variant, juvenile T waves
- ☐ c. Nonspecific ST and/or T wave abnormalities
- ☐ d. ST and/or T wave abnormalities suggesting myocardial ischemia
- ☐ e. ST and/or T wave abnormalities suggesting myocardial injury
- ☐ f. ST and/or T wave abnormalities suggesting acute pericarditis
- ☐ g. ST-T segment abnormalities secondary to intraventricular conduction disturbance or hypertrophy
- ☐ h. Post-extrasystolic T wave abnormality
- ☐ i. Isolated J point depression
- ☐ j. Peaked T waves
- ☐ k. Prolonged QT interval
- ☐ l. Prominent U waves

13. PACEMAKER FUNCTION AND RHYTHM

- ☐ a. Atrial or coronary sinus pacing
- ☐ b. Ventricular demand pacing
- ☐ c. AV sequential pacing
- ☐ d. Ventricular pacing, complete control
- ☐ e. Dual chamber, atrial sensing pacemaker
- ☐ f. Pacemaker malfunction, not constantly capturing (atrium or ventricle)
- ☐ g. Pacemaker malfunction, not constantly sensing (atrium or ventricle)
- ☐ h. Pacemaker malfunction, not firing
- ☐ i. Pacemaker malfunction, slowing

14. SUGGESTED OR PROBABLE CLINICAL DISORDERS

- ☐ a. Digitalis effect
- ☐ b. Digitalis toxicity
- ☐ c. Antiarrhythmic drug effect
- ☐ d. Antiarrhythmic drug toxicity
- ☐ e. Hyperkalemia
- ☐ f. Hypokalemia
- ☐ g. Hypercalcemia
- ☐ h. Hypocalcemia
- ☐ i. Atrial septal defect, secundum
- ☐ j. Atrial septal defect, primum
- ☐ k. Dextrocardia, mirror image
- ☐ l. Mitral valve disease
- ☐ m. Chronic lung disease
- ☐ n. Acute cor pulmonale, including pulmonary embolus
- ☐ o. Pericardial effusion
- ☐ p. Acute pericarditis
- ☐ q. Hypertrophic cardiomyopathy
- ☐ r. Coronary artery disease
- ☐ s. Central nervous system disorder
- ☐ t. Myxedema
- ☐ u. Hypothermia
- ☐ v. Sick sinus syndrome

ECG 66 was obtained from a 46-year-old female with a history of rheumatic fever, who presented with dyspnea on exertion. The ECG shows sinus rhythm and RBBB (arrows mark a wide rSR' complex in V_1 and wide slurred S waves in I, V_5, V_6) with secondary ST-T abnormalities. Right atrial abnormality (asterisk), left atrial abnormality (arrowhead), and left axis deviation are evident. These findings are compatible with mitral valve disease.

Codes:

2a	Sinus rhythm
7b	RBBB, complete
8a	Right atrial abnormality
8b	Left atrial abnormality
9c	Left axis deviation (>-30°)
12g	ST-T segment abnormalities secondary to IVCD or hypertrophy
14l	Mitral valve disease

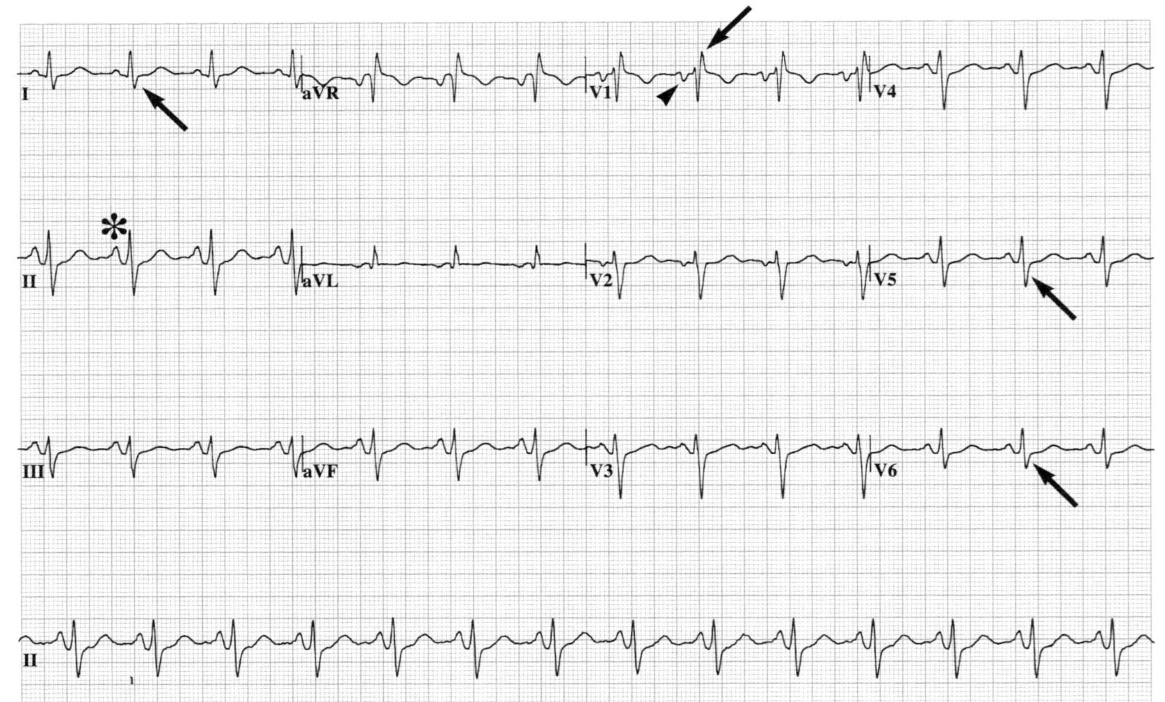

Questions: ECG 66

1 Which of the following statements about the P wave are true?

a. The P wave is normally upright in leads I, II and aVF, and inverted in aVR
b. The right atrium is responsible for the electrical potential inscription in the late portion of the P wave
c. Anatomical left atrial enlargement can exist with normal P wave amplitude, duration, and contour
d. Right atrial abnormality is a common finding in mitral valve disease
e. There is a good correlation between the amplitude of the P wave and right atrial pressure
f. Left atrial enlargement can cause a P pulmonale pattern

2. P pulmonale can be seen in:

a. Pulmonary embolism
b. COPD without cor pulmonale
c. Tetralogy of Fallot
d. Normal variant

3. Notching and widening of the P wave (P mitrale) may be caused by:

a. Atrial hypertrophy
b. Atrial dilatation
c. Intra-atrial conduction delay

4. Which of the following statements about the PR interval/segment are true?

a. The PR interval correlates with the period of atrial repolarization
b. PR depression can be a normal finding
c. PR elevation can be a normal finding
d. Leads with tall P waves are more likely to have PR depression than leads with smaller P waves

Answers: ECG 66

1. The right and left atria are responsible for the electrical potential inscription in the early and late portions of the P wave, respectively. The P wave amplitude, duration, and contour lack sensitivity and specificity for left atrial enlargement (i.e., left

atrial enlargement can exist with a normal P wave, and P mitrale may be present in the absence of left atrial enlargement). Increased amplitude of the late portion of the P wave from left atrial enlargement can result in a P-pulmonale pattern in the absence of right atrial enlargement (pseudo-P-pulmonale). (Answer: a, c, f)

2. P pulmonale, defined as a tall and peaked P wave (amplitude ≥ 2.5 mm in leads II, III, and aVF) of normal duration, may be seen in pulmonary embolism (usually transient), COPD with or without cor pulmonale, and as a normal variant in patients with a thin body habitus and/or verticle heart. P pulmonale can also be seen in tetralogy of Fallot and other forms of congenital heart disease, including Eisenmenger's physiology, tricuspid atresia, pulmonary hypertension, and pulmonic stenosis. (Answer: All)

3. P mitrale is defined by the presence of a notched and widened (≥ 0.12 seconds) P wave. While minor notching is common, pronounced notching (peak-to-peak interval > 0.04 seconds) is unusual. Mechanisms responsible for P mitrale include left atrial hypertrophy or dilatation, intra-atrial conduction delay, increased left atrial volume, and an acute rise in left atrial pressure. (Answer: All)

4. The PR segment, which represents the time from the onset of atrial depolarization to the onset of ventricular depolarization, is usually oriented in polarity opposite to that of the P wave, and is most pronounced in leads with taller P waves. PR depression < 0.8 mm is present on many normal ECGs, but PR depression > 0.8 mm is often abnormal. PR elevation is abnormal if present in any lead other than aVR. (Answer: b, d)

— Quick Review 66 —

Mitral valve disease	
• Mitral stenosis: Combination of (right/left) ventricular hypertrophy and (right/left) atrial abnormality is suggestive	right left
• Mitral valve prolapse:	
▸ Flattened or inverted ___ waves in leads II, III and aVF (and sometimes in right precordial leads) ± ST segment depression in the left precordial leads	T
▸ Prominent ___ waves	U
▸ Prolonged ___ interval	QT

— Comic Relief —

Who said there's nothing funny about managed care?

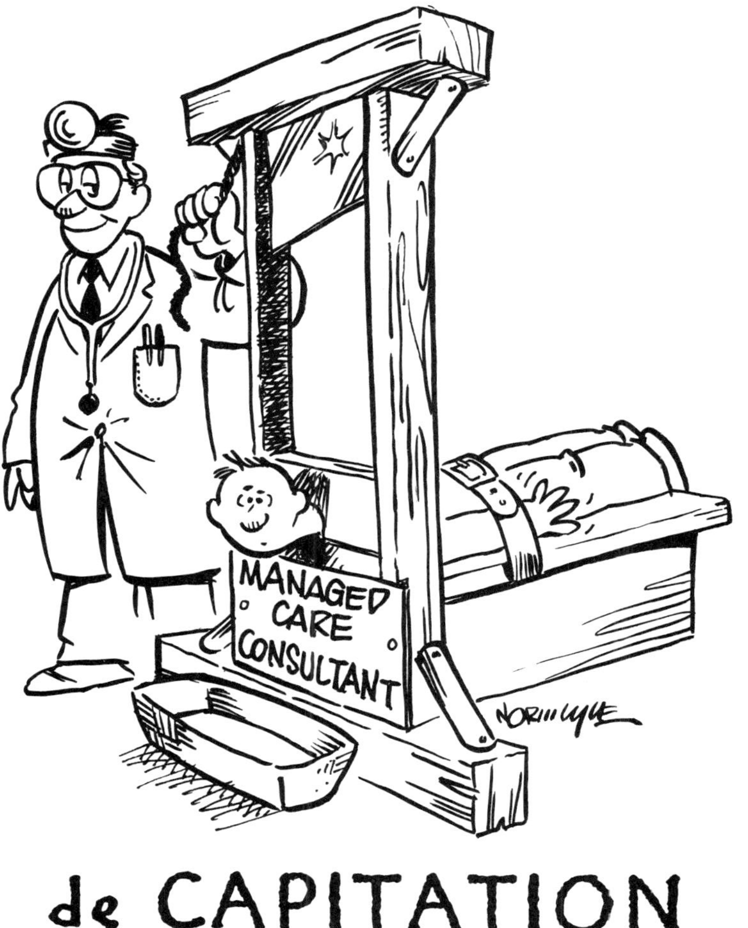

de CAPITATION

ECG 67. 39-year-old male with cardiomyopathy and syncope:

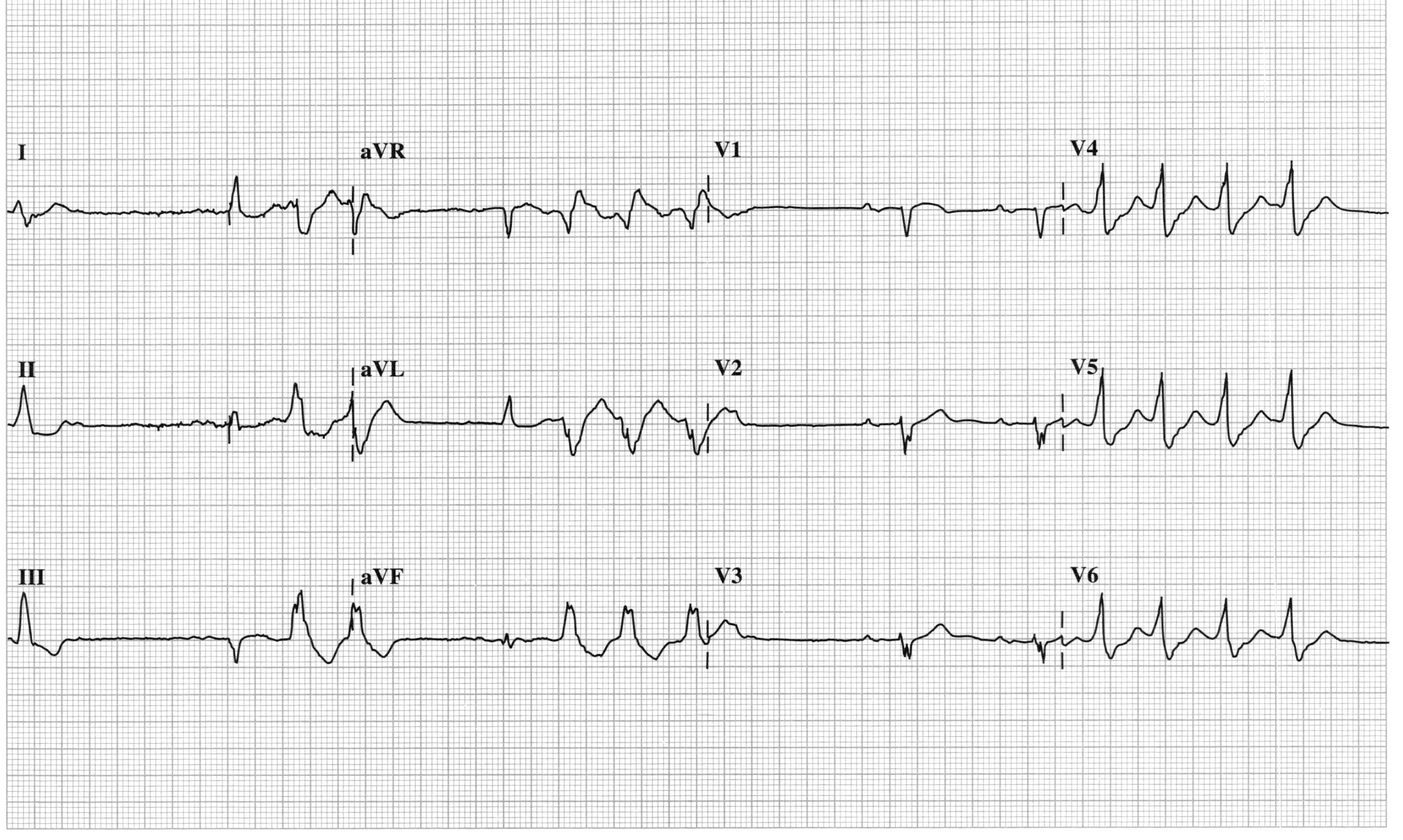

1. GENERAL FEATURES

☐ a. Normal ECG
☐ b. Borderline normal ECG or normal variant
☐ c. Incorrect electrode placement
☐ d. Artifact due to tremor

2. ATRIAL RHYTHMS

☐ a. Sinus rhythm
☐ b. Sinus arrhythmia
☐ c. Sinus bradycardia (< 60)
☐ d. Sinus tachycardia (> 100)
☐ e. Sinus pause or arrest
☐ f. Sinoatrial exit block
☐ g. Ecoptic atrial rhythm
☐ h. Wandering atrial pacemaker
☐ i. Atrial premature complexes, normally conducted
☐ j. Atrial premature complexes, nonconducted
☐ k. Atrial premature complexes with aberrant intraventricular conduction
☐ l. Atrial tachycardia (regular, sustained, 1:1 conduction)
☐ m. Atrial tachycardia, repetitive (short paroxysms)
☐ n. Atrial tachycardia, multifocal
☐ o. Atrial tachycardia with AV block
☐ p. Supraventricular tachycardia, unspecific
☐ q. Supraventricular tachycardia, paroxysmal
☐ r. Atrial flutter
☐ s. Atrial fibrillation
☐ t. Retrograde atrial activation

3. AV JUNCTIONAL RHYTHMS

☐ a. AV junctional premature complexes
☐ b. AV junctional escape complexes
☐ c. AV junctional rhythm, accelerated
☐ d. AV junctional rhythm

4. VENTRICULAR RHYTHMS

☐ a. Ventricular premature complex(es), uniform, fixed coupling
☐ b. Ventricular premature complex(es), uniform, nonfixed coupling
☐ c. Ventricular premature complexes(es), multiform
☐ d. Ventricular premature complexes, in pairs
☐ e. Ventricular parasystole
☐ f. Ventricular tachycardia (≥ 3 consecutive complexes)
☐ g. Accelerated idioventricular rhythm
☐ h. Ventricular escape complexes or rhythm
☐ i. Ventricular fibrillation

5. ATRIAL-VENTRICULAR INTERACTIONS IN ARRHYTHMIAS

☐ a. Fusion complexes
☐ b. Reciprocal (echo) complexes
☐ c. Ventricular capture complexes
☐ d. AV dissociation
☐ e. Ventriculophasic sinus arrhythmia

6. AV CONDUCTION ABNORMALITIES

☐ a. AV block, 1°
☐ b. AV block, 2° - Mobitz type I (Wenckebach)
☐ c. AV block, 2° - Mobitz type II
☐ d. AV block, 2:1
☐ e. AV block, 3°
☐ f. AV block, variable
☐ g. Short PR interval (with sinus rhythm and normal QRS duration)
☐ h. Wolff-Parkinson-White pattern

7. INTRAVENTRICULAR CONDUCTION DISTURBANCES

☐ a. RBBB, incomplete
☐ b. RBBB, complete
☐ c. Left anterior fascicular block
☐ d. Left posterior fascicular block
☐ e. LBBB, with ST-T wave suggestive of acute myocardial injury or infarction
☐ f. LBBB, complete
☐ g. LBBB, intermittent
☐ h. Intraventricular conduction disturbance, nonspecific
☐ i. Aberrant intraventricular conduction with supraventricular arrhythmia

8. P WAVE ABNORMALITIES

☐ a. Right atrial abnormality
☐ b. Left atrial abnormalities
☐ c. Nonspecific atrial abnormality

9. ABNORMALITIES OF QRS VOLTAGE OR AXIS

☐ a. Low voltage, limb leads only
☐ b. Low voltage, limb and precordial leads
☐ c. Left axis deviation (> - 30%)
☐ d. Right axis deviation (> + 100)
☐ e. Electrical alternans

10. VENTRICULAR HYPERTROPHY

☐ a. LVH by voltage only
☐ b. LVH by voltage and ST-T segment abnormalities
☐ c. RVH
☐ d. Combined ventricular hypertrophy

11. Q WAVE MYOCARDIAL INFARCTION

	Probably Acute or Recent	Probably Old or Age Indeterminate
Anterolateral	☐ a.	☐ g.
Anterior	☐ b.	☐ h.
Anteroseptal	☐ c.	☐ i.
Lateral/High lateral	☐ d.	☐ j.
Inferior	☐ e.	☐ k.
Posterior	☐ f.	☐ l.

☐ m. Probably ventricular aneurysm

12. ST, T, U, WAVE ABNORMALITIES

☐ a. Normal variant, early repolarization
☐ b. Normal variant, juvenile T waves
☐ c. Nonspecific ST and/or T wave abnormalities
☐ d. ST and/or T wave abnormalities suggesting myocardial ischemia
☐ e. ST and/or T wave abnormalities suggesting myocardial injury
☐ f. ST and/or T wave abnormalities suggesting acute pericarditis
☐ g. ST-T segment abnormalities secondary to intraventricular conduction disturbance or hypertrophy
☐ h. Post-extrasystolic T wave abnormality
☐ i. Isolated J point depression
☐ j. Peaked T waves
☐ k. Prolonged QT interval
☐ l. Prominent U waves

13. PACEMAKER FUNCTION AND RHYTHM

☐ a. Atrial or coronary sinus pacing
☐ b. Ventricular demand pacing
☐ c. AV sequential pacing
☐ d. Ventricular pacing, complete control
☐ e. Dual chamber, atrial sensing pacemaker
☐ f. Pacemaker malfunction, not constantly capturing (atrium or ventricle)
☐ g. Pacemaker malfunction, not constantly sensing (atrium or ventricle)
☐ h. Pacemaker malfunction, not firing
☐ i. Pacemaker malfunction, slowing

14. SUGGESTED OR PROBABLE CLINICAL DISORDERS

☐ a. Digitalis effect
☐ b. Digitalis toxicity
☐ c. Antiarrhythmic drug effect
☐ d. Antiarrhythmic drug toxicity
☐ e. Hyperkalemia
☐ f. Hypokalemia
☐ g. Hypercalcemia
☐ h. Hypocalcemia
☐ i. Atrial septal defect, secundum
☐ j. Atrial septal defect, primum
☐ k. Dextrocardia, mirror image
☐ l. Mitral valve disease
☐ m. Chronic lung disease
☐ n. Acute cor pulmonale, including pulmonary embolus
☐ o. Pericardial effusion
☐ p. Acute pericarditis
☐ q. Hypertrophic cardiomyopathy
☐ r. Coronary artery disease
☐ s. Central nervous system disorder
☐ t. Myxedema
☐ u. Hypothermia
☐ v. Sick sinus syndrome

ECG 67 was obtained in a 39-year-old male with a history of cardiomyopathy, who was being evaluated for syncope. Sinus rhythm at approximately 60 beats/minute (arrowheads mark P waves in V_1) and first-degree AV block are noted. Recurring runs of nonsustained ventricular tachycardia (asterisks) are initiated by repeated R on T occurrences. Intermittent pauses following the VT are due to AV block from concealed conduction, which on one occasion results in appropriate demand pacing (arrow). The fine baseline irregularity in the limb leads (double asterisk) is due to artifact.

Codes:

1d	Artifact due to tremor
2a	Sinus rhythm
4f	Ventricular tachycardia (≥ 3 consecutive complexes)
6a	AV block, 1°
13b	Ventricular demand pacing

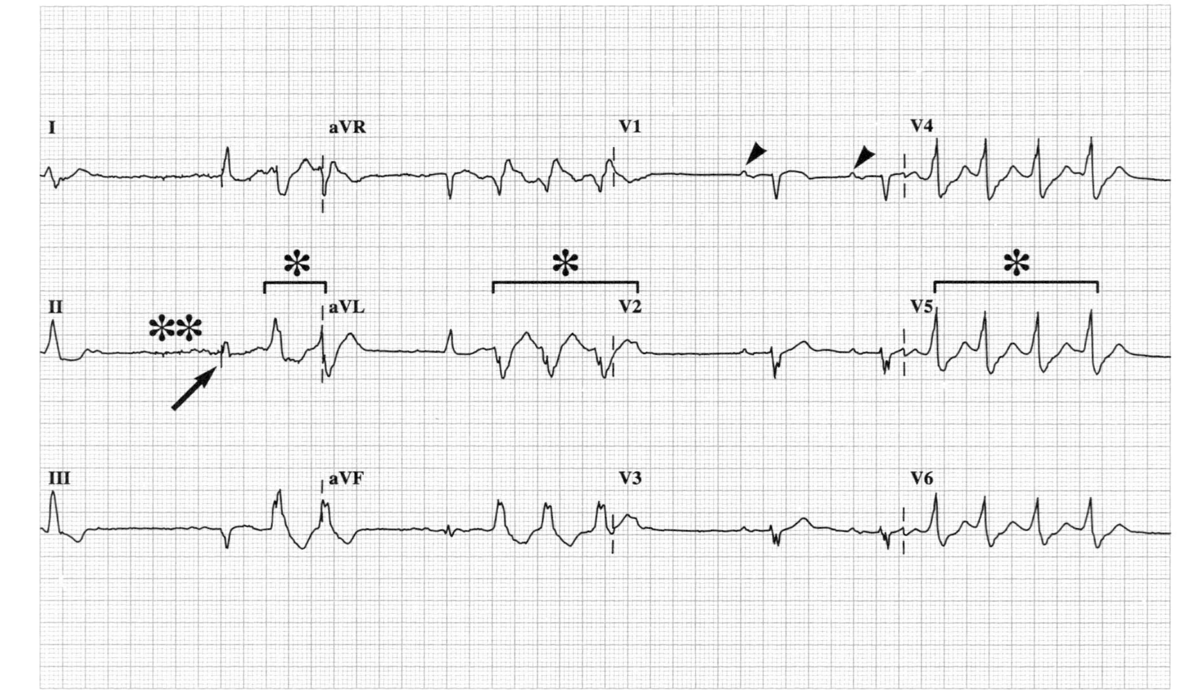

Questions: ECG 67

1. The differential diagnosis of a pause without a P wave includes:

   a. Sinus arrhythmia
   b. Mobitz Type I second-degree AV block
   c. Sinus arrest
   d. Blocked APC
   e. Sinoatrial exit block

2. Ventricular tachycardia is associated with:

   a. Capture beats
   b. Fusion beats
   c. AV dissociation
   d. Triggering by an APC

Answers: ECG 67

1. A pause without a P wave can be due to a number of different causes including sinus arrhythmia, sinus arrest, a blocked atrial premature complex, and sinoatrial exit block. Mobitz Type I second-degree AV block results in a nonconducted (but electrocardiographically apparent) P wave. (Answer: All except b)

2. The differentiation of supraventricular tachycardia with aberration from ventricular tachycardia is an important and common dilemma when confronted with a wide QRS tachycardia. The presence of capture beats, fusion beats, and ventricular concordance favor a ventricular origin for the arrhythmia. (Answer: a, b, c)

— Quick Review —	
Ventricular tachycardia	
• Rapid succession of three or more premature ventricular beats at a rate > ____ per minute	100
• RR intervals are usually regular but may be irregular (true/false)	true
• (Abrupt/gradual) onset and termination are evident	Abrupt
• AV ____ is common	dissociation
• Look for ventricular ____ complexes and ____ beats as markers for VT	capture, fusion
AV block, 1°	
• PR interval ≥ ____ seconds	0.20
Ventricular demand pacing	
• Pacemaker stimulus followed by a QRS complex that has (the same/different) morphology compared to the intrinsic QRS	different
• Must demonstrate ____ of pacemaker output in response to intrinsic QRS	inhibition

ECG 68. 71-year-old female with orthopnea and pedal edema:

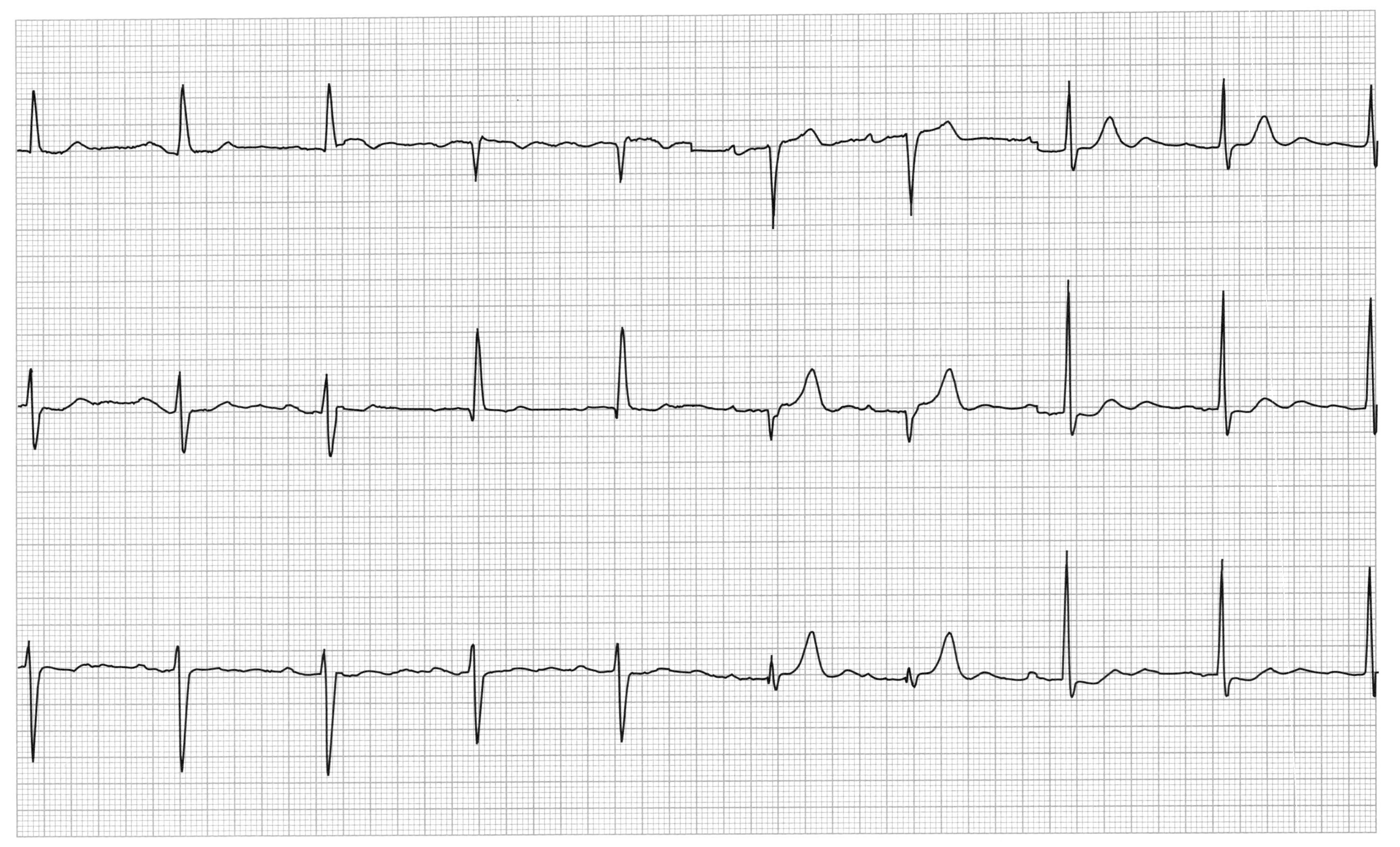

1. GENERAL FEATURES

☐ a. Normal ECG
☐ b. Borderline normal ECG or normal variant
☐ c. Incorrect electrode placement
☐ d. Artifact due to tremor

2. ATRIAL RHYTHMS

☐ a. Sinus rhythm
☐ b. Sinus arrhythmia
☐ c. Sinus bradycardia (< 60)
☐ d. Sinus tachycardia (> 100)
☐ e. Sinus pause or arrest
☐ f. Sinoatrial exit block
☐ g. Ecoptic atrial rhythm
☐ h. Wandering atrial pacemaker
☐ i. Atrial premature complexes, normally conducted
☐ j. Atrial premature complexes, nonconducted
☐ k. Atrial premature complexes with aberrant intraventricular conduction
☐ l. Atrial tachycardia (regular, sustained, 1:1 conduction)
☐ m. Atrial tachycardia, repetitive (short paroxysms)
☐ n. Atrial tachycardia, multifocal
☐ o. Atrial tachycardia with AV block
☐ p. Supraventricular tachycardia, unspecific
☐ q. Supraventricular tachycardia, paroxysmal
☐ r. Atrial flutter
☐ s. Atrial fibrillation
☐ t. Retrograde atrial activation

3. AV JUNCTIONAL RHYTHMS

☐ a. AV junctional premature complexes
☐ b. AV junctional escape complexes
☐ c. AV junctional rhythm, accelerated
☐ d. AV junctional rhythm

4. VENTRICULAR RHYTHMS

☐ a. Ventricular premature complex(es), uniform, fixed coupling
☐ b. Ventricular premature complex(es), uniform, nonfixed coupling
☐ c. Ventricular premature complexes(es), multiform
☐ d. Ventricular premature complexes, in pairs
☐ e. Ventricular parasystole
☐ f. Ventricular tachycardia (≥ 3 consecutive complexes)
☐ g. Accelerated idioventricular rhythm
☐ h. Ventricular escape complexes or rhythm
☐ i. Ventricular fibrillation

5. ATRIAL-VENTRICULAR INTERACTIONS IN ARRHYTHMIAS

☐ a. Fusion complexes
☐ b. Reciprocal (echo) complexes
☐ c. Ventricular capture complexes
☐ d. AV dissociation

☐ e. Ventriculophasic sinus arrhythmia

6. AV CONDUCTION ABNORMALITIES

☐ a. AV block, 1°
☐ b. AV block, 2° - Mobitz type I (Wenckebach)
☐ c. AV block, 2° - Mobitz type II
☐ d. AV block, 2:1
☐ e. AV block, 3°
☐ f. AV block, variable
☐ g. Short PR interval (with sinus rhythm and normal QRS duration)
☐ h. Wolff-Parkinson-White pattern

7. INTRAVENTRICULAR CONDUCTION DISTURBANCES

☐ a. RBBB, incomplete
☐ b. RBBB, complete
☐ c. Left anterior fascicular block
☐ d. Left posterior fascicular block
☐ e. LBBB, with ST-T wave suggestive of acute myocardial injury or infarction
☐ f. LBBB, complete
☐ g. LBBB, intermittent
☐ h. Intraventricular conduction disturbance, nonspecific
☐ i. Aberrant intraventricular conduction with supraventricular arrhythmia

8. P WAVE ABNORMALITIES

☐ a. Right atrial abnormality
☐ b. Left atrial abnormalities
☐ c. Nonspecific atrial abnormality

9. ABNORMALITIES OF QRS VOLTAGE OR AXIS

☐ a. Low voltage, limb leads only
☐ b. Low voltage, limb and precordial leads
☐ c. Left axis deviation (> - 30%)
☐ d. Right axis deviation (> + 100)
☐ e. Electrical alternans

10. VENTRICULAR HYPERTROPHY

☐ a. LVH by voltage only
☐ b. LVH by voltage and ST-T segment abnormalities
☐ c. RVH
☐ d. Combined ventricular hypertrophy

11. Q WAVE MYOCARDIAL INFARCTION

	Probably Acute or Recent	Probably Old or Age Indeterminate
Anterolateral	☐ a.	☐ g.
Anterior	☐ b.	☐ h.
Anteroseptal	☐ c.	☐ i.
Lateral/High lateral	☐ d.	☐ j.
Inferior	☐ e.	☐ k.
Posterior	☐ f.	☐ l.

☐ m. Probably ventricular aneurysm

12. ST, T, U, WAVE ABNORMALITIES

☐ a. Normal variant, early repolarization
☐ b. Normal variant, juvenile T waves
☐ c. Nonspecific ST and/or T wave abnormalities
☐ d. ST and/or T wave abnormalities suggesting myocardial ischemia
☐ e. ST and/or T wave abnormalities suggesting myocardial injury
☐ f. ST and/or T wave abnormalities suggesting acute pericarditis
☐ g. ST-T segment abnormalities secondary to intraventricular conduction disturbance or hypertrophy
☐ h. Post-extrasystolic T wave abnormality
☐ i. Isolated J point depression
☐ j. Peaked T waves
☐ k. Prolonged QT interval
☐ l. Prominent U waves

13. PACEMAKER FUNCTION AND RHYTHM

☐ a. Atrial or coronary sinus pacing
☐ b. Ventricular demand pacing
☐ c. AV sequential pacing
☐ d. Ventricular pacing, complete control
☐ e. Dual chamber, atrial sensing pacemaker
☐ f. Pacemaker malfunction, not constantly capturing (atrium or ventricle)
☐ g. Pacemaker malfunction, not constantly sensing (atrium or ventricle)
☐ h. Pacemaker malfunction, not firing
☐ i. Pacemaker malfunction, slowing

14. SUGGESTED OR PROBABLE CLINICAL DISORDERS

☐ a. Digitalis effect
☐ b. Digitalis toxicity
☐ c. Antiarrhythmic drug effect
☐ d. Antiarrhythmic drug toxicity
☐ e. Hyperkalemia
☐ f. Hypokalemia
☐ g. Hypercalcemia
☐ h. Hypocalcemia
☐ i. Atrial septal defect, secundum
☐ j. Atrial septal defect, primum
☐ k. Dextrocardia, mirror image
☐ l. Mitral valve disease
☐ m. Chronic lung disease
☐ n. Acute cor pulmonale, including pulmonary embolus
☐ o. Pericardial effusion
☐ p. Acute pericarditis
☐ q. Hypertrophic cardiomyopathy
☐ r. Coronary artery disease
☐ s. Central nervous system disorder
☐ t. Myxedema
☐ u. Hypothermia
☐ v. Sick sinus syndrome

ECG 68 was obtained in a 71-year-old female with complaints of orthopnea and pedal edema. The ECG shows sinus bradycardia at 55 beats/minute with first-degree AV block, left atrial abnormality, and left axis deviation. Voltage criteria for LVH (especially notable in aVL, where the R wave is 15 mm; arrow) with secondary ST-T changes and prominent U waves (asterisk) are also evident. Anteroseptal MI should not be coded since a Q wave is absent in V_3; the Q waves in V_1 and V_2 are probably due to LVH.

Codes:

2c	Sinus bradycardia (< 60)
6a	AV block, 1 °
8b	Left atrial abnormality
9c	Left axis deviation (> -30°)
10b	LVH by both voltage and ST-T segment abnormalities
12g	ST-T segment abnormalities secondary to IVCD or hypertrophy
12l	Prominent U waves

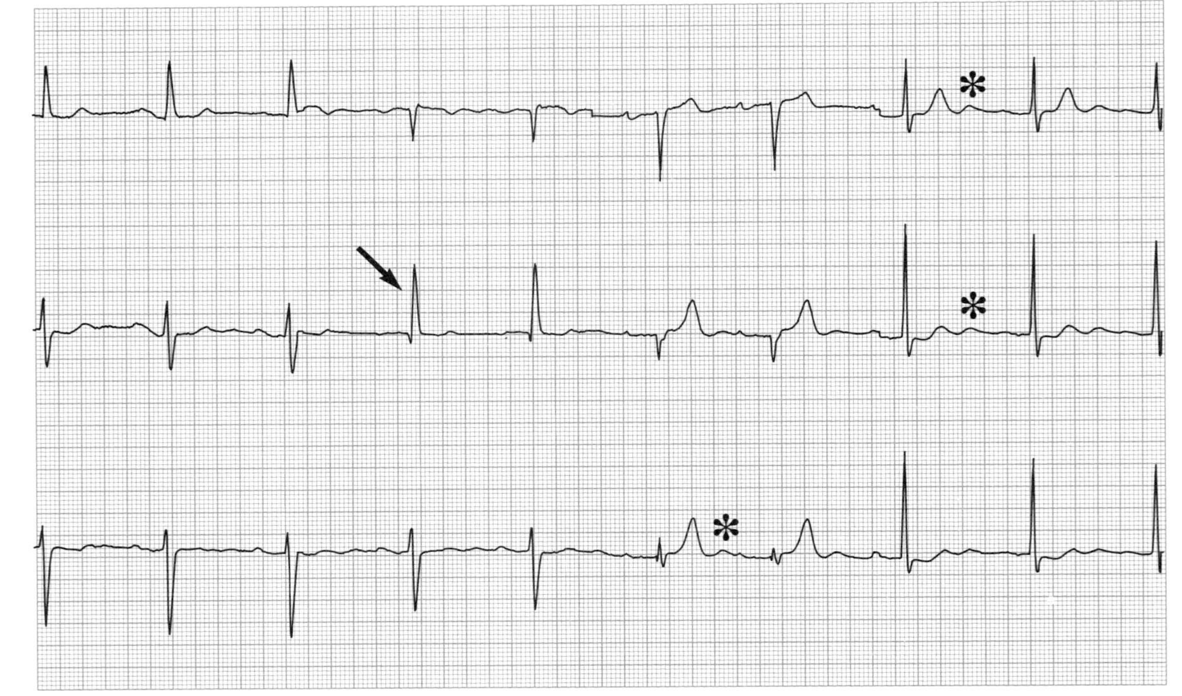

Questions: ECG 68

1. If the PR interval is prolonged and the QRS is narrow, where is the site of block:

   a. SA node
   b. AV node
   c. His bundle
   d. His-Purkinje system

2. Which of the following statements about left anterior fascicular block (LAFB) are true:

   a. LAFB always signifies the presence of structural heart disease
   b. LAFB reduces the specificity for the diagnosis of LVH by voltage criteria
   c. The most common cause of LAFB is coronary artery disease
   d. In the presence of inferior MI, the specificity of ECG criteria for the diagnosis of LAFB is reduced

3. Aside from left anterior fascicular block, other causes of left axis deviation include:

   a. Hyperkalemia
   b. Pulmonary emphysema
   c. Ostium secundum atrial septal defect
   d. Inferior MI
   e. LVH
   f. Left posterior fascicular block
   g. Lateral MI

Answers: ECG 68

1. The PR interval represents the time from the onset of atrial depolarization to the onset of ventricular depolarization (i.e., conduction time from the atrium → AV node → His bundle → Purkinje system → ventricles). It does not reflect conduction from the sinus node to the atrial tissue. Therefore, a prolonged PR interval with a narrow QRS complex identifies the site of block in the AV node. If the QRS is wide, conduction delay or block typically occurs in the His-Purkinje system (although block in the AV node can manifest as a prolonged PR and wide QRS if preexisting bundle branch block or rate-dependant aberrancy is present). (Answer: b)

2. The left bundle branch supplies the Purkinje fibers to the left ventricle via an anterior fascicle (anterior and lateral ventricle) and a posterior fascicle (inferior and posterior ventricle). Block in the left anterior fascicle results in late activation of the anterior

and lateral ventricular walls, shifting the mean QRS axis to the left. The most common cause of left anterior fascicular block (LAFB) is coronary artery disease, but this conduction abnormality can be seen in patients without structural heart disease. LAFB reduces the specificity for the diagnosis of LVH based on voltage criteria in leads I and aVL. Inferior myocardial infarction (MI), which can shift the mean QRS axis superior and leftward (from unopposed anterior and lateral forces), can cause left axis deviation despite normal conduction down the left anterior fascicle. When QS complexes are present in the inferior leads, inferior MI and LAFB may both be present. (Answer: b, c)

3. Left axis deviation may occur in hyperkalemia, pulmonary emphysema, inferior myocardial infarction, and left ventricular hypertrophy. Ostium secundum ASD, left posterior fascicular block, and lateral MI shift the mean QRS axis rightward (i.e., right axis deviation). (Answer: a, b, d, e)

— Quick Review 68 —

Sinus bradycardia	
• Rate < ____ per minute	60
• If rate is < 40 per minute, think of 2:1 ____	sinoatrial exit block
AV block, 1°	
• PR interval ≥ ____ seconds	0.20
Left atrial abnormality	
• Notched P wave with a duration ≥ ____ seconds in leads II, III or aVF, *or*	0.12
• Terminal negative portion of the P wave in lead V_1 ≥ 1 mm deep and ≥ ____ seconds in duration	0.04
Prominent U waves	
• Amplitude ≥ ____ mm	1.5
• The U wave is normally ____% the height of the T wave, and is largest in leads ____	5-25 V_2, V_3

Common Dilemmas in ECG Interpretation

Problem

A dominant junctional or ventricular rhythm is present. Is it necessary to code the underlying atrial rhythm if one is present?

Recommendation

Yes. If in addition to the presence of a dominant junctional or ventricular rhythm, an atrial rhythm is also apparent, the atrial rhythm should also be coded (e.g., ventricular tachycardia and sinus rhythm). This applies to significant AV block as well (e.g., sinus tachycardia with third-degree AV block).

ECG 69. 76-year-old asymptomatic female:

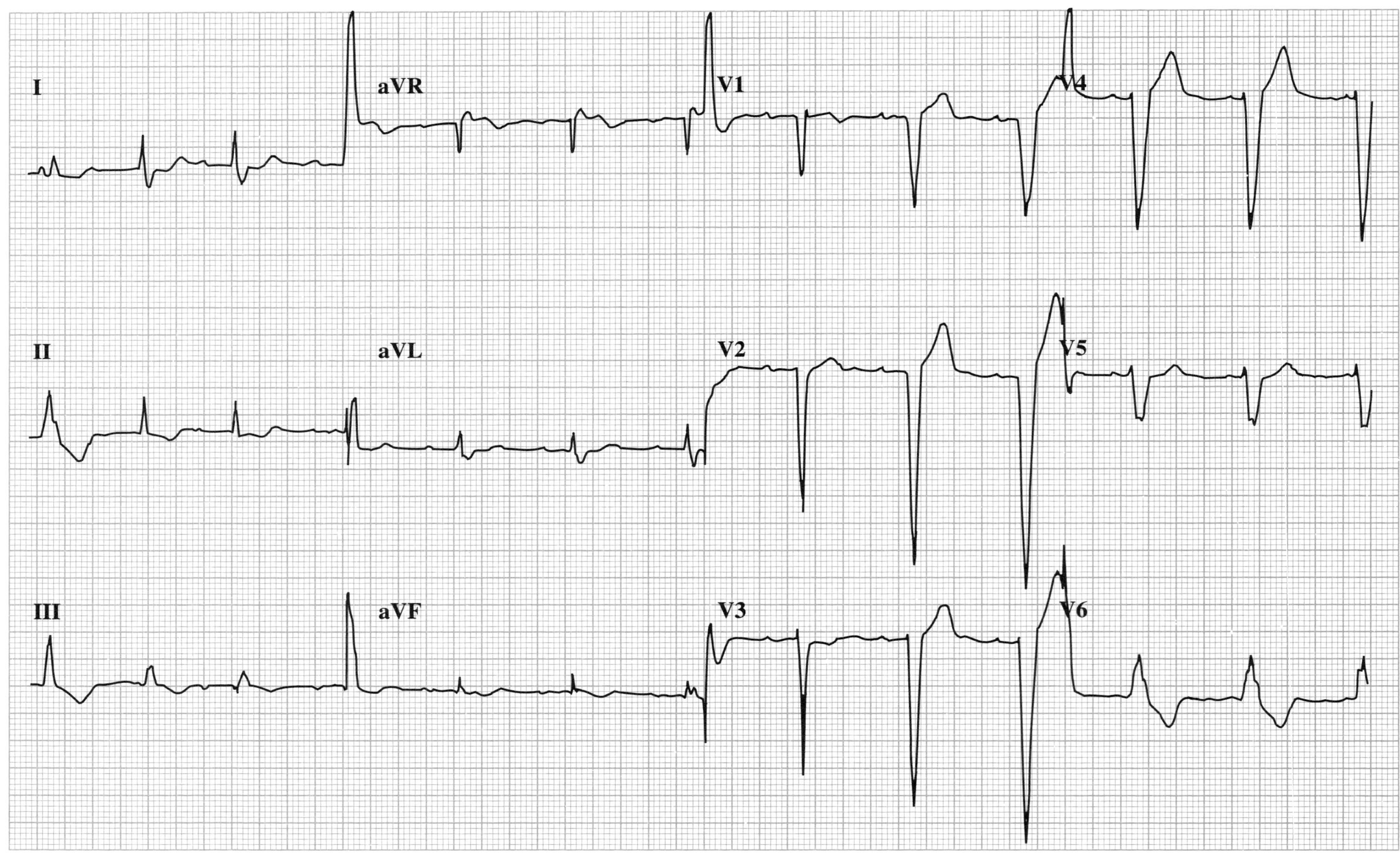

1. GENERAL FEATURES
- ☐ a. Normal ECG
- ☐ b. Borderline normal ECG or normal variant
- ☐ c. Incorrect electrode placement
- ☐ d. Artifact due to tremor

2. ATRIAL RHYTHMS
- ☐ a. Sinus rhythm
- ☐ b. Sinus arrhythmia
- ☐ c. Sinus bradycardia (< 60)
- ☐ d. Sinus tachycardia (> 100)
- ☐ e. Sinus pause or arrest
- ☐ f. Sinoatrial exit block
- ☐ g. Ecoptic atrial rhythm
- ☐ h. Wandering atrial pacemaker
- ☐ i. Atrial premature complexes, normally conducted
- ☐ j. Atrial premature complexes, nonconducted
- ☐ k. Atrial premature complexes with aberrant intraventricular conduction
- ☐ l. Atrial tachycardia (regular, sustained, 1:1 conduction)
- ☐ m. Atrial tachycardia, repetitive (short paroxysms)
- ☐ n. Atrial tachycardia, multifocal
- ☐ o. Atrial tachycardia with AV block
- ☐ p. Supraventricular tachycardia, unspecific
- ☐ q. Supraventricular tachycardia, paroxysmal
- ☐ r. Atrial flutter
- ☐ s. Atrial fibrillation
- ☐ t. Retrograde atrial activation

3. AV JUNCTIONAL RHYTHMS
- ☐ a. AV junctional premature complexes
- ☐ b. AV junctional escape complexes
- ☐ c. AV junctional rhythm, accelerated
- ☐ d. AV junctional rhythm

4. VENTRICULAR RHYTHMS
- ☐ a. Ventricular premature complex(es), uniform, fixed coupling
- ☐ b. Ventricular premature complex(es), uniform, nonfixed coupling
- ☐ c. Ventricular premature complexes(es), multiform
- ☐ d. Ventricular premature complexes, in pairs
- ☐ e. Ventricular parasystole
- ☐ f. Ventricular tachycardia (≥ 3 consecutive complexes)
- ☐ g. Accelerated idioventricular rhythm
- ☐ h. Ventricular escape complexes or rhythm
- ☐ i. Ventricular fibrillation

5. ATRIAL-VENTRICULAR INTERACTIONS IN ARRHYTHMIAS
- ☐ a. Fusion complexes
- ☐ b. Reciprocal (echo) complexes
- ☐ c. Ventricular capture complexes
- ☐ d. AV dissociation
- ☐ e. Ventriculophasic sinus arrhythmia

6. AV CONDUCTION ABNORMALITIES
- ☐ a. AV block, 1°
- ☐ b. AV block, 2° - Mobitz type I (Wenckebach)
- ☐ c. AV block, 2° - Mobitz type II
- ☐ d. AV block, 2:1
- ☐ e. AV block, 3°
- ☐ f. AV block, variable
- ☐ g. Short PR interval (with sinus rhythm and normal QRS duration)
- ☐ h. Wolff-Parkinson-White pattern

7. INTRAVENTRICULAR CONDUCTION DISTURBANCES
- ☐ a. RBBB, incomplete
- ☐ b. RBBB, complete
- ☐ c. Left anterior fascicular block
- ☐ d. Left posterior fascicular block
- ☐ e. LBBB, with ST-T wave suggestive of acute myocardial injury or infarction
- ☐ f. LBBB, complete
- ☐ g. LBBB, intermittent
- ☐ h. Intraventricular conduction disturbance, nonspecific
- ☐ i. Aberrant intraventricular conduction with supraventricular arrhythmia

8. P WAVE ABNORMALITIES
- ☐ a. Right atrial abnormality
- ☐ b. Left atrial abnormalities
- ☐ c. Nonspecific atrial abnormality

9. ABNORMALITIES OF QRS VOLTAGE OR AXIS
- ☐ a. Low voltage, limb leads only
- ☐ b. Low voltage, limb and precordial leads
- ☐ c. Left axis deviation (> - 30%)
- ☐ d. Right axis deviation (> + 100)
- ☐ e. Electrical alternans

10. VENTRICULAR HYPERTROPHY
- ☐ a. LVH by voltage only
- ☐ b. LVH by voltage and ST-T segment abnormalities
- ☐ c. RVH
- ☐ d. Combined ventricular hypertrophy

11. Q WAVE MYOCARDIAL INFARCTION

	Probably Acute or Recent	Probably Old or Age Indeterminate
Anterolateral	☐ a.	☐ g.
Anterior	☐ b.	☐ h.
Anteroseptal	☐ c.	☐ i.
Lateral/High lateral	☐ d.	☐ j.
Inferior	☐ e.	☐ k.
Posterior	☐ f.	☐ l.

☐ m. Probably ventricular aneurysm

12. ST, T, U, WAVE ABNORMALITIES
- ☐ a. Normal variant, early repolarization
- ☐ b. Normal variant, juvenile T waves
- ☐ c. Nonspecific ST and/or T wave abnormalities
- ☐ d. ST and/or T wave abnormalities suggesting myocardial ischemia
- ☐ e. ST and/or T wave abnormalities suggesting myocardial injury
- ☐ f. ST and/or T wave abnormalities suggesting acute pericarditis
- ☐ g. ST-T segment abnormalities secondary to intraventricular conduction disturbance or hypertrophy
- ☐ h. Post-extrasystolic T wave abnormality
- ☐ i. Isolated J point depression
- ☐ j. Peaked T waves
- ☐ k. Prolonged QT interval
- ☐ l. Prominent U waves

13. PACEMAKER FUNCTION AND RHYTHM
- ☐ a. Atrial or coronary sinus pacing
- ☐ b. Ventricular demand pacing
- ☐ c. AV sequential pacing
- ☐ d. Ventricular pacing, complete control
- ☐ e. Dual chamber, atrial sensing pacemaker
- ☐ f. Pacemaker malfunction, not constantly capturing (atrium or ventricle)
- ☐ g. Pacemaker malfunction, not constantly sensing (atrium or ventricle)
- ☐ h. Pacemaker malfunction, not firing
- ☐ i. Pacemaker malfunction, slowing

14. SUGGESTED OR PROBABLE CLINICAL DISORDERS
- ☐ a. Digitalis effect
- ☐ b. Digitalis toxicity
- ☐ c. Antiarrhythmic drug effect
- ☐ d. Antiarrhythmic drug toxicity
- ☐ e. Hyperkalemia
- ☐ f. Hypokalemia
- ☐ g. Hypercalcemia
- ☐ h. Hypocalcemia
- ☐ i. Atrial septal defect, secundum
- ☐ j. Atrial septal defect, primum
- ☐ k. Dextrocardia, mirror image
- ☐ l. Mitral valve disease
- ☐ m. Chronic lung disease
- ☐ n. Acute cor pulmonale, including pulmonary embolus
- ☐ o. Pericardial effusion
- ☐ p. Acute pericarditis
- ☐ q. Hypertrophic cardiomyopathy
- ☐ r. Coronary artery disease
- ☐ s. Central nervous system disorder
- ☐ t. Myxedema
- ☐ u. Hypothermia
- ☐ v. Sick sinus syndrome

ECG 69 was obtained in a 76-year-old asymptomatic female. During the first half of the ECG, sinus rhythm with first-degree AV block is present. This is overridden by an accelerated idioventricular rhythm (arrows) resulting in isorhythmic AV dissociation and fusion complexes (QRS with asterisk is intermediate in morphology between the QRS complexes labeled 1 and 2). A nonspecific intraventricular conduction defect (QRS in sinus rhythm = 116 msec) with secondary ST-T abnormalities is also present.

Codes:

2a	Sinus rhythm
4g	Accelerated idioventricular rhythm
5a	Fusion complexes
5d	AV dissociation
6a	AV block, 1°
7h	IVCD, nonspecific type
12g	ST-T segment abnormalities secondary to IVCD or hypertrophy

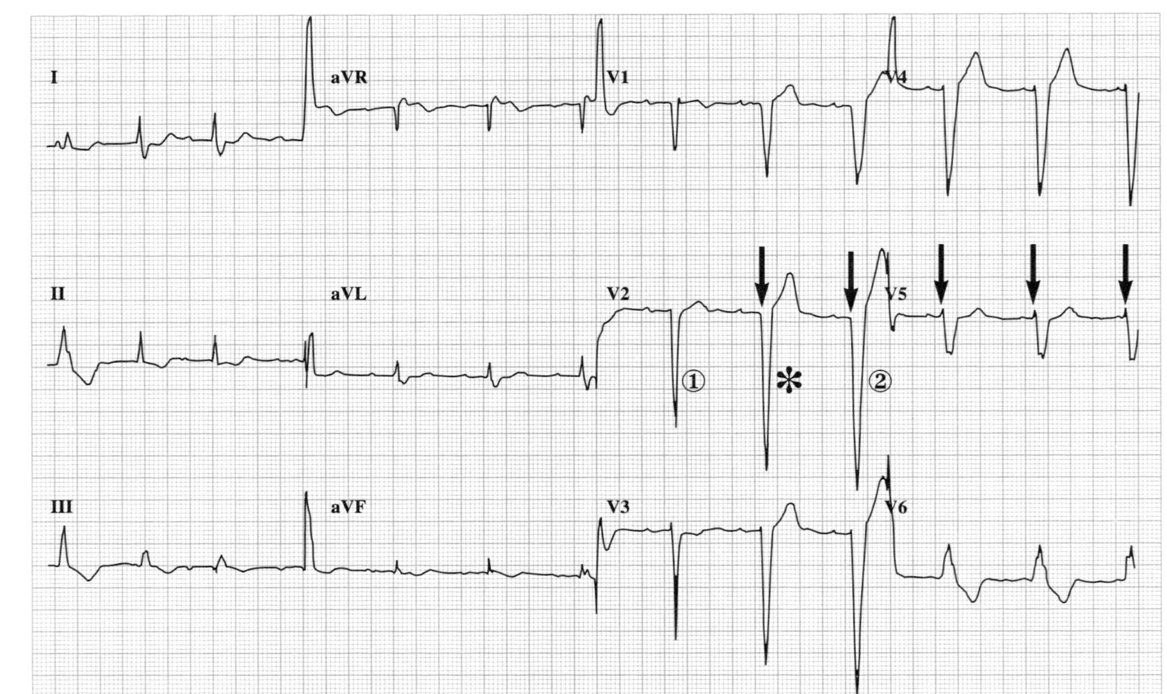

Questions: ECG 69

1. AV dissociation is characterized by an atrial rate that is ___ the ventricular rate:

   a. Slower than
   b. Faster than
   c. Equal to

2. By definition, the rate of an accelerated idioventricular rhythm is:

   a. 30-50 bpm
   b. 60-110 bpm
   c. 40-60 bpm
   d. < 30 bpm

3. Secondary repolarization abnormalities are usually seen with:

   a. Coronary artery spasm
   b. RBBB
   c. LVH
   d. LBBB
   e. RVH

Answers: ECG 69

1. AV dissociation occurs when the atrial and ventricular activities are independent of each other, and the atrial rate is ***slower*** than the ventricular rate. This generally occurs in the setting of extreme sinus bradycardia or normal sinus rhythm with a faster (escape or accelerated) junctional or idioventricular rhythm. (Answer: a)

2. Accelerated idioventricular rhythm is a regular rhythm characterized by wide QRS complexes occurring at a rate of 60-110 BPM. AV dissociation, capture complexes, and fusion beats are common during AIVR because of the competition between the normal sinus and ectopic ventricular rhythms. AIVR does not have the same adverse impact on prognosis that ventricular tachycardia does. (Answer: b)

3. Secondary repolarization (ST-T) changes occur with ventricular hypertrophy and bundle branch blocks. The ST-T changes associated with coronary spasm are due to ischemia and/or injury — they are considered "primary," not "secondary." (Answer: All except a)

— Quick Review 69 —

Accelerated idioventricular rhythm	
• Highly irregular ventricular rhythm (true/false)	false
• Ventricular rate of ____ per minute	60-110
• QRS morphology is similar to ____	VPCs
• Ventricular ____ complexes, ____ beats, and AV ____ are common	capture, fusion dissociation
AV dissociation	
• Atrial and ventricular rhythms are ____ of each other	independent
• Ventricular rate is (</≥) than the atrial rate	≥

Differential Diagnosis

LEFT AXIS DEVIATION (>-30°)

- Left anterior fascicular block (if axis > -45°, item 7c)
- Inferior wall MI (item 11e, k)
- LBBB (item f)
- LVH (items 10 a, b)
- Ostium primum ASD (item 14j)
- COPD (item 14m)
- Hyperkalemia (item 14e)

ECG 70. 72-year-old male with previous myocardial infarction who is currently asymptomatic:

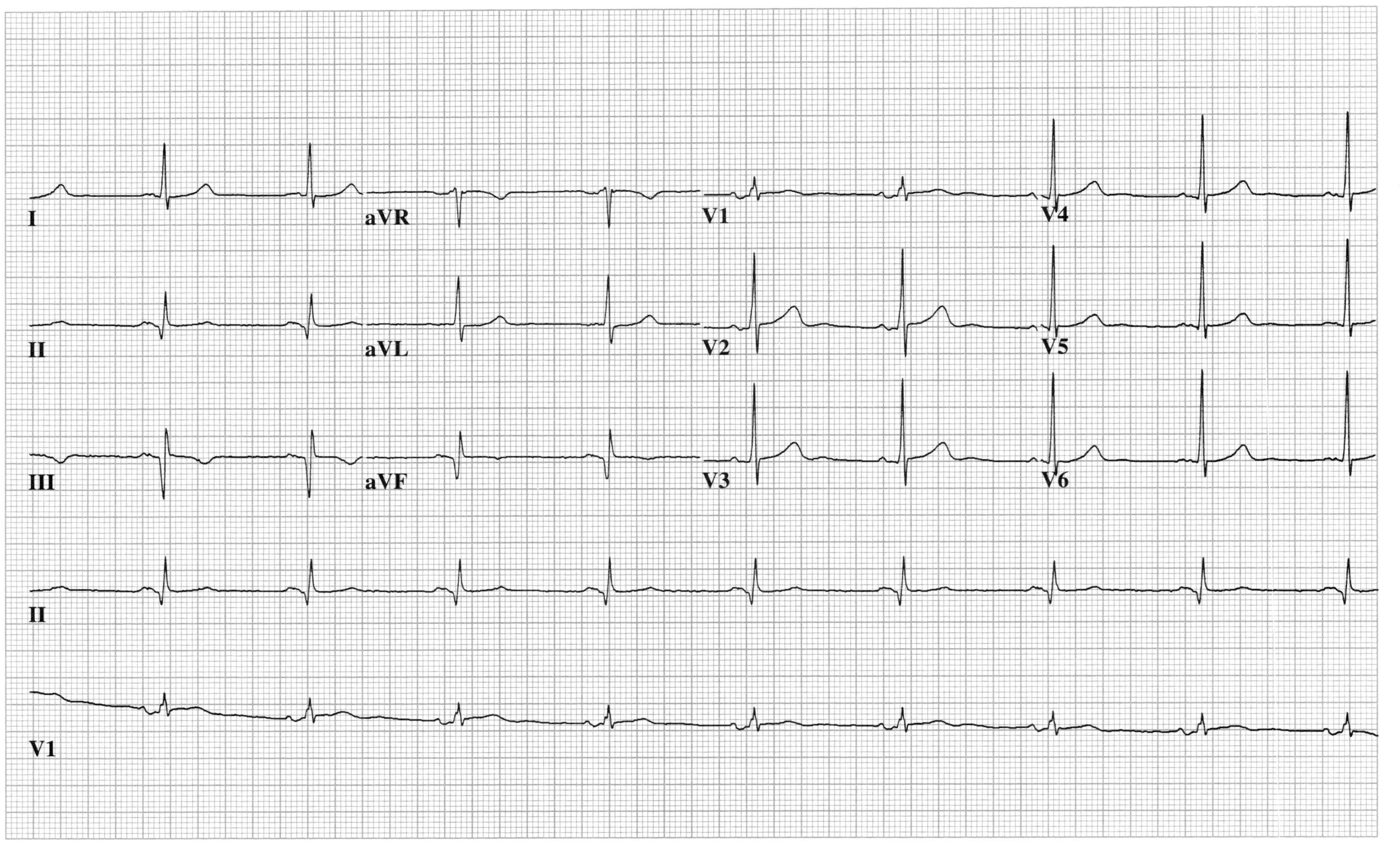

1. GENERAL FEATURES
- ☐ a. Normal ECG
- ☐ b. Borderline normal ECG or normal variant
- ☐ c. Incorrect electrode placement
- ☐ d. Artifact due to tremor

2. ATRIAL RHYTHMS
- ☐ a. Sinus rhythm
- ☐ b. Sinus arrhythmia
- ☐ c. Sinus bradycardia (< 60)
- ☐ d. Sinus tachycardia (> 100)
- ☐ e. Sinus pause or arrest
- ☐ f. Sinoatrial exit block
- ☐ g. Ecoptic atrial rhythm
- ☐ h. Wandering atrial pacemaker
- ☐ i. Atrial premature complexes, normally conducted
- ☐ j. Atrial premature complexes, nonconducted
- ☐ k. Atrial premature complexes with aberrant intraventricular conduction
- ☐ l. Atrial tachycardia (regular, sustained, 1:1 conduction)
- ☐ m. Atrial tachycardia, repetitive (short paroxysms)
- ☐ n. Atrial tachycardia, multifocal
- ☐ o. Atrial tachycardia with AV block
- ☐ p. Supraventricular tachycardia, unspecific
- ☐ q. Supraventricular tachycardia, paroxysmal
- ☐ r. Atrial flutter
- ☐ s. Atrial fibrillation
- ☐ t. Retrograde atrial activation

3. AV JUNCTIONAL RHYTHMS
- ☐ a. AV junctional premature complexes
- ☐ b. AV junctional escape complexes
- ☐ c. AV junctional rhythm, accelerated
- ☐ d. AV junctional rhythm

4. VENTRICULAR RHYTHMS
- ☐ a. Ventricular premature complex(es), uniform, fixed coupling
- ☐ b. Ventricular premature complex(es), uniform, nonfixed coupling
- ☐ c. Ventricular premature complexes(es), multiform
- ☐ d. Ventricular premature complexes, in pairs
- ☐ e. Ventricular parasystole
- ☐ f. Ventricular tachycardia (≥ 3 consecutive complexes)
- ☐ g. Accelerated idioventricular rhythm
- ☐ h. Ventricular escape complexes or rhythm
- ☐ i. Ventricular fibrillation

5. ATRIAL-VENTRICULAR INTERACTIONS IN ARRHYTHMIAS
- ☐ a. Fusion complexes
- ☐ b. Reciprocal (echo) complexes
- ☐ c. Ventricular capture complexes
- ☐ d. AV dissociation
- ☐ e. Ventriculophasic sinus arrhythmia

6. AV CONDUCTION ABNORMALITIES
- ☐ a. AV block, 1°
- ☐ b. AV block, 2° - Mobitz type I (Wenckebach)
- ☐ c. AV block, 2° - Mobitz type II
- ☐ d. AV block, 2:1
- ☐ e. AV block, 3°
- ☐ f. AV block, variable
- ☐ g. Short PR interval (with sinus rhythm and normal QRS duration)
- ☐ h. Wolff-Parkinson-White pattern

7. INTRAVENTRICULAR CONDUCTION DISTURBANCES
- ☐ a. RBBB, incomplete
- ☐ b. RBBB, complete
- ☐ c. Left anterior fascicular block
- ☐ d. Left posterior fascicular block
- ☐ e. LBBB, with ST-T wave suggestive of acute myocardial injury or infarction
- ☐ f. LBBB, complete
- ☐ g. LBBB, intermittent
- ☐ h. Intraventricular conduction disturbance, nonspecific
- ☐ i. Aberrant intraventricular conduction with supraventricular arrhythmia

8. P WAVE ABNORMALITIES
- ☐ a. Right atrial abnormality
- ☐ b. Left atrial abnormalities
- ☐ c. Nonspecific atrial abnormality

9. ABNORMALITIES OF QRS VOLTAGE OR AXIS
- ☐ a. Low voltage, limb leads only
- ☐ b. Low voltage, limb and precordial leads
- ☐ c. Left axis deviation (> - 30%)
- ☐ d. Right axis deviation (> + 100)
- ☐ e. Electrical alternans

10. VENTRICULAR HYPERTROPHY
- ☐ a. LVH by voltage only
- ☐ b. LVH by voltage and ST-T segment abnormalities
- ☐ c. RVH
- ☐ d. Combined ventricular hypertrophy

11. Q WAVE MYOCARDIAL INFARCTION

	Probably Acute or Recent	Probably Old or Age Indeterminate
Anterolateral	☐ a.	☐ g.
Anterior	☐ b.	☐ h.
Anteroseptal	☐ c.	☐ i.
Lateral/High lateral	☐ d.	☐ j.
Inferior	☐ e.	☐ k.
Posterior	☐ f.	☐ l.

☐ m. Probably ventricular aneurysm

12. ST, T, U, WAVE ABNORMALITIES
- ☐ a. Normal variant, early repolarization
- ☐ b. Normal variant, juvenile T waves
- ☐ c. Nonspecific ST and/or T wave abnormalities
- ☐ d. ST and/or T wave abnormalities suggesting myocardial ischemia
- ☐ e. ST and/or T wave abnormalities suggesting myocardial injury
- ☐ f. ST and/or T wave abnormalities suggesting acute pericarditis
- ☐ g. ST-T segment abnormalities secondary to intraventricular conduction disturbance or hypertrophy
- ☐ h. Post-extrasystolic T wave abnormality
- ☐ i. Isolated J point depression
- ☐ j. Peaked T waves
- ☐ k. Prolonged QT interval
- ☐ l. Prominent U waves

13. PACEMAKER FUNCTION AND RHYTHM
- ☐ a. Atrial or coronary sinus pacing
- ☐ b. Ventricular demand pacing
- ☐ c. AV sequential pacing
- ☐ d. Ventricular pacing, complete control
- ☐ e. Dual chamber, atrial sensing pacemaker
- ☐ f. Pacemaker malfunction, not constantly capturing (atrium or ventricle)
- ☐ g. Pacemaker malfunction, not constantly sensing (atrium or ventricle)
- ☐ h. Pacemaker malfunction, not firing
- ☐ i. Pacemaker malfunction, slowing

14. SUGGESTED OR PROBABLE CLINICAL DISORDERS
- ☐ a. Digitalis effect
- ☐ b. Digitalis toxicity
- ☐ c. Antiarrhythmic drug effect
- ☐ d. Antiarrhythmic drug toxicity
- ☐ e. Hyperkalemia
- ☐ f. Hypokalemia
- ☐ g. Hypercalcemia
- ☐ h. Hypocalcemia
- ☐ i. Atrial septal defect, secundum
- ☐ j. Atrial septal defect, primum
- ☐ k. Dextrocardia, mirror image
- ☐ l. Mitral valve disease
- ☐ m. Chronic lung disease
- ☐ n. Acute cor pulmonale, including pulmonary embolus
- ☐ o. Pericardial effusion
- ☐ p. Acute pericarditis
- ☐ q. Hypertrophic cardiomyopathy
- ☐ r. Coronary artery disease
- ☐ s. Central nervous system disorder
- ☐ t. Myxedema
- ☐ u. Hypothermia
- ☐ v. Sick sinus syndrome

ECG 70 was obtained in a 72-year-old asymptomatic male with a history of myocardial infarction. This tracing shows a sinus bradycardia at 54 beats/minute. The abnormal Q waves and nonspecific ST-T changes in leads II, III and aVF (arrows), and the prominent R wave in leads V_1 and V_2 (arrowheads) are consistent with prior inferoposterior infarction. Coronary artery disease should also be coded.

Codes:

2c	Sinus bradycardia
11k	Inferior Q wave MI, probably old or age indeterminate
11l	Posterior MI, probably old and age indeterminate
12c	Nonspecific ST and/or T wave abnormalities
14r	Coronary artery disease

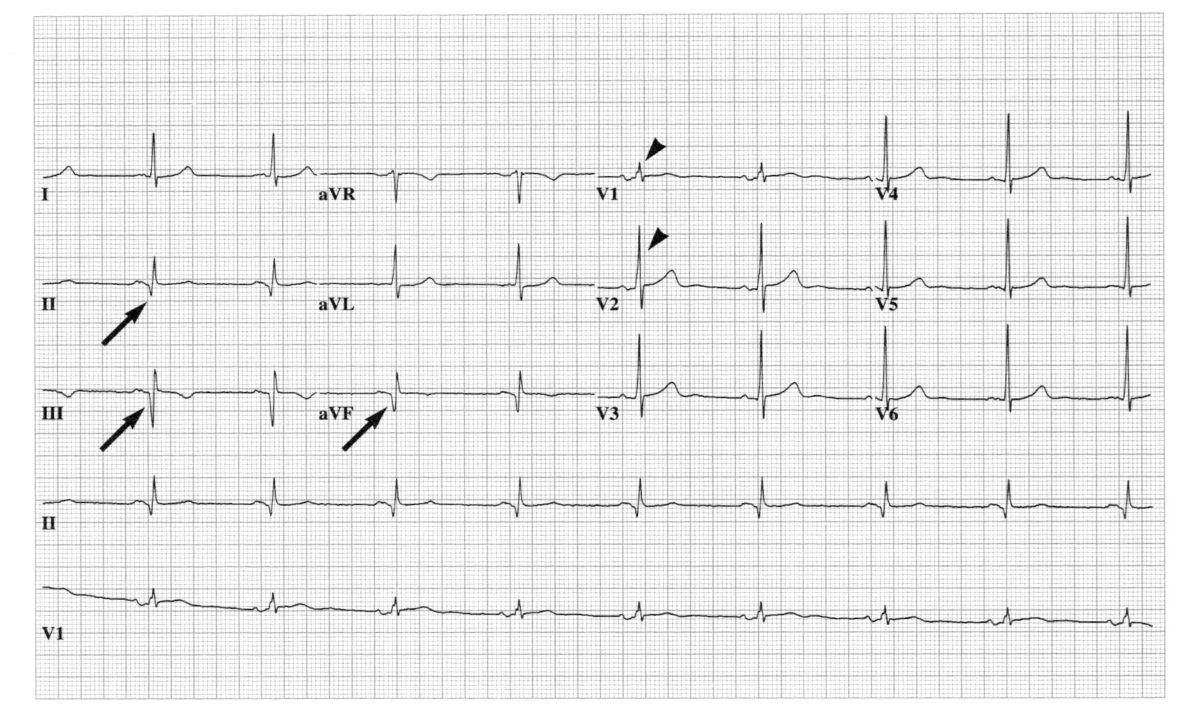

Questions: ECG 70

1. Conditions that interfere with the ECG diagnosis of posterior myocardial infarction include:

   a. Right ventricular hypertrophy
   b. Inferior MI
   c. Wolff-Parkinson-White syndrome
   d. Right bundle branch block

Answers: ECG 70

1. Posterior myocardial infarction is diagnosed when R wave amplitude is greater than S wave amplitude in leads V_1 and V_2, and the R wave exceeds 0.04 seconds in duration in these same leads. This diagnosis is difficult to make in the setting of RVH, WPW, and RBBB, all of which can manifest a dominant R wave in the right precordial leads. Posterior MI typically occurs in the setting of inferior MI, and is often accompanied by pathological Q waves in leads II, III, and aVF. (Answer: a, c, d)

— Quick Review 70 —	
Inferior MI, age indeterminate or probably old	
• Abnormal Q waves (with/without) ST elevation in at least two of leads ____	without II, III, aVF
Posterior MI, age indeterminate or probably old	
• Initial R wave ≥ ____ seconds in leads ____ and ____ with:	0.04, V_1 - V_2
▸ R wave amplitude (greater than/less than) S wave amplitude	greater than

ECG 71. 6-year-old female with congenital heart disease:

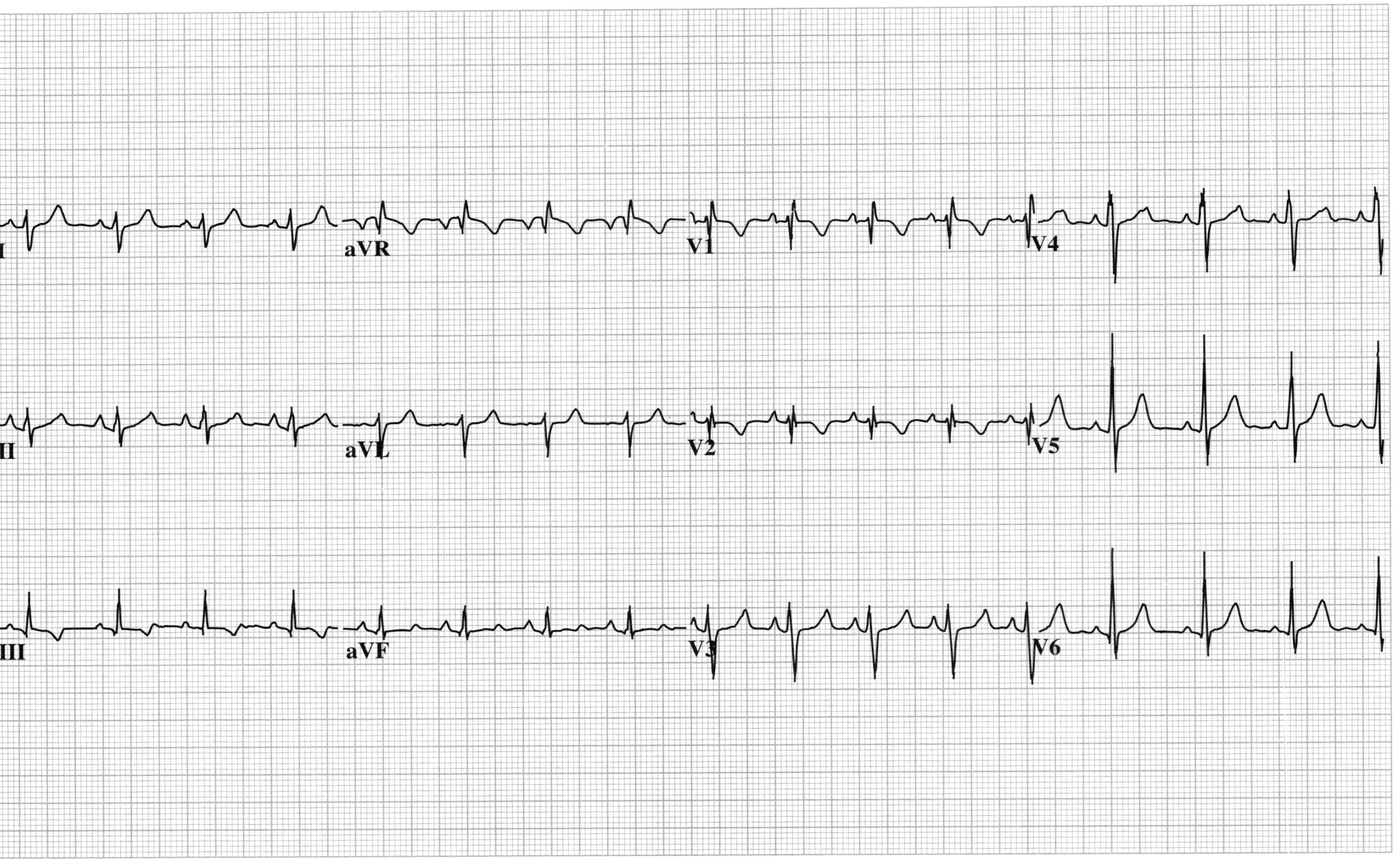

1. GENERAL FEATURES

☐ a. Normal ECG
☐ b. Borderline normal ECG or normal variant
☐ c. Incorrect electrode placement
☐ d. Artifact due to tremor

2. ATRIAL RHYTHMS

☐ a. Sinus rhythm
☐ b. Sinus arrhythmia
☐ c. Sinus bradycardia (< 60)
☐ d. Sinus tachycardia (> 100)
☐ e. Sinus pause or arrest
☐ f. Sinoatrial exit block
☐ g. Ecoptic atrial rhythm
☐ h. Wandering atrial pacemaker
☐ i. Atrial premature complexes, normally conducted
☐ j. Atrial premature complexes, nonconducted
☐ k. Atrial premature complexes with aberrant intraventricular conduction
☐ l. Atrial tachycardia (regular, sustained, 1:1 conduction)
☐ m. Atrial tachycardia, repetitive (short paroxysms)
☐ n. Atrial tachycardia, multifocal
☐ o. Atrial tachycardia with AV block
☐ p. Supraventricular tachycardia, unspecific
☐ q. Supraventricular tachycardia, paroxysmal
☐ r. Atrial flutter
☐ s. Atrial fibrillation
☐ t. Retrograde atrial activation

3. AV JUNCTIONAL RHYTHMS

☐ a. AV junctional premature complexes
☐ b. AV junctional escape complexes
☐ c. AV junctional rhythm, accelerated
☐ d. AV junctional rhythm

4. VENTRICULAR RHYTHMS

☐ a. Ventricular premature complex(es), uniform, fixed coupling
☐ b. Ventricular premature complex(es), uniform, nonfixed coupling
☐ c. Ventricular premature complexes(es), multiform
☐ d. Ventricular premature complexes, in pairs
☐ e. Ventricular parasystole
☐ f. Ventricular tachycardia (≥ 3 consecutive complexes)
☐ g. Accelerated idioventricular rhythm
☐ h. Ventricular escape complexes or rhythm
☐ i. Ventricular fibrillation

5. ATRIAL-VENTRICULAR INTERACTIONS IN ARRHYTHMIAS

☐ a. Fusion complexes
☐ b. Reciprocal (echo) complexes
☐ c. Ventricular capture complexes
☐ d. AV dissociation
☐ e. Ventriculophasic sinus arrhythmia

6. AV CONDUCTION ABNORMALITIES

☐ a. AV block, 1°
☐ b. AV block, 2° - Mobitz type I (Wenckebach)
☐ c. AV block, 2° - Mobitz type II
☐ d. AV block, 2:1
☐ e. AV block, 3°
☐ f. AV block, variable
☐ g. Short PR interval (with sinus rhythm and normal QRS duration)
☐ h. Wolff-Parkinson-White pattern

7. INTRAVENTRICULAR CONDUCTION DISTURBANCES

☐ a. RBBB, incomplete
☐ b. RBBB, complete
☐ c. Left anterior fascicular block
☐ d. Left posterior fascicular block
☐ e. LBBB, with ST-T wave suggestive of acute myocardial injury or infarction
☐ f. LBBB, complete
☐ g. LBBB, intermittent
☐ h. Intraventricular conduction disturbance, nonspecific
☐ i. Aberrant intraventricular conduction with supraventricular arrhythmia

8. P WAVE ABNORMALITIES

☐ a. Right atrial abnormality
☐ b. Left atrial abnormalities
☐ c. Nonspecific atrial abnormality

9. ABNORMALITIES OF QRS VOLTAGE OR AXIS

☐ a. Low voltage, limb leads only
☐ b. Low voltage, limb and precordial leads
☐ c. Left axis deviation (> - 30%)
☐ d. Right axis deviation (> + 100)
☐ e. Electrical alternans

10. VENTRICULAR HYPERTROPHY

☐ a. LVH by voltage only
☐ b. LVH by voltage and ST-T segment abnormalities
☐ c. RVH
☐ d. Combined ventricular hypertrophy

11. Q WAVE MYOCARDIAL INFARCTION

	Probably Acute or Recent	Probably Old or Age Indeterminate
Anterolateral	☐ a.	☐ g.
Anterior	☐ b.	☐ h.
Anteroseptal	☐ c.	☐ i.
Lateral/High lateral	☐ d.	☐ j.
Inferior	☐ e.	☐ k.
Posterior	☐ f.	☐ l.

☐ m. Probably ventricular aneurysm

12. ST, T, U, WAVE ABNORMALITIES

☐ a. Normal variant, early repolarization
☐ b. Normal variant, juvenile T waves
☐ c. Nonspecific ST and/or T wave abnormalities
☐ d. ST and/or T wave abnormalities suggesting myocardial ischemia
☐ e. ST and/or T wave abnormalities suggesting myocardial injury
☐ f. ST and/or T wave abnormalities suggesting acute pericarditis
☐ g. ST-T segment abnormalities secondary to intraventricular conduction disturbance or hypertrophy
☐ h. Post-extrasystolic T wave abnormality
☐ i. Isolated J point depression
☐ j. Peaked T waves
☐ k. Prolonged QT interval
☐ l. Prominent U waves

13. PACEMAKER FUNCTION AND RHYTHM

☐ a. Atrial or coronary sinus pacing
☐ b. Ventricular demand pacing
☐ c. AV sequential pacing
☐ d. Ventricular pacing, complete control
☐ e. Dual chamber, atrial sensing pacemaker
☐ f. Pacemaker malfunction, not constantly capturing (atrium or ventricle)
☐ g. Pacemaker malfunction, not constantly sensing (atrium or ventricle)
☐ h. Pacemaker malfunction, not firing
☐ i. Pacemaker malfunction, slowing

14. SUGGESTED OR PROBABLE CLINICAL DISORDERS

☐ a. Digitalis effect
☐ b. Digitalis toxicity
☐ c. Antiarrhythmic drug effect
☐ d. Antiarrhythmic drug toxicity
☐ e. Hyperkalemia
☐ f. Hypokalemia
☐ g. Hypercalcemia
☐ h. Hypocalcemia
☐ i. Atrial septal defect, secundum
☐ j. Atrial septal defect, primum
☐ k. Dextrocardia, mirror image
☐ l. Mitral valve disease
☐ m. Chronic lung disease
☐ n. Acute cor pulmonale, including pulmonary embolus
☐ o. Pericardial effusion
☐ p. Acute pericarditis
☐ q. Hypertrophic cardiomyopathy
☐ r. Coronary artery disease
☐ s. Central nervous system disorder
☐ t. Myxedema
☐ u. Hypothermia
☐ v. Sick sinus syndrome

ECG 71 was obtained in a 6-year-old female with congenital heart disease. The tracing shows sinus rhythm at 98 beats/minute. Also present are incomplete RBBB (asterisk marks the rSR' complex in V_1, which is 0.10 seconds in duration) with secondary ST-T changes, right atrial abnormality (arrow), and right axis deviation. These findings are all consistent with a secundum atrial septal defect, which was confirmed by echocardiography.

Codes:

2a	Sinus rhythm
7a	RBBB, incomplete
8a	Right atrial abnormality
9d	Right axis deviation (> + 100°)
12g	ST-T segment abnormalities secondary to IVCD or hypertrophy
14i	Atrial septal defect, secundum

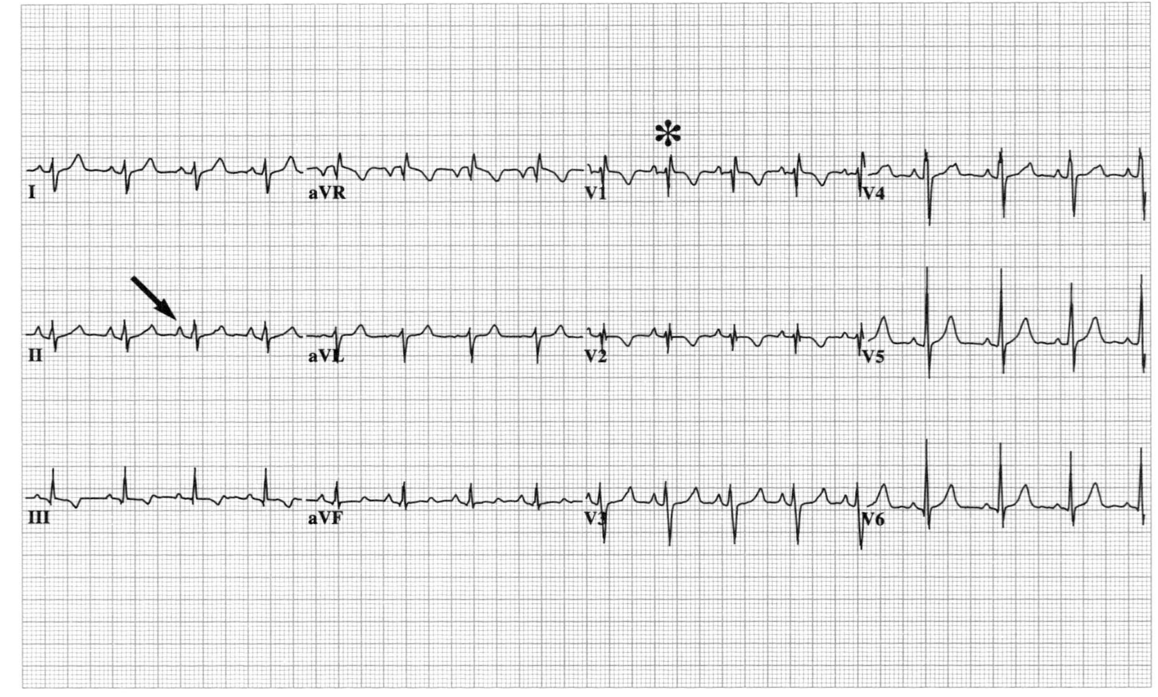

Questions: ECG 71

1. Secundum atrial septal defect results in ____ axis deviation:

   a. Right
   b. Left

2. The QRS conduction defect most commonly associated with secundum ASD is:

   a. LBBB
   b. Incomplete LBBB
   c. RBBB
   d. Incomplete RBBB

Answers: ECG 71

1. Secundum atrial septal defect is typically associated with right axis deviation, incomplete RBBB, and right atrial enlargement. (Answer: a)

2. The QRS conduction defect most commonly associated with secundum ASD is incomplete RBBB. The QRS duration is typically < 0.11 seconds in duration and has a typical rSr' configuration. (Answer: d)

— Quick Review 71 —

Atrial septal defect, secundum	
• Incomplete (RBBB/LBBB)	RBBB
• (Right/left) axis deviation ± (right/left) ventricular hypertrophy	Right, right
• (Right/left) atrial abnormality in ~ 30%	Right
• ____ degree AV block in < 20%	First
• Secundum ASDs represent 70% of all ASDs, and are due to deficient tissue in the region of the____	fossa ovalis

ECG 72. 79-year-old male with renal failure:

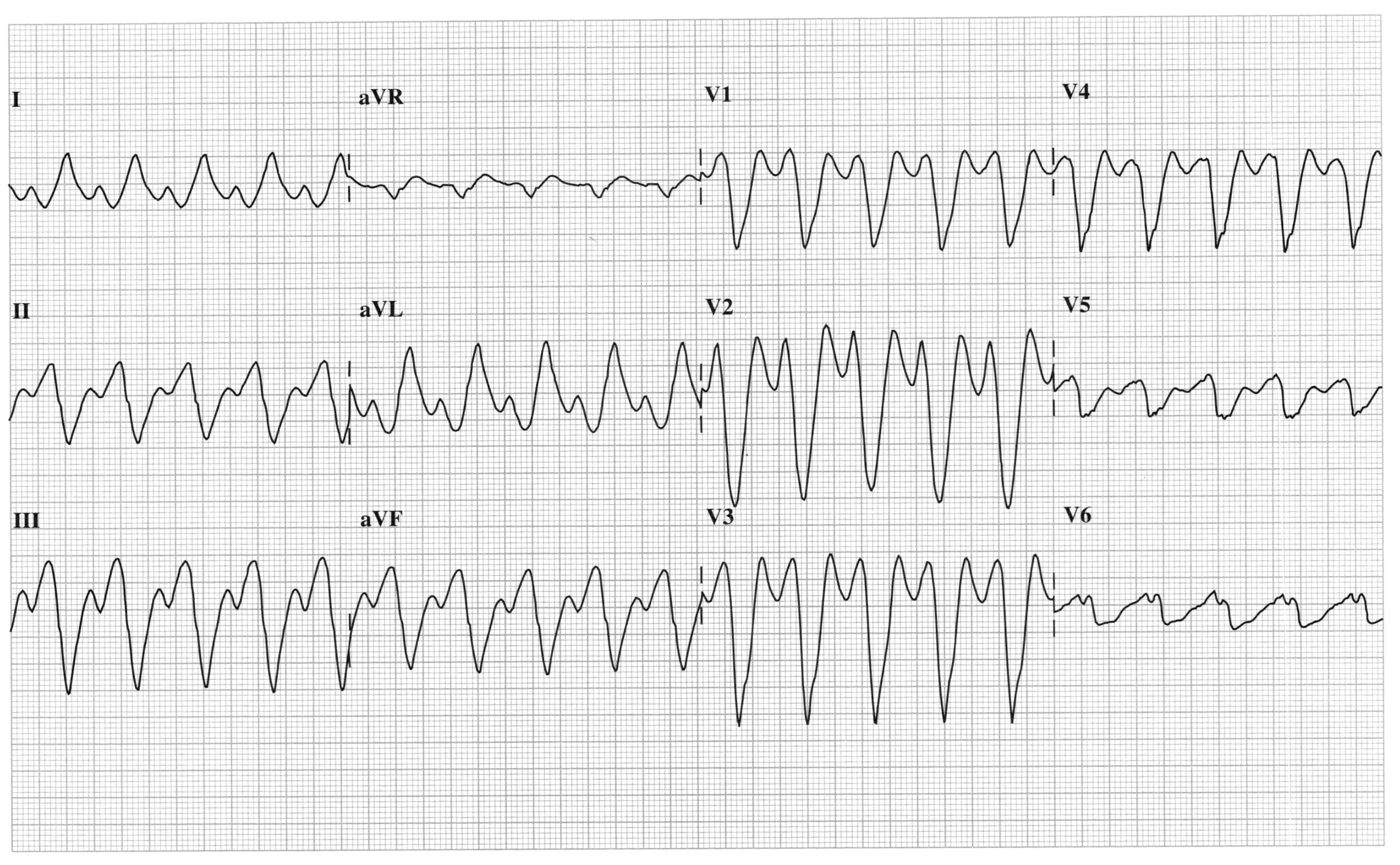

1. GENERAL FEATURES
- ☐ a. Normal ECG
- ☐ b. Borderline normal ECG or normal variant
- ☐ c. Incorrect electrode placement
- ☐ d. Artifact due to tremor

2. ATRIAL RHYTHMS
- ☐ a. Sinus rhythm
- ☐ b. Sinus arrhythmia
- ☐ c. Sinus bradycardia (< 60)
- ☐ d. Sinus tachycardia (> 100)
- ☐ e. Sinus pause or arrest
- ☐ f. Sinoatrial exit block
- ☐ g. Ecoptic atrial rhythm
- ☐ h. Wandering atrial pacemaker
- ☐ i. Atrial premature complexes, normally conducted
- ☐ j. Atrial premature complexes, nonconducted
- ☐ k. Atrial premature complexes with aberrant intraventricular conduction
- ☐ l. Atrial tachycardia (regular, sustained, 1:1 conduction)
- ☐ m. Atrial tachycardia, repetitive (short paroxysms)
- ☐ n. Atrial tachycardia, multifocal
- ☐ o. Atrial tachycardia with AV block
- ☐ p. Supraventricular tachycardia, unspecific
- ☐ q. Supraventricular tachycardia, paroxysmal
- ☐ r. Atrial flutter
- ☐ s. Atrial fibrillation
- ☐ t. Retrograde atrial activation

3. AV JUNCTIONAL RHYTHMS
- ☐ a. AV junctional premature complexes
- ☐ b. AV junctional escape complexes
- ☐ c. AV junctional rhythm, accelerated
- ☐ d. AV junctional rhythm

4. VENTRICULAR RHYTHMS
- ☐ a. Ventricular premature complex(es), uniform, fixed coupling
- ☐ b. Ventricular premature complex(es), uniform, nonfixed coupling
- ☐ c. Ventricular premature complexes(es), multiform
- ☐ d. Ventricular premature complexes, in pairs
- ☐ e. Ventricular parasystole
- ☐ f. Ventricular tachycardia (≥ 3 consecutive complexes)
- ☐ g. Accelerated idioventricular rhythm
- ☐ h. Ventricular escape complexes or rhythm
- ☐ i. Ventricular fibrillation

5. ATRIAL-VENTRICULAR INTERACTIONS IN ARRHYTHMIAS
- ☐ a. Fusion complexes
- ☐ b. Reciprocal (echo) complexes
- ☐ c. Ventricular capture complexes
- ☐ d. AV dissociation
- ☐ e. Ventriculophasic sinus arrhythmia

6. AV CONDUCTION ABNORMALITIES
- ☐ a. AV block, 1°
- ☐ b. AV block, 2° - Mobitz type I (Wenckebach)
- ☐ c. AV block, 2° - Mobitz type II
- ☐ d. AV block, 2:1
- ☐ e. AV block, 3°
- ☐ f. AV block, variable
- ☐ g. Short PR interval (with sinus rhythm and normal QRS duration)
- ☐ h. Wolff-Parkinson-White pattern

7. INTRAVENTRICULAR CONDUCTION DISTURBANCES
- ☐ a. RBBB, incomplete
- ☐ b. RBBB, complete
- ☐ c. Left anterior fascicular block
- ☐ d. Left posterior fascicular block
- ☐ e. LBBB, with ST-T wave suggestive of acute myocardial injury or infarction
- ☐ f. LBBB, complete
- ☐ g. LBBB, intermittent
- ☐ h. Intraventricular conduction disturbance, nonspecific
- ☐ i. Aberrant intraventricular conduction with supraventricular arrhythmia

8. P WAVE ABNORMALITIES
- ☐ a. Right atrial abnormality
- ☐ b. Left atrial abnormalities
- ☐ c. Nonspecific atrial abnormality

9. ABNORMALITIES OF QRS VOLTAGE OR AXIS
- ☐ a. Low voltage, limb leads only
- ☐ b. Low voltage, limb and precordial leads
- ☐ c. Left axis deviation (> - 30%)
- ☐ d. Right axis deviation (> + 100)
- ☐ e. Electrical alternans

10. VENTRICULAR HYPERTROPHY
- ☐ a. LVH by voltage only
- ☐ b. LVH by voltage and ST-T segment abnormalities
- ☐ c. RVH
- ☐ d. Combined ventricular hypertrophy

11. Q WAVE MYOCARDIAL INFARCTION

	Probably Acute or Recent	Probably Old or Age Indeterminate
Anterolateral	☐ a.	☐ g.
Anterior	☐ b.	☐ h.
Anteroseptal	☐ c.	☐ i.
Lateral/High lateral	☐ d.	☐ j.
Inferior	☐ e.	☐ k.
Posterior	☐ f.	☐ l.

- ☐ m. Probably ventricular aneurysm

12. ST, T, U, WAVE ABNORMALITIES
- ☐ a. Normal variant, early repolarization
- ☐ b. Normal variant, juvenile T waves
- ☐ c. Nonspecific ST and/or T wave abnormalities
- ☐ d. ST and/or T wave abnormalities suggesting myocardial ischemia
- ☐ e. ST and/or T wave abnormalities suggesting myocardial injury
- ☐ f. ST and/or T wave abnormalities suggesting acute pericarditis
- ☐ g. ST-T segment abnormalities secondary to intraventricular conduction disturbance or hypertrophy
- ☐ h. Post-extrasystolic T wave abnormality
- ☐ i. Isolated J point depression
- ☐ j. Peaked T waves
- ☐ k. Prolonged QT interval
- ☐ l. Prominent U waves

13. PACEMAKER FUNCTION AND RHYTHM
- ☐ a. Atrial or coronary sinus pacing
- ☐ b. Ventricular demand pacing
- ☐ c. AV sequential pacing
- ☐ d. Ventricular pacing, complete control
- ☐ e. Dual chamber, atrial sensing pacemaker
- ☐ f. Pacemaker malfunction, not constantly capturing (atrium or ventricle)
- ☐ g. Pacemaker malfunction, not constantly sensing (atrium or ventricle)
- ☐ h. Pacemaker malfunction, not firing
- ☐ i. Pacemaker malfunction, slowing

14. SUGGESTED OR PROBABLE CLINICAL DISORDERS
- ☐ a. Digitalis effect
- ☐ b. Digitalis toxicity
- ☐ c. Antiarrhythmic drug effect
- ☐ d. Antiarrhythmic drug toxicity
- ☐ e. Hyperkalemia
- ☐ f. Hypokalemia
- ☐ g. Hypercalcemia
- ☐ h. Hypocalcemia
- ☐ i. Atrial septal defect, secundum
- ☐ j. Atrial septal defect, primum
- ☐ k. Dextrocardia, mirror image
- ☐ l. Mitral valve disease
- ☐ m. Chronic lung disease
- ☐ n. Acute cor pulmonale, including pulmonary embolus
- ☐ o. Pericardial effusion
- ☐ p. Acute pericarditis
- ☐ q. Hypertrophic cardiomyopathy
- ☐ r. Coronary artery disease
- ☐ s. Central nervous system disorder
- ☐ t. Myxedema
- ☐ u. Hypothermia
- ☐ v. Sick sinus syndrome

ECG 72 was obtained in a 79-year-old male with a history of renal failure. The ECG shows a wide complex tachycardia with probable atrial activity (arrows) preceding each QRS complex (consistent with a sinus tachycardia). A markedly widened QRS complex is noted, most consistent with LBBB. Left axis deviation is noted with ST-T abnormalities secondary to the intraventricular conduction defect. This constellation of findings is suggestive of hyperkalemia, especially in a patient with chronic renal failure. Subsequent blood testing did show a markedly elevated potassium at the time this tracing was taken.

Codes:

2d	Sinus tachycardia
7f	LBBB, complete
9c	Left axis deviation (>-30°)
12g	ST-T segment abnormalities secondary to IVCD or hypertrophy
14e	Hyperkalemia

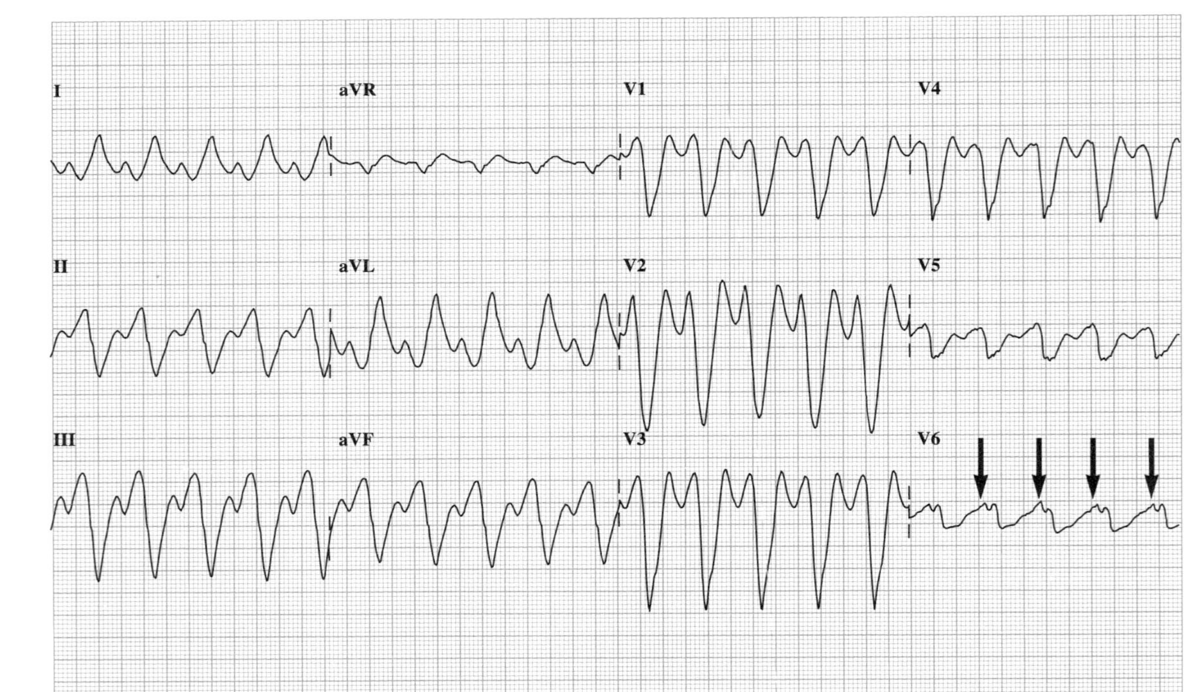

Questions: ECG 72

1. Findings in this ECG consistent with the diagnosis of severe hyperkalemia include:

   a. Wide QRS complex
   b. Prominent P wave
   c. Sinus tachycardia
   d. Left axis deviation

2. Could the upward (positive) deflections in lead V_1 be flutter waves?

   a. Yes
   b. No

3. Which of the following statements about left bundle branch block (LBBB) are true?

   a. LBBB often interferes with the ECG diagnosis of LVH
   b. LBBB often interferes with the ECG diagnosis of RVH
   c. LBBB does not interfere with the ECG diagnosis of myocardial infarction
   d. Left axis deviation is often present and is not necessarily due to coexistent left anterior fascicular block

4. Is tachycardia-dependant bundle branch block more likely to have a left or right bundle branch block morphology?

   a. Left
   b. Right

Answers: ECG 72

1. Hyperkalemia can cause widening of the QRS complex, and on occasion, left (or right) axis deviation. As serum potassium levels rise, P waves often get smaller and may disappear (sinoventricular conduction). Sinus tachycardia is not a manifestation of hyperkalemia per se, but is often associated with conditions causing hyperkalemia (e.g., diabetic ketoacidosis, shock, sepsis). (Answer: a, d)

2. Since the peak-to-peak intervals are not regular, atrial flutter is excluded. (Answer: b)

3. Left bundle branch block (LBBB) often obscures the ECG diagnosis of ventricular hypertrophy (right and left) and acute MI. Criteria for the diagnosis of acute MI in the presence of LBBB have been proposed, but lack predictive accuracy, including serial changes in the ST segments during the first 2-5 days following MI; ST segment elevation (> 1 mm concordant

or > 5 mm discondant to the main QRS complex); pathological Q waves in leads I, aVL and V_6, or III and aVF; and notching in the rising limb of the S wave in leads V_3 or V_4 (Cabrera's sign). (Answer: a, b, d)

4. Since the right bundle has a longer refractory period than the left bundle, premature atrial impulses and rapid atrial rhythms are more likely to find the right bundle refractory and the left bundle able to conduct. Thus, tachycardia-dependent bundle branch block is more likely to manifest right bundle branch block morphology. (Answer: b)

— Quick Review 72 —

LBBB, complete	
• QRS duration ≥ ____ seconds	0.12
• Onset of intrinsicoid deflection in leads I, V_5, V_6 > ____ seconds	0.05
• Broad monophasic R waves in leads ____, which are usually notched or slurred	I, V_5, V_6
• Secondary ST & T wave changes in the (same/opposite) direction to the major QRS deflection	opposite
• ____ or ____ complex in the right precordial leads	rS or QS
• LBBB (does/does not) interfere with determination of QRS axis and the diagnoses of ventricular hypertrophy and acute MI	does
Hyperkalemia	
• ***K^+ = 5.5 - 6.5 mEq/L***	
▸ Tall, peaked, narrow based ____ waves	T
▸ QT interval (shortening/lengthening)	shortening
▸ (Reversible/irreversible) left anterior or posterior fascicular block	Reversible
• ***K^+ = 6.5 - 7.5 mEq/L***	
▸ ____ degree AV block	First
▸ Flattening and widening of the ____ wave	P
▸ ST segment (depression/elevation)	depression
▸ ____widening	QRS
• ***K^+ > 7.5 mEq/L***	
▸ Disappearance of ____ waves	P
▸ LBBB, RBBB, or markedly widened and diffuse intraventricular conduction delay resembling a ____ wave pattern	sine
▸ Arrhythmias and conduction disturbances including VT, VF, idioventricular rhythm, asystole (true/false)	true

— POP QUIZ —

Find The Mistake

Instructions: Identify the incorrect ECG feature(s) for each of the ECG diagnoses listed below

ECG Features	Answer
Pericarditis • Classic evolutionary ST-T pattern consists of 4 stages: 1) Diffuse upwardly concave ST elevation; 2) T waves invert; 3) ST junction returns to baseline & T wave amplitude decreases; 4) ECG returns to normal • Other clues include sinus tachycardia, PR depression late, and low voltage QRS	ST junction returns to baseline before (not after) the T waves invert; PR depression occurs early (not late)
Digitalis effect • Sagging ST segment depression with upward convexity • T wave flat, inverted, or biphasic • QT interval shortened • U wave amplitude increased • PR interval lengthened	ST segments have upward concavity (not convexity)
Digitalis toxicity • Typical abnormalities include paroxysmal atrial tachycardia with block, atrial fibrillation with complete heart block, second- or third-degree AV block, complete heart block with accelerated junctional or idioventricular rhythm, and bundle branch block	Isolated bundle branch block is not a manifestation of digitalis toxicity
Antiarrhythmic drug effect • Prominent U waves (one of the earliest findings) • Prolonged QT interval • Nonspecific ST and/or T wave changes • Widening of the QRS complex and QT interval • Various degrees of AV block	Widening of the QRS complex & QT interval, and AV block are consistent with drug toxicity (not drug effect)

ECG 73. 85-year-old female with recent onset of chest pain:

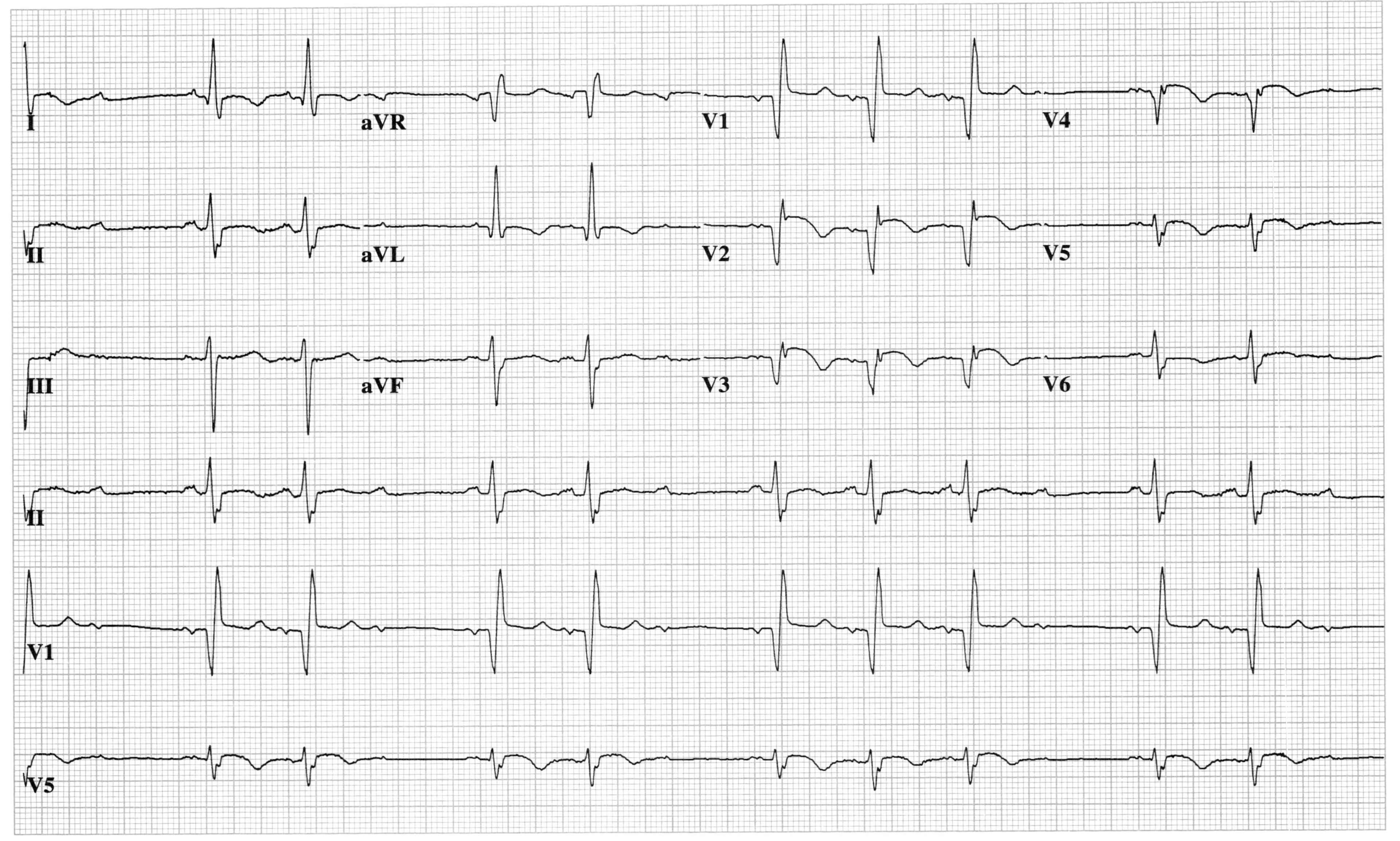

1. GENERAL FEATURES

- ☐ a. Normal ECG
- ☐ b. Borderline normal ECG or normal variant
- ☐ c. Incorrect electrode placement
- ☐ d. Artifact due to tremor

2. ATRIAL RHYTHMS

- ☐ a. Sinus rhythm
- ☐ b. Sinus arrhythmia
- ☐ c. Sinus bradycardia (< 60)
- ☐ d. Sinus tachycardia (> 100)
- ☐ e. Sinus pause or arrest
- ☐ f. Sinoatrial exit block
- ☐ g. Ecoptic atrial rhythm
- ☐ h. Wandering atrial pacemaker
- ☐ i. Atrial premature complexes, normally conducted
- ☐ j. Atrial premature complexes, nonconducted
- ☐ k. Atrial premature complexes with aberrant intraventricular conduction
- ☐ l. Atrial tachycardia (regular, sustained, 1:1 conduction)
- ☐ m. Atrial tachycardia, repetitive (short paroxysms)
- ☐ n. Atrial tachycardia, multifocal
- ☐ o. Atrial tachycardia with AV block
- ☐ p. Supraventricular tachycardia, unspecific
- ☐ q. Supraventricular tachycardia, paroxysmal
- ☐ r. Atrial flutter
- ☐ s. Atrial fibrillation
- ☐ t. Retrograde atrial activation

3. AV JUNCTIONAL RHYTHMS

- ☐ a. AV junctional premature complexes
- ☐ b. AV junctional escape complexes
- ☐ c. AV junctional rhythm, accelerated
- ☐ d. AV junctional rhythm

4. VENTRICULAR RHYTHMS

- ☐ a. Ventricular premature complex(es), uniform, fixed coupling
- ☐ b. Ventricular premature complex(es), uniform, nonfixed coupling
- ☐ c. Ventricular premature complexes(es), multiform
- ☐ d. Ventricular premature complexes, in pairs
- ☐ e. Ventricular parasystole
- ☐ f. Ventricular tachycardia ($\geq$ 3 consecutive complexes)
- ☐ g. Accelerated idioventricular rhythm
- ☐ h. Ventricular escape complexes or rhythm
- ☐ i. Ventricular fibrillation

5. ATRIAL-VENTRICULAR INTERACTIONS IN ARRHYTHMIAS

- ☐ a. Fusion complexes
- ☐ b. Reciprocal (echo) complexes
- ☐ c. Ventricular capture complexes
- ☐ d. AV dissociation
- ☐ e. Ventriculophasic sinus arrhythmia

6. AV CONDUCTION ABNORMALITIES

- ☐ a. AV block, 1°
- ☐ b. AV block, 2° - Mobitz type I (Wenckebach)
- ☐ c. AV block, 2° - Mobitz type II
- ☐ d. AV block, 2:1
- ☐ e. AV block, 3°
- ☐ f. AV block, variable
- ☐ g. Short PR interval (with sinus rhythm and normal QRS duration)
- ☐ h. Wolff-Parkinson-White pattern

7. INTRAVENTRICULAR CONDUCTION DISTURBANCES

- ☐ a. RBBB, incomplete
- ☐ b. RBBB, complete
- ☐ c. Left anterior fascicular block
- ☐ d. Left posterior fascicular block
- ☐ e. LBBB, with ST-T wave suggestive of acute myocardial injury or infarction
- ☐ f. LBBB, complete
- ☐ g. LBBB, intermittent
- ☐ h. Intraventricular conduction disturbance, nonspecific
- ☐ i. Aberrant intraventricular conduction with supraventricular arrhythmia

8. P WAVE ABNORMALITIES

- ☐ a. Right atrial abnormality
- ☐ b. Left atrial abnormalities
- ☐ c. Nonspecific atrial abnormality

9. ABNORMALITIES OF QRS VOLTAGE OR AXIS

- ☐ a. Low voltage, limb leads only
- ☐ b. Low voltage, limb and precordial leads
- ☐ c. Left axis deviation (> - 30%)
- ☐ d. Right axis deviation (> + 100)
- ☐ e. Electrical alternans

10. VENTRICULAR HYPERTROPHY

- ☐ a. LVH by voltage only
- ☐ b. LVH by voltage and ST-T segment abnormalities
- ☐ c. RVH
- ☐ d. Combined ventricular hypertrophy

11. Q WAVE MYOCARDIAL INFARCTION

	Probably Acute or Recent	Probably Old or Age Indeterminate
Anterolateral	☐ a.	☐ g.
Anterior	☐ b.	☐ h.
Anteroseptal	☐ c.	☐ i.
Lateral/High lateral	☐ d.	☐ j.
Inferior	☐ e.	☐ k.
Posterior	☐ f.	☐ l.

☐ m. Probably ventricular aneurysm

12. ST, T, U, WAVE ABNORMALITIES

- ☐ a. Normal variant, early repolarization
- ☐ b. Normal variant, juvenile T waves
- ☐ c. Nonspecific ST and/or T wave abnormalities
- ☐ d. ST and/or T wave abnormalities suggesting myocardial ischemia
- ☐ e. ST and/or T wave abnormalities suggesting myocardial injury
- ☐ f. ST and/or T wave abnormalities suggesting acute pericarditis
- ☐ g. ST-T segment abnormalities secondary to intraventricular conduction disturbance or hypertrophy
- ☐ h. Post-extrasystolic T wave abnormality
- ☐ i. Isolated J point depression
- ☐ j. Peaked T waves
- ☐ k. Prolonged QT interval
- ☐ l. Prominent U waves

13. PACEMAKER FUNCTION AND RHYTHM

- ☐ a. Atrial or coronary sinus pacing
- ☐ b. Ventricular demand pacing
- ☐ c. AV sequential pacing
- ☐ d. Ventricular pacing, complete control
- ☐ e. Dual chamber, atrial sensing pacemaker
- ☐ f. Pacemaker malfunction, not constantly capturing (atrium or ventricle)
- ☐ g. Pacemaker malfunction, not constantly sensing (atrium or ventricle)
- ☐ h. Pacemaker malfunction, not firing
- ☐ i. Pacemaker malfunction, slowing

14. SUGGESTED OR PROBABLE CLINICAL DISORDERS

- ☐ a. Digitalis effect
- ☐ b. Digitalis toxicity
- ☐ c. Antiarrhythmic drug effect
- ☐ d. Antiarrhythmic drug toxicity
- ☐ e. Hyperkalemia
- ☐ f. Hypokalemia
- ☐ g. Hypercalcemia
- ☐ h. Hypocalcemia
- ☐ i. Atrial septal defect, secundum
- ☐ j. Atrial septal defect, primum
- ☐ k. Dextrocardia, mirror image
- ☐ l. Mitral valve disease
- ☐ m. Chronic lung disease
- ☐ n. Acute cor pulmonale, including pulmonary embolus
- ☐ o. Pericardial effusion
- ☐ p. Acute pericarditis
- ☐ q. Hypertrophic cardiomyopathy
- ☐ r. Coronary artery disease
- ☐ s. Central nervous system disorder
- ☐ t. Myxedema
- ☐ u. Hypothermia
- ☐ v. Sick sinus syndrome

ECG 73 was obtained in an 85-year-old female with recent onset of chest pain. The ECG shows sinus rhythm and Mobitz Type II second-degree AV block with 3:2 AV conduction (3 P waves [arrows] for every 2 QRS complexes [asterisks]). Also noted are right bundle branch block, left atrial enlargement, left ventricular hypertrophy (R wave in aVL ≥ 12mm), and acute or recent anteroseptal myocardial infarction (arrowheads) with ST and T wave abnormalities suggesting myocardial injury. The T wave inversions in the lateral leads (I, aVL, V_5, V_6) are consistent with repolarization abnormality secondary to LVH; however, in the setting of evolving myocardial infarction, they are most likely due to myocardial ischemia.

Codes:

2a	Sinus rhythm
6c	AV block, second-degree Mobitz Type II
7b	RBBB, complete
8b	Left atrial abnormality
10a	Left ventricular hypertrophy by voltage only
11c	Anteroseptal myocardial infarction, probably acute or recent
12d	ST and/or T wave abnormality suggesting myocardial ischemia
12e	ST and/or T wave abnormality suggesting myocardial injury
14r	Coronary artery disease

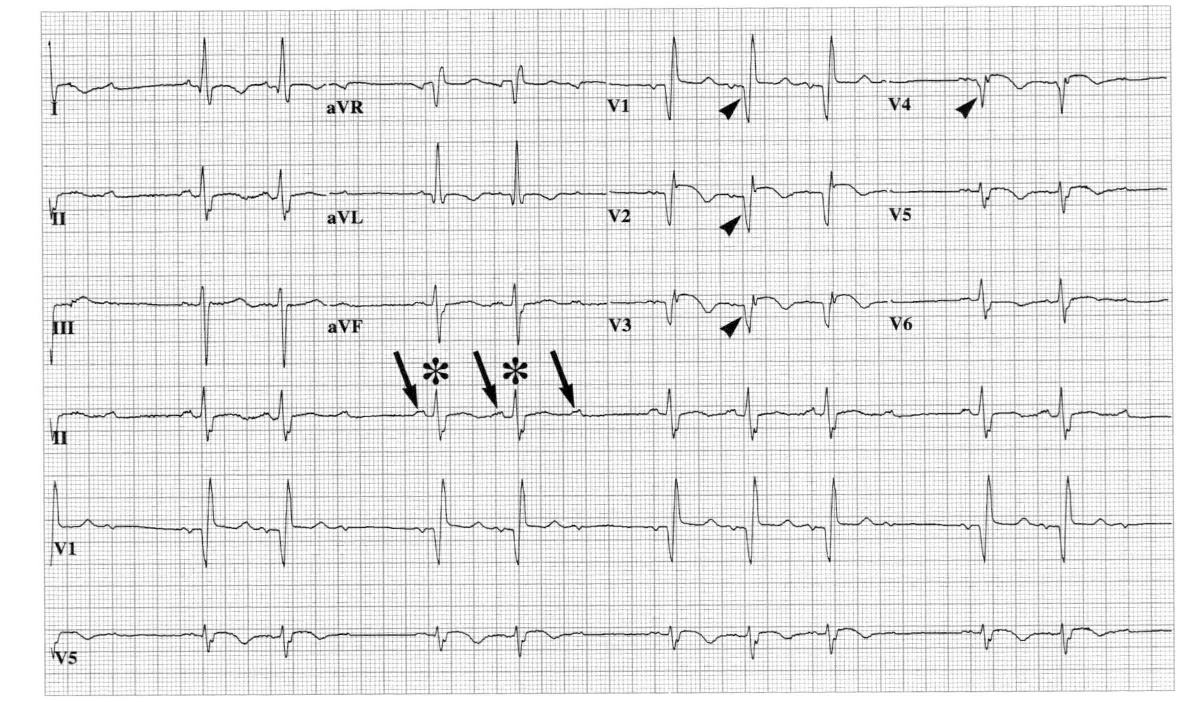

Questions: ECG 73

1. The diagnosis of Mobitz Type II second-degree AV block requires all of the following except:

   a. Constant PR interval in the conducted beats
   b. RR interval containing the nonconducted P wave is less than two PP intervals
   c. Intermittently nonconducted P waves without evidence of atrial prematurity
   d. RR interval containing the nonconducted P wave equals two PP intervals
   e. Atrial rate is less than the ventricular rate

2. Which of the following features favor Mobitz I (Wenckebach) over Mobitz II AV block in patients with 2:1 AV conduction:

   a. Increasing the heart rate and PR conduction with exercise improves AV conduction
   b. Classic Mobitz I AV block is present on another part of the ECG
   c. Abnormal QRS conduction (due to bifascicular block) is present

Answers: ECG 73

1. This 85-year-old female presenting with an acute anteroseptal myocardial infarction has damaged her AV and His-Purkinje conduction systems, resulting in right bundle branch block and Mobitz II AV block. The diagnosis of Mobitz Type II second-degree AV block requires that the PR interval remains constant in the conducted beats, that there are intermittently nonconducted P waves without evidence of premature atrial complexes, and that the RR interval containing the nonconducted P wave equals two PP intervals. If the RR interval containing the nonconducted P wave is less than two PP intervals, Mobitz Type I second-degree AV block is suggested, and evidence for PR interval prolongation should be assessed. The atrial rate is always faster than the ventricular rate in second-degree AV block. (Answer: b, e)

2. Patients with 2:1 AV block can have either a Mobitz Type I (Wenckebach) or Mobitz Type II mechanism. Maneuvers that increase heart rate and PR conduction (e.g., exercise, atropine) will improve AV conduction and decrease heart block in patients with Mobitz I block at the level of the AV node. In contrast, patients with Mobitz II and block in the His-Purkinje system will often have worsening AV block as heart rate and PR

conduction improve. If classic Mobitz I AV block is seen on another part of the ECG, then the episode of 2:1 AV block is most likely based on a Mobitz I mechanism. The presence of bundle branch block or bifascicular block indicates disease of the Purkinje system and suggests that 2:1 AV block is due to a Mobitz II mechanism. (Answer: a, b)

— Quick Review 73 —

AV block, 2° - Mobitz Type II	
• Regular sinus or atrial rhythm with intermittent nonconducted ____ waves (with/without) evidence for atrial prematurity	P, without
• PR interval in the conducted beats is (constant/variable)	constant
• RR interval containing the nonconducted P wave is (less than/equal to/greater than) two PP intervals	equal to
ST and/or T wave abnormalities suggesting myocardial ischemia	
• Abnormally tall, symmetrical, (upright/inverted) T waves	inverted
• Horizontal or ____ ST segments with or without T wave inversion	downsloping
• Associated ECG findings:	
▸ QT interval is usually (normal/prolonged)	prolonged
▸ Reciprocal ____ wave changes may be evident	T
▸ Prominent U waves are often present and may be upright or inverted (true/false)	true

— Quick Review 73 —

LVH by voltage only	
• **Cornell Criteria** (most accurate): R wave in aVL + S wave in V_3 > ____ mm in males or > ____ mm in females	24, 20
• **Other voltage-based criteria**	
▸ Precordial leads (one or more)	
(1) R wave in V_5 or V_6 + S wave in V_1	
▸ > ____ mm if age > 30 years	35
▸ > ____ mm if age 20-30 years	40
▸ > ____ mm if age 16-19 years	60
(2) Maximum R wave + S wave in precordial leads > ____ mm	45
(3) R wave in V_5 > ____ mm	26
(4) R wave in V_6 > ____ mm	20
▸ Limb leads (one or more)	
(1) R wave in lead I + S wave in lead II ≥ ____ mm	26
(2) R wave in lead I ≥ ____ mm	14
(3) S wave in aVR ≥ ____ mm	15
(4) R wave in aVL ≥ ____ mm	12
(5) R wave in aVF ≥ ____ mm	21
• **Non-voltage related criteria for LVH**	
▸ (Left/right) atrial abnormality	left
▸ (Left/right) axis deviation	left
▸ Onset of intrinsicoid deflection > ____ seconds	0.05
▸ Small or absent R waves in leads ____	V_1-V_3
▸ Absent ____ waves in leads I, V_5, V_6	Q
▸ Abnormal ____ waves in leads II, III, aVF	Q
▸ Prominent ____ waves, especially in leads with large R and T waves	U
▸ R wave amplitude in V_6 (greater than/less than) V_5, provided there are dominant R waves in these leads	greater than

— ECG CROSSWORD PUZZLE —

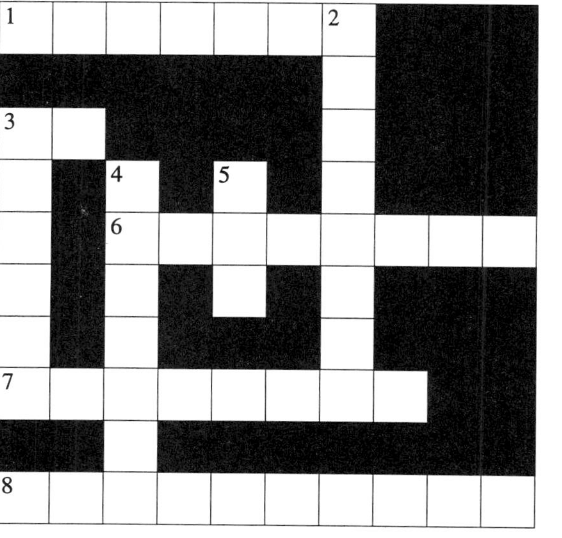

ACROSS

1. Hyper_____ is associated with QT shortening, a sine wave QRS pattern, and sinoventricular conduction
3. WPW results in a PR interval < 0.12 seconds and a constant _____ interval that is ≤ 0.26 seconds
6. Reversal of right and left arm leads results in P-QRS-T complexes that are _____ in I and aVL
7. Associated findings include low QRS voltage, sinus bradycardia, and pericardial effusion
8. Mobitz Type I _____ exit block demonstrates shortening of the PP interval up to PP pause, a constant PR interval, and a PP pause less than twice the normal PP interval

DOWN

2. Suggested by ST elevation ≥ 1 mm persisting 4 or more weeks after acute MI in leads with abnormal Q waves
3. Type of atrial septal defect associated with left axis deviation
4. _____ toxicity can cause atrial fibrillation with a regular ventricular response due to complete heart block and junctional tachycardia
5. Associated with right axis deviation, a dominant R wave in V_1, secondary ST-T changes, and right atrial abnormality

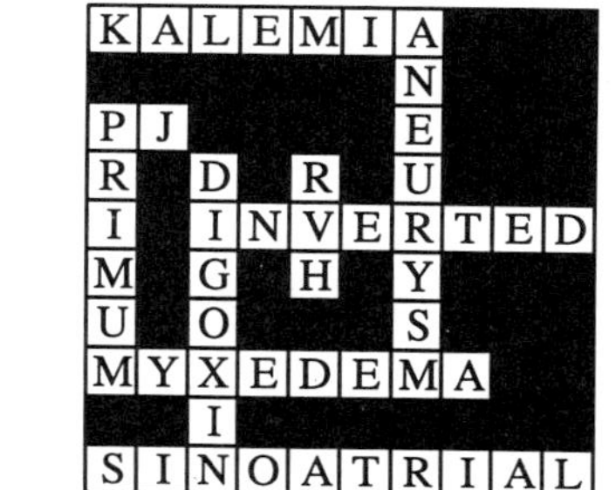

ECG 74. 80-year-old male with a recent episode of chest tightness:

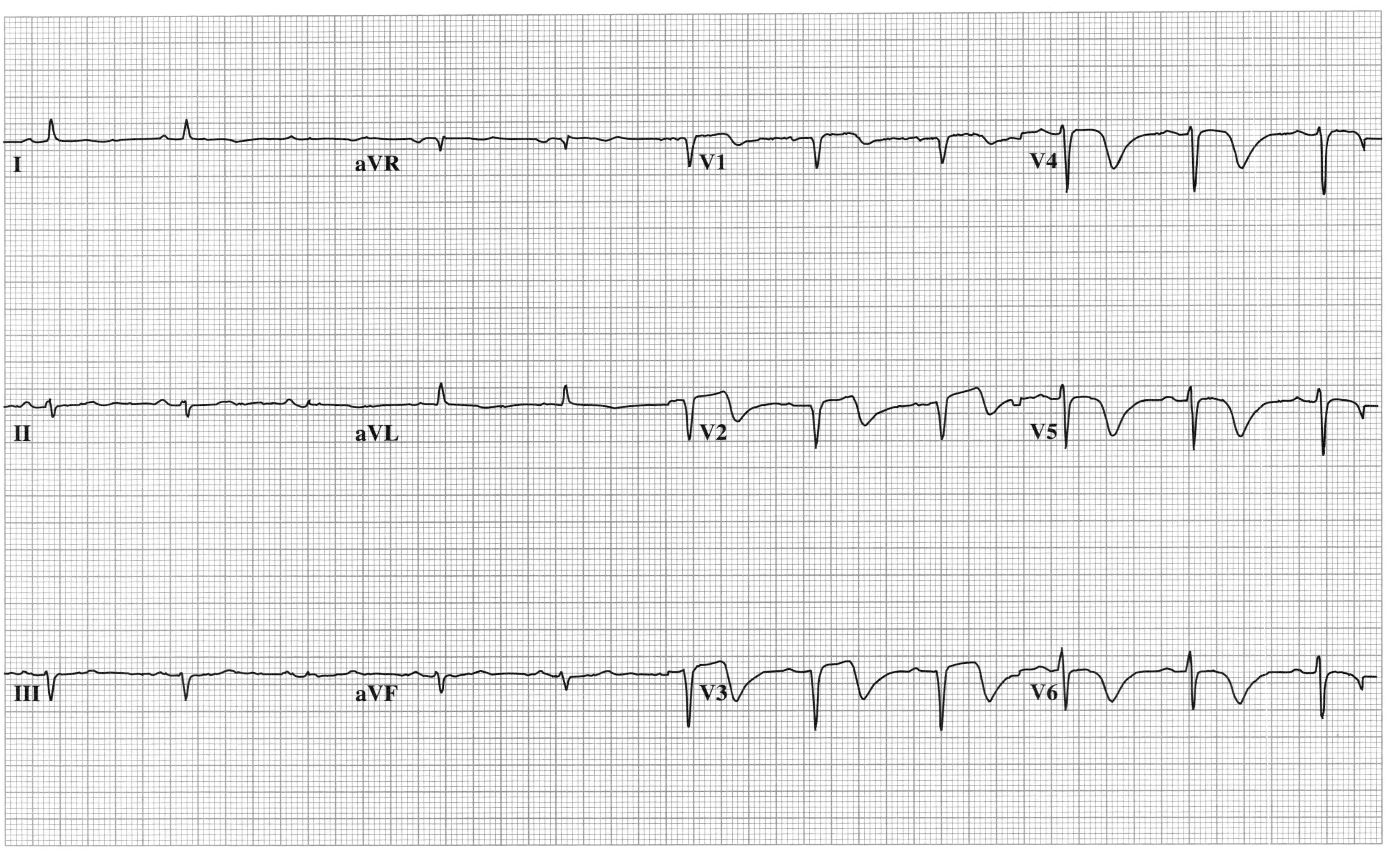

1. GENERAL FEATURES

- ☐ a. Normal ECG
- ☐ b. Borderline normal ECG or normal variant
- ☐ c. Incorrect electrode placement
- ☐ d. Artifact due to tremor

2. ATRIAL RHYTHMS

- ☐ a. Sinus rhythm
- ☐ b. Sinus arrhythmia
- ☐ c. Sinus bradycardia (< 60)
- ☐ d. Sinus tachycardia (> 100)
- ☐ e. Sinus pause or arrest
- ☐ f. Sinoatrial exit block
- ☐ g. Ecoptic atrial rhythm
- ☐ h. Wandering atrial pacemaker
- ☐ i. Atrial premature complexes, normally conducted
- ☐ j. Atrial premature complexes, nonconducted
- ☐ k. Atrial premature complexes with aberrant intraventricular conduction
- ☐ l. Atrial tachycardia (regular, sustained, 1:1 conduction)
- ☐ m. Atrial tachycardia, repetitive (short paroxysms)
- ☐ n. Atrial tachycardia, multifocal
- ☐ o. Atrial tachycardia with AV block
- ☐ p. Supraventricular tachycardia, unspecific
- ☐ q. Supraventricular tachycardia, paroxysmal
- ☐ r. Atrial flutter
- ☐ s. Atrial fibrillation
- ☐ t. Retrograde atrial activation

3. AV JUNCTIONAL RHYTHMS

- ☐ a. AV junctional premature complexes
- ☐ b. AV junctional escape complexes
- ☐ c. AV junctional rhythm, accelerated
- ☐ d. AV junctional rhythm

4. VENTRICULAR RHYTHMS

- ☐ a. Ventricular premature complex(es), uniform, fixed coupling
- ☐ b. Ventricular premature complex(es), uniform, nonfixed coupling
- ☐ c. Ventricular premature complexes(es), multiform
- ☐ d. Ventricular premature complexes, in pairs
- ☐ e. Ventricular parasystole
- ☐ f. Ventricular tachycardia (≥ 3 consecutive complexes)
- ☐ g. Accelerated idioventricular rhythm
- ☐ h. Ventricular escape complexes or rhythm
- ☐ i. Ventricular fibrillation

5. ATRIAL-VENTRICULAR INTERACTIONS IN ARRHYTHMIAS

- ☐ a. Fusion complexes
- ☐ b. Reciprocal (echo) complexes
- ☐ c. Ventricular capture complexes
- ☐ d. AV dissociation
- ☐ e. Ventriculophasic sinus arrhythmia

6. AV CONDUCTION ABNORMALITIES

- ☐ a. AV block, 1°
- ☐ b. AV block, 2° - Mobitz type I (Wenckebach)
- ☐ c. AV block, 2° - Mobitz type II
- ☐ d. AV block, 2:1
- ☐ e. AV block, 3°
- ☐ f. AV block, variable
- ☐ g. Short PR interval (with sinus rhythm and normal QRS duration)
- ☐ h. Wolff-Parkinson-White pattern

7. INTRAVENTRICULAR CONDUCTION DISTURBANCES

- ☐ a. RBBB, incomplete
- ☐ b. RBBB, complete
- ☐ c. Left anterior fascicular block
- ☐ d. Left posterior fascicular block
- ☐ e. LBBB, with ST-T wave suggestive of acute myocardial injury or infarction
- ☐ f. LBBB, complete
- ☐ g. LBBB, intermittent
- ☐ h. Intraventricular conduction disturbance, nonspecific
- ☐ i. Aberrant intraventricular conduction with supraventricular arrhythmia

8. P WAVE ABNORMALITIES

- ☐ a. Right atrial abnormality
- ☐ b. Left atrial abnormalities
- ☐ c. Nonspecific atrial abnormality

9. ABNORMALITIES OF QRS VOLTAGE OR AXIS

- ☐ a. Low voltage, limb leads only
- ☐ b. Low voltage, limb and precordial leads
- ☐ c. Left axis deviation (> - 30%)
- ☐ d. Right axis deviation (> + 100)
- ☐ e. Electrical alternans

10. VENTRICULAR HYPERTROPHY

- ☐ a. LVH by voltage only
- ☐ b. LVH by voltage and ST-T segment abnormalities
- ☐ c. RVH
- ☐ d. Combined ventricular hypertrophy

11. Q WAVE MYOCARDIAL INFARCTION

	Probably Acute or Recent	Probably Old or Age Indeterminate
Anterolateral	☐ a.	☐ g.
Anterior	☐ b.	☐ h.
Anteroseptal	☐ c.	☐ i.
Lateral/High lateral	☐ d.	☐ j.
Inferior	☐ e.	☐ k.
Posterior	☐ f.	☐ l.

- ☐ m. Probably ventricular aneurysm

12. ST, T, U, WAVE ABNORMALITIES

- ☐ a. Normal variant, early repolarization
- ☐ b. Normal variant, juvenile T waves
- ☐ c. Nonspecific ST and/or T wave abnormalities
- ☐ d. ST and/or T wave abnormalities suggesting myocardial ischemia
- ☐ e. ST and/or T wave abnormalities suggesting myocardial injury
- ☐ f. ST and/or T wave abnormalities suggesting acute pericarditis
- ☐ g. ST-T segment abnormalities secondary to intraventricular conduction disturbance or hypertrophy
- ☐ h. Post-extrasystolic T wave abnormality
- ☐ i. Isolated J point depression
- ☐ j. Peaked T waves
- ☐ k. Prolonged QT interval
- ☐ l. Prominent U waves

13. PACEMAKER FUNCTION AND RHYTHM

- ☐ a. Atrial or coronary sinus pacing
- ☐ b. Ventricular demand pacing
- ☐ c. AV sequential pacing
- ☐ d. Ventricular pacing, complete control
- ☐ e. Dual chamber, atrial sensing pacemaker
- ☐ f. Pacemaker malfunction, not constantly capturing (atrium or ventricle)
- ☐ g. Pacemaker malfunction, not constantly sensing (atrium or ventricle)
- ☐ h. Pacemaker malfunction, not firing
- ☐ i. Pacemaker malfunction, slowing

14. SUGGESTED OR PROBABLE CLINICAL DISORDERS

- ☐ a. Digitalis effect
- ☐ b. Digitalis toxicity
- ☐ c. Antiarrhythmic drug effect
- ☐ d. Antiarrhythmic drug toxicity
- ☐ e. Hyperkalemia
- ☐ f. Hypokalemia
- ☐ g. Hypercalcemia
- ☐ h. Hypocalcemia
- ☐ i. Atrial septal defect, secundum
- ☐ j. Atrial septal defect, primum
- ☐ k. Dextrocardia, mirror image
- ☐ l. Mitral valve disease
- ☐ m. Chronic lung disease
- ☐ n. Acute cor pulmonale, including pulmonary embolus
- ☐ o. Pericardial effusion
- ☐ p. Acute pericarditis
- ☐ q. Hypertrophic cardiomyopathy
- ☐ r. Coronary artery disease
- ☐ s. Central nervous system disorder
- ☐ t. Myxedema
- ☐ u. Hypothermia
- ☐ v. Sick sinus syndrome

ECG 74 was obtained in an 80-year-old male who was hospitalized with a recent episode of chest tightness. The tracing shows a sinus rhythm at 65 beats/minute. Left axis deviation is present although it does not meet criteria (i.e., > - 45°) for the diagnosis of left anterior fascicular block. An acute or recent anteroseptal myocardial infarction is present with ST-T changes suggesting myocardial injury (asterisks). The T wave inversions in V_4 - V_6 are consistent with lateral wall ischemia. QT prolongation is most apparent in the lateral precordial leads. Coronary artery disease should also be coded.

Codes:

2a	Sinus rhythm
9c	Left axis deviation (>-30°)
11c	Anteroseptal Q wave MI, probably acute or recent
12d	ST and/or T wave abnormalities suggesting myocardial ischemia
12e	ST and/or T wave abnormalities suggesting myocardial injury
12k	Prolonged QT interval
14r	Coronary artery disease

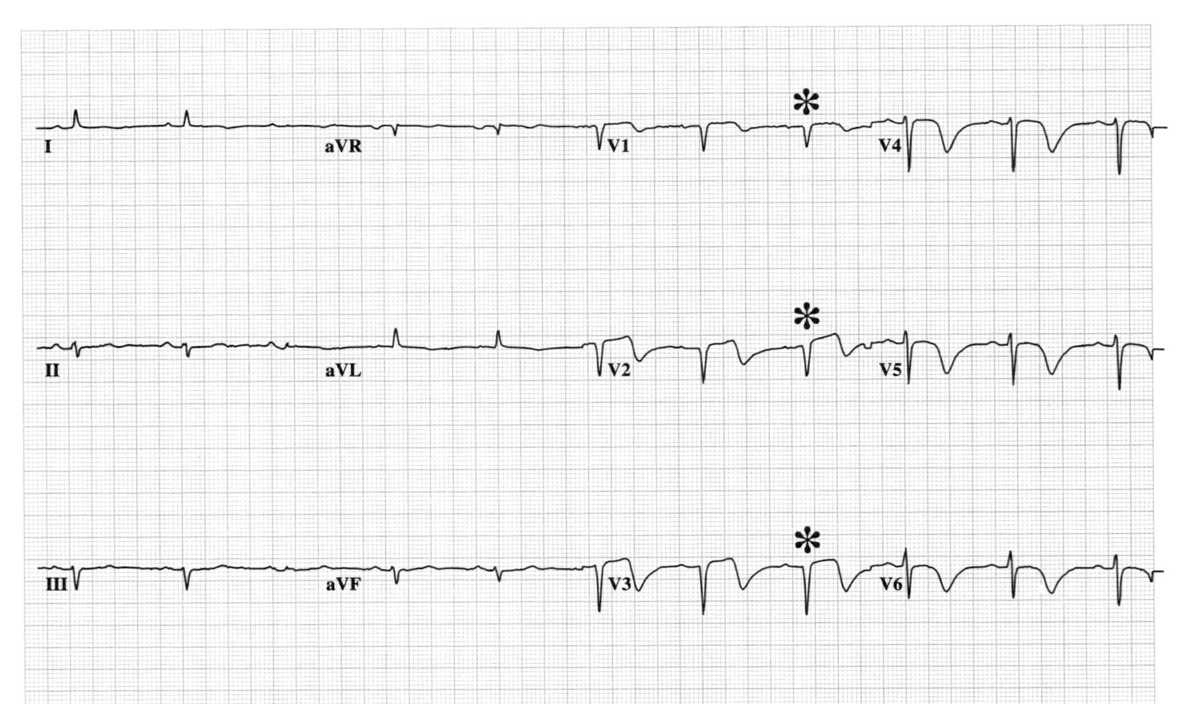

Questions: ECG 74

1. All of the following conditions can cause deep T wave inversion except:

   a. Subarachnoid hemorrhage
   b. Acute myocardial ischemia
   c. Left ventricular hypertrophy
   d. Right ventricular hypertrophy
   e. Digitalis effect
   f. Hyperkalemia
   g. Post tachycardia (after SVT or VT)
   h. Post pacemaker
   i. Mitral valve prolapse
   j. Pericarditis
   k. Pulmonary embolism
   l. Pneumothorax
   m. Myocardial contusion
   n. Stokes-Adams attack due to complete heart block

2. For each of the following conditions, indicate whether the QT interval is typically prolonged, shortened, or remains unchanged:

   a. Myocardial ischemia
   b. Mitral valve prolapse
   c. Central nervous system disorders (e.g., cerebrovascular accident)
   d. Hypercalcemia
   e. Hypocalcemia
   f. Digitalis
   g. Type I antiarrhythmics (quinidine, procainamide, disopyramide)
   h. Type III antiarrhythmics (sotalol, amiodarone)
   I. Hypomagnesemia
   j. Hypothermia
   k. Hypothyroidism

3. What is the age of the myocardial infarction on this ECG:

   a. Hours-to-days
   b. Days-to-weeks
   c. Weeks-to-months

Answers: ECG 74

1. Deep T wave inversions can be seen in CNS disorders (e.g., subarachnoid hemorrhage), cardiac disorders (e.g., myocardial ischemia, ventricular hypertrophy, pericarditis, myocardial contusion), pulmonary disorders (e.g., pulmonary embolism,

neumothorax), and in patients taking digitalis (T waves are more often upright or diphasic). Hyperkalemia is associated with tall upright T waves, not T wave inversion. (Answer: f)

2. Answer:

QT interval prolongation:	a, c, e, g, h, i, j, k
QT interval unchanged:	b (may be slightly prolonged)
QT interval shortening:	d, f

3. ***Q waves*** usually develop in the hours to days after MI and may persist indefinitely, regress, or infrequently disappear. ***ST elevation*** usually develops in seconds-to-minutes after MI and resolves in minutes-to-hours after reperfusion of the infarct artery. If reperfusion is not achieved, ST elevation resolves slowly over hours-to-days. ST elevation persisting beyond 48 hours post-MI is an adverse prognostic marker. ***T wave inversion*** begins before the ST segment returns to baseline. The present ECG shows Q waves, ST elevation, and T wave inversion, suggesting an infarct that is either hours to days old, or an older infarct complicated by ventricular aneurysm. The clinical history of chest pain 2 days earlier makes the diagnosis of recent MI most likely. (Answer: a)

— Quick Review 74 —

Anteroseptal MI, recent or probably acute	
• Abnormal Q or QS deflection and ST elevation in leads ____ (and sometimes V_4)	V_1-V_3
• The presence of a Q wave in lead ____ distinguishes anteroseptal from anterior infarction	V_1
ST and/or T wave changes suggesting myocardial injury	
• Acute ST segment (elevation/depression) with upward (convexity/concavity) in the leads representing the area of infarction	elevation convexity
• T waves invert (before/after) ST segments return to baseline	before
• Associated ST (elevation/depression) in the noninfarct leads is common	depression
• Acute ____ wall injury often has horizontal or downsloping ST segment depression with upright T waves in V_1-V_3, with or without a prominent R wave in these same leads	posterior
Prolonged QT interval	
• Corrected QT interval (QTc) ≥ ____ seconds, where QTc = QT interval divided by the square root of the preceding ____ interval	0.42-0.46 RR
• QT interval varies (directly/inversely) with heart rate	inversely
• The normal QT interval should be (less than/greater than) 50% of the RR interval	less than

Don't Forget!

- In RBBB, mean QRS axis is determined by the initial unblocked 0.06-0.08 seconds of QRS, and should be normal unless left anterior (item 7c) or posterior fascicular block (item 7d) is present
- RBBB does not interfere with the ECG diagnosis of ventricular hypertrophy or Q-wave MI
- LAFB may result in a false-positive diagnosis of LVH based on voltage criteria using leads I or aVL
- Left anterior fascicular block can mask the presence of inferior wall MI
- Left posterior fascicular block can mask the presence of lateral wall MI
- LBBB interferes with QRS axis and the ECG diagnoses of ventricular hypertrophy and acute MI
- Intermittent LBBB is more commonly seen at high rates (tachycardia-dependent) but may be bradycardia-dependent as well
- In up to 30% of cases, P pulmonale may actually manisfest as left atrial enlargement. Suspect this possibility when left atrial abnormality (item 8b) is present in lead V_1.

ECG 75. 1-year-old male with a heart murmur:

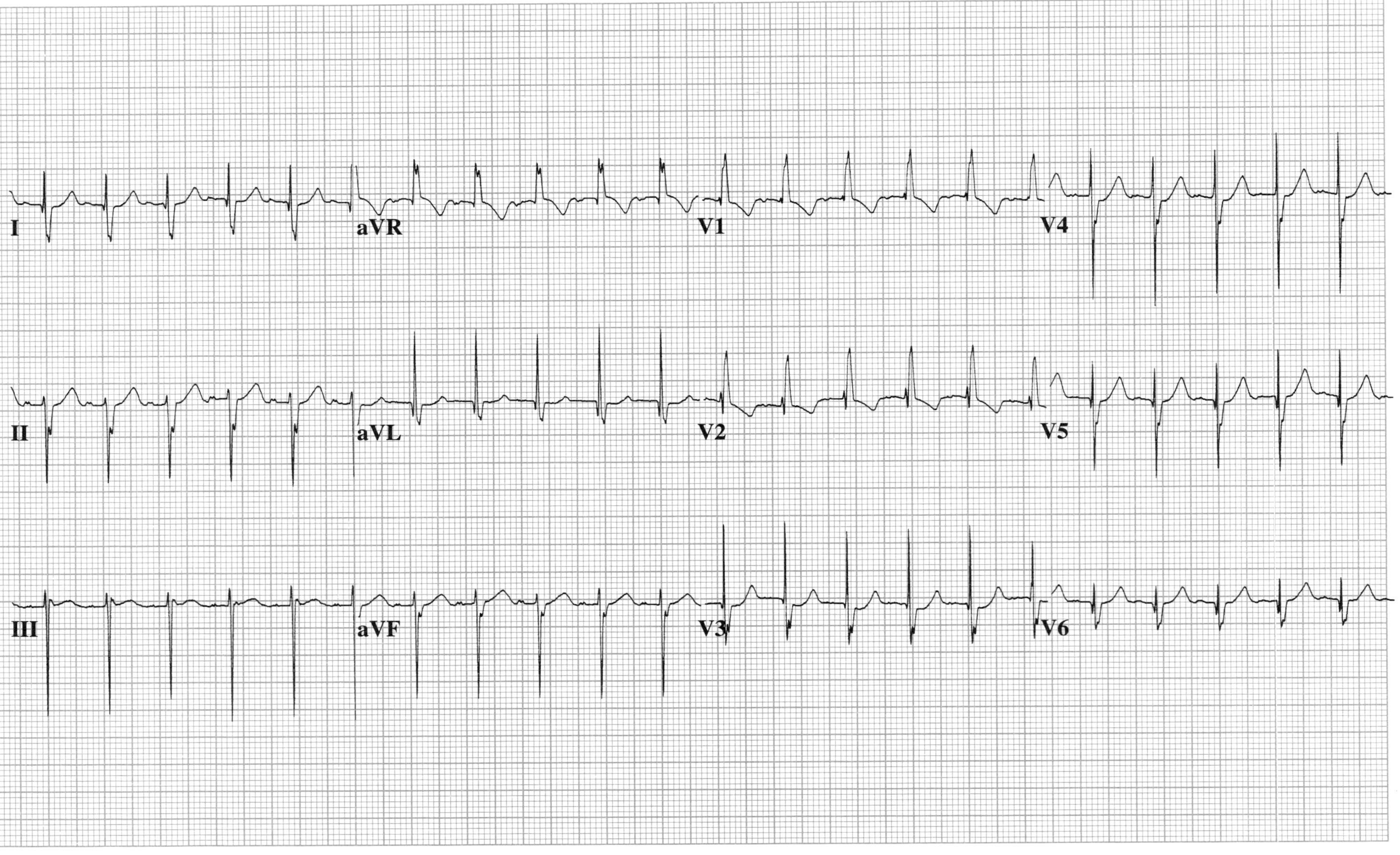

1. GENERAL FEATURES

☐ a. Normal ECG
☐ b. Borderline normal ECG or normal variant
☐ c. Incorrect electrode placement
☐ d. Artifact due to tremor

2. ATRIAL RHYTHMS

☐ a. Sinus rhythm
☐ b. Sinus arrhythmia
☐ c. Sinus bradycardia (< 60)
☐ d. Sinus tachycardia (> 100)
☐ e. Sinus pause or arrest
☐ f. Sinoatrial exit block
☐ g. Ecoptic atrial rhythm
☐ h. Wandering atrial pacemaker
☐ i. Atrial premature complexes, normally conducted
☐ j. Atrial premature complexes, nonconducted
☐ k. Atrial premature complexes with aberrant intraventricular conduction
☐ l. Atrial tachycardia (regular, sustained, 1:1 conduction)
☐ m. Atrial tachycardia, repetitive (short paroxysms)
☐ n. Atrial tachycardia, multifocal
☐ o. Atrial tachycardia with AV block
☐ p. Supraventricular tachycardia, unspecific
☐ q. Supraventricular tachycardia, paroxysmal
☐ r. Atrial flutter
☐ s. Atrial fibrillation
☐ t. Retrograde atrial activation

3. AV JUNCTIONAL RHYTHMS

☐ a. AV junctional premature complexes
☐ b. AV junctional escape complexes
☐ c. AV junctional rhythm, accelerated
☐ d. AV junctional rhythm

4. VENTRICULAR RHYTHMS

☐ a. Ventricular premature complex(es), uniform, fixed coupling
☐ b. Ventricular premature complex(es), uniform, nonfixed coupling
☐ c. Ventricular premature complexes(es), multiform
☐ d. Ventricular premature complexes, in pairs
☐ e. Ventricular parasystole
☐ f. Ventricular tachycardia (≥ 3 consecutive complexes)
☐ g. Accelerated idioventricular rhythm
☐ h. Ventricular escape complexes or rhythm
☐ i. Ventricular fibrillation

5. ATRIAL-VENTRICULAR INTERACTIONS IN ARRHYTHMIAS

☐ a. Fusion complexes
☐ b. Reciprocal (echo) complexes
☐ c. Ventricular capture complexes
☐ d. AV dissociation

☐ e. Ventriculophasic sinus arrhythmia

6. AV CONDUCTION ABNORMALITIES

☐ a. AV block, 1°
☐ b. AV block, 2° - Mobitz type I (Wenckebach)
☐ c. AV block, 2° - Mobitz type II
☐ d. AV block, 2:1
☐ e. AV block, 3°
☐ f. AV block, variable
☐ g. Short PR interval (with sinus rhythm and normal QRS duration)
☐ h. Wolff-Parkinson-White pattern

7. INTRAVENTRICULAR CONDUCTION DISTURBANCES

☐ a. RBBB, incomplete
☐ b. RBBB, complete
☐ c. Left anterior fascicular block
☐ d. Left posterior fascicular block
☐ e. LBBB, with ST-T wave suggestive of acute myocardial injury or infarction
☐ f. LBBB, complete
☐ g. LBBB, intermittent
☐ h. Intraventricular conduction disturbance, nonspecific
☐ i. Aberrant intraventricular conduction with supraventricular arrhythmia

8. P WAVE ABNORMALITIES

☐ a. Right atrial abnormality
☐ b. Left atrial abnormalities
☐ c. Nonspecific atrial abnormality

9. ABNORMALITIES OF QRS VOLTAGE OR AXIS

☐ a. Low voltage, limb leads only
☐ b. Low voltage, limb and precordial leads
☐ c. Left axis deviation (> - 30%)
☐ d. Right axis deviation (> + 100)
☐ e. Electrical alternans

10. VENTRICULAR HYPERTROPHY

☐ a. LVH by voltage only
☐ b. LVH by voltage and ST-T segment abnormalities
☐ c. RVH
☐ d. Combined ventricular hypertrophy

11. Q WAVE MYOCARDIAL INFARCTION

	Probably Acute or Recent	Probably Old or Age Indeterminate
Anterolateral	☐ a.	☐ g.
Anterior	☐ b.	☐ h.
Anteroseptal	☐ c.	☐ i.
Lateral/High lateral	☐ d.	☐ j.
Inferior	☐ e.	☐ k.
Posterior	☐ f.	☐ l.

☐ m. Probably ventricular aneurysm

12. ST, T, U, WAVE ABNORMALITIES

☐ a. Normal variant, early repolarization
☐ b. Normal variant, juvenile T waves
☐ c. Nonspecific ST and/or T wave abnormalities
☐ d. ST and/or T wave abnormalities suggesting myocardial ischemia
☐ e. ST and/or T wave abnormalities suggesting myocardial injury
☐ f. ST and/or T wave abnormalities suggesting acute pericarditis
☐ g. ST-T segment abnormalities secondary to intraventricular conduction disturbance or hypertrophy
☐ h. Post-extrasystolic T wave abnormality
☐ i. Isolated J point depression
☐ j. Peaked T waves
☐ k. Prolonged QT interval
☐ l. Prominent U waves

13. PACEMAKER FUNCTION AND RHYTHM

☐ a. Atrial or coronary sinus pacing
☐ b. Ventricular demand pacing
☐ c. AV sequential pacing
☐ d. Ventricular pacing, complete control
☐ e. Dual chamber, atrial sensing pacemaker
☐ f. Pacemaker malfunction, not constantly capturing (atrium or ventricle)
☐ g. Pacemaker malfunction, not constantly sensing (atrium or ventricle)
☐ h. Pacemaker malfunction, not firing
☐ i. Pacemaker malfunction, slowing

14. SUGGESTED OR PROBABLE CLINICAL DISORDERS

☐ a. Digitalis effect
☐ b. Digitalis toxicity
☐ c. Antiarrhythmic drug effect
☐ d. Antiarrhythmic drug toxicity
☐ e. Hyperkalemia
☐ f. Hypokalemia
☐ g. Hypercalcemia
☐ h. Hypocalcemia
☐ i. Atrial septal defect, secundum
☐ j. Atrial septal defect, primum
☐ k. Dextrocardia, mirror image
☐ l. Mitral valve disease
☐ m. Chronic lung disease
☐ n. Acute cor pulmonale, including
☐ o. Pericardial effusion
☐ p. Acute pericarditis
☐ q. Hypertrophic cardiomy
☐ r. Coronary artery dise
☐ s. Central nervous s
☐ t. Myxedema
☐ u. Hypothermi
☐ v. Sick sinus

ECG 75 was obtained in a 1-year-old male with a heart murmur. The ECG shows sinus tachycardia deviation. This constellation of findings is typical for a primum atrial septal defect. Electrical alternans subsequently underwent cardiac surgery to repair a large primum ASD.

Codes:

2d	Sinus tachycardia
7a	RBBB, incomplete
9c	Left axis deviation (>-30°)
9e	Electrical alternans
14j	Atrial septal defect, primum

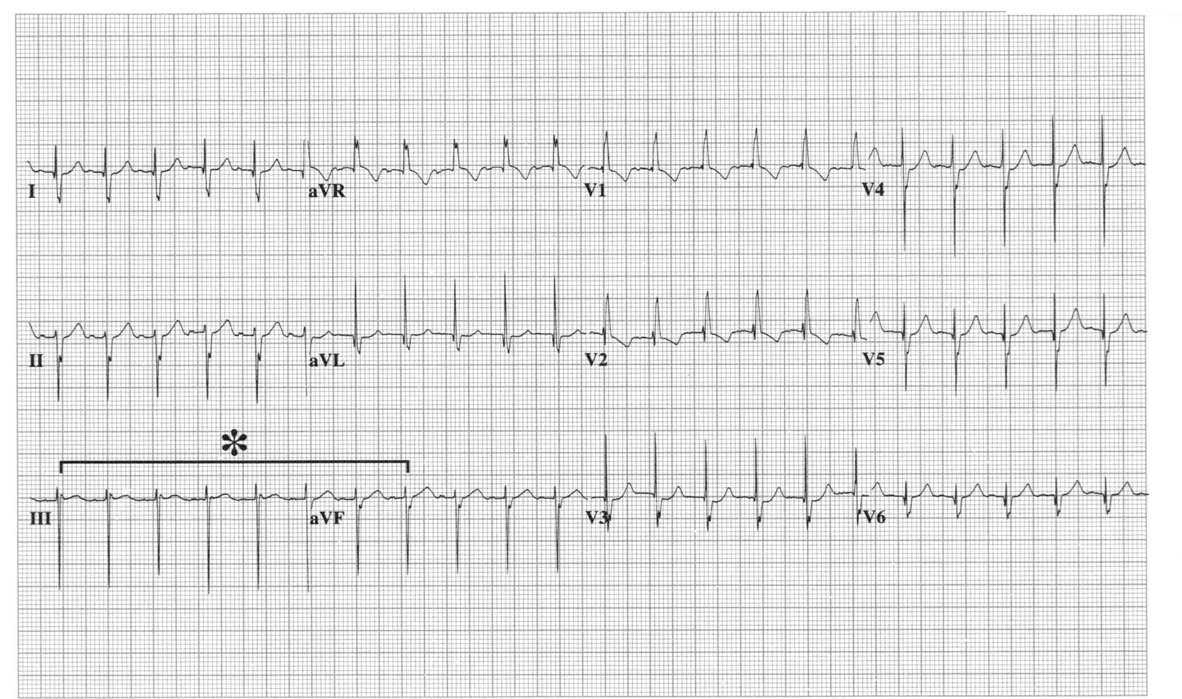

Questions: ECG 75

1. Primum atrial septal defect results in ___ axis deviation:

   a. Right
   b. Left

2. First-degree AV block is seen in 15-40% of patients with primum ASD:

   a. True
   b. False

3. ECG findings suggestive of RVH include:

   a. Left axis deviation
   b. Right atrial abnormality
   c. R > S in V_1
   d. R in aVL > 12 mm
   e. Downsloping ST segments and T wave inversion in V_1-V_3

Answers: ECG 75

1. Primum atrial septal defect is associated with an rSr' complex in V_1 and left axis deviation. Advanced cases may also demonstrate biventricular hypertrophy. (Answer: b)

2. (Answer: a)

3. ECG findings associated with right ventricular hypertrophy include right axis deviation, a dominant R wave in lead V_1 (which is greater than the S wave), and repolarization abnormalities in the right precordial leads. An R wave in lead aVL > 12 mm suggests left rather than right ventricular hypertrophy. (Answer: b, c, e)

— Quick Review 75 —

Sinus tachycardia	
• Rate > ____ per minute	100
• P wave amplitude often (increases/decreases) and PR interval often (increases/decreases) with increasing heart rate	increases shortens
Atrial septal defect, primum	
• RSR' complex in lead ____	V_1
• (Right/left) axis deviation, in contrast to (right/left) axis deviation in secundum ASD	Left, right
• ____ degree AV block in 15-40%	First
• Advanced cases have ____ hypertrophy	biventricular
• Primum ASDs represent 15% of all ASDs, and are due to deficient tissue in the lower portion of the ____. These ASDs are usually (small/large), may be accompanied by anomalous ____ venous drainage, and are associated with a cleft anterior ____ valve leaflet	septum, large pulmonary mitral

— POP QUIZ —

Make The Diagnosis

Instructions: Determine the clinical disorder that best corresponds to the ECG features listed below (see item 14 of score sheet for options)

ECG Features	Answer
• Tall, peaked, narrow based T waves • QT interval shortening • Reversible left anterior or posterior fascicular block • QRS widening • Disappearance of P waves	Hyperkalemia
• Prominent U waves • ST segment depression • Flattened T waves • Prolonged QT interval • Arrhythmias and conduction disturbances, including paroxysmal atrial tachycardia with block, first-degree AV block, Type I second-degree AV block, AV dissociation, VPCs, ventricular tachycardia, and ventricular fibrillation	Hypokalemia
• QT interval shortening • May see PR prolongation • No effect on P, QRS, and T wave	Hypercalcemia
• Earliest and most common finding is prolonged QT interval • Occasional flattening, peaking, or inversion of T waves	Hypocalcemia
• Typical RSR' or rSR' complex in lead V_1 with a QRS duration < 0.11 seconds • Incomplete RBBB • Right axis deviation ± right ventricular hypertrophy • Right atrial abnormality in ~ 30% • First-degree AV block in < 20%	Atrial septal defect, secundum

ECG 76. 43-year-old male in the emergency department with chest pain:

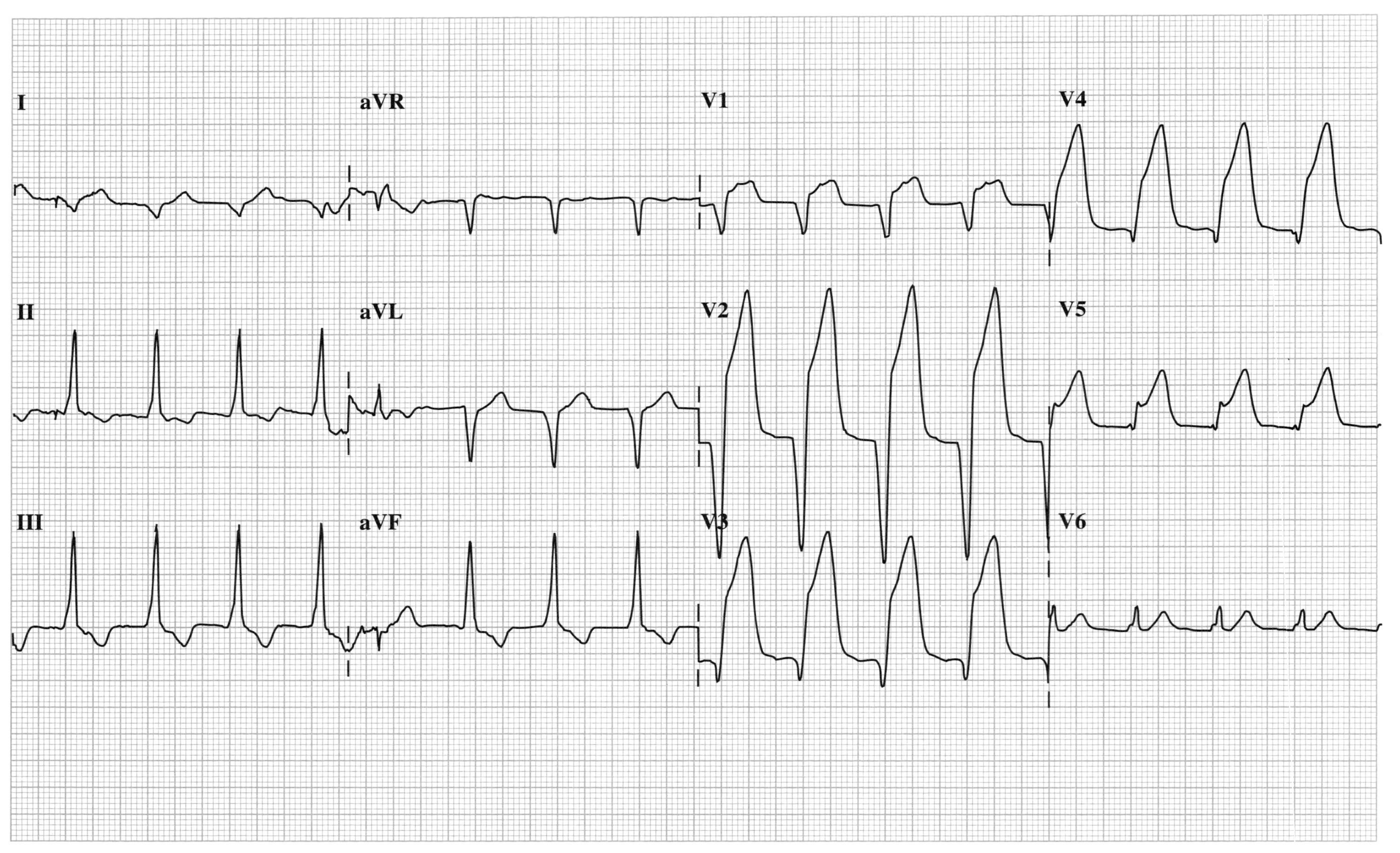

1. GENERAL FEATURES

☐ a. Normal ECG
☐ b. Borderline normal ECG or normal variant
☐ c. Incorrect electrode placement
☐ d. Artifact due to tremor

2. ATRIAL RHYTHMS

☐ a. Sinus rhythm
☐ b. Sinus arrhythmia
☐ c. Sinus bradycardia (< 60)
☐ d. Sinus tachycardia (> 100)
☐ e. Sinus pause or arrest
☐ f. Sinoatrial exit block
☐ g. Ecoptic atrial rhythm
☐ h. Wandering atrial pacemaker
☐ i. Atrial premature complexes, normally conducted
☐ j. Atrial premature complexes, nonconducted
☐ k. Atrial premature complexes with aberrant intraventricular conduction
☐ l. Atrial tachycardia (regular, sustained, 1:1 conduction)
☐ m. Atrial tachycardia, repetitive (short paroxysms)
☐ n. Atrial tachycardia, multifocal
☐ o. Atrial tachycardia with AV block
☐ p. Supraventricular tachycardia, unspecific
☐ q. Supraventricular tachycardia, paroxysmal
☐ r. Atrial flutter
☐ s. Atrial fibrillation
☐ t. Retrograde atrial activation

3. AV JUNCTIONAL RHYTHMS

☐ a. AV junctional premature complexes
☐ b. AV junctional escape complexes
☐ c. AV junctional rhythm, accelerated
☐ d. AV junctional rhythm

4. VENTRICULAR RHYTHMS

☐ a. Ventricular premature complex(es), uniform, fixed coupling
☐ b. Ventricular premature complex(es), uniform, nonfixed coupling
☐ c. Ventricular premature complexes(es), multiform
☐ d. Ventricular premature complexes, in pairs
☐ e. Ventricular parasystole
☐ f. Ventricular tachycardia (≥ 3 consecutive complexes)
☐ g. Accelerated idioventricular rhythm
☐ h. Ventricular escape complexes or rhythm
☐ i. Ventricular fibrillation

5. ATRIAL-VENTRICULAR INTERACTIONS IN ARRHYTHMIAS

☐ a. Fusion complexes
☐ b. Reciprocal (echo) complexes
☐ c. Ventricular capture complexes
☐ d. AV dissociation
☐ e. Ventriculophasic sinus arrhythmia

6. AV CONDUCTION ABNORMALITIES

☐ a. AV block, 1°
☐ b. AV block, 2° - Mobitz type I (Wenckebach)
☐ c. AV block, 2° - Mobitz type II
☐ d. AV block, 2:1
☐ e. AV block, 3°
☐ f. AV block, variable
☐ g. Short PR interval (with sinus rhythm and normal QRS duration)
☐ h. Wolff-Parkinson-White pattern

7. INTRAVENTRICULAR CONDUCTION DISTURBANCES

☐ a. RBBB, incomplete
☐ b. RBBB, complete
☐ c. Left anterior fascicular block
☐ d. Left posterior fascicular block
☐ e. LBBB, with ST-T wave suggestive of acute myocardial injury or infarction
☐ f. LBBB, complete
☐ g. LBBB, intermittent
☐ h. Intraventricular conduction disturbance, nonspecific
☐ i. Aberrant intraventricular conduction with supraventricular arrhythmia

8. P WAVE ABNORMALITIES

☐ a. Right atrial abnormality
☐ b. Left atrial abnormalities
☐ c. Nonspecific atrial abnormality

9. ABNORMALITIES OF QRS VOLTAGE OR AXIS

☐ a. Low voltage, limb leads only
☐ b. Low voltage, limb and precordial leads
☐ c. Left axis deviation (> - 30%)
☐ d. Right axis deviation (> + 100)
☐ e. Electrical alternans

10. VENTRICULAR HYPERTROPHY

☐ a. LVH by voltage only
☐ b. LVH by voltage and ST-T segment abnormalities
☐ c. RVH
☐ d. Combined ventricular hypertrophy

11. Q WAVE MYOCARDIAL INFARCTION

	Probably Acute or Recent	Probably Old or Age Indeterminate
Anterolateral	☐ a.	☐ g.
Anterior	☐ b.	☐ h.
Anteroseptal	☐ c.	☐ i.
Lateral/High lateral	☐ d.	☐ j.
Inferior	☐ e.	☐ k.
Posterior	☐ f.	☐ l.

☐ m. Probably ventricular aneurysm

12. ST, T, U, WAVE ABNORMALITIES

☐ a. Normal variant, early repolarization
☐ b. Normal variant, juvenile T waves
☐ c. Nonspecific ST and/or T wave abnormalities
☐ d. ST and/or T wave abnormalities suggesting myocardial ischemia
☐ e. ST and/or T wave abnormalities suggesting myocardial injury
☐ f. ST and/or T wave abnormalities suggesting acute pericarditis
☐ g. ST-T segment abnormalities secondary to intraventricular conduction disturbance or hypertrophy
☐ h. Post-extrasystolic T wave abnormality
☐ i. Isolated J point depression
☐ j. Peaked T waves
☐ k. Prolonged QT interval
☐ l. Prominent U waves

13. PACEMAKER FUNCTION AND RHYTHM

☐ a. Atrial or coronary sinus pacing
☐ b. Ventricular demand pacing
☐ c. AV sequential pacing
☐ d. Ventricular pacing, complete control
☐ e. Dual chamber, atrial sensing pacemaker
☐ f. Pacemaker malfunction, not constantly capturing (atrium or ventricle)
☐ g. Pacemaker malfunction, not constantly sensing (atrium or ventricle)
☐ h. Pacemaker malfunction, not firing
☐ i. Pacemaker malfunction, slowing

14. SUGGESTED OR PROBABLE CLINICAL DISORDERS

☐ a. Digitalis effect
☐ b. Digitalis toxicity
☐ c. Antiarrhythmic drug effect
☐ d. Antiarrhythmic drug toxicity
☐ e. Hyperkalemia
☐ f. Hypokalemia
☐ g. Hypercalcemia
☐ h. Hypocalcemia
☐ i. Atrial septal defect, secundum
☐ j. Atrial septal defect, primum
☐ k. Dextrocardia, mirror image
☐ l. Mitral valve disease
☐ m. Chronic lung disease
☐ n. Acute cor pulmonale, including pulmonary embolus
☐ o. Pericardial effusion
☐ p. Acute pericarditis
☐ q. Hypertrophic cardiomyopathy
☐ r. Coronary artery disease
☐ s. Central nervous system disorder
☐ t. Myxedema
☐ u. Hypothermia
☐ v. Sick sinus syndrome

ECG 76 was obtained from a 43-year-old male who presented to the emergency department with chest pain. The tracing shows an accelerated junctional rhythm at 99 beats/minute with retrograde P waves (most apparent in the first portion of the T wave in lead V_1; arrow). The fifth beat in the tracing is a VPC (arrowhead). The most striking finding on the ECG is the marked ST segment elevation (approximately 15 mm) and hyperacute peaking of the T waves (asterisks), consistent with an acute extensive myocardial infarction involving the anteroseptal and anterolateral walls. While it is likely that the high lateral wall is involved in the acute process (given the extensive nature of the infarct), acute lateral infarction should *not* be coded since the ST segments and T waves are normal in leads I and aVL. Also noted are right axis deviation (due to the high-lateral infarction) and a nonspecific intraventricular conduction defect. The findings are consistent with coronary artery disease.

Codes:				
	2t	Retrograde atrial activation	11c	Anteroseptal Q wave MI, probably acute or recent
	3c	AV junctional rhythm, accelerated	11j	Lateral or high lateral Q wave MI, probably old or age indeterminate
	4a	VPCs, uniform, fixed coupling	12d	ST and/or T wave abnormalities suggesting myocardial ischemia
	7h	IVCD, nonspecific type	12e	ST and/or T wave abnormalities suggesting myocardial injury
	9d	Right axis deviation	12j	Peaked T waves
	11a	Anterolateral Q wave MI, probably acute or recent	14r	Coronary artery disease

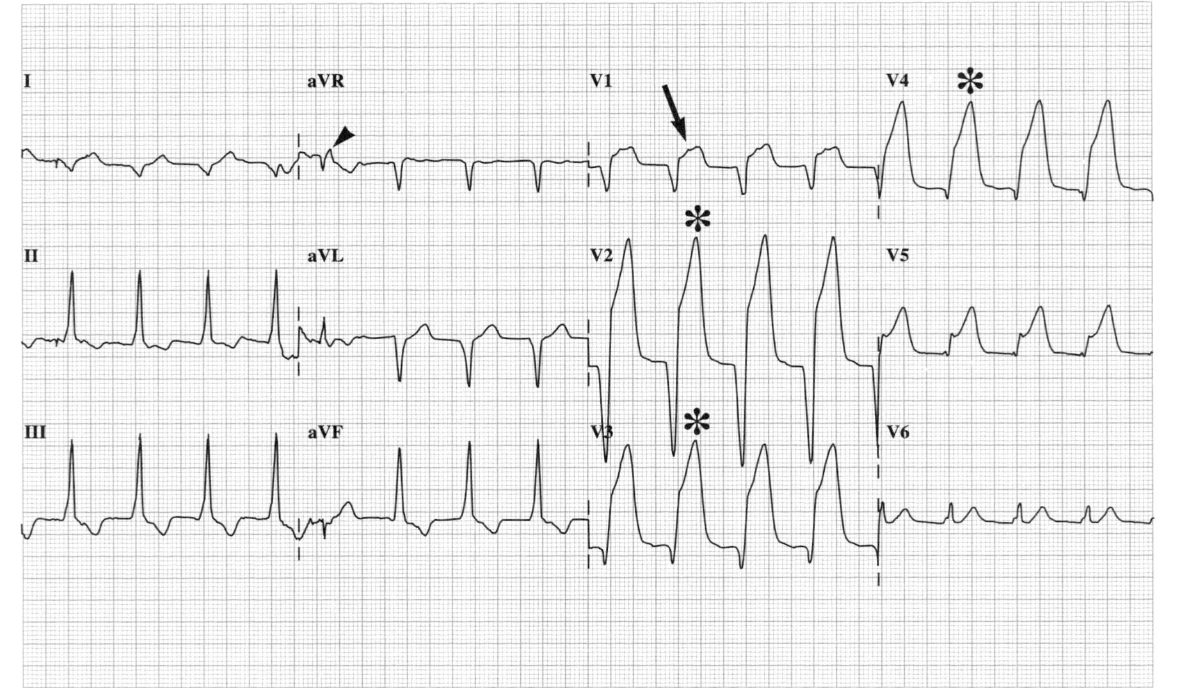

Questions: ECG 76

1. The most likely cause of the ST and T wave changes in leads II, III, and aVF is:

   a. Inferior wall myocardial ischemia
   b. Reciprocal changes secondary to acute MI
   c. WPW
   d. LVH
   e. Digitalis effect

2. What is responsible for the small positive deflection appearing 0.08 seconds after the QRS in leads II, III, and aVF?

   a. Actually part of the QRS complex and due to intraventricular conduction delay
   b. Artifact
   c. Blocked premature atrial contraction
   d. Retrograde atrial activation

3. Retrograde atrial activation from junctional tachycardia can manifest as a P wave that precedes the QRS complex:

   a. True
   b. False

4. Giant T waves can be seen in:

   a. Left ventricular hypertrophy
   b. Acute myocardial infarction
   c. Cerebrovascular accident
   d. Normal patients
   e. Hyperkalemia
   f. Hypocalcemia

5. Could the slurred initial portion of the QRS complex (best seen in leads II and III) be due to WPW?

   a. Yes
   b. No

6. Junctional tachycardia can be seen in:

   a. Acute myocardial infarction
   b. Digitalis toxicity
   c. Myocarditis
   d. Following open heart surgery

Answers: ECG 76

1. The ST segment depression and T wave inversion in the inferior leads are most likely due myocardial ischemia, although reciprocal changes are possible. The diagnosis of WPW is excluded since there is no evidence for a sinus or atrial rhythm present. The deep ST and T wave changes are not typical of digitalis effect. (Answer: a)

2. The small deflection appearing 0.08 seconds after the QRS complex in the inferior leads is due to retrograde atrial activation from a junctional pacemaker. The deflection, also seen in lead V_1, clearly deforms the ST segment, and is therefore not due to intraventricular conduction delay. (Answer: d)

3. A junctional beat may result in a P wave that precedes, is buried in, or follows the QRS complex. In the present tracing, antegrade ventricular activation from the junctional focus occurs prior to retrograde atrial activation, resulting in a QRS complex that precedes the P wave. (Answer: a)

4. Tall upright T waves may be seen in normal patients, and in a variety of cardiac, metabolic, and CNS conditions. These include ventricular hypertrophy (right and left), acute MI, angina pectoris, hyperkalemia, and cerebrovascular accident. In left ventricular hypertrophy, tall upright T waves are often seen in leads containing predominantly negative QRS complexes (i.e., V_1 - V_3). In angina and acute myocardial infarction, tall upright T waves may be the earliest manifestation of transmural myocardial ischemia. Patients with acute cerebrovascular accidents, especially with intracranial hemorrhage, may present with giant T waves that can be upright or inverted; ST elevation or depression, large U waves, marked QT prolongation, and abnormal Q waves can also occur. Tall upright T waves are occasionally seen in normal patients, especially in leads V_2 and V_3 in young adults; peaked T waves are often an early finding in hyperkalemia, especially when the rise in serum potassium is acute. Hypocalcemia results in QT prolongation, but does not typically produce giant T waves. (Answer: All except f)

5. In the WPW syndrome, atrial impulses conduct to the ventricles via the bundle of Kent, bypassing the AV node (and normal AV nodal delay) and resulting in a short PR interval. Premature activation of the ventricles produces an abnormal pattern of ventricular depolarization characterized by slurring of the initial QRS complex (delta wave), and repolarization abnormalities consisting of secondary ST and T wave changes. The lack of a sinus or atrial mechanism in the present tracing excludes the diagnosis of WPW. (Answer: b)

6. Junctional tachycardia can be seen in acute myocardial infarction (usually inferior), myocarditis, and following open heart surgery. Digitalis toxicity may also induce junctional tachycardia; when atrial fibrillation is present, junctional tachycardia often manifests as regularization of the ventricular rate. (Answer: All)

— Quick Review 76 —

Anterolateral MI, probably acute or recent	
• Abnormal Q waves (duration ≥ 0.03 seconds) and ST segment elevation in leads ____	V_4-V_6
Anteroseptal MI, probably acute or recent	
• Abnormal Q or QS deflection and ST elevation in leads ____ (and sometimes V_4)	V_1-V_3
• The presence of a Q wave in lead ____ distinguishes anteroseptal from anterior infarction	V_1
Lateral or high lateral MI, probably acute or recent	
• Abnormal Q waves and ST elevation in leads I and ____	aVL
• An isolated Q wave in aVL (does/does not) qualify as a lateral MI	does not
Peaked T waves	
• T wave > ____ mm in the limb leads or > ____ mm in the precordial leads	6, 10

ECG 77. Asymptomatic 61-year-old female:

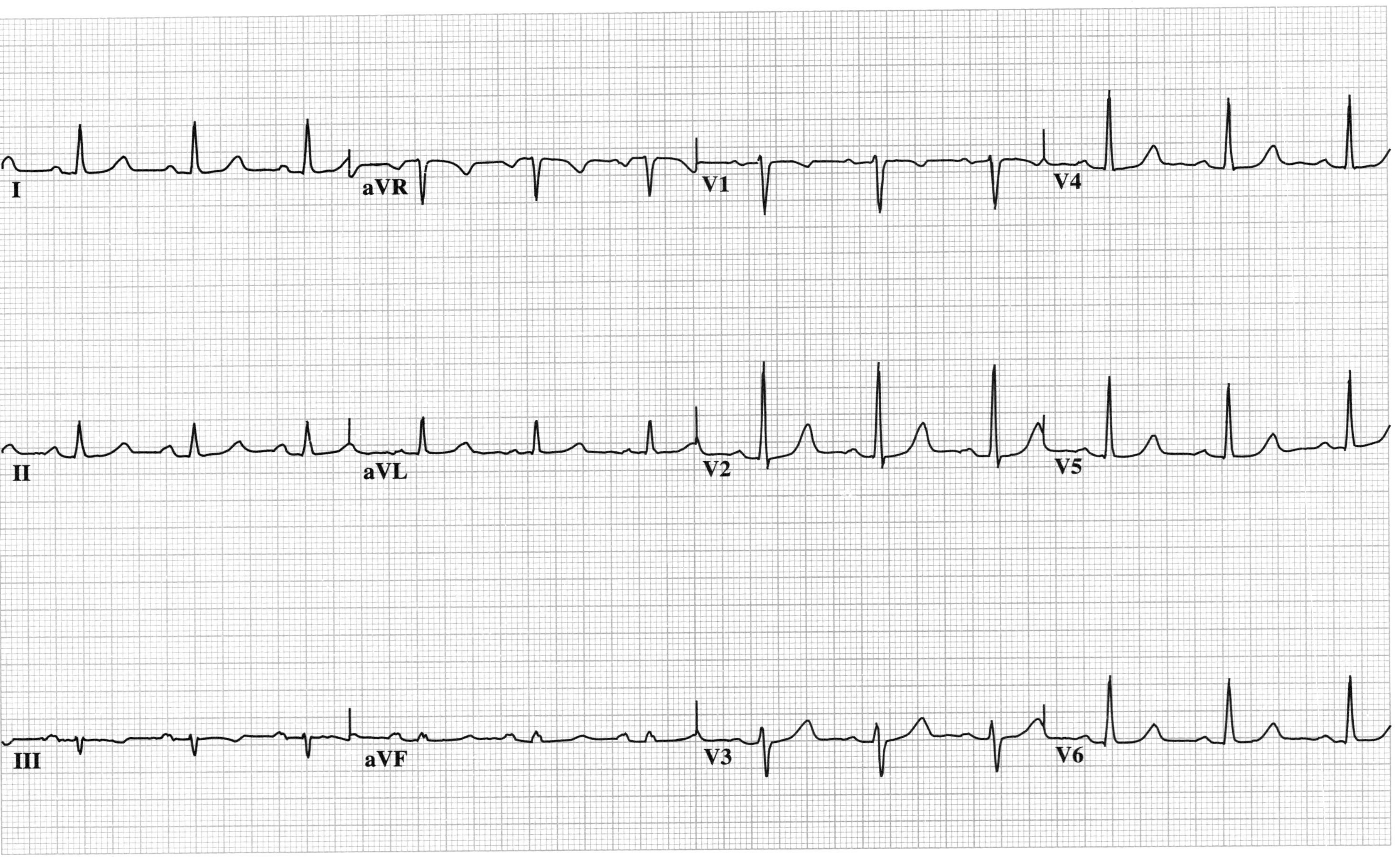

1. GENERAL FEATURES

- ☐ a. Normal ECG
- ☐ b. Borderline normal ECG or normal variant
- ☐ c. Incorrect electrode placement
- ☐ d. Artifact due to tremor

2. ATRIAL RHYTHMS

- ☐ a. Sinus rhythm
- ☐ b. Sinus arrhythmia
- ☐ c. Sinus bradycardia (< 60)
- ☐ d. Sinus tachycardia (> 100)
- ☐ e. Sinus pause or arrest
- ☐ f. Sinoatrial exit block
- ☐ g. Ecoptic atrial rhythm
- ☐ h. Wandering atrial pacemaker
- ☐ i. Atrial premature complexes, normally conducted
- ☐ j. Atrial premature complexes, nonconducted
- ☐ k. Atrial premature complexes with aberrant intraventricular conduction
- ☐ l. Atrial tachycardia (regular, sustained, 1:1 conduction)
- ☐ m. Atrial tachycardia, repetitive (short paroxysms)
- ☐ n. Atrial tachycardia, multifocal
- ☐ o. Atrial tachycardia with AV block
- ☐ p. Supraventricular tachycardia, unspecific
- ☐ q. Supraventricular tachycardia, paroxysmal
- ☐ r. Atrial flutter
- ☐ s. Atrial fibrillation
- ☐ t. Retrograde atrial activation

3. AV JUNCTIONAL RHYTHMS

- ☐ a. AV junctional premature complexes
- ☐ b. AV junctional escape complexes
- ☐ c. AV junctional rhythm, accelerated
- ☐ d. AV junctional rhythm

4. VENTRICULAR RHYTHMS

- ☐ a. Ventricular premature complex(es), uniform, fixed coupling
- ☐ b. Ventricular premature complex(es), uniform, nonfixed coupling
- ☐ c. Ventricular premature complexes(es), multiform
- ☐ d. Ventricular premature complexes, in pairs
- ☐ e. Ventricular parasystole
- ☐ f. Ventricular tachycardia (≥ 3 consecutive complexes)
- ☐ g. Accelerated idioventricular rhythm
- ☐ h. Ventricular escape complexes or rhythm
- ☐ i. Ventricular fibrillation

5. ATRIAL-VENTRICULAR INTERACTIONS IN ARRHYTHMIAS

- ☐ a. Fusion complexes
- ☐ b. Reciprocal (echo) complexes
- ☐ c. Ventricular capture complexes
- ☐ d. AV dissociation
- ☐ e. Ventriculophasic sinus arrhythmia

6. AV CONDUCTION ABNORMALITIES

- ☐ a. AV block, 1°
- ☐ b. AV block, 2° - Mobitz type I (Wenckebach)
- ☐ c. AV block, 2° - Mobitz type II
- ☐ d. AV block, 2:1
- ☐ e. AV block, 3°
- ☐ f. AV block, variable
- ☐ g. Short PR interval (with sinus rhythm and normal QRS duration)
- ☐ h. Wolff-Parkinson-White pattern

7. INTRAVENTRICULAR CONDUCTION DISTURBANCES

- ☐ a. RBBB, incomplete
- ☐ b. RBBB, complete
- ☐ c. Left anterior fascicular block
- ☐ d. Left posterior fascicular block
- ☐ e. LBBB, with ST-T wave suggestive of acute myocardial injury or infarction
- ☐ f. LBBB, complete
- ☐ g. LBBB, intermittent
- ☐ h. Intraventricular conduction disturbance, nonspecific
- ☐ i. Aberrant intraventricular conduction with supraventricular arrhythmia

8. P WAVE ABNORMALITIES

- ☐ a. Right atrial abnormality
- ☐ b. Left atrial abnormalities
- ☐ c. Nonspecific atrial abnormality

9. ABNORMALITIES OF QRS VOLTAGE OR AXIS

- ☐ a. Low voltage, limb leads only
- ☐ b. Low voltage, limb and precordial leads
- ☐ c. Left axis deviation (> - 30%)
- ☐ d. Right axis deviation (> + 100)
- ☐ e. Electrical alternans

10. VENTRICULAR HYPERTROPHY

- ☐ a. LVH by voltage only
- ☐ b. LVH by voltage and ST-T segment abnormalities
- ☐ c. RVH
- ☐ d. Combined ventricular hypertrophy

11. Q WAVE MYOCARDIAL INFARCTION

	Probably Acute or Recent	Probably Old or Age Indeterminate
Anterolateral	☐ a.	☐ g.
Anterior	☐ b.	☐ h.
Anteroseptal	☐ c.	☐ i.
Lateral/High lateral	☐ d.	☐ j.
Inferior	☐ e.	☐ k.
Posterior	☐ f.	☐ l.

☐ m. Probably ventricular aneurysm

12. ST, T, U, WAVE ABNORMALITIES

- ☐ a. Normal variant, early repolarization
- ☐ b. Normal variant, juvenile T waves
- ☐ c. Nonspecific ST and/or T wave abnormalities
- ☐ d. ST and/or T wave abnormalities suggesting myocardial ischemia
- ☐ e. ST and/or T wave abnormalities suggesting myocardial injury
- ☐ f. ST and/or T wave abnormalities suggesting acute pericarditis
- ☐ g. ST-T segment abnormalities secondary to intraventricular conduction disturbance or hypertrophy
- ☐ h. Post-extrasystolic T wave abnormality
- ☐ i. Isolated J point depression
- ☐ j. Peaked T waves
- ☐ k. Prolonged QT interval
- ☐ l. Prominent U waves

13. PACEMAKER FUNCTION AND RHYTHM

- ☐ a. Atrial or coronary sinus pacing
- ☐ b. Ventricular demand pacing
- ☐ c. AV sequential pacing
- ☐ d. Ventricular pacing, complete control
- ☐ e. Dual chamber, atrial sensing pacemaker
- ☐ f. Pacemaker malfunction, not constantly capturing (atrium or ventricle)
- ☐ g. Pacemaker malfunction, not constantly sensing (atrium or ventricle)
- ☐ h. Pacemaker malfunction, not firing
- ☐ i. Pacemaker malfunction, slowing

14. SUGGESTED OR PROBABLE CLINICAL DISORDERS

- ☐ a. Digitalis effect
- ☐ b. Digitalis toxicity
- ☐ c. Antiarrhythmic drug effect
- ☐ d. Antiarrhythmic drug toxicity
- ☐ e. Hyperkalemia
- ☐ f. Hypokalemia
- ☐ g. Hypercalcemia
- ☐ h. Hypocalcemia
- ☐ i. Atrial septal defect, secundum
- ☐ j. Atrial septal defect, primum
- ☐ k. Dextrocardia, mirror image
- ☐ l. Mitral valve disease
- ☐ m. Chronic lung disease
- ☐ n. Acute cor pulmonale, including pulmonary embolus
- ☐ o. Pericardial effusion
- ☐ p. Acute pericarditis
- ☐ q. Hypertrophic cardiomyopathy
- ☐ r. Coronary artery disease
- ☐ s. Central nervous system disorder
- ☐ t. Myxedema
- ☐ u. Hypothermia
- ☐ v. Sick sinus syndrome

ECG 77 was obtained in an asymptomatic 61-year-old female. The ECG shows a normal sinus rhythm with a PR interval at the upper limits of normal (0.20 seconds). A prominent R wave is noted in lead V_2 (asterisk) with subsequent loss in R wave voltage from V_2 to V_3. Upon closer inspection, this is due to V_2-V_3 electrode switch. This is otherwise a normal tracing.

Codes:

1c	Incorrect electrode placement
2a	Sinus rhythm

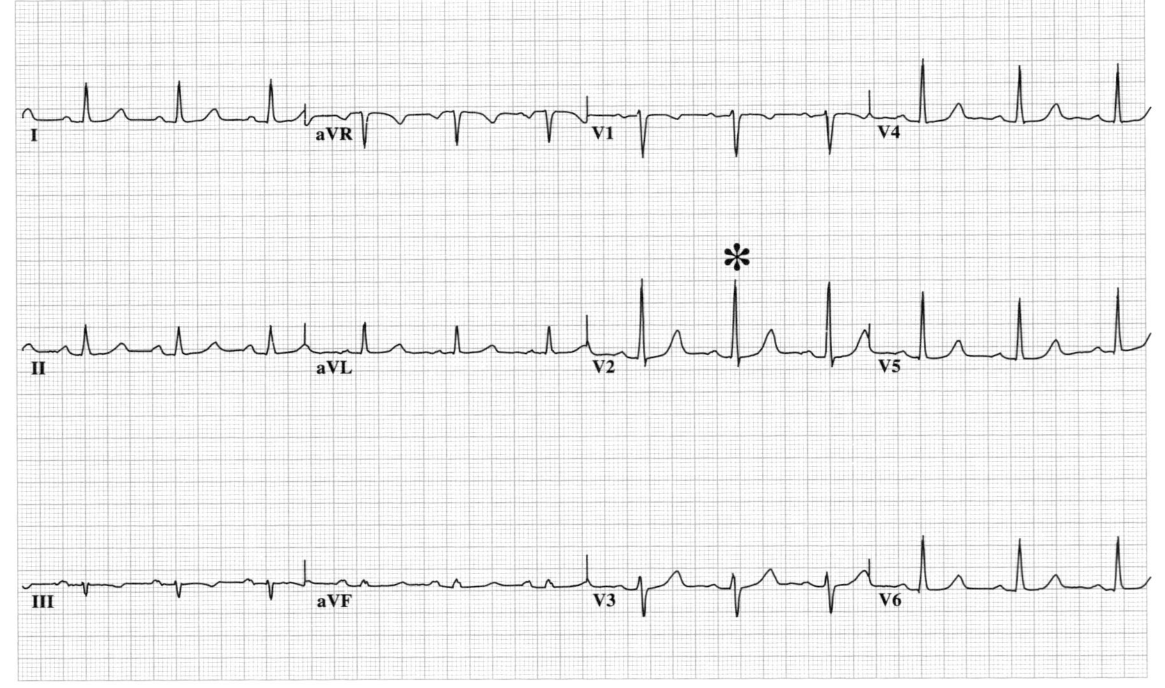

Questions: ECG 77

1. Limb lead electrode switch and dextrocardia both demonstrate:

   a. Inversion of the P-QRS-T in leads I and aVL
   b. Abnormal R wave progression in V_1-V_6
   c. Right ventricular hypertrophy
   d. Right atrial abnormality

2. Incorrect electrode placement of one of the precordial leads often manifests as unexplained loss of R wave voltage in the affected lead:

   a. True
   b. False

Answers: ECG 77

1. Limb lead electrode switch can be mistaken for dextrocardia. Both conditions manifest inversion the P-QRS-T in leads I and aVL. Dextrocardia is associated with reverse R wave progression in leads V_1-V_6, right ventricular hypertrophy, and right atrial abnormality, none of which are present in limb lead electrode switch. (Answer: a)

2. Incorrect electrode placement in one of the precordial leads usually manifests as unexplained loss of R wave voltage in the affected lead. (Answer: a)

— Quick Review 77 —

Incorrect electrode placement	
Limb lead reversal (reversal of right and left arm leads)	
• Resultant ECG mimics dextrocardia with ____ of the P-QRS-T in leads ____ and aVL	inversion I
• To distinguish between these conditions, look at precordial leads: dextrocardia shows (reverse/normal) R wave progression, while limb lead reversal shows (reverse/normal) R wave progression.	reverse normal
Precordial lead reversal: Unexplained decrease in ____ voltage in two consecutive leads (e.g., V_1, V_2) with a return to normal progression in the following leads	R wave

ECG 78. 66-year-old male in the emergency room with palpitations and syncope:

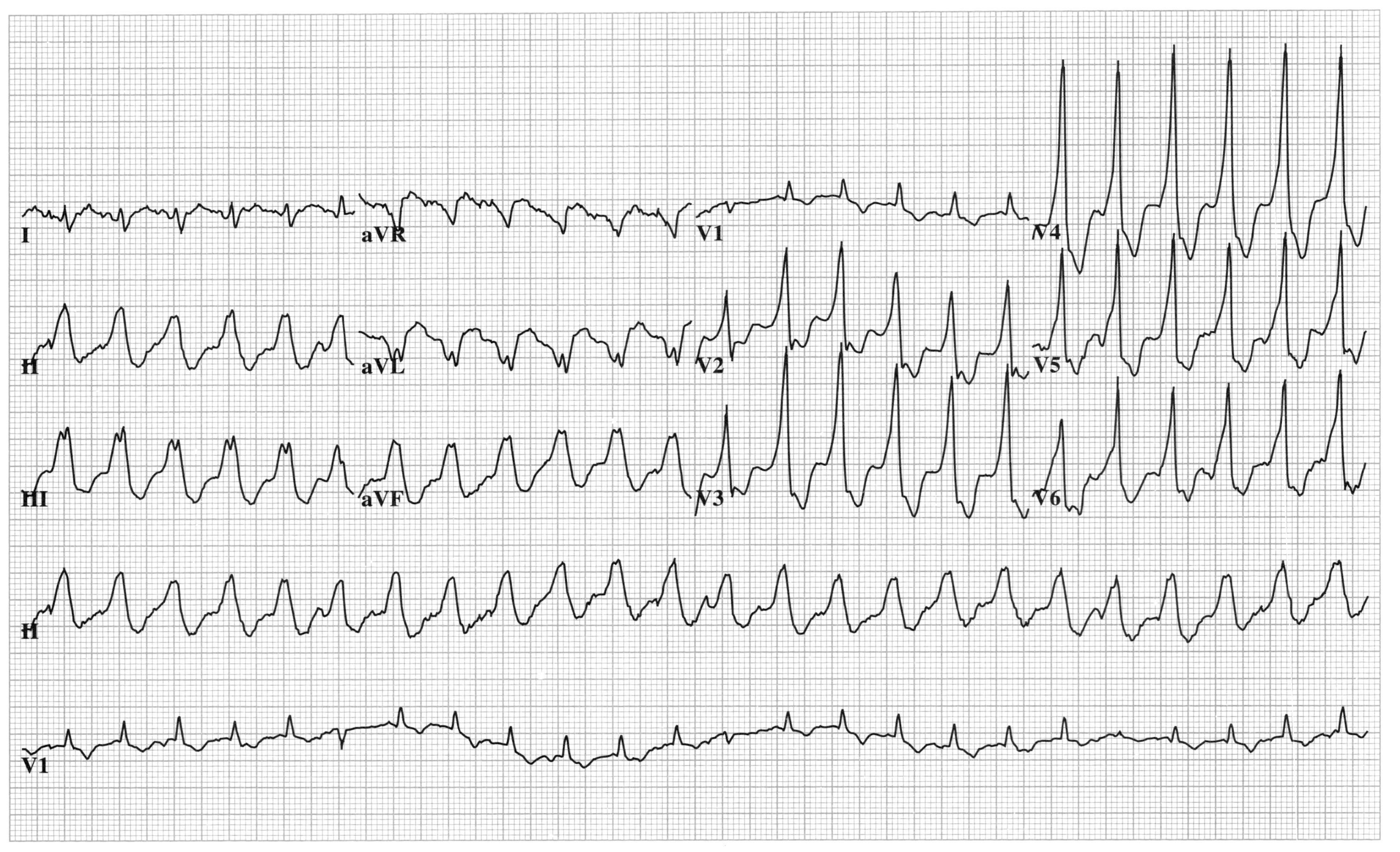

1. GENERAL FEATURES

☐ a. Normal ECG
☐ b. Borderline normal ECG or normal variant
☐ c. Incorrect electrode placement
☐ d. Artifact due to tremor

2. ATRIAL RHYTHMS

☐ a. Sinus rhythm
☐ b. Sinus arrhythmia
☐ c. Sinus bradycardia (< 60)
☐ d. Sinus tachycardia (> 100)
☐ e. Sinus pause or arrest
☐ f. Sinoatrial exit block
☐ g. Ecoptic atrial rhythm
☐ h. Wandering atrial pacemaker
☐ i. Atrial premature complexes, normally conducted
☐ j. Atrial premature complexes, nonconducted
☐ k. Atrial premature complexes with aberrant intraventricular conduction
☐ l. Atrial tachycardia (regular, sustained, 1:1 conduction)
☐ m. Atrial tachycardia, repetitive (short paroxysms)
☐ n. Atrial tachycardia, multifocal
☐ o. Atrial tachycardia with AV block
☐ p. Supraventricular tachycardia, unspecific
☐ q. Supraventricular tachycardia, paroxysmal
☐ r. Atrial flutter
☐ s. Atrial fibrillation
☐ t. Retrograde atrial activation

3. AV JUNCTIONAL RHYTHMS

☐ a. AV junctional premature complexes
☐ b. AV junctional escape complexes
☐ c. AV junctional rhythm, accelerated
☐ d. AV junctional rhythm

4. VENTRICULAR RHYTHMS

☐ a. Ventricular premature complex(es), uniform, fixed coupling
☐ b. Ventricular premature complex(es), uniform, nonfixed coupling
☐ c. Ventricular premature complexes(es), multiform
☐ d. Ventricular premature complexes, in pairs
☐ e. Ventricular parasystole
☐ f. Ventricular tachycardia (≥ 3 consecutive complexes)
☐ g. Accelerated idioventricular rhythm
☐ h. Ventricular escape complexes or rhythm
☐ i. Ventricular fibrillation

5. ATRIAL-VENTRICULAR INTERACTIONS IN ARRHYTHMIAS

☐ a. Fusion complexes
☐ b. Reciprocal (echo) complexes
☐ c. Ventricular capture complexes
☐ d. AV dissociation
☐ e. Ventriculophasic sinus arrhythmia

6. AV CONDUCTION ABNORMALITIES

☐ a. AV block, 1°
☐ b. AV block, 2° - Mobitz type I (Wenckebach)
☐ c. AV block, 2° - Mobitz type II
☐ d. AV block, 2:1
☐ e. AV block, 3°
☐ f. AV block, variable
☐ g. Short PR interval (with sinus rhythm and normal QRS duration)
☐ h. Wolff-Parkinson-White pattern

7. INTRAVENTRICULAR CONDUCTION DISTURBANCES

☐ a. RBBB, incomplete
☐ b. RBBB, complete
☐ c. Left anterior fascicular block
☐ d. Left posterior fascicular block
☐ e. LBBB, with ST-T wave suggestive of acute myocardial injury or infarction
☐ f. LBBB, complete
☐ g. LBBB, intermittent
☐ h. Intraventricular conduction disturbance, nonspecific
☐ i. Aberrant intraventricular conduction with supraventricular arrhythmia

8. P WAVE ABNORMALITIES

☐ a. Right atrial abnormality
☐ b. Left atrial abnormalities
☐ c. Nonspecific atrial abnormality

9. ABNORMALITIES OF QRS VOLTAGE OR AXIS

☐ a. Low voltage, limb leads only
☐ b. Low voltage, limb and precordial leads
☐ c. Left axis deviation (> - 30%)
☐ d. Right axis deviation (> + 100)
☐ e. Electrical alternans

10. VENTRICULAR HYPERTROPHY

☐ a. LVH by voltage only
☐ b. LVH by voltage and ST-T segment abnormalities
☐ c. RVH
☐ d. Combined ventricular hypertrophy

11. Q WAVE MYOCARDIAL INFARCTION

	Probably Acute or Recent	Probably Old or Age Indeterminate
Anterolateral	☐ a.	☐ g.
Anterior	☐ b.	☐ h.
Anteroseptal	☐ c.	☐ i.
Lateral/High lateral	☐ d.	☐ j.
Inferior	☐ e.	☐ k.
Posterior	☐ f.	☐ l.

☐ m. Probably ventricular aneurysm

12. ST, T, U, WAVE ABNORMALITIES

☐ a. Normal variant, early repolarization
☐ b. Normal variant, juvenile T waves
☐ c. Nonspecific ST and/or T wave abnormalities
☐ d. ST and/or T wave abnormalities suggesting myocardial ischemia
☐ e. ST and/or T wave abnormalities suggesting myocardial injury
☐ f. ST and/or T wave abnormalities suggesting acute pericarditis
☐ g. ST-T segment abnormalities secondary to intraventricular conduction disturbance or hypertrophy
☐ h. Post-extrasystolic T wave abnormality
☐ i. Isolated J point depression
☐ j. Peaked T waves
☐ k. Prolonged QT interval
☐ l. Prominent U waves

13. PACEMAKER FUNCTION AND RHYTHM

☐ a. Atrial or coronary sinus pacing
☐ b. Ventricular demand pacing
☐ c. AV sequential pacing
☐ d. Ventricular pacing, complete control
☐ e. Dual chamber, atrial sensing pacemaker
☐ f. Pacemaker malfunction, not constantly capturing (atrium or ventricle)
☐ g. Pacemaker malfunction, not constantly sensing (atrium or ventricle)
☐ h. Pacemaker malfunction, not firing
☐ i. Pacemaker malfunction, slowing

14. SUGGESTED OR PROBABLE CLINICAL DISORDERS

☐ a. Digitalis effect
☐ b. Digitalis toxicity
☐ c. Antiarrhythmic drug effect
☐ d. Antiarrhythmic drug toxicity
☐ e. Hyperkalemia
☐ f. Hypokalemia
☐ g. Hypercalcemia
☐ h. Hypocalcemia
☐ i. Atrial septal defect, secundum
☐ j. Atrial septal defect, primum
☐ k. Dextrocardia, mirror image
☐ l. Mitral valve disease
☐ m. Chronic lung disease
☐ n. Acute cor pulmonale, including pulmonary embolus
☐ o. Pericardial effusion
☐ p. Acute pericarditis
☐ q. Hypertrophic cardiomyopathy
☐ r. Coronary artery disease
☐ s. Central nervous system disorder
☐ t. Myxedema
☐ u. Hypothermia
☐ v. Sick sinus syndrome

ECG 78 was obtained in a 66-year-old male who was taken to the emergency room with palpitations and syncope. The ECG shows a rapid wide complex tachycardia at 146 beats/minute. The wide QRS duration (152 msec) suggests a ventricular origin for the tachycardia; this is confirmed by the presence of an underlying sinus tachycardia at approximately 120 beats/minute (arrows mark the P waves) resulting in AV dissociation, and the presence of ventricular capture complexes manifesting as fusion complexes in the sixth beat on the rhythm strip and every seventh beat thereafter (asterisks). The QRS axis is rightward (measuring 98° by the computer), but does not meet criteria for right axis deviation (> 100°). Irregularity in the baseline in leads I and aVR is due to artifact.

Codes:

1d	Sinus tachycardia
4f	Ventricular tachycardia (≥ 3 consecutive complexes)
5a	Fusion complexes
5c	Ventricular capture complexes
5d	AV dissociation

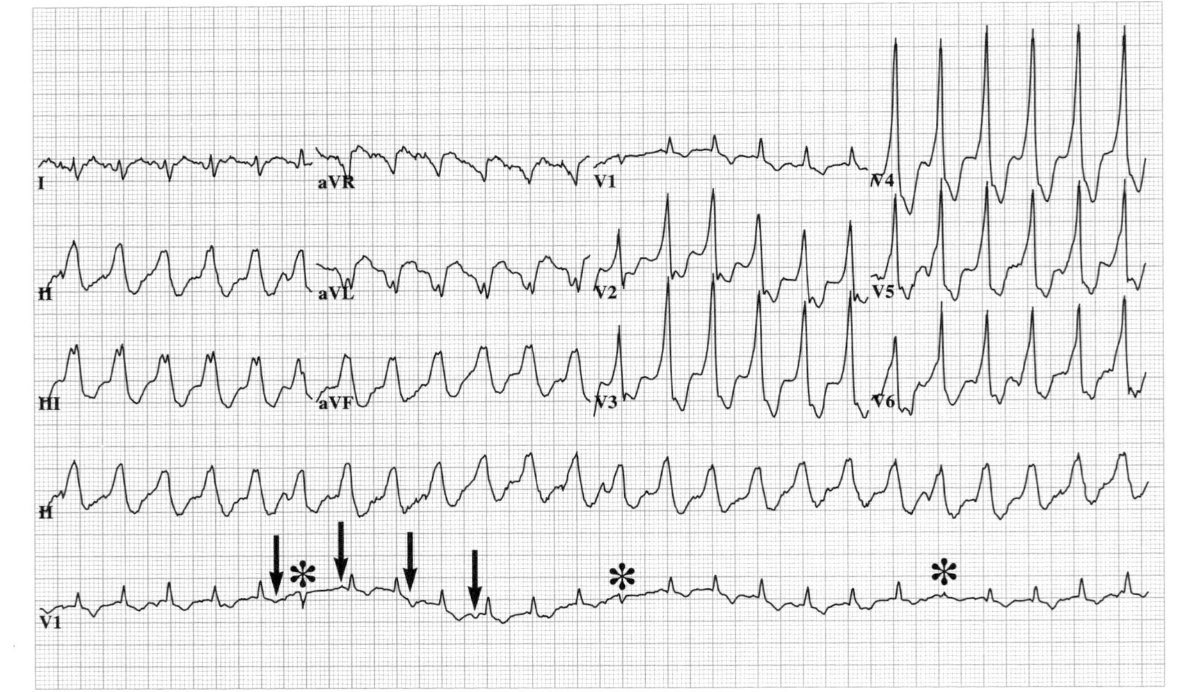

Questions: ECG 78

1. ECG findings in this tracing favoring the diagnosis of ventricular tachycardia over supraventricular tachycardia include:

   a. QRS > 0.14 seconds
   b. Concordance of QRS complexes in V_1 - V_6
   c. Ventricular fusion
   d. Right axis deviation
   e. Monophasic right bundle branch block pattern in V_1
   f. AV dissociation

2. The presence of a fusion complex is a common ECG finding during ventricular tachycardia:

   a. True
   b. False

3. The origin of the ventricular tachycardia in this tracing is:

   a. Left ventricle
   b. Right ventricle
   c. Right ventricular outflow tract
   d. Unable to determine

Answers: ECG 78

1. Answer: All

2. Although not commonly seen, the presence of a fusion complex in the setting of a wide QRS tachycardia strongly suggests ventricular tachycardia. (Answer: b)

3. In general, a positive QRS defection in lead V_1 suggests a left ventricular focus for ventricular tachycardia, while a negative QRS in lead V_1 suggests a right ventricular origin. (Answer: a)

— Quick Review 78 —

Ventricular tachycardia	
• Rapid succession of three or more premature ventricular beats at a rate > ____ per minute	100
• RR intervals are usually regular but may be irregular (true/false)	true
• (Abrupt/gradual) onset and termination are evident	Abrupt
• AV ____ is common	dissociation
• Look for ventricular ____ complexes and ____ beats as markers for VT	capture, fusion
Fusion complexes	
• Due to simultaneous activation of the ventricle from ____ sources, resulting in a QRS complex that is ____ in morphology between each source	2 intermediate
AV dissociation	
• Atrial and ventricular rhythms are ____ of each other	independent
• Ventricular rate is (</≥) than the atrial rate	≥

Differential Diagnosis

Low Voltage, Limb and Precordial Leads

(Amplitude of the entire QRS complex (R+S) < 10 mm in each precordial lead, *and* amplitude of R+S < 5 mm in all limb leads)

- Chronic lung disease (item 14m)
- Pericardial effusion (item 14o)
- Myxedema (item 14t)
- Obesity
- Pleural effusion
- Restrictive or infiltrative cardiomyopathies
- Diffuse coronary disease

ECG 79. 83-year-old female with chest pressure:

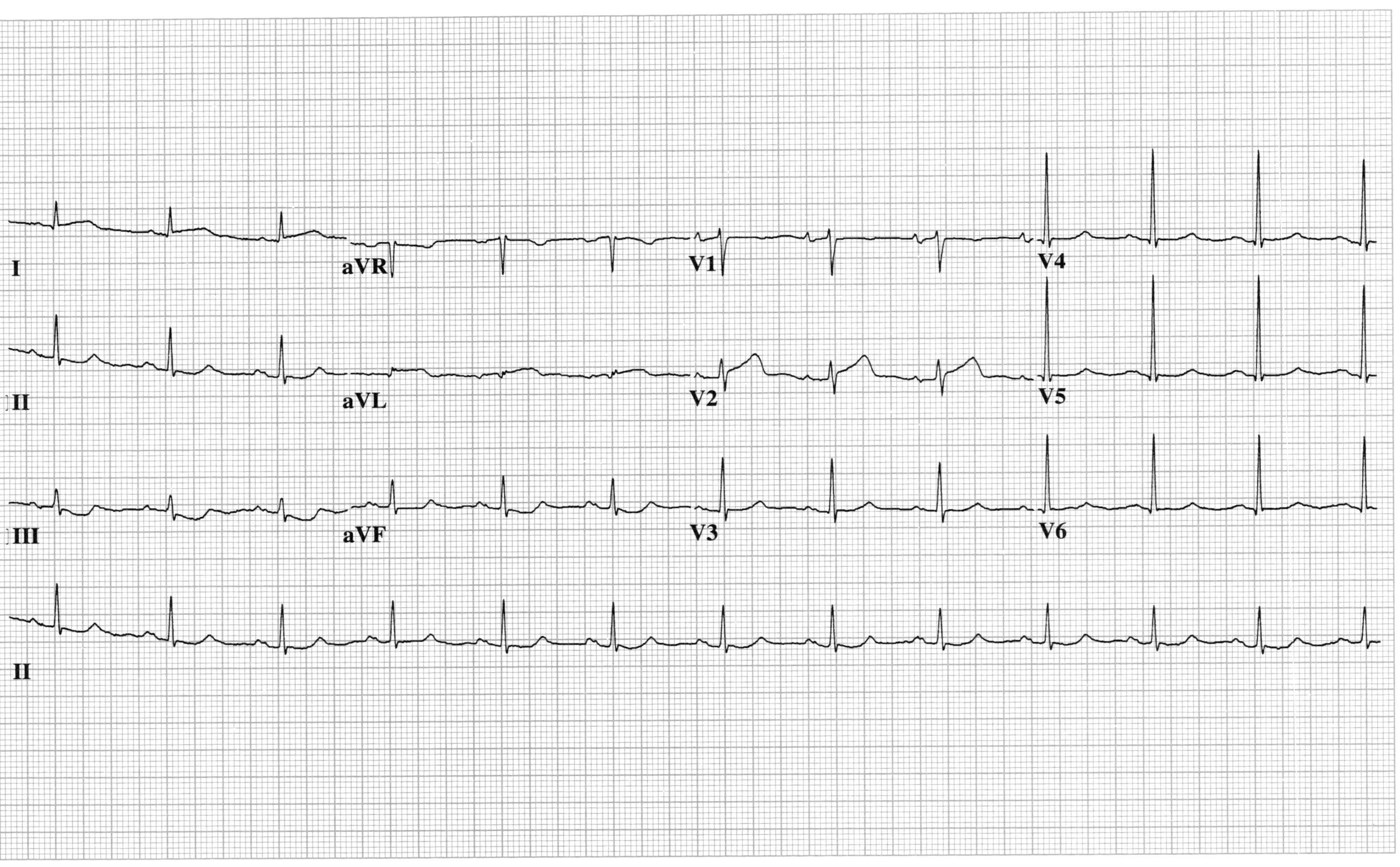

1. GENERAL FEATURES

☐ a. Normal ECG
☐ b. Borderline normal ECG or normal variant
☐ c. Incorrect electrode placement
☐ d. Artifact due to tremor

2. ATRIAL RHYTHMS

☐ a. Sinus rhythm
☐ b. Sinus arrhythmia
☐ c. Sinus bradycardia (< 60)
☐ d. Sinus tachycardia (> 100)
☐ e. Sinus pause or arrest
☐ f. Sinoatrial exit block
☐ g. Ecoptic atrial rhythm
☐ h. Wandering atrial pacemaker
☐ i. Atrial premature complexes, normally conducted
☐ j. Atrial premature complexes, nonconducted
☐ k. Atrial premature complexes with aberrant intraventricular conduction
☐ l. Atrial tachycardia (regular, sustained, 1:1 conduction)
☐ m. Atrial tachycardia, repetitive (short paroxysms)
☐ n. Atrial tachycardia, multifocal
☐ o. Atrial tachycardia with AV block
☐ p. Supraventricular tachycardia, unspecific
☐ q. Supraventricular tachycardia, paroxysmal
☐ r. Atrial flutter
☐ s. Atrial fibrillation
☐ t. Retrograde atrial activation

3. AV JUNCTIONAL RHYTHMS

☐ a. AV junctional premature complexes
☐ b. AV junctional escape complexes
☐ c. AV junctional rhythm, accelerated
☐ d. AV junctional rhythm

4. VENTRICULAR RHYTHMS

☐ a. Ventricular premature complex(es), uniform, fixed coupling
☐ b. Ventricular premature complex(es), uniform, nonfixed coupling
☐ c. Ventricular premature complexes(es), multiform
☐ d. Ventricular premature complexes, in pairs
☐ e. Ventricular parasystole
☐ f. Ventricular tachycardia (≥ 3 consecutive complexes)
☐ g. Accelerated idioventricular rhythm
☐ h. Ventricular escape complexes or rhythm
☐ i. Ventricular fibrillation

5. ATRIAL-VENTRICULAR INTERACTIONS IN ARRHYTHMIAS

☐ a. Fusion complexes
☐ b. Reciprocal (echo) complexes
☐ c. Ventricular capture complexes
☐ d. AV dissociation
☐ e. Ventriculophasic sinus arrhythmia

6. AV CONDUCTION ABNORMALITIES

☐ a. AV block, 1°
☐ b. AV block, 2° - Mobitz type I (Wenckebach)
☐ c. AV block, 2° - Mobitz type II
☐ d. AV block, 2:1
☐ e. AV block, 3°
☐ f. AV block, variable
☐ g. Short PR interval (with sinus rhythm and normal QRS duration)
☐ h. Wolff-Parkinson-White pattern

7. INTRAVENTRICULAR CONDUCTION DISTURBANCES

☐ a. RBBB, incomplete
☐ b. RBBB, complete
☐ c. Left anterior fascicular block
☐ d. Left posterior fascicular block
☐ e. LBBB, with ST-T wave suggestive of acute myocardial injury or infarction
☐ f. LBBB, complete
☐ g. LBBB, intermittent
☐ h. Intraventricular conduction disturbance, nonspecific
☐ i. Aberrant intraventricular conduction with supraventricular arrhythmia

8. P WAVE ABNORMALITIES

☐ a. Right atrial abnormality
☐ b. Left atrial abnormalities
☐ c. Nonspecific atrial abnormality

9. ABNORMALITIES OF QRS VOLTAGE OR AXIS

☐ a. Low voltage, limb leads only
☐ b. Low voltage, limb and precordial leads
☐ c. Left axis deviation (> - 30%)
☐ d. Right axis deviation (> + 100)
☐ e. Electrical alternans

10. VENTRICULAR HYPERTROPHY

☐ a. LVH by voltage only
☐ b. LVH by voltage and ST-T segment abnormalities
☐ c. RVH
☐ d. Combined ventricular hypertrophy

11. Q WAVE MYOCARDIAL INFARCTION

	Probably Acute or Recent	Probably Old or Age Indeterminate
Anterolateral	☐ a.	☐ g.
Anterior	☐ b.	☐ h.
Anteroseptal	☐ c.	☐ i.
Lateral/High lateral	☐ d.	☐ j.
Inferior	☐ e.	☐ k.
Posterior	☐ f.	☐ l.

☐ m. Probably ventricular aneurysm

12. ST, T, U, WAVE ABNORMALITIES

☐ a. Normal variant, early repolarization
☐ b. Normal variant, juvenile T waves
☐ c. Nonspecific ST and/or T wave abnormalities
☐ d. ST and/or T wave abnormalities suggesting myocardial ischemia
☐ e. ST and/or T wave abnormalities suggesting myocardial injury
☐ f. ST and/or T wave abnormalities suggesting acute pericarditis
☐ g. ST-T segment abnormalities secondary to intraventricular conduction disturbance or hypertrophy
☐ h. Post-extrasystolic T wave abnormality
☐ i. Isolated J point depression
☐ j. Peaked T waves
☐ k. Prolonged QT interval
☐ l. Prominent U waves

13. PACEMAKER FUNCTION AND RHYTHM

☐ a. Atrial or coronary sinus pacing
☐ b. Ventricular demand pacing
☐ c. AV sequential pacing
☐ d. Ventricular pacing, complete control
☐ e. Dual chamber, atrial sensing pacemaker
☐ f. Pacemaker malfunction, not constantly capturing (atrium or ventricle)
☐ g. Pacemaker malfunction, not constantly sensing (atrium or ventricle)
☐ h. Pacemaker malfunction, not firing
☐ i. Pacemaker malfunction, slowing

14. SUGGESTED OR PROBABLE CLINICAL DISORDERS

☐ a. Digitalis effect
☐ b. Digitalis toxicity
☐ c. Antiarrhythmic drug effect
☐ d. Antiarrhythmic drug toxicity
☐ e. Hyperkalemia
☐ f. Hypokalemia
☐ g. Hypercalcemia
☐ h. Hypocalcemia
☐ i. Atrial septal defect, secundum
☐ j. Atrial septal defect, primum
☐ k. Dextrocardia, mirror image
☐ l. Mitral valve disease
☐ m. Chronic lung disease
☐ n. Acute cor pulmonale, including pulmonary embolus
☐ o. Pericardial effusion
☐ p. Acute pericarditis
☐ q. Hypertrophic cardiomyopathy
☐ r. Coronary artery disease
☐ s. Central nervous system disorder
☐ t. Myxedema
☐ u. Hypothermia
☐ v. Sick sinus syndrome

ECG 79 was obtained in an 83-year-old female with complaints of chest pressure. The ECG shows a sinus rhythm with left atrial abnormality (arrow) and high lateral wall myocardial injury, manifesting as ST segment elevation leads I and aVL (asterisks). An abnormal Q wave is present in aVL, but not in lead I, so lateral Q wave MI should not be coded. Subtle ST segment elevation is noted in lead V_2, but other criteria for the diagnosis of acute anteroseptal myocardial infarction are absent. These findings are consistent with coronary artery disease.

Codes:

2a	Sinus rhythm
8b	Left atrial abnormality
12e	ST and/or T wave abnormalities suggesting myocardial injury
14r	Coronary artery disease

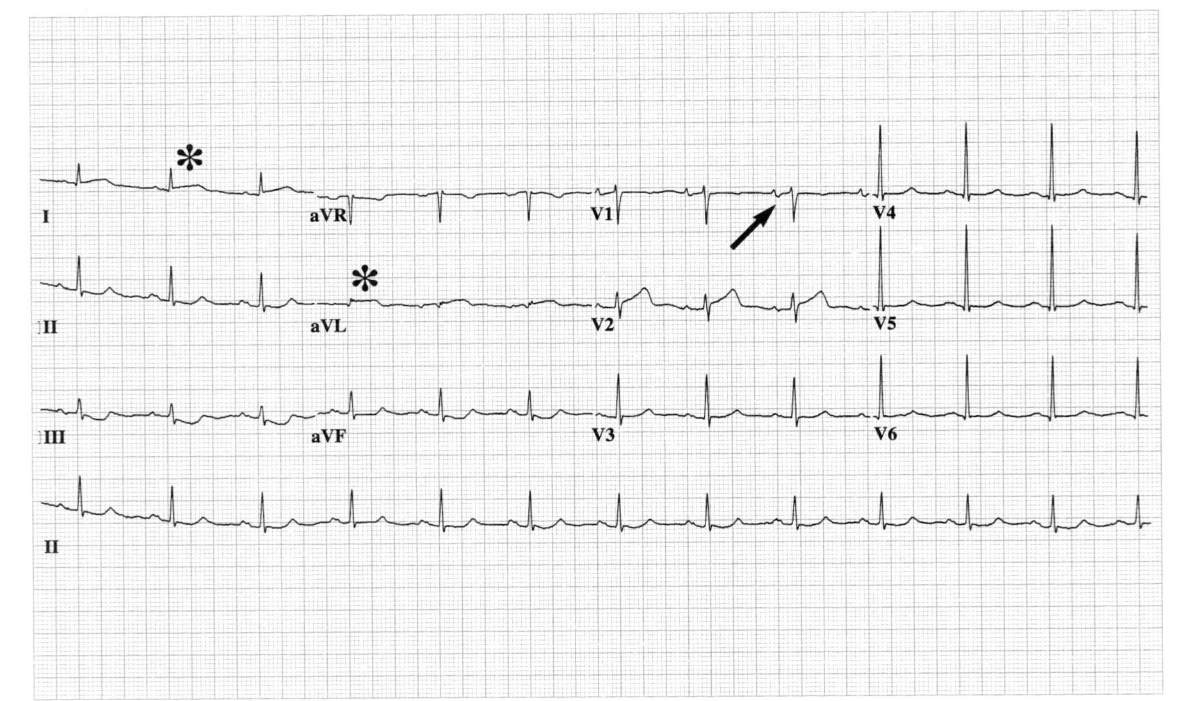

Questions: ECG 79

1. The ECG equivalent of a pathological Q wave in posterior myocardial infarction:

   a. Tall R wave in V_1-V_3
   b. ST depression in V_1-V_3
   c. Deep S wave in V_1-V_3

2. The duration of a pathological Q wave in leads III, aVL, aVF and V_1 is ≥ ___ seconds, and ≥ ___ seconds in all other leads.

   a. 0.03 and 0.04
   b. 0.04 and 0.03
   c. 0.04 and 0.04
   d. 0.03 and 0.03

Answers: ECG 79

1. The posterior wall of the left ventricular differs from the anterior, inferior, and lateral walls by not having ECG leads directly overly it. Instead of Q waves and ST elevation, acute posterior MI presents with mirror-image changes in the anterior precordial leads (V_1-V_3), including dominant R waves (the mirror-image of abnormal Q waves), and horizontal ST segment depression (the mirror-image of ST elevation). Acute posterior infarction is often associated with ECG changes of acute inferior or inferolateral myocardial infarction, but may occur in isolation. (Answer: a)

2. For a Q wave to be considered pathological, it must be at least 0.04 seconds in duration in leads III, aVL, aVF, and V_1, and at least 0.03 seconds in duration in all other leads. (Answer: b)

— Quick Review 79 —

Left atrial abnormality	
• Notched P wave with a duration ≥ ____ seconds in leads II, III or aVF, *or*	0.12
• Terminal negative portion of the P wave in lead V_1 ≥ 1 mm deep and ≥ ____ seconds in duration	0.04
ST and/or T wave changes suggesting myocardial injury	
• Acute ST segment (elevation/depression) with upward (convexity/concavity) in the leads representing the area of infarction	elevation convexity
• T waves invert (before/after) ST segments return to baseline	before
• Associated ST (elevation/depression) in the noninfarct leads is common	depression
• Acute ____ wall injury often has horizontal or downsloping ST segment depression with upright T waves in V_1-V_3, with or without a prominent R wave in these same leads	posterior

ECG 80. 23-year-old female with fatigue and dizziness:

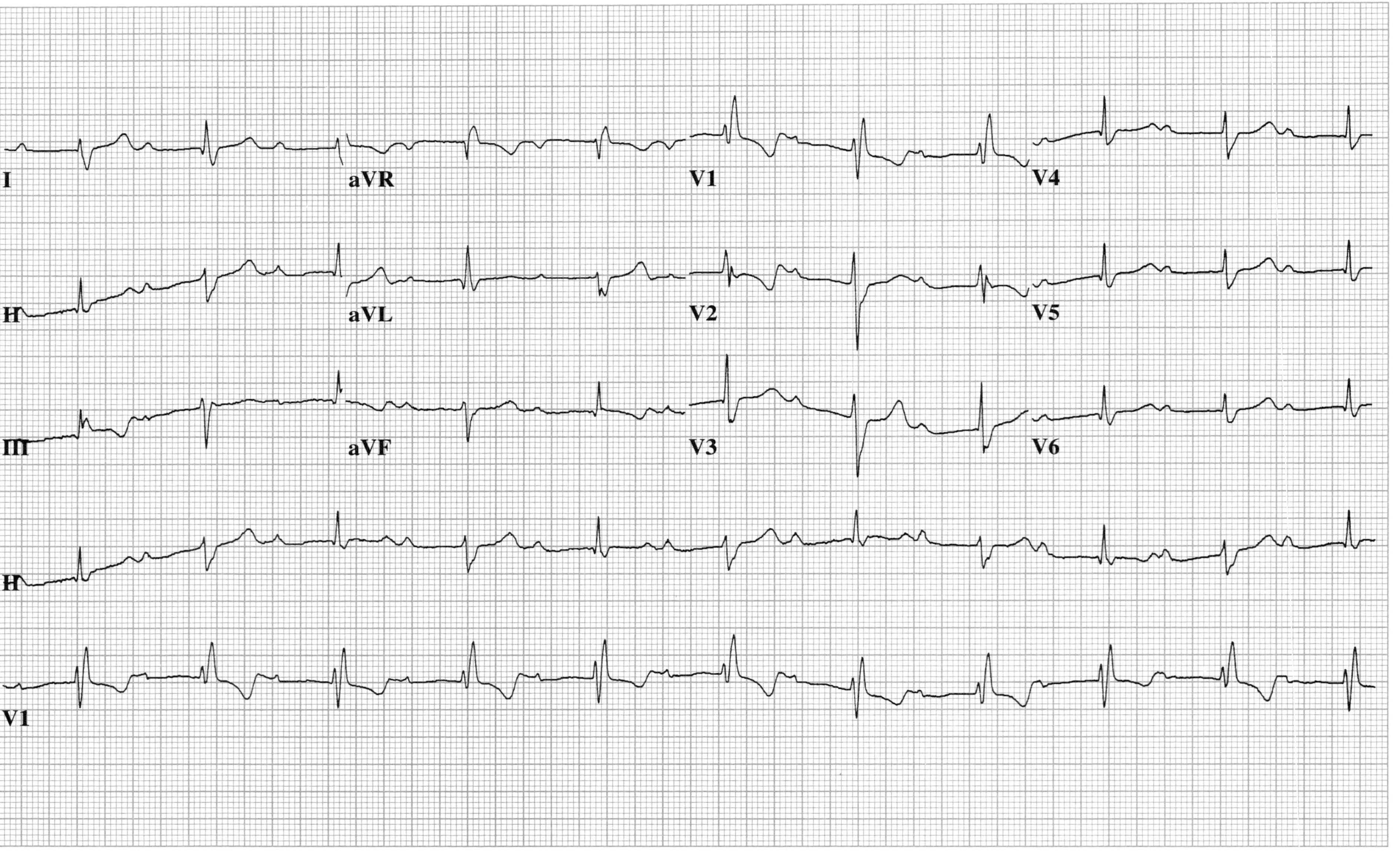

1. GENERAL FEATURES

- ☐ a. Normal ECG
- ☐ b. Borderline normal ECG or normal variant
- ☐ c. Incorrect electrode placement
- ☐ d. Artifact due to tremor

2. ATRIAL RHYTHMS

- ☐ a. Sinus rhythm
- ☐ b. Sinus arrhythmia
- ☐ c. Sinus bradycardia (< 60)
- ☐ d. Sinus tachycardia (> 100)
- ☐ e. Sinus pause or arrest
- ☐ f. Sinoatrial exit block
- ☐ g. Ecoptic atrial rhythm
- ☐ h. Wandering atrial pacemaker
- ☐ i. Atrial premature complexes, normally conducted
- ☐ j. Atrial premature complexes, nonconducted
- ☐ k. Atrial premature complexes with aberrant intraventricular conduction
- ☐ l. Atrial tachycardia (regular, sustained, 1:1 conduction)
- ☐ m. Atrial tachycardia, repetitive (short paroxysms)
- ☐ n. Atrial tachycardia, multifocal
- ☐ o. Atrial tachycardia with AV block
- ☐ p. Supraventricular tachycardia, unspecific
- ☐ q. Supraventricular tachycardia, paroxysmal
- ☐ r. Atrial flutter
- ☐ s. Atrial fibrillation
- ☐ t. Retrograde atrial activation

3. AV JUNCTIONAL RHYTHMS

- ☐ a. AV junctional premature complexes
- ☐ b. AV junctional escape complexes
- ☐ c. AV junctional rhythm, accelerated
- ☐ d. AV junctional rhythm

4. VENTRICULAR RHYTHMS

- ☐ a. Ventricular premature complex(es), uniform, fixed coupling
- ☐ b. Ventricular premature complex(es), uniform, nonfixed coupling
- ☐ c. Ventricular premature complexes(es), multiform
- ☐ d. Ventricular premature complexes, in pairs
- ☐ e. Ventricular parasystole
- ☐ f. Ventricular tachycardia (≥ 3 consecutive complexes)
- ☐ g. Accelerated idioventricular rhythm
- ☐ h. Ventricular escape complexes or rhythm
- ☐ i. Ventricular fibrillation

5. ATRIAL-VENTRICULAR INTERACTIONS IN ARRHYTHMIAS

- ☐ a. Fusion complexes
- ☐ b. Reciprocal (echo) complexes
- ☐ c. Ventricular capture complexes
- ☐ d. AV dissociation
- ☐ e. Ventriculophasic sinus arrhythmia

6. AV CONDUCTION ABNORMALITIES

- ☐ a. AV block, 1°
- ☐ b. AV block, 2° - Mobitz type I (Wenckebach)
- ☐ c. AV block, 2° - Mobitz type II
- ☐ d. AV block, 2:1
- ☐ e. AV block, 3°
- ☐ f. AV block, variable
- ☐ g. Short PR interval (with sinus rhythm and normal QRS duration)
- ☐ h. Wolff-Parkinson-White pattern

7. INTRAVENTRICULAR CONDUCTION DISTURBANCES

- ☐ a. RBBB, incomplete
- ☐ b. RBBB, complete
- ☐ c. Left anterior fascicular block
- ☐ d. Left posterior fascicular block
- ☐ e. LBBB, with ST-T wave suggestive of acute myocardial injury or infarction
- ☐ f. LBBB, complete
- ☐ g. LBBB, intermittent
- ☐ h. Intraventricular conduction disturbance, nonspecific
- ☐ i. Aberrant intraventricular conduction with supraventricular arrhythmia

8. P WAVE ABNORMALITIES

- ☐ a. Right atrial abnormality
- ☐ b. Left atrial abnormalities
- ☐ c. Nonspecific atrial abnormality

9. ABNORMALITIES OF QRS VOLTAGE OR AXIS

- ☐ a. Low voltage, limb leads only
- ☐ b. Low voltage, limb and precordial leads
- ☐ c. Left axis deviation (> - 30%)
- ☐ d. Right axis deviation (> + 100)
- ☐ e. Electrical alternans

10. VENTRICULAR HYPERTROPHY

- ☐ a. LVH by voltage only
- ☐ b. LVH by voltage and ST-T segment abnormalities
- ☐ c. RVH
- ☐ d. Combined ventricular hypertrophy

11. Q WAVE MYOCARDIAL INFARCTION

	Probably Acute or Recent	Probably Old or Age Indeterminate
Anterolateral	☐ a.	☐ g.
Anterior	☐ b.	☐ h.
Anteroseptal	☐ c.	☐ i.
Lateral/High lateral	☐ d.	☐ j.
Inferior	☐ e.	☐ k.
Posterior	☐ f.	☐ l.

- ☐ m. Probably ventricular aneurysm

12. ST, T, U, WAVE ABNORMALITIES

- ☐ a. Normal variant, early repolarization
- ☐ b. Normal variant, juvenile T waves
- ☐ c. Nonspecific ST and/or T wave abnormalities
- ☐ d. ST and/or T wave abnormalities suggesting myocardial ischemia
- ☐ e. ST and/or T wave abnormalities suggesting myocardial injury
- ☐ f. ST and/or T wave abnormalities suggesting acute pericarditis
- ☐ g. ST-T segment abnormalities secondary to intraventricular conduction disturbance or hypertrophy
- ☐ h. Post-extrasystolic T wave abnormality
- ☐ i. Isolated J point depression
- ☐ j. Peaked T waves
- ☐ k. Prolonged QT interval
- ☐ l. Prominent U waves

13. PACEMAKER FUNCTION AND RHYTHM

- ☐ a. Atrial or coronary sinus pacing
- ☐ b. Ventricular demand pacing
- ☐ c. AV sequential pacing
- ☐ d. Ventricular pacing, complete control
- ☐ e. Dual chamber, atrial sensing pacemaker
- ☐ f. Pacemaker malfunction, not constantly capturing (atrium or ventricle)
- ☐ g. Pacemaker malfunction, not constantly sensing (atrium or ventricle)
- ☐ h. Pacemaker malfunction, not firing
- ☐ i. Pacemaker malfunction, slowing

14. SUGGESTED OR PROBABLE CLINICAL DISORDERS

- ☐ a. Digitalis effect
- ☐ b. Digitalis toxicity
- ☐ c. Antiarrhythmic drug effect
- ☐ d. Antiarrhythmic drug toxicity
- ☐ e. Hyperkalemia
- ☐ f. Hypokalemia
- ☐ g. Hypercalcemia
- ☐ h. Hypocalcemia
- ☐ i. Atrial septal defect, secundum
- ☐ j. Atrial septal defect, primum
- ☐ k. Dextrocardia, mirror image
- ☐ l. Mitral valve disease
- ☐ m. Chronic lung disease
- ☐ n. Acute cor pulmonale, including pulmonary embolus
- ☐ o. Pericardial effusion
- ☐ p. Acute pericarditis
- ☐ q. Hypertrophic cardiomyopathy
- ☐ r. Coronary artery disease
- ☐ s. Central nervous system disorder
- ☐ t. Myxedema
- ☐ u. Hypothermia
- ☐ v. Sick sinus syndrome

ECG 80 was obtained in a 23-year-old female who was being evaluated for fatigue and dizziness. Sinus rhythm with first-degree AV block is present. Also noted is RBBB with secondary ST-T abnormalities and alternating right axis deviation (due to left posterior fascicular block) (asterisks) and left axis deviation (due left anterior fascicular block) (arrowheads).

Codes:

2a	Sinus rhythm
6a	AV block, 1°
7b	RBBB, complete
7c	Left anterior fascicular block
7d	Left posterior fascicular block
9c	Left axis deviation
9d	Right axis deviation (> + 100°)
12g	ST-T segment abnormalities secondary to IVCD or hypertrophy

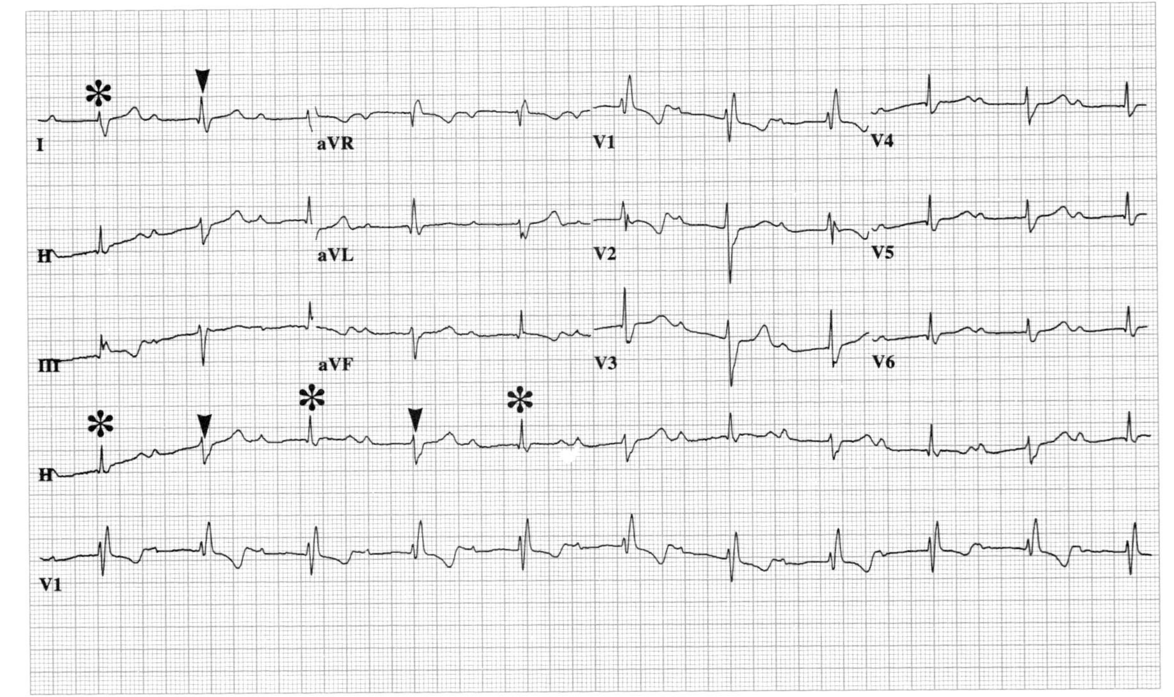

Questions: ECG 80

1. Which of the following statements about left posterior fascicular block (LPFB) are true?

   a. Isolated LPFB is rare
   b. LPFB is the least common conduction disturbance to occur during acute myocardial infarction
   c. LPFB routinely results in prolongation of the QRS to more than 0.10 seconds

2. The ECG criteria for the diagnosis of right bundle branch block + left posterior fascicular block (a form of bifascicular block) include all except:

   a. RSR' in lead V_1
   b. QRS $\geq$ 0.12 seconds
   c. Wide S waves in leads I, V_5, and V_6
   d. Mean QRS axis > 90°
   e. qR pattern in lead I and rS pattern in leads II, III, and aVF

Answers: ECG 80

1. The left bundle divides into anterior and posterior divisions. Compared to the left anterior fascicle, the left posterior fascicle is shorter, thicker, and receives blood supply from both left and right coronary arteries. Isolated left posterior fascicular block (LPFB) is much less prevalent than left bundle branch block, right bundle branch block, or left anterior fascicular block. Coronary artery disease is the most common cause of LPFB; when it develops during acute MI, multivessel coronary disease and extensive infarction are usually present, and the prognosis is poor. Diagnostic criteria for LPFB include a mean QRS axis of +100° to +180°, an rS in lead I and qR in lead III, and a normal or slightly prolonged ($\leq$ 0.10 seconds) QRS. LPFB is a diagnosis of exclusion; other causes of right axis deviation (e.g., right ventricular hypertrophy, COPD, lateral wall myocardial infarction, vertical heart) must be ruled out before right axis deviation can be attributed to LPFB. (Answer: a, b)

2. The diagnosis of right bundle branch block + left posterior fascicular block (a form of bifascicular block) is established when: (1) ECG findings of LPFB are evident in the first portion of the QRS (QRS axis > +90°, rS in lead I and qR in leads II, III, and aVF); and (2) ECG findings of RBBB are evident in the latter half of the QRS (RSR' in lead V_1, QRS duration $\geq$ 0.12 seconds, wide S waves in leads I, V_5, and V_6). This form of bifascicular block is most commonly due to multivessel coronary

artery disease and complicates < 1% of acute myocardial infarctions. The likelihood of progression from this type of chronic bifascicular block to complete heart block ranges from 10-60% over 2-4 years. A qR pattern in lead I and an rS pattern in leads II, III, and aVF is consistent with left anterior fascicular block. (Answer: e)

— Quick Review 80 —

RBBB, complete	
• QRS duration ≥ ____ seconds	0.12
• Secondary R wave (R') in lead ____ is usually (shorter/taller) than the initial R wave	V_1 taller
• Onset of intrinsicoid deflection in leads V_1 and V_2 > ____ seconds	0.05
• ST segment (depression/elevation) and (upright/inverted) T wave in V_1, V_2	depression inverted
• Wide slurred S wave in leads ____	I, V_5, V_6
• QRS axis is usually (normal/leftward/rightward)	normal
• RBBB (does/does not) interfere with the ECG diagnosis of ventricular hypertrophy or Q wave MI	does not
Left posterior fascicular block	
• ____ axis deviation with a mean QRS axis between ___ and ____ degrees	Right +100, +180
• ____ wave in lead I and ____ wave in lead III	S, Q
• Normal or slightly prolonged QRS duration (true/false)	true
• No other cause for right axis deviation should be present (true/false)	true

— POP QUIZ —

VT or Not VT: That is the Question

Instructions: In the setting of a wide QRS tachycardia, decide whether the ECG findings below favor a diagnosis of ventricular tachycardia or SVT with aberrancy

ECG Feature	VT or SVT with Aberrancy
QRS morphology similar to VPCs	VT
Tachycardia initiated by APCs	SVT
AV dissociation absent	SVT
Capture beats present	VT
Fusion beats absent	SVT
QRS duration during tachycardia > 0.14 sec. if RBBB morphology (or > 0.16 sec. if LBBB morphology (assuming QRS is narrow during sinus rhythm)	VT
QRS deflection in precordial leads are all positive or negative (concordance)	VT
RSR' in V_1: R wave shorter than R'	SVT

ECG 81. 48-year-old female with recent throat tightness and diaphoresis:

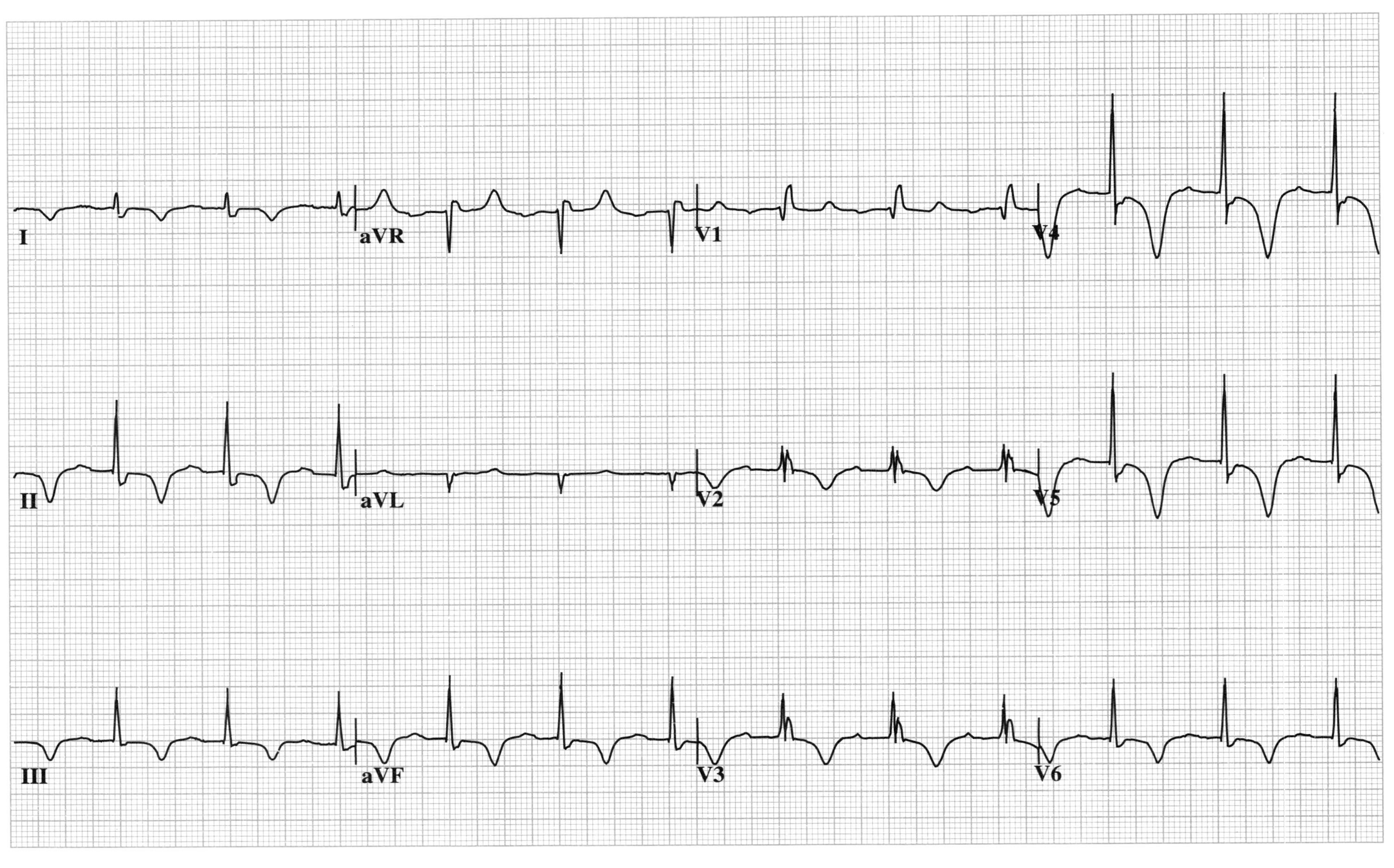

1. GENERAL FEATURES

- ☐ a. Normal ECG
- ☐ b. Borderline normal ECG or normal variant
- ☐ c. Incorrect electrode placement
- ☐ d. Artifact due to tremor

2. ATRIAL RHYTHMS

- ☐ a. Sinus rhythm
- ☐ b. Sinus arrhythmia
- ☐ c. Sinus bradycardia (< 60)
- ☐ d. Sinus tachycardia (> 100)
- ☐ e. Sinus pause or arrest
- ☐ f. Sinoatrial exit block
- ☐ g. Ecoptic atrial rhythm
- ☐ h. Wandering atrial pacemaker
- ☐ i. Atrial premature complexes, normally conducted
- ☐ j. Atrial premature complexes, nonconducted
- ☐ k. Atrial premature complexes with aberrant intraventricular conduction
- ☐ l. Atrial tachycardia (regular, sustained, 1:1 conduction)
- ☐ m. Atrial tachycardia, repetitive (short paroxysms)
- ☐ n. Atrial tachycardia, multifocal
- ☐ o. Atrial tachycardia with AV block
- ☐ p. Supraventricular tachycardia, unspecific
- ☐ q. Supraventricular tachycardia, paroxysmal
- ☐ r. Atrial flutter
- ☐ s. Atrial fibrillation
- ☐ t. Retrograde atrial activation

3. AV JUNCTIONAL RHYTHMS

- ☐ a. AV junctional premature complexes
- ☐ b. AV junctional escape complexes
- ☐ c. AV junctional rhythm, accelerated
- ☐ d. AV junctional rhythm

4. VENTRICULAR RHYTHMS

- ☐ a. Ventricular premature complex(es), uniform, fixed coupling
- ☐ b. Ventricular premature complex(es), uniform, nonfixed coupling
- ☐ c. Ventricular premature complexes(es), multiform
- ☐ d. Ventricular premature complexes, in pairs
- ☐ e. Ventricular parasystole
- ☐ f. Ventricular tachycardia (≥ 3 consecutive complexes)
- ☐ g. Accelerated idioventricular rhythm
- ☐ h. Ventricular escape complexes or rhythm
- ☐ i. Ventricular fibrillation

5. ATRIAL-VENTRICULAR INTERACTIONS IN ARRHYTHMIAS

- ☐ a. Fusion complexes
- ☐ b. Reciprocal (echo) complexes
- ☐ c. Ventricular capture complexes
- ☐ d. AV dissociation
- ☐ e. Ventriculophasic sinus arrhythmia

6. AV CONDUCTION ABNORMALITIES

- ☐ a. AV block, 1°
- ☐ b. AV block, 2° - Mobitz type I (Wenckebach)
- ☐ c. AV block, 2° - Mobitz type II
- ☐ d. AV block, 2:1
- ☐ e. AV block, 3°
- ☐ f. AV block, variable
- ☐ g. Short PR interval (with sinus rhythm and normal QRS duration)
- ☐ h. Wolff-Parkinson-White pattern

7. INTRAVENTRICULAR CONDUCTION DISTURBANCES

- ☐ a. RBBB, incomplete
- ☐ b. RBBB, complete
- ☐ c. Left anterior fascicular block
- ☐ d. Left posterior fascicular block
- ☐ e. LBBB, with ST-T wave suggestive of acute myocardial injury or infarction
- ☐ f. LBBB, complete
- ☐ g. LBBB, intermittent
- ☐ h. Intraventricular conduction disturbance, nonspecific
- ☐ i. Aberrant intraventricular conduction with supraventricular arrhythmia

8. P WAVE ABNORMALITIES

- ☐ a. Right atrial abnormality
- ☐ b. Left atrial abnormalities
- ☐ c. Nonspecific atrial abnormality

9. ABNORMALITIES OF QRS VOLTAGE OR AXIS

- ☐ a. Low voltage, limb leads only
- ☐ b. Low voltage, limb and precordial leads
- ☐ c. Left axis deviation (> - 30%)
- ☐ d. Right axis deviation (> + 100)
- ☐ e. Electrical alternans

10. VENTRICULAR HYPERTROPHY

- ☐ a. LVH by voltage only
- ☐ b. LVH by voltage and ST-T segment abnormalities
- ☐ c. RVH
- ☐ d. Combined ventricular hypertrophy

11. Q WAVE MYOCARDIAL INFARCTION

	Probably Acute or Recent	Probably Old or Age Indeterminate
Anterolateral	☐ a.	☐ g.
Anterior	☐ b.	☐ h.
Anteroseptal	☐ c.	☐ i.
Lateral/High lateral	☐ d.	☐ j.
Inferior	☐ e.	☐ k.
Posterior	☐ f.	☐ l.

- ☐ m. Probably ventricular aneurysm

12. ST, T, U, WAVE ABNORMALITIES

- ☐ a. Normal variant, early repolarization
- ☐ b. Normal variant, juvenile T waves
- ☐ c. Nonspecific ST and/or T wave abnormalities
- ☐ d. ST and/or T wave abnormalities suggesting myocardial ischemia
- ☐ e. ST and/or T wave abnormalities suggesting myocardial injury
- ☐ f. ST and/or T wave abnormalities suggesting acute pericarditis
- ☐ g. ST-T segment abnormalities secondary to intraventricular conduction disturbance or hypertrophy
- ☐ h. Post-extrasystolic T wave abnormality
- ☐ i. Isolated J point depression
- ☐ j. Peaked T waves
- ☐ k. Prolonged QT interval
- ☐ l. Prominent U waves

13. PACEMAKER FUNCTION AND RHYTHM

- ☐ a. Atrial or coronary sinus pacing
- ☐ b. Ventricular demand pacing
- ☐ c. AV sequential pacing
- ☐ d. Ventricular pacing, complete control
- ☐ e. Dual chamber, atrial sensing pacemaker
- ☐ f. Pacemaker malfunction, not constantly capturing (atrium or ventricle)
- ☐ g. Pacemaker malfunction, not constantly sensing (atrium or ventricle)
- ☐ h. Pacemaker malfunction, not firing
- ☐ i. Pacemaker malfunction, slowing

14. SUGGESTED OR PROBABLE CLINICAL DISORDERS

- ☐ a. Digitalis effect
- ☐ b. Digitalis toxicity
- ☐ c. Antiarrhythmic drug effect
- ☐ d. Antiarrhythmic drug toxicity
- ☐ e. Hyperkalemia
- ☐ f. Hypokalemia
- ☐ g. Hypercalcemia
- ☐ h. Hypocalcemia
- ☐ i. Atrial septal defect, secundum
- ☐ j. Atrial septal defect, primum
- ☐ k. Dextrocardia, mirror image
- ☐ l. Mitral valve disease
- ☐ m. Chronic lung disease
- ☐ n. Acute cor pulmonale, including pulmonary embolus
- ☐ o. Pericardial effusion
- ☐ p. Acute pericarditis
- ☐ q. Hypertrophic cardiomyopathy
- ☐ r. Coronary artery disease
- ☐ s. Central nervous system disorder
- ☐ t. Myxedema
- ☐ u. Hypothermia
- ☐ v. Sick sinus syndrome

ECG 81 was obtained in a 48-year-old female with recent complaints of throat tightness and diaphoresis. The ECG shows sinus rhythm with first-degree AV block, RBBB (widened rSR' complex in V_1 - V_2, and wide S waves in I, $_5V$, $_6V$), and striking T wave inversion and QT prolongation throughout most of the tracing but most prominently in the lateral precordial leads (asterisks). The deep T wave inversions in V_4-V_6, especially in a patient with chest pain, suggest myocardial ischemia or even a recent non-Q-wave myocardial infarction (note: secondary T waves of RBBB should be upright in these leads). Myocardial infarction should not be coded since abnormal Q waves are not present.

Codes:

2a	Sinus rhythm
6a	AV block, 1°
7b	RBBB, complete
12d	ST and/or T wave abnormalities suggesting myocardial ischemia
12k	Prolonged QT interval

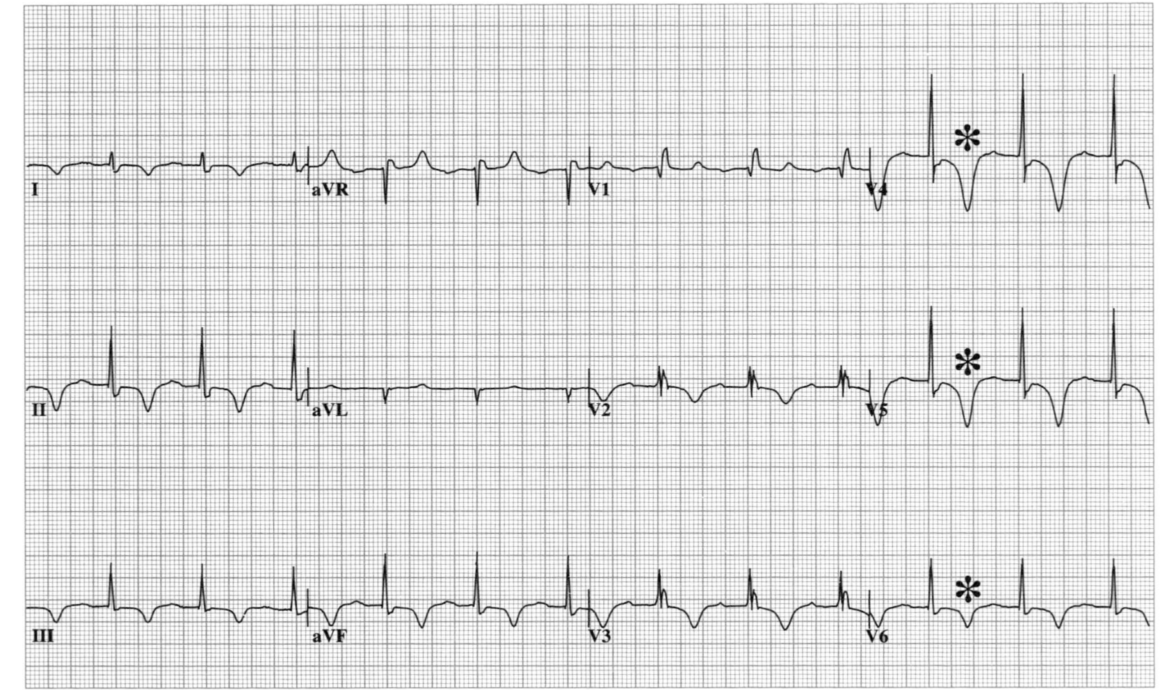

Questions: ECG 81

1. Deep T wave inversion in the precordial leads may be seen in:

   a. Non-Q-wave anterior MI
   b. Normal variant
   c. Hypertrophic cardiomyopathy
   d. Subarachnoid bleeding

2. QT prolongation can be seen in:

   a. CNS injury
   b. Hypercalcemia
   c. Quinidine effect
   d. Myocardial ischemia or injury

Answers: ECG 81

1. Deep T wave inversion in the precordial leads can be seen with non-Q-wave anterior MI, hypertrophic cardiomyopathy (especially the apical variant), subarachnoid hemorrhage, and following ventricular pacing. Normal variant T wave inversion is shallow, not deep, and unlike the conditions mentioned above, is not associated with QT prolongation. (Answer: a, c, d)

2. QT prolongation can be seen in a variety of conditions including CNS injury (e.g., subarachnoid bleed), hypothermia, quinidine and other antiarrhythmic drugs, and myocardial ischemia or injury. Among electrolyte disturbances, hypocalcemia and hypokalemia can cause QT prolongation, whereas hypercalcemia results in shortening of the QT interval. (Answer: All except b)

— Quick Review 81 —

ST and/or T wave abnormalities suggesting myocardial ischemia	
• Abnormally tall, symmetrical, (upright/inverted) T waves	inverted
• Horizontal or ____ ST segments with or without T wave inversion	downsloping
• Associated ECG findings:	
▸ QT interval is usually (normal/prolonged)	prolonged
▸ Reciprocal ____ wave changes may be evident	T
▸ Prominent U waves are often present and may be upright or inverted (true/false)	true
Prolonged QT interval	
• Corrected QT interval (QTc) ≥ ____ seconds, where QTc = QT interval divided by the square root of the preceding ____ interval	0.42-0.46 RR
• QT interval varies (directly/inversely) with heart rate	inversely
• The normal QT interval should be (less than/greater than) 50% of the RR interval	less than

ECG 82. 64-year-old male found unconscious lying outside in a Minnesota winter:

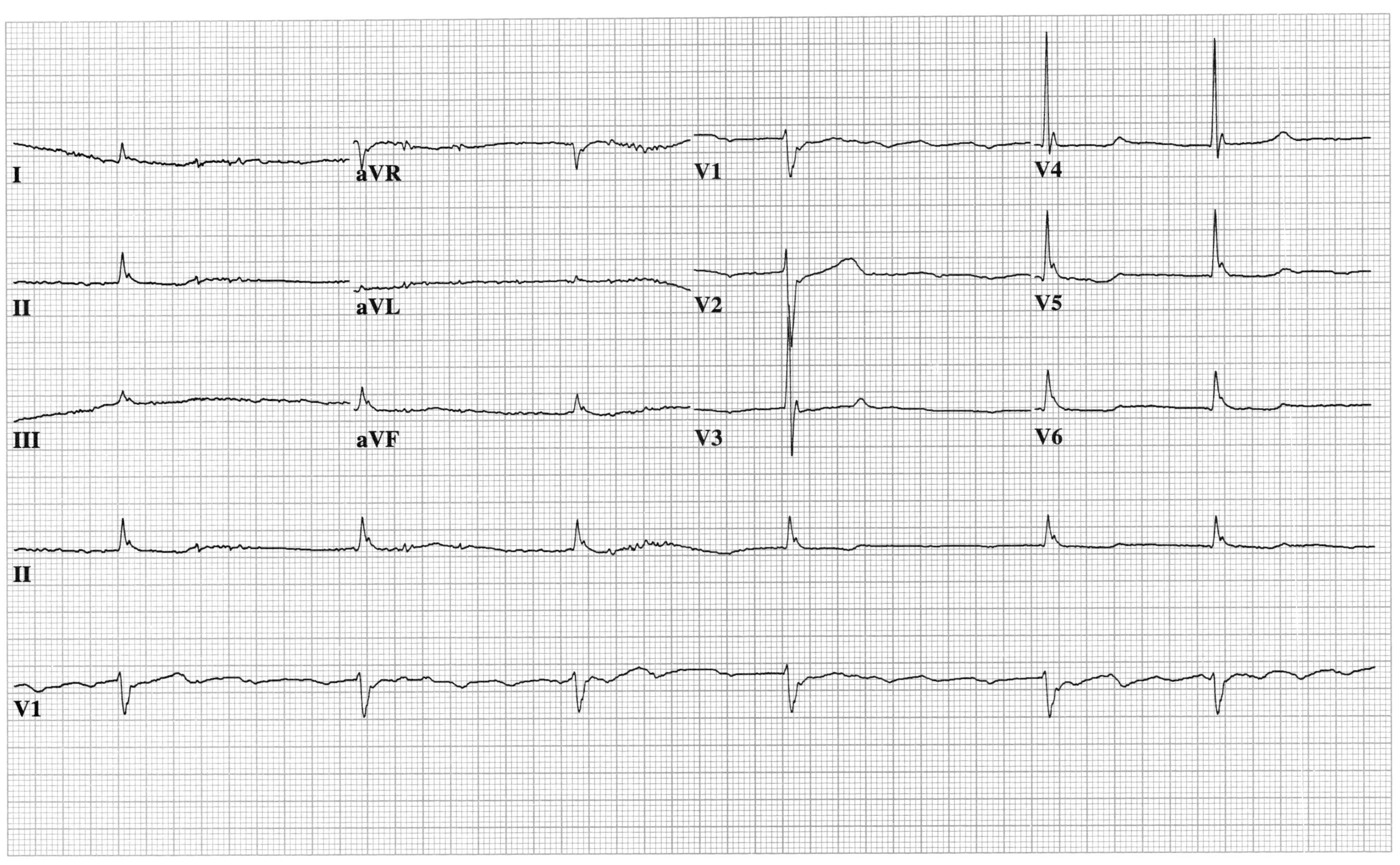

1. GENERAL FEATURES

☐ a. Normal ECG
☐ b. Borderline normal ECG or normal variant
☐ c. Incorrect electrode placement
☐ d. Artifact due to tremor

2. ATRIAL RHYTHMS

☐ a. Sinus rhythm
☐ b. Sinus arrhythmia
☐ c. Sinus bradycardia (< 60)
☐ d. Sinus tachycardia (> 100)
☐ e. Sinus pause or arrest
☐ f. Sinoatrial exit block
☐ g. Ecoptic atrial rhythm
☐ h. Wandering atrial pacemaker
☐ i. Atrial premature complexes, normally conducted
☐ j. Atrial premature complexes, nonconducted
☐ k. Atrial premature complexes with aberrant intraventricular conduction
☐ l. Atrial tachycardia (regular, sustained, 1:1 conduction)
☐ m. Atrial tachycardia, repetitive (short paroxysms)
☐ n. Atrial tachycardia, multifocal
☐ o. Atrial tachycardia with AV block
☐ p. Supraventricular tachycardia, unspecific
☐ q. Supraventricular tachycardia, paroxysmal
☐ r. Atrial flutter
☐ s. Atrial fibrillation
☐ t. Retrograde atrial activation

3. AV JUNCTIONAL RHYTHMS

☐ a. AV junctional premature complexes
☐ b. AV junctional escape complexes
☐ c. AV junctional rhythm, accelerated
☐ d. AV junctional rhythm

4. VENTRICULAR RHYTHMS

☐ a. Ventricular premature complex(es), uniform, fixed coupling
☐ b. Ventricular premature complex(es), uniform, nonfixed coupling
☐ c. Ventricular premature complexes(es), multiform
☐ d. Ventricular premature complexes, in pairs
☐ e. Ventricular parasystole
☐ f. Ventricular tachycardia (≥ 3 consecutive complexes)
☐ g. Accelerated idioventricular rhythm
☐ h. Ventricular escape complexes or rhythm
☐ i. Ventricular fibrillation

5. ATRIAL-VENTRICULAR INTERACTIONS IN ARRHYTHMIAS

☐ a. Fusion complexes
☐ b. Reciprocal (echo) complexes
☐ c. Ventricular capture complexes
☐ d. AV dissociation
☐ e. Ventriculophasic sinus arrhythmia

6. AV CONDUCTION ABNORMALITIES

☐ a. AV block, 1°
☐ b. AV block, 2° - Mobitz type I (Wenckebach)
☐ c. AV block, 2° - Mobitz type II
☐ d. AV block, 2:1
☐ e. AV block, 3°
☐ f. AV block, variable
☐ g. Short PR interval (with sinus rhythm and normal QRS duration)
☐ h. Wolff-Parkinson-White pattern

7. INTRAVENTRICULAR CONDUCTION DISTURBANCES

☐ a. RBBB, incomplete
☐ b. RBBB, complete
☐ c. Left anterior fascicular block
☐ d. Left posterior fascicular block
☐ e. LBBB, with ST-T wave suggestive of acute myocardial injury or infarction
☐ f. LBBB, complete
☐ g. LBBB, intermittent
☐ h. Intraventricular conduction disturbance, nonspecific
☐ i. Aberrant intraventricular conduction with supraventricular arrhythmia

8. P WAVE ABNORMALITIES

☐ a. Right atrial abnormality
☐ b. Left atrial abnormalities
☐ c. Nonspecific atrial abnormality

9. ABNORMALITIES OF QRS VOLTAGE OR AXIS

☐ a. Low voltage, limb leads only
☐ b. Low voltage, limb and precordial leads
☐ c. Left axis deviation (> - 30%)
☐ d. Right axis deviation (> + 100)
☐ e. Electrical alternans

10. VENTRICULAR HYPERTROPHY

☐ a. LVH by voltage only
☐ b. LVH by voltage and ST-T segment abnormalities
☐ c. RVH
☐ d. Combined ventricular hypertrophy

11. Q WAVE MYOCARDIAL INFARCTION

	Probably Acute or Recent	Probably Old or Age Indeterminate
Anterolateral	☐ a.	☐ g.
Anterior	☐ b.	☐ h.
Anteroseptal	☐ c.	☐ i.
Lateral/High lateral	☐ d.	☐ j.
Inferior	☐ e.	☐ k.
Posterior	☐ f.	☐ l.

☐ m. Probably ventricular aneurysm

12. ST, T, U, WAVE ABNORMALITIES

☐ a. Normal variant, early repolarization
☐ b. Normal variant, juvenile T waves
☐ c. Nonspecific ST and/or T wave abnormalities
☐ d. ST and/or T wave abnormalities suggesting myocardial ischemia
☐ e. ST and/or T wave abnormalities suggesting myocardial injury
☐ f. ST and/or T wave abnormalities suggesting acute pericarditis
☐ g. ST-T segment abnormalities secondary to intraventricular conduction disturbance or hypertrophy
☐ h. Post-extrasystolic T wave abnormality
☐ i. Isolated J point depression
☐ j. Peaked T waves
☐ k. Prolonged QT interval
☐ l. Prominent U waves

13. PACEMAKER FUNCTION AND RHYTHM

☐ a. Atrial or coronary sinus pacing
☐ b. Ventricular demand pacing
☐ c. AV sequential pacing
☐ d. Ventricular pacing, complete control
☐ e. Dual chamber, atrial sensing pacemaker
☐ f. Pacemaker malfunction, not constantly capturing (atrium or ventricle)
☐ g. Pacemaker malfunction, not constantly sensing (atrium or ventricle)
☐ h. Pacemaker malfunction, not firing
☐ i. Pacemaker malfunction, slowing

14. SUGGESTED OR PROBABLE CLINICAL DISORDERS

☐ a. Digitalis effect
☐ b. Digitalis toxicity
☐ c. Antiarrhythmic drug effect
☐ d. Antiarrhythmic drug toxicity
☐ e. Hyperkalemia
☐ f. Hypokalemia
☐ g. Hypercalcemia
☐ h. Hypocalcemia
☐ i. Atrial septal defect, secundum
☐ j. Atrial septal defect, primum
☐ k. Dextrocardia, mirror image
☐ l. Mitral valve disease
☐ m. Chronic lung disease
☐ n. Acute cor pulmonale, including pulmonary embolus
☐ o. Pericardial effusion
☐ p. Acute pericarditis
☐ q. Hypertrophic cardiomyopathy
☐ r. Coronary artery disease
☐ s. Central nervous system disorder
☐ t. Myxedema
☐ u. Hypothermia
☐ v. Sick sinus syndrome

ECG 82 was obtained in a 64-year-old male who was found unconscious lying outside in a Minnesota winter. The tracing shows atrial fibrillation with a very slow ventricular response, prominent J ("Osborne") waves (arrows), and nonspecific QRS widening. Artifact due to tremor (shivering), apparent on the rhythm strip (asterisks), is superimposed on the atrial fibrillation. All of these findings are consistent with hypothermia.

Codes:

1d	Artifact due to tremor
2s	Atrial fibrillation
7h	IVCD, nonspecific type
14u	Hypothermia

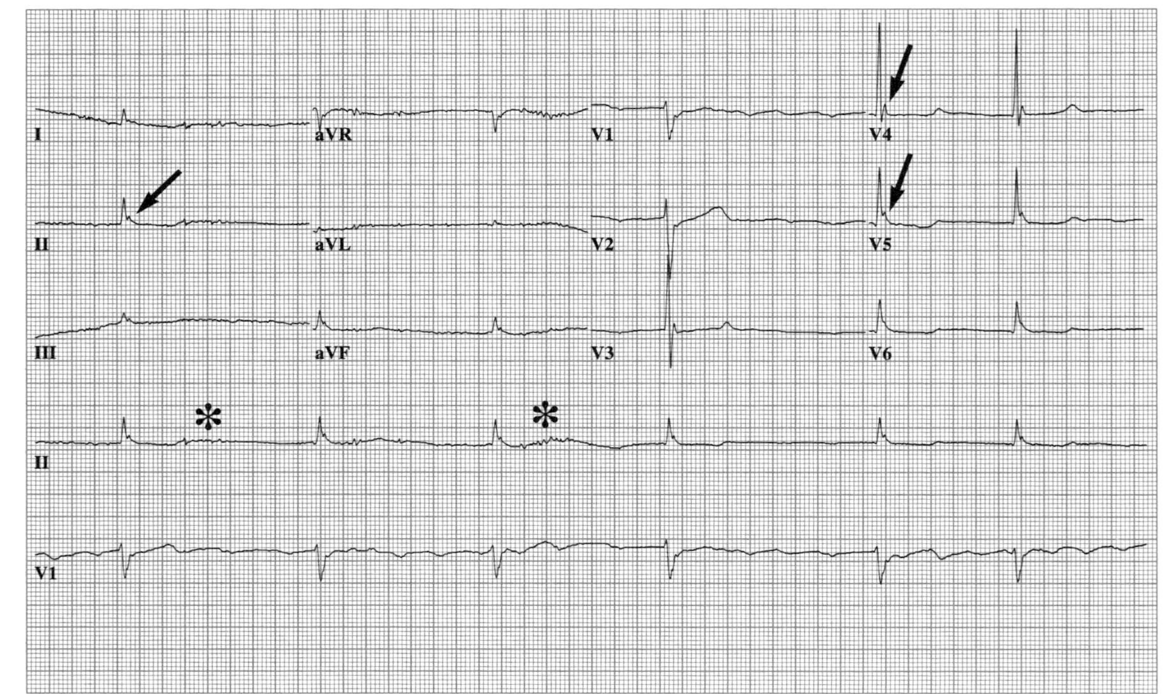

Questions: ECG 82

1. ECG findings consistent with hypothermia include:

   a. Sinus bradycardia
   b. Junctional rhythm
   c. Atrial fibrillation with slow ventricular response
   d. Prolonged PR, QRS, and QT intervals
   e. Osborne wave
   f. T-wave inversions

2. The oscillations in the baseline seen in the present tracing are most likely due to:

   a. Fibrillation waves
   b. Muscle tremor
   c. Artifact
   d. Parkinson's disease

Answers: ECG 82

1. Profound hypothermia (core temperature < 32° C) causes peripheral vasoconstriction, impaired enzymatic activity, and decreased cardiac output and respirations. Complications include aspiration pneumonia, adult respiratory distress syndrome, pulmonary edema, rhabdomyolysis, acute tubular necrosis, gastric dilitation, upper GI bleed, hyperviscosity syndrome, and disseminated intravascular coagulation. The classic ECG finding of hypothermia is the Osborne wave (or J wave), which is an extra positive deflection between the terminal portion of the QRS complex and the beginning of ST segment. The Osborne wave is usually positive in the left precordial leads, and has an amplitude that is inversely proportional to body temperature. Other ECG changes caused by hypothermia include prolongation of the PR, QRS, and QT intervals; T wave inversion; and bradyarrhythmias consisting of sinus bradycardia, junctional rhythm, and atrial fibrillation with a slow ventricular response. (Answer: All)

2. Signals unrelated to cardiac conduction are seen frequently on the ECG. Muscle tremor (e.g., shivering or Parkinson disease) can be continuous or intermittent, and in some instances, crescendo-decrescendo in character (e.g., scratching). Electrical interference, particularly 60-cycle oscillations, are occasionally seen. Such interference can be severe in intensive care units operating rooms, and cardiac catheterization laboratories.

(Answer: b)

— Quick Review 82 —

Atrial fibrillation	
• ____ waves are absent	P
• Atrial activity is totally ____ and represented by fibrillatory (f) waves of varying amplitudes, duration and morphology	irregular
• Atrial activity is best seen in the ____ and ____ leads	right precordial, inferior
• Ventricular rhythm is (regularly/irregularly) irregular	irregularly
• ____ toxicity may result in regularization of the RR interval due to complete heart block with junctional tachycardia	Digitalis
• Ventricular rate is usually ____ per minute in the absence of drugs	100-180
▸ Think ____ if the ventricular rate is > 200 per minute and the QRS is > 0.12 seconds	Wolff-Parkinson-White
Hypothermia	
• Sinus (tachycardia/bradycardia)	bradycardia
• PR, QRS, and QT prolonged (true/false)	true
• Osborne ("J") wave: late upright terminal deflection of QRS complex; amplitude (increases/decreases) as temperature declines	increases
• Atrial ____ in 50-60%	fibrillation
• Other arrhythmias include AV junctional rhythm, ventricular tachycardia, ventricular fibrillation (true/false)	true

Don't Get Confused!

Wandering Atrial Pacemaker

P waves with $\geq$ 3 morphologies; rate <100 per minute; varying PR, RR, and RP intervals

May be confused with:

Sinus rhythm with multifocal APCs

Sinus rhythm with multifocal APCs demonstrates one dominant atrial pacemaker (i.e., the sinus node); in wandering atrial pacemaker, *no* dominant atrial pacemaker (i.e., no dominant P wave morphology) is present.

Atrial fibrillation/flutter

In atrial fibrillation/flutter, there is lack of an isoelectric baseline; in wandering atrial pacemaker, a distinct isoelectric baseline is present.

ECG 83. 72-year-old male with hypertension and diabetes:

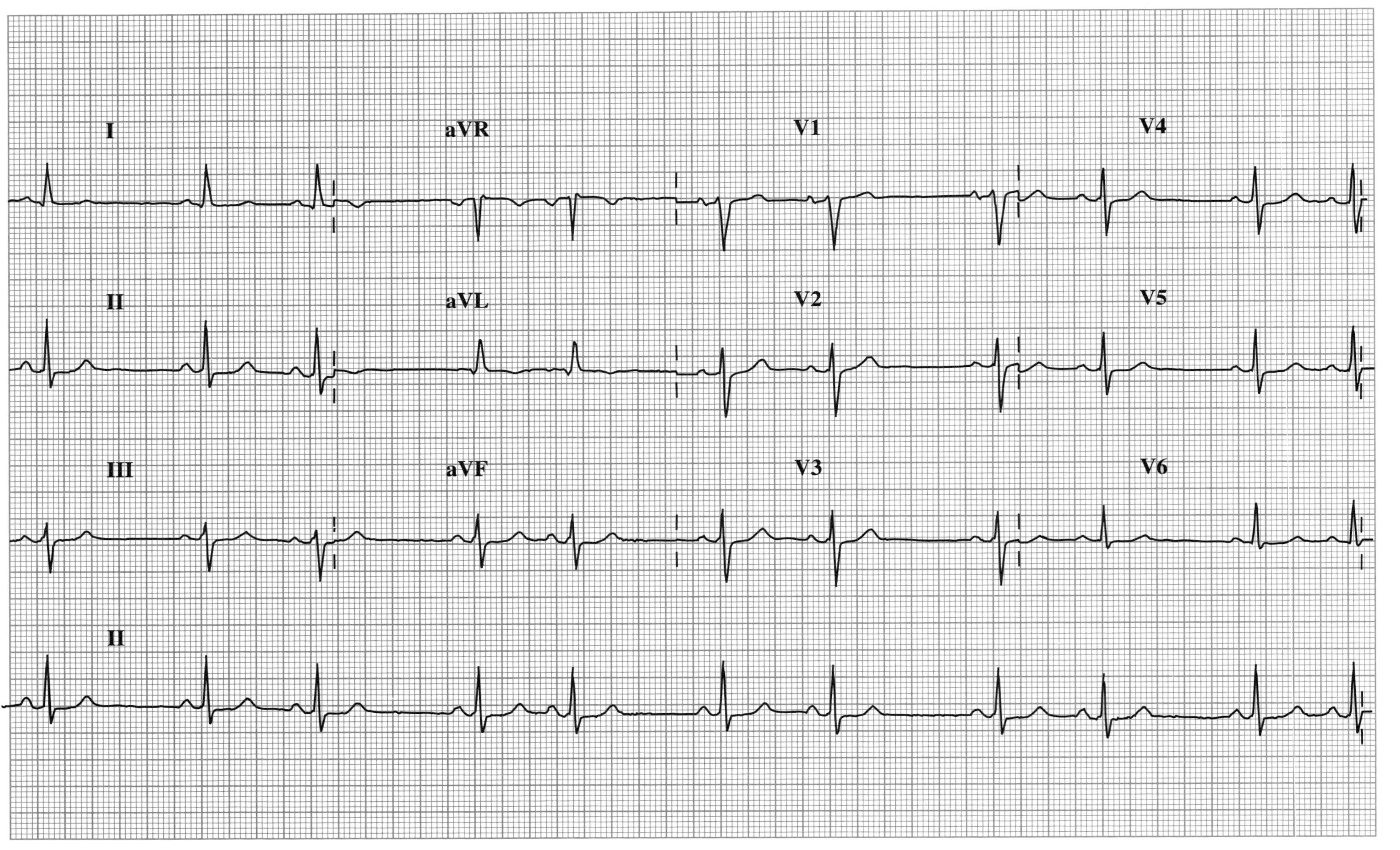

1. GENERAL FEATURES
- ☐ a. Normal ECG
- ☐ b. Borderline normal ECG or normal variant
- ☐ c. Incorrect electrode placement
- ☐ d. Artifact due to tremor

2. ATRIAL RHYTHMS
- ☐ a. Sinus rhythm
- ☐ b. Sinus arrhythmia
- ☐ c. Sinus bradycardia (< 60)
- ☐ d. Sinus tachycardia (> 100)
- ☐ e. Sinus pause or arrest
- ☐ f. Sinoatrial exit block
- ☐ g. Ecoptic atrial rhythm
- ☐ h. Wandering atrial pacemaker
- ☐ i. Atrial premature complexes, normally conducted
- ☐ j. Atrial premature complexes, nonconducted
- ☐ k. Atrial premature complexes with aberrant intraventricular conduction
- ☐ l. Atrial tachycardia (regular, sustained, 1:1 conduction)
- ☐ m. Atrial tachycardia, repetitive (short paroxysms)
- ☐ n. Atrial tachycardia, multifocal
- ☐ o. Atrial tachycardia with AV block
- ☐ p. Supraventricular tachycardia, unspecific
- ☐ q. Supraventricular tachycardia, paroxysmal
- ☐ r. Atrial flutter
- ☐ s. Atrial fibrillation
- ☐ t. Retrograde atrial activation

3. AV JUNCTIONAL RHYTHMS
- ☐ a. AV junctional premature complexes
- ☐ b. AV junctional escape complexes
- ☐ c. AV junctional rhythm, accelerated
- ☐ d. AV junctional rhythm

4. VENTRICULAR RHYTHMS
- ☐ a. Ventricular premature complex(es), uniform, fixed coupling
- ☐ b. Ventricular premature complex(es), uniform, nonfixed coupling
- ☐ c. Ventricular premature complexes(es), multiform
- ☐ d. Ventricular premature complexes, in pairs
- ☐ e. Ventricular parasystole
- ☐ f. Ventricular tachycardia (≥ 3 consecutive complexes)
- ☐ g. Accelerated idioventricular rhythm
- ☐ h. Ventricular escape complexes or rhythm
- ☐ i. Ventricular fibrillation

5. ATRIAL-VENTRICULAR INTERACTIONS IN ARRHYTHMIAS
- ☐ a. Fusion complexes
- ☐ b. Reciprocal (echo) complexes
- ☐ c. Ventricular capture complexes
- ☐ d. AV dissociation
- ☐ e. Ventriculophasic sinus arrhythmia

6. AV CONDUCTION ABNORMALITIES
- ☐ a. AV block, 1°
- ☐ b. AV block, 2° - Mobitz type I (Wenckebach)
- ☐ c. AV block, 2° - Mobitz type II
- ☐ d. AV block, 2:1
- ☐ e. AV block, 3°
- ☐ f. AV block, variable
- ☐ g. Short PR interval (with sinus rhythm and normal QRS duration)
- ☐ h. Wolff-Parkinson-White pattern

7. INTRAVENTRICULAR CONDUCTION DISTURBANCES
- ☐ a. RBBB, incomplete
- ☐ b. RBBB, complete
- ☐ c. Left anterior fascicular block
- ☐ d. Left posterior fascicular block
- ☐ e. LBBB, with ST-T wave suggestive of acute myocardial injury or infarction
- ☐ f. LBBB, complete
- ☐ g. LBBB, intermittent
- ☐ h. Intraventricular conduction disturbance, nonspecific
- ☐ i. Aberrant intraventricular conduction with supraventricular arrhythmia

8. P WAVE ABNORMALITIES
- ☐ a. Right atrial abnormality
- ☐ b. Left atrial abnormalities
- ☐ c. Nonspecific atrial abnormality

9. ABNORMALITIES OF QRS VOLTAGE OR AXIS
- ☐ a. Low voltage, limb leads only
- ☐ b. Low voltage, limb and precordial leads
- ☐ c. Left axis deviation (> - 30%)
- ☐ d. Right axis deviation (> + 100)
- ☐ e. Electrical alternans

10. VENTRICULAR HYPERTROPHY
- ☐ a. LVH by voltage only
- ☐ b. LVH by voltage and ST-T segment abnormalities
- ☐ c. RVH
- ☐ d. Combined ventricular hypertrophy

11. Q WAVE MYOCARDIAL INFARCTION

	Probably Acute or Recent	Probably Old or Age Indeterminate
Anterolateral	☐ a.	☐ g.
Anterior	☐ b.	☐ h.
Anteroseptal	☐ c.	☐ i.
Lateral/High lateral	☐ d.	☐ j.
Inferior	☐ e.	☐ k.
Posterior	☐ f.	☐ l.

☐ m. Probably ventricular aneurysm

12. ST, T, U, WAVE ABNORMALITIES
- ☐ a. Normal variant, early repolarization
- ☐ b. Normal variant, juvenile T waves
- ☐ c. Nonspecific ST and/or T wave abnormalities
- ☐ d. ST and/or T wave abnormalities suggesting myocardial ischemia
- ☐ e. ST and/or T wave abnormalities suggesting myocardial injury
- ☐ f. ST and/or T wave abnormalities suggesting acute pericarditis
- ☐ g. ST-T segment abnormalities secondary to intraventricular conduction disturbance or hypertrophy
- ☐ h. Post-extrasystolic T wave abnormality
- ☐ i. Isolated J point depression
- ☐ j. Peaked T waves
- ☐ k. Prolonged QT interval
- ☐ l. Prominent U waves

13. PACEMAKER FUNCTION AND RHYTHM
- ☐ a. Atrial or coronary sinus pacing
- ☐ b. Ventricular demand pacing
- ☐ c. AV sequential pacing
- ☐ d. Ventricular pacing, complete control
- ☐ e. Dual chamber, atrial sensing pacemaker
- ☐ f. Pacemaker malfunction, not constantly capturing (atrium or ventricle)
- ☐ g. Pacemaker malfunction, not constantly sensing (atrium or ventricle)
- ☐ h. Pacemaker malfunction, not firing
- ☐ i. Pacemaker malfunction, slowing

14. SUGGESTED OR PROBABLE CLINICAL DISORDERS
- ☐ a. Digitalis effect
- ☐ b. Digitalis toxicity
- ☐ c. Antiarrhythmic drug effect
- ☐ d. Antiarrhythmic drug toxicity
- ☐ e. Hyperkalemia
- ☐ f. Hypokalemia
- ☐ g. Hypercalcemia
- ☐ h. Hypocalcemia
- ☐ i. Atrial septal defect, secundum
- ☐ j. Atrial septal defect, primum
- ☐ k. Dextrocardia, mirror image
- ☐ l. Mitral valve disease
- ☐ m. Chronic lung disease
- ☐ n. Acute cor pulmonale, including pulmonary embolus
- ☐ o. Pericardial effusion
- ☐ p. Acute pericarditis
- ☐ q. Hypertrophic cardiomyopathy
- ☐ r. Coronary artery disease
- ☐ s. Central nervous system disorder
- ☐ t. Myxedema
- ☐ u. Hypothermia
- ☐ v. Sick sinus syndrome

ECG 83 was obtained in a 72-year-old male with hypertension and diabetes. The tracing shows a sinus rhythm at approximately 75 beats/minute with "group beating." The recurring sequence throughout the tracing is two normally conducted P waves (which all have the same morphology; arrowheads mark the P waves) followed by a pause (asterisks) that is somewhat less than two times the usual PP interval. These findings are consistent with the diagnosis of 3:2 SA node exit block (a manifestation of sick sinus syndrome). Sinus arrhythmia should also be coded.

Codes:

2a	Sinus rhythm
2b	Sinus arrhythmia
2f	Sinoatrial exit block
14v	Sick sinus syndrome

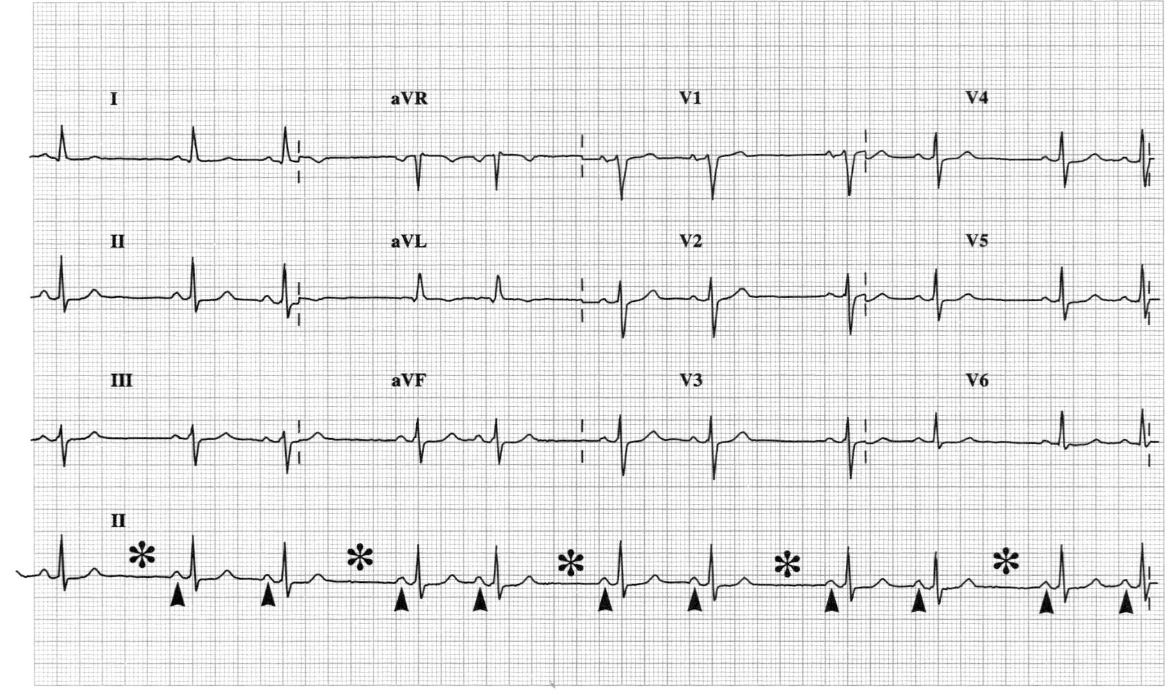

Questions: ECG 83

1. ECG features of Mobitz Type I SA exit block include:

   a. Shortening of the PP interval
   b. Group beating
   c. PP pause less than 2 times the normal PP interval
   d. Constant PR interval

2. Mobitz Type II SA exit block results in a PP pause that is ___ times the usual PP interval:

   a. 2
   b. 3
   c. 4
   d. Any of the above

Answers: ECG 83

1. Mobitz Type I SA exit block results in intermittent failure of the sinus impulse to capture the atria, resulting in a pause without a P wave. Additional ECG manifestations include shortening of the PP interval leading up to the pause, group beating, a PP pause that is somewhat less than two times the normal PP interval, and a constant PR interval. (Answer: All)

2. Mobitz Type II SA exit block results in a PP pause that is a multiple of the usual PP interval. PP pauses that are two times, three times, four times, etc. the basic PP interval are often due to Mobitz Type II SA exit block. (Answer: d)

— Quick Review 83 —

Sinus arrhythmia	
• (Sinus/nonsinus) P wave	Sinus
• Longest and shortest PP intervals vary by > ____ seconds or 10%	0.16
• Sinus arrhythmia differs from "ventriculophasic" sinus arrhythmia, the latter of which occurs in the setting of ____	heart block
Sinoatrial (SA) exit block	
First-degree: Conduction of sinus impulses to the atrium is (normal/delayed), but ____:1 response is maintained	delayed, 1
• First-degree SA exit block (is/is not) detectable on the surface ECG	is not
Second-degree: Some sinus impulses fail to ____ the atria	capture
• Type I (Mobitz I):	
▸ Sinus P wave (true/false)	true
▸ "____ beating" with:	Group
(1) (Shortening/lengthening) of the PP interval prior to absent P wave	Shortening
(2) (Constant/variable) PR interval	Constant
(3) PP pause < ____ normal PP interval	2
• Type II (Mobitz II): Constant PP interval followed by a pause that (is/is not) a multiple (2x, 3x, etc.) of the normal PP interval	is
Third-degree:	
• Complete failure of ____ conduction	sinoatrial
• Cannot be differentiated from ____	complete sinus arrest

— Comic Relief —

Hope you've been reading your ECGs more carefully than our young doctor read his employment contract!

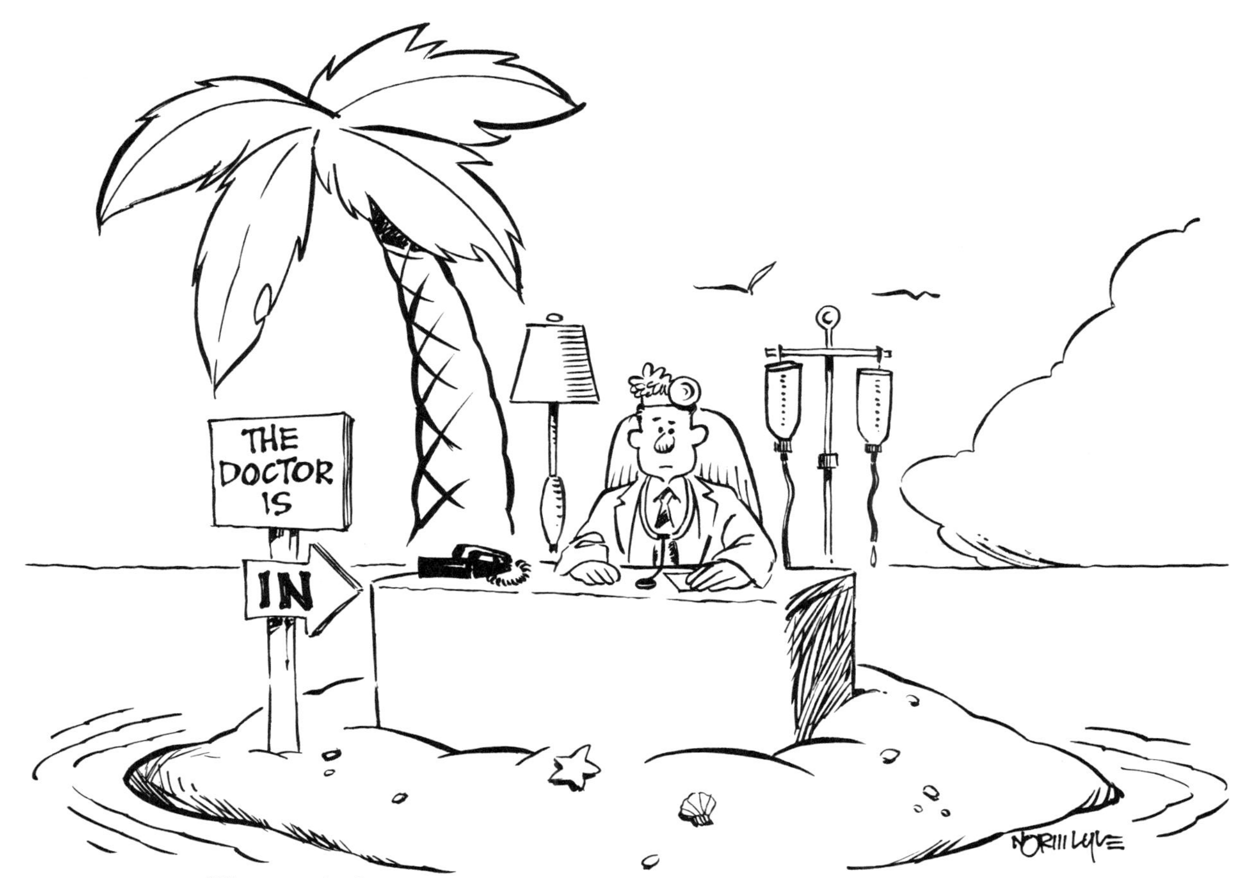

His restrictive covenant was a little more "restrictive" than Milo had originally thought.

ECG 84. 83-year-old female with hypertension and chronic dyspnea on exertion:

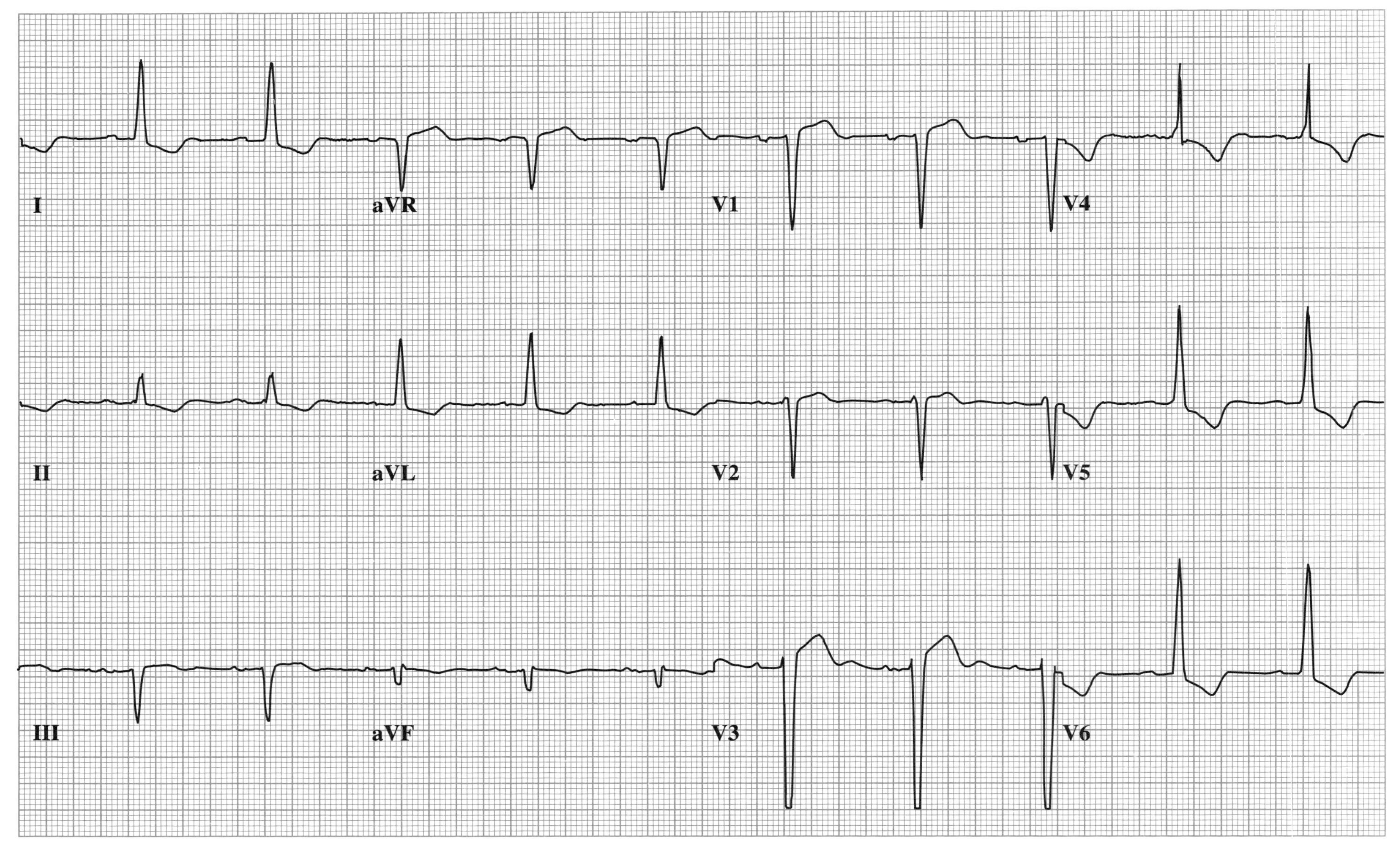

1. GENERAL FEATURES

☐ a. Normal ECG
☐ b. Borderline normal ECG or normal variant
☐ c. Incorrect electrode placement
☐ d. Artifact due to tremor

2. ATRIAL RHYTHMS

☐ a. Sinus rhythm
☐ b. Sinus arrhythmia
☐ c. Sinus bradycardia (< 60)
☐ d. Sinus tachycardia (> 100)
☐ e. Sinus pause or arrest
☐ f. Sinoatrial exit block
☐ g. Ecoptic atrial rhythm
☐ h. Wandering atrial pacemaker
☐ i. Atrial premature complexes, normally conducted
☐ j. Atrial premature complexes, nonconducted
☐ k. Atrial premature complexes with aberrant intraventricular conduction
☐ l. Atrial tachycardia (regular, sustained, 1:1 conduction)
☐ m. Atrial tachycardia, repetitive (short paroxysms)
☐ n. Atrial tachycardia, multifocal
☐ o. Atrial tachycardia with AV block
☐ p. Supraventricular tachycardia, unspecific
☐ q. Supraventricular tachycardia, paroxysmal
☐ r. Atrial flutter
☐ s. Atrial fibrillation
☐ t. Retrograde atrial activation

3. AV JUNCTIONAL RHYTHMS

☐ a. AV junctional premature complexes
☐ b. AV junctional escape complexes
☐ c. AV junctional rhythm, accelerated
☐ d. AV junctional rhythm

4. VENTRICULAR RHYTHMS

☐ a. Ventricular premature complex(es), uniform, fixed coupling
☐ b. Ventricular premature complex(es), uniform, nonfixed coupling
☐ c. Ventricular premature complexes(es), multiform
☐ d. Ventricular premature complexes, in pairs
☐ e. Ventricular parasystole
☐ f. Ventricular tachycardia (≥ 3 consecutive complexes)
☐ g. Accelerated idioventricular rhythm
☐ h. Ventricular escape complexes or rhythm
☐ i. Ventricular fibrillation

5. ATRIAL-VENTRICULAR INTERACTIONS IN ARRHYTHMIAS

☐ a. Fusion complexes
☐ b. Reciprocal (echo) complexes
☐ c. Ventricular capture complexes
☐ d. AV dissociation
☐ e. Ventriculophasic sinus arrhythmia

6. AV CONDUCTION ABNORMALITIES

☐ a. AV block, 1°
☐ b. AV block, 2° - Mobitz type I (Wenckebach)
☐ c. AV block, 2° - Mobitz type II
☐ d. AV block, 2:1
☐ e. AV block, 3°
☐ f. AV block, variable
☐ g. Short PR interval (with sinus rhythm and normal QRS duration)
☐ h. Wolff-Parkinson-White pattern

7. INTRAVENTRICULAR CONDUCTION DISTURBANCES

☐ a. RBBB, incomplete
☐ b. RBBB, complete
☐ c. Left anterior fascicular block
☐ d. Left posterior fascicular block
☐ e. LBBB, with ST-T wave suggestive of acute myocardial injury or infarction
☐ f. LBBB, complete
☐ g. LBBB, intermittent
☐ h. Intraventricular conduction disturbance, nonspecific
☐ i. Aberrant intraventricular conduction with supraventricular arrhythmia

8. P WAVE ABNORMALITIES

☐ a. Right atrial abnormality
☐ b. Left atrial abnormalities
☐ c. Nonspecific atrial abnormality

9. ABNORMALITIES OF QRS VOLTAGE OR AXIS

☐ a. Low voltage, limb leads only
☐ b. Low voltage, limb and precordial leads
☐ c. Left axis deviation (> - 30%)
☐ d. Right axis deviation (> + 100)
☐ e. Electrical alternans

10. VENTRICULAR HYPERTROPHY

☐ a. LVH by voltage only
☐ b. LVH by voltage and ST-T segment abnormalities
☐ c. RVH
☐ d. Combined ventricular hypertrophy

11. Q WAVE MYOCARDIAL INFARCTION

	Probably Acute or Recent	Probably Old or Age Indeterminate
Anterolateral	☐ a.	☐ g.
Anterior	☐ b.	☐ h.
Anteroseptal	☐ c.	☐ i.
Lateral/High lateral	☐ d.	☐ j.
Inferior	☐ e.	☐ k.
Posterior	☐ f.	☐ l.

☐ m. Probably ventricular aneurysm

12. ST, T, U, WAVE ABNORMALITIES

☐ a. Normal variant, early repolarization
☐ b. Normal variant, juvenile T waves
☐ c. Nonspecific ST and/or T wave abnormalities
☐ d. ST and/or T wave abnormalities suggesting myocardial ischemia
☐ e. ST and/or T wave abnormalities suggesting myocardial injury
☐ f. ST and/or T wave abnormalities suggesting acute pericarditis
☐ g. ST-T segment abnormalities secondary to intraventricular conduction disturbance or hypertrophy
☐ h. Post-extrasystolic T wave abnormality
☐ i. Isolated J point depression
☐ j. Peaked T waves
☐ k. Prolonged QT interval
☐ l. Prominent U waves

13. PACEMAKER FUNCTION AND RHYTHM

☐ a. Atrial or coronary sinus pacing
☐ b. Ventricular demand pacing
☐ c. AV sequential pacing
☐ d. Ventricular pacing, complete control
☐ e. Dual chamber, atrial sensing pacemaker
☐ f. Pacemaker malfunction, not constantly capturing (atrium or ventricle)
☐ g. Pacemaker malfunction, not constantly sensing (atrium or ventricle)
☐ h. Pacemaker malfunction, not firing
☐ i. Pacemaker malfunction, slowing

14. SUGGESTED OR PROBABLE CLINICAL DISORDERS

☐ a. Digitalis effect
☐ b. Digitalis toxicity
☐ c. Antiarrhythmic drug effect
☐ d. Antiarrhythmic drug toxicity
☐ e. Hyperkalemia
☐ f. Hypokalemia
☐ g. Hypercalcemia
☐ h. Hypocalcemia
☐ i. Atrial septal defect, secundum
☐ j. Atrial septal defect, primum
☐ k. Dextrocardia, mirror image
☐ l. Mitral valve disease
☐ m. Chronic lung disease
☐ n. Acute cor pulmonale, including pulmonary embolus
☐ o. Pericardial effusion
☐ p. Acute pericarditis
☐ q. Hypertrophic cardiomyopathy
☐ r. Coronary artery disease
☐ s. Central nervous system disorder
☐ t. Myxedema
☐ u. Hypothermia
☐ v. Sick sinus syndrome

ECG 84 was obtained in an 83-year-old female with hypertension and chronic dyspnea on exertion. The tracing shows sinus rhythm, first-degree AV block, and LVH with secondary ST-T changes. The rS pattern in leads III and aVF (arrowheads) is consistent with previous inferior MI, but does not meet formal criteria for the diagnosis. The low R wave voltage in V_2-V_3 and ST segment elevation in V_1-V_3 (asterisks) can be attributed to LVH. Voltage criteria for LVH satisfied in this tracing include: an R wave in aVL + S wave in $V_3 > 20$ mm; an R wave in V_6 + S wave in $V_1 > 35$ mm; an R wave in $V_6 > 20$ mm; an R wave in I > 14 mm; and an R wave in AVL ≥ 12 mm. Coronary artery disease should also be coded.

Codes:

2a	Sinus rhythm
6a	AV block, 1 °
10b	LVH by both voltage and ST-T segment abnormalities
12g	ST-T segment abnormalities secondary to IVCD or hypertrophy
14r	Coronary artery disease

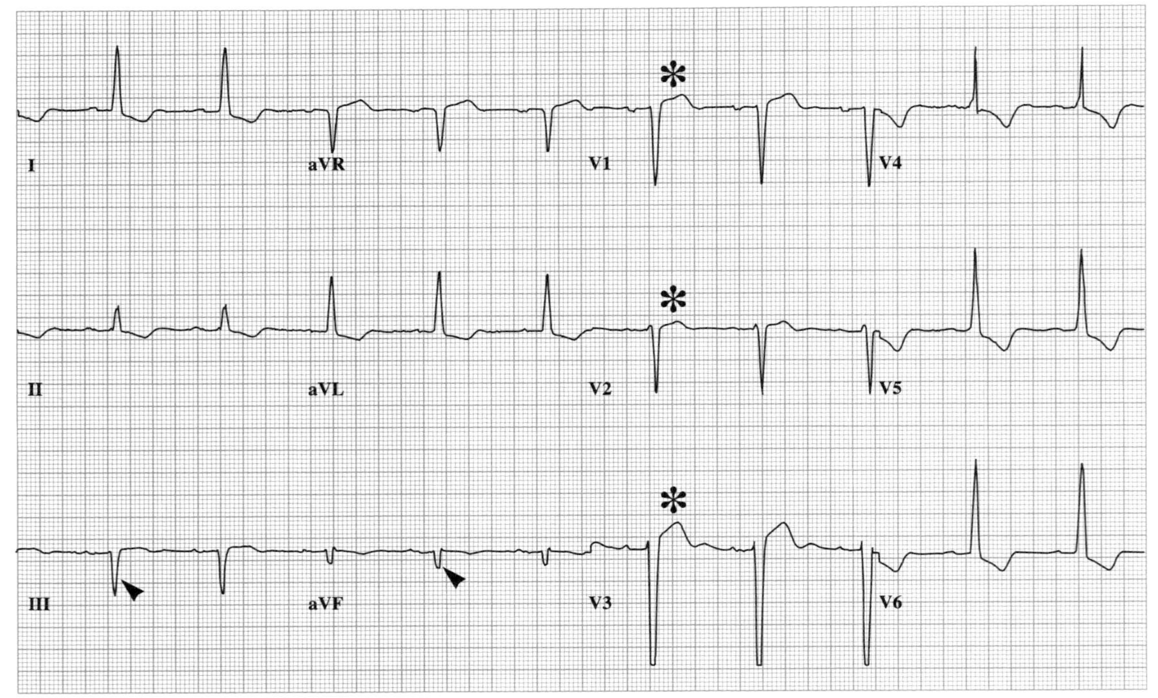

Questions: ECG 84

1. Can the diagnosis of inferior myocardial infarction be excluded in this ECG:

    a. Yes
    b. No

2. Which of the following statements about ST segment elevation are true:

    a The degree of ST elevation in patients with early repolarization may vary between ECGs
    b. In acute MI, T waves begin to invert before the ST segment returns to baseline
    c. In acute pericarditis, T waves begin to invert before the ST segment returns to baseline
    d. ST elevation is common in LVH
    e. ST elevation is common in RVH
    f. ST elevation of 1-2 mm in the right precordial leads (especially in V_2 and V_3) may be a normal variant in patients > 40 years old

3. Which of the following conditions is associated with poor R-wave progression:

    a. Anterior MI
    b. LVH
    c. COPD
    d. Left bundle branch block

Answers: ECG 84

1. The formal criteria for inferior myocardial infarction are not met and should not be scored on the answer sheet. Nevertheless, it is possible that this patient has had an inferior infarct in the past: While Q-waves representing areas of infarction may persist indefinitely, a small percentage may regress or disappear completely; at times, an rS pattern, as in the present tracing, may be seen. (Answer: b)

2. (Answer: a, b, d, f)

3. Poor R wave progression has been defined as a precordial transition zone (i.e., lead with R:S = 1) at V_5 or V_6, or an R:S < 1 in V_5 or V_6. Poor R wave progression can be seen in normals, anterior MI, dilated or hypertrophic cardiomyopathy, left

ventricular hypertrophy, COPD with or without cor pulmonale, left anterior fascicular block, and WPW syndrome. Left bundle branch block sometimes causes poor R wave progression as well. (Answer: All)

— Quick Review 84 —	
AV block, 1°	
• PR interval ≥ ____ seconds	0.20
LVH by both voltage and ST-T segment abnormalities	
• Voltage criteria for LVH and one or more ST-T abnormalities:	
▸ ST segment and T wave deviation in (same/opposite) direction to the major deflection of QRS	opposite
▸ ST segment (elevation/depression) in leads I, aVL, III, aVF, and/or V_4-V_6	depression
▸ Subtle (< 1-2 mm) ST (elevation/depression) in leads V_1-V_3	elevation
▸ Inverted ____ waves in leads I, aVL, V_4-V_6	T
▸ (Absent/prominent) U waves	prominent

— POP QUIZ —

Make The Diagnosis

Instructions: Determine the clinical disorder that best corresponds to the ECG features listed below (see item 14 of score sheet for options)

ECG Features	Answer
• Typical RSR' or rSR' complex in lead V_1 with a QRS duration < 0.11 seconds • Incomplete RBBB • Right axis deviation ± right ventricular hypertrophy • Right atrial abnormality in ~ 30% • First-degree AV block in < 20%	Atrial septal defect, secundum
• RSR' complex in lead V_1 • Left axis deviation • First-degree AV block in 15-40% • Advanced cases have biventricular hypertrophy	Atrial septal defect, primum
• P-QRS-T in leads I and aVL are inverted or "upside down" • Decreasing R wave amplitude from leads V_1-V_6	Dextrocardia, mirror image
• Right ventricular hypertrophy • Right axis deviation • Right atrial abnormality • Shift of transitional zone counterclockwise • Low voltage QRS • Pseudoinfarct pattern in the anteroseptal leads • S_1 S_2 S_3 pattern • May also see sinus tachycardia, junctional rhythm, various degrees of AV block, IVCD, and bundle branch block	Chronic lung disease

ECG 85. 62-year-old female with chest discomfort:

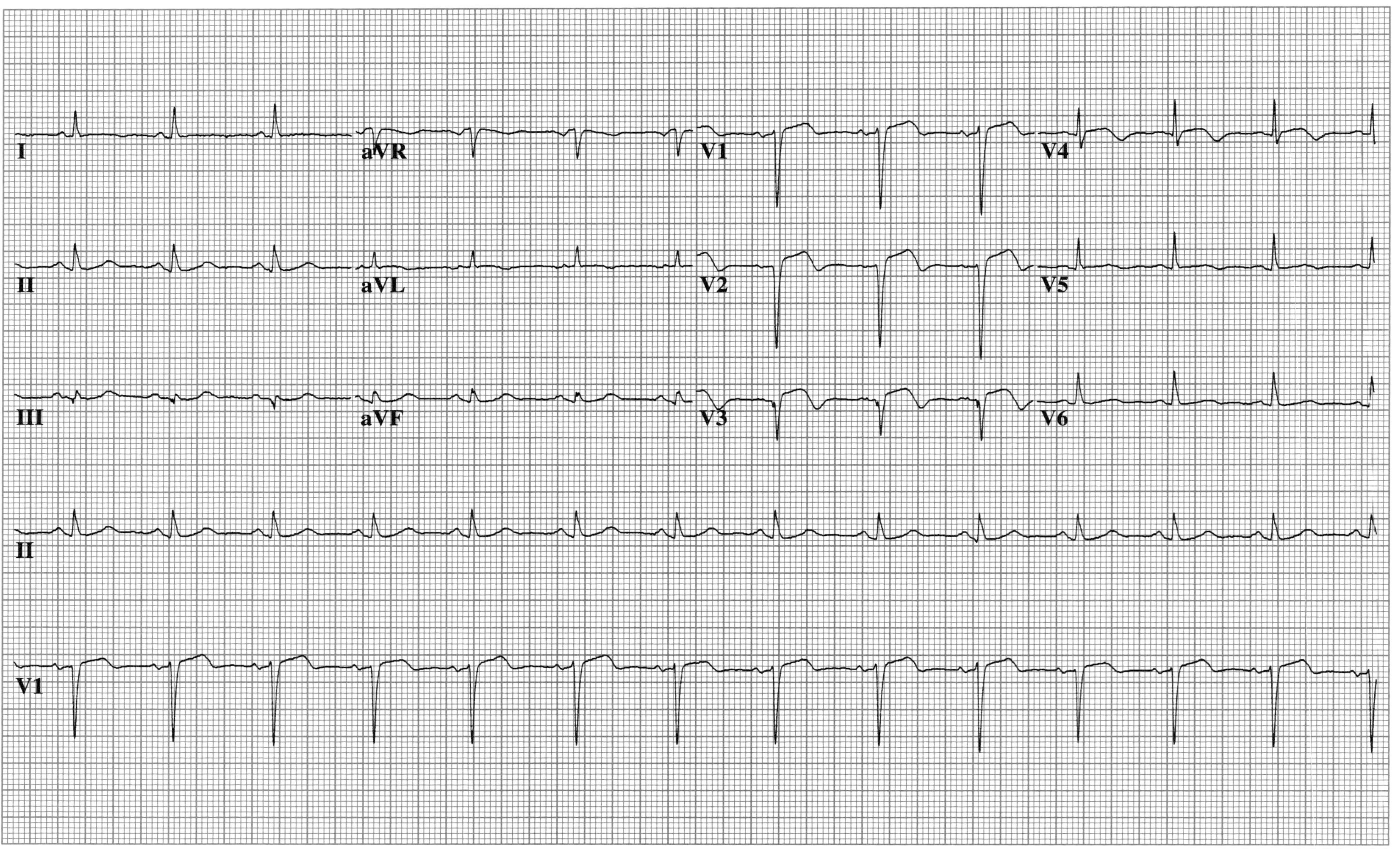

1. GENERAL FEATURES

- ☐ a. Normal ECG
- ☐ b. Borderline normal ECG or normal variant
- ☐ c. Incorrect electrode placement
- ☐ d. Artifact due to tremor

2. ATRIAL RHYTHMS

- ☐ a. Sinus rhythm
- ☐ b. Sinus arrhythmia
- ☐ c. Sinus bradycardia (< 60)
- ☐ d. Sinus tachycardia (> 100)
- ☐ e. Sinus pause or arrest
- ☐ f. Sinoatrial exit block
- ☐ g. Ecoptic atrial rhythm
- ☐ h. Wandering atrial pacemaker
- ☐ i. Atrial premature complexes, normally conducted
- ☐ j. Atrial premature complexes, nonconducted
- ☐ k. Atrial premature complexes with aberrant intraventricular conduction
- ☐ l. Atrial tachycardia (regular, sustained, 1:1 conduction)
- ☐ m. Atrial tachycardia, repetitive (short paroxysms)
- ☐ n. Atrial tachycardia, multifocal
- ☐ o. Atrial tachycardia with AV block
- ☐ p. Supraventricular tachycardia, unspecific
- ☐ q. Supraventricular tachycardia, paroxysmal
- ☐ r. Atrial flutter
- ☐ s. Atrial fibrillation
- ☐ t. Retrograde atrial activation

3. AV JUNCTIONAL RHYTHMS

- ☐ a. AV junctional premature complexes
- ☐ b. AV junctional escape complexes
- ☐ c. AV junctional rhythm, accelerated
- ☐ d. AV junctional rhythm

4. VENTRICULAR RHYTHMS

- ☐ a. Ventricular premature complex(es), uniform, fixed coupling
- ☐ b. Ventricular premature complex(es), uniform, nonfixed coupling
- ☐ c. Ventricular premature complexes(es), multiform
- ☐ d. Ventricular premature complexes, in pairs
- ☐ e. Ventricular parasystole
- ☐ f. Ventricular tachycardia (≥ 3 consecutive complexes)
- ☐ g. Accelerated idioventricular rhythm
- ☐ h. Ventricular escape complexes or rhythm
- ☐ i. Ventricular fibrillation

5. ATRIAL-VENTRICULAR INTERACTIONS IN ARRHYTHMIAS

- ☐ a. Fusion complexes
- ☐ b. Reciprocal (echo) complexes
- ☐ c. Ventricular capture complexes
- ☐ d. AV dissociation
- ☐ e. Ventriculophasic sinus arrhythmia

6. AV CONDUCTION ABNORMALITIES

- ☐ a. AV block, 1°
- ☐ b. AV block, 2° - Mobitz type I (Wenckebach)
- ☐ c. AV block, 2° - Mobitz type II
- ☐ d. AV block, 2:1
- ☐ e. AV block, 3°
- ☐ f. AV block, variable
- ☐ g. Short PR interval (with sinus rhythm and normal QRS duration)
- ☐ h. Wolff-Parkinson-White pattern

7. INTRAVENTRICULAR CONDUCTION DISTURBANCES

- ☐ a. RBBB, incomplete
- ☐ b. RBBB, complete
- ☐ c. Left anterior fascicular block
- ☐ d. Left posterior fascicular block
- ☐ e. LBBB, with ST-T wave suggestive of acute myocardial injury or infarction
- ☐ f. LBBB, complete
- ☐ g. LBBB, intermittent
- ☐ h. Intraventricular conduction disturbance, nonspecific
- ☐ i. Aberrant intraventricular conduction with supraventricular arrhythmia

8. P WAVE ABNORMALITIES

- ☐ a. Right atrial abnormality
- ☐ b. Left atrial abnormalities
- ☐ c. Nonspecific atrial abnormality

9. ABNORMALITIES OF QRS VOLTAGE OR AXIS

- ☐ a. Low voltage, limb leads only
- ☐ b. Low voltage, limb and precordial leads
- ☐ c. Left axis deviation (> - 30%)
- ☐ d. Right axis deviation (> + 100)
- ☐ e. Electrical alternans

10. VENTRICULAR HYPERTROPHY

- ☐ a. LVH by voltage only
- ☐ b. LVH by voltage and ST-T segment abnormalities
- ☐ c. RVH
- ☐ d. Combined ventricular hypertrophy

11. Q WAVE MYOCARDIAL INFARCTION

	Probably Acute or Recent	Probably Old or Age Indeterminate
Anterolateral	☐ a.	☐ g.
Anterior	☐ b.	☐ h.
Anteroseptal	☐ c.	☐ i.
Lateral/High lateral	☐ d.	☐ j.
Inferior	☐ e.	☐ k.
Posterior	☐ f.	☐ l.

- ☐ m. Probably ventricular aneurysm

12. ST, T, U, WAVE ABNORMALITIES

- ☐ a. Normal variant, early repolarization
- ☐ b. Normal variant, juvenile T waves
- ☐ c. Nonspecific ST and/or T wave abnormalities
- ☐ d. ST and/or T wave abnormalities suggesting myocardial ischemia
- ☐ e. ST and/or T wave abnormalities suggesting myocardial injury
- ☐ f. ST and/or T wave abnormalities suggesting acute pericarditis
- ☐ g. ST-T segment abnormalities secondary to intraventricular conduction disturbance or hypertrophy
- ☐ h. Post-extrasystolic T wave abnormality
- ☐ i. Isolated J point depression
- ☐ j. Peaked T waves
- ☐ k. Prolonged QT interval
- ☐ l. Prominent U waves

13. PACEMAKER FUNCTION AND RHYTHM

- ☐ a. Atrial or coronary sinus pacing
- ☐ b. Ventricular demand pacing
- ☐ c. AV sequential pacing
- ☐ d. Ventricular pacing, complete control
- ☐ e. Dual chamber, atrial sensing pacemaker
- ☐ f. Pacemaker malfunction, not constantly capturing (atrium or ventricle)
- ☐ g. Pacemaker malfunction, not constantly sensing (atrium or ventricle)
- ☐ h. Pacemaker malfunction, not firing
- ☐ i. Pacemaker malfunction, slowing

14. SUGGESTED OR PROBABLE CLINICAL DISORDERS

- ☐ a. Digitalis effect
- ☐ b. Digitalis toxicity
- ☐ c. Antiarrhythmic drug effect
- ☐ d. Antiarrhythmic drug toxicity
- ☐ e. Hyperkalemia
- ☐ f. Hypokalemia
- ☐ g. Hypercalcemia
- ☐ h. Hypocalcemia
- ☐ i. Atrial septal defect, secundum
- ☐ j. Atrial septal defect, primum
- ☐ k. Dextrocardia, mirror image
- ☐ l. Mitral valve disease
- ☐ m. Chronic lung disease
- ☐ n. Acute cor pulmonale, including pulmonary embolus
- ☐ o. Pericardial effusion
- ☐ p. Acute pericarditis
- ☐ q. Hypertrophic cardiomyopathy
- ☐ r. Coronary artery disease
- ☐ s. Central nervous system disorder
- ☐ t. Myxedema
- ☐ u. Hypothermia
- ☐ v. Sick sinus syndrome

ECG 85 was obtained in a 62-year-old female with chest discomfort. Sinus rhythm with acute or recent anterior myocardial infarction is present (asterisks). Because a Q wave is absent in lead V_1 (arrow), the infarct should be identified as anterior rather than anteroseptal. Coronary artery disease should also be coded.

Codes:

2a	Sinus rhythm
11b	Anterior Q wave MI, probably acute or recent
12e	ST and/or T wave abnormalities suggesting myocardial injury
14r	Coronary artery disease

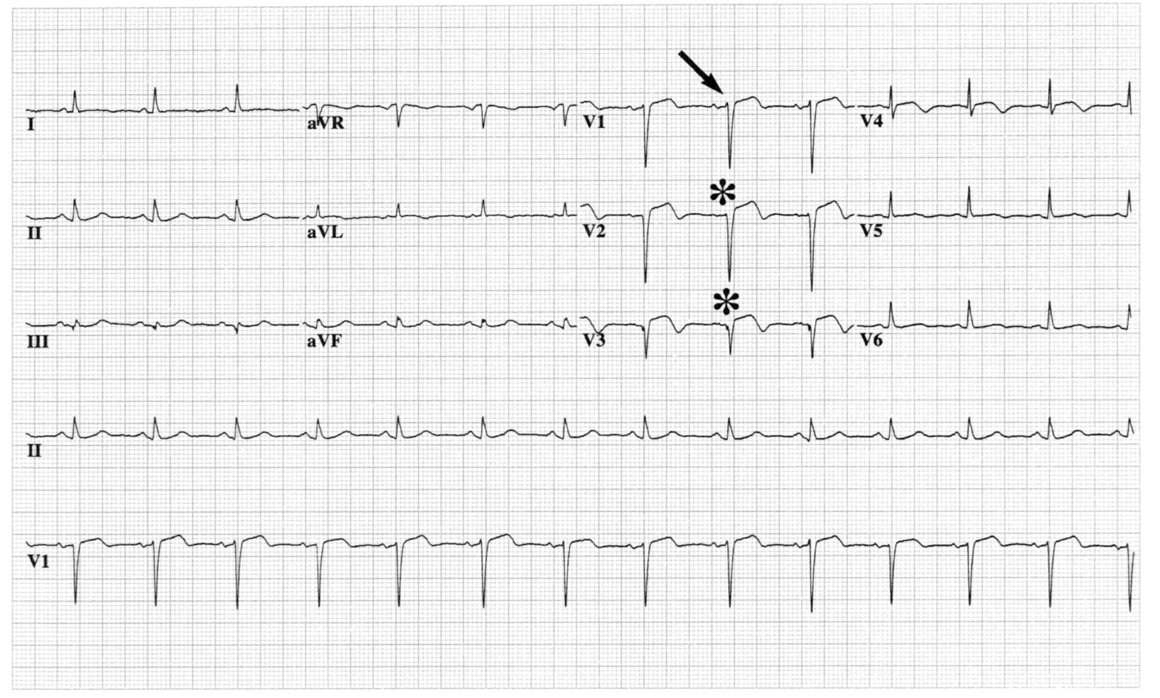

Questions: ECG 85

1. Conditions that can mimic anterior myocardial infarction include:

   a. Amyloid heart disease
   b. Right ventricular hypertrophy
   c. Left ventricular hypertrophy
   d. Left anterior fascicular block

2. To diagnose anteroseptal myocardial infarction, a pathological Q wave must be present in lead V_1:

   a. True
   b. False

Answers: ECG 85

1. Many conditions can result in low or absent anterior forces on the 12-lead ECG and mimic anterior myocardial infarction, including amyloid heart disease, left ventricular hypertrophy, left anterior fascicular block, WPW, chronic lung disease, and LBBB. (Answer: a, c, d)

2. Anteroseptal myocardial infarction requires a pathological Q wave in lead V_1. If Q waves are present in leads V_2-V_4, but not in V_1, anterior rather than anteroseptal myocardial infarction should be coded. (Answer: a)

— *Quick Review* —	
Anterior MI, recent or probably acute	
• rS in lead ____, *followed by* QS or QR complexes (Q wave duration ≥ 0.03 seconds) and ST segment elevation in two of leads ____, *or* (increasing/decreasing) R wave amplitude from V_2-V_5	V_1 V_2-V_4, decreasing
ST and/or T wave changes suggesting myocardial injury	
• Acute ST segment (elevation/depression) with upward (convexity/concavity) in the leads representing the area of infarction	elevation convexity
• T waves invert (before/after) ST segments return to baseline	before
• Associated ST (elevation/depression) in the noninfarct leads is common	depression
• Acute ____ wall injury often has horizontal or downsloping ST segment depression with upright T waves in V_1-V_3, with or without a prominent R wave in these same leads	posterior

ECG 86. 46-year-old female with chest pain:

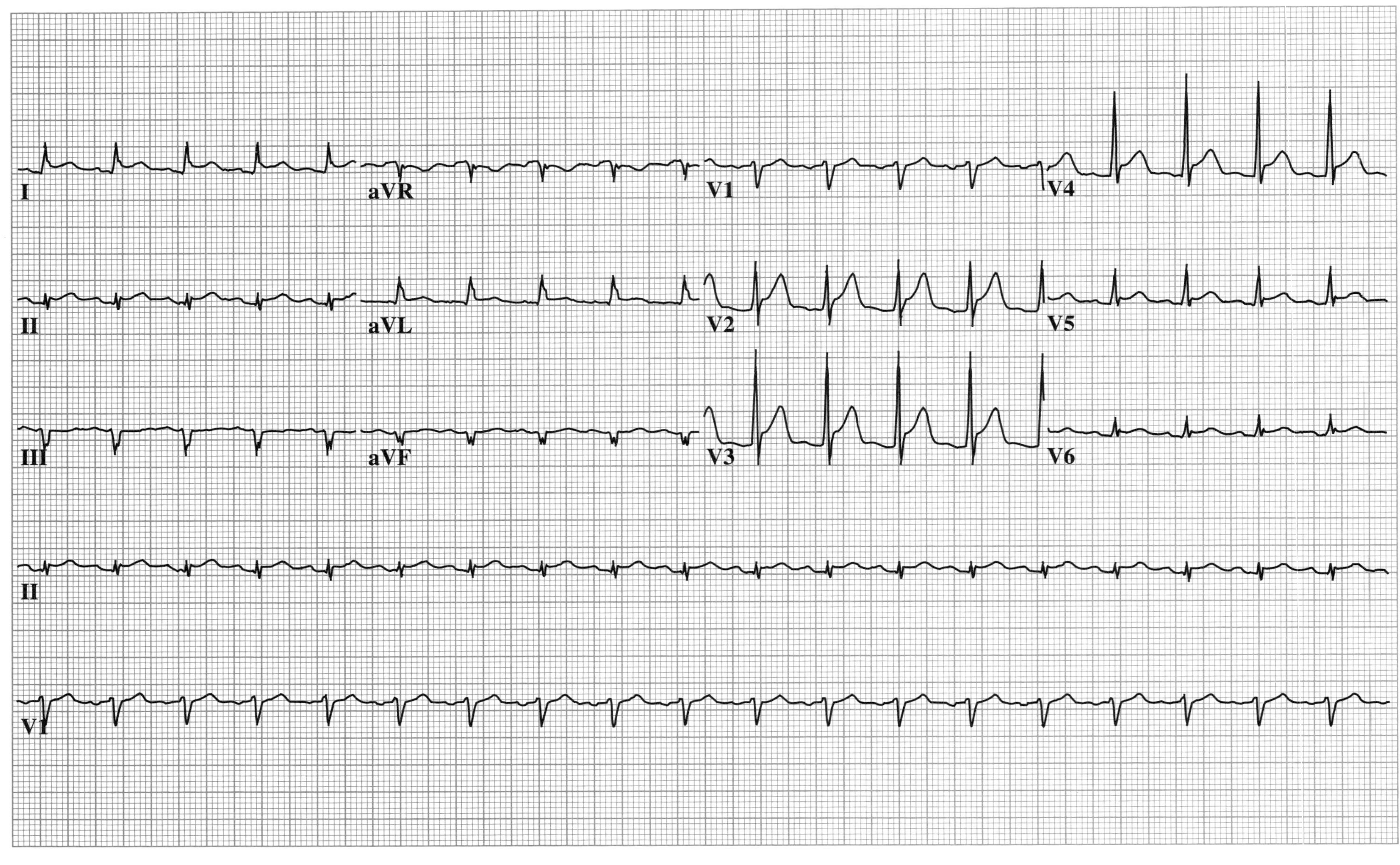

1. GENERAL FEATURES

- ☐ a. Normal ECG
- ☐ b. Borderline normal ECG or normal variant
- ☐ c. Incorrect electrode placement
- ☐ d. Artifact due to tremor

2. ATRIAL RHYTHMS

- ☐ a. Sinus rhythm
- ☐ b. Sinus arrhythmia
- ☐ c. Sinus bradycardia (< 60)
- ☐ d. Sinus tachycardia (> 100)
- ☐ e. Sinus pause or arrest
- ☐ f. Sinoatrial exit block
- ☐ g. Ecoptic atrial rhythm
- ☐ h. Wandering atrial pacemaker
- ☐ i. Atrial premature complexes, normally conducted
- ☐ j. Atrial premature complexes, nonconducted
- ☐ k. Atrial premature complexes with aberrant intraventricular conduction
- ☐ l. Atrial tachycardia (regular, sustained, 1:1 conduction)
- ☐ m. Atrial tachycardia, repetitive (short paroxysms)
- ☐ n. Atrial tachycardia, multifocal
- ☐ o. Atrial tachycardia with AV block
- ☐ p. Supraventricular tachycardia, unspecific
- ☐ q. Supraventricular tachycardia, paroxysmal
- ☐ r. Atrial flutter
- ☐ s. Atrial fibrillation
- ☐ t. Retrograde atrial activation

3. AV JUNCTIONAL RHYTHMS

- ☐ a. AV junctional premature complexes
- ☐ b. AV junctional escape complexes
- ☐ c. AV junctional rhythm, accelerated
- ☐ d. AV junctional rhythm

4. VENTRICULAR RHYTHMS

- ☐ a. Ventricular premature complex(es), uniform, fixed coupling
- ☐ b. Ventricular premature complex(es), uniform, nonfixed coupling
- ☐ c. Ventricular premature complexes(es), multiform
- ☐ d. Ventricular premature complexes, in pairs
- ☐ e. Ventricular parasystole
- ☐ f. Ventricular tachycardia (≥ 3 consecutive complexes)
- ☐ g. Accelerated idioventricular rhythm
- ☐ h. Ventricular escape complexes or rhythm
- ☐ i. Ventricular fibrillation

5. ATRIAL-VENTRICULAR INTERACTIONS IN ARRHYTHMIAS

- ☐ a. Fusion complexes
- ☐ b. Reciprocal (echo) complexes
- ☐ c. Ventricular capture complexes
- ☐ d. AV dissociation
- ☐ e. Ventriculophasic sinus arrhythmia

6. AV CONDUCTION ABNORMALITIES

- ☐ a. AV block, 1°
- ☐ b. AV block, 2° - Mobitz type I (Wenckebach)
- ☐ c. AV block, 2° - Mobitz type II
- ☐ d. AV block, 2:1
- ☐ e. AV block, 3°
- ☐ f. AV block, variable
- ☐ g. Short PR interval (with sinus rhythm and normal QRS duration)
- ☐ h. Wolff-Parkinson-White pattern

7. INTRAVENTRICULAR CONDUCTION DISTURBANCES

- ☐ a. RBBB, incomplete
- ☐ b. RBBB, complete
- ☐ c. Left anterior fascicular block
- ☐ d. Left posterior fascicular block
- ☐ e. LBBB, with ST-T wave suggestive of acute myocardial injury or infarction
- ☐ f. LBBB, complete
- ☐ g. LBBB, intermittent
- ☐ h. Intraventricular conduction disturbance, nonspecific
- ☐ i. Aberrant intraventricular conduction with supraventricular arrhythmia

8. P WAVE ABNORMALITIES

- ☐ a. Right atrial abnormality
- ☐ b. Left atrial abnormalities
- ☐ c. Nonspecific atrial abnormality

9. ABNORMALITIES OF QRS VOLTAGE OR AXIS

- ☐ a. Low voltage, limb leads only
- ☐ b. Low voltage, limb and precordial leads
- ☐ c. Left axis deviation (> - 30%)
- ☐ d. Right axis deviation (> + 100)
- ☐ e. Electrical alternans

10. VENTRICULAR HYPERTROPHY

- ☐ a. LVH by voltage only
- ☐ b. LVH by voltage and ST-T segment abnormalities
- ☐ c. RVH
- ☐ d. Combined ventricular hypertrophy

11. Q WAVE MYOCARDIAL INFARCTION

	Probably Acute or Recent	Probably Old or Age Indeterminate
Anterolateral	☐ a.	☐ g.
Anterior	☐ b.	☐ h.
Anteroseptal	☐ c.	☐ i.
Lateral/High lateral	☐ d.	☐ j.
Inferior	☐ e.	☐ k.
Posterior	☐ f.	☐ l.

- ☐ m. Probably ventricular aneurysm

12. ST, T, U, WAVE ABNORMALITIES

- ☐ a. Normal variant, early repolarization
- ☐ b. Normal variant, juvenile T waves
- ☐ c. Nonspecific ST and/or T wave abnormalities
- ☐ d. ST and/or T wave abnormalities suggesting myocardial ischemia
- ☐ e. ST and/or T wave abnormalities suggesting myocardial injury
- ☐ f. ST and/or T wave abnormalities suggesting acute pericarditis
- ☐ g. ST-T segment abnormalities secondary to intraventricular conduction disturbance or hypertrophy
- ☐ h. Post-extrasystolic T wave abnormality
- ☐ i. Isolated J point depression
- ☐ j. Peaked T waves
- ☐ k. Prolonged QT interval
- ☐ l. Prominent U waves

13. PACEMAKER FUNCTION AND RHYTHM

- ☐ a. Atrial or coronary sinus pacing
- ☐ b. Ventricular demand pacing
- ☐ c. AV sequential pacing
- ☐ d. Ventricular pacing, complete control
- ☐ e. Dual chamber, atrial sensing pacemaker
- ☐ f. Pacemaker malfunction, not constantly capturing (atrium or ventricle)
- ☐ g. Pacemaker malfunction, not constantly sensing (atrium or ventricle)
- ☐ h. Pacemaker malfunction, not firing
- ☐ i. Pacemaker malfunction, slowing

14. SUGGESTED OR PROBABLE CLINICAL DISORDERS

- ☐ a. Digitalis effect
- ☐ b. Digitalis toxicity
- ☐ c. Antiarrhythmic drug effect
- ☐ d. Antiarrhythmic drug toxicity
- ☐ e. Hyperkalemia
- ☐ f. Hypokalemia
- ☐ g. Hypercalcemia
- ☐ h. Hypocalcemia
- ☐ i. Atrial septal defect, secundum
- ☐ j. Atrial septal defect, primum
- ☐ k. Dextrocardia, mirror image
- ☐ l. Mitral valve disease
- ☐ m. Chronic lung disease
- ☐ n. Acute cor pulmonale, including pulmonary embolus
- ☐ o. Pericardial effusion
- ☐ p. Acute pericarditis
- ☐ q. Hypertrophic cardiomyopathy
- ☐ r. Coronary artery disease
- ☐ s. Central nervous system disorder
- ☐ t. Myxedema
- ☐ u. Hypothermia
- ☐ v. Sick sinus syndrome

ECG 86 was obtained in a 46-year-old female with complaints of chest pain. The ECG shows sinus tachycardia with diffuse ST segment elevation (arrows) and some associated PR depression (relative to the TP segment; arrowheads mark PR depression). These findings are consistent with acute pericarditis. The diffuse nature of the ST segment elevation in the absence of Q waves, the upwardly concave configuration of the ST segments, and the PR depression (most noticeable in leads V_2 and V_3) all suggest a pericardial process rather than an acute ischemic process. Subtle electrical alternans is noted in lead V_4 (asterisk), which is likely due to pericardial effusion.

Codes:

2d	Sinus tachycardia
9e	Electrical alternans
12f	ST and/or T wave abnormalities suggesting acute pericarditis
14o	Pericardial effusion
14p	Acute pericarditis

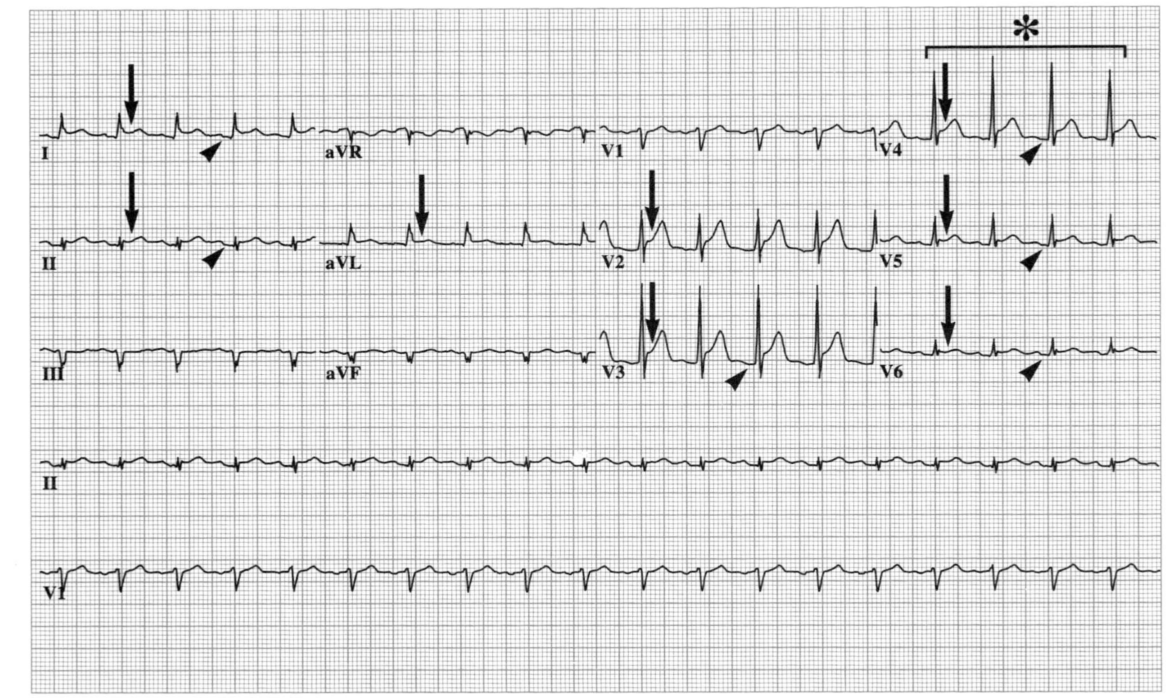

Questions: ECG 86

1. Is the present ECG consistent with the diagnosis of early repolarization?

   a. Yes
   b. No

2. Which of the following statements about pericarditis are true?

   a. The P wave usually diminishes in amplitude
   b. PR segment depression is common, and is usually present in all leads
   c. Electrical alternans is a common and specific finding for pericardial effusion
   d. T wave inversion begins while the ST segments are still elevated

Answers: ECG 86

1. The tracing is consistent with early repolarization (neither the PR depression, which can sometimes be seen on normal ECGs, nor the sinus tachycardia excludes this diagnosis). However, acute pericarditis is far and away the most likely diagnosis in a patient with pleuritic chest pain. (Answer: a)

2. The typical evolutionary pattern of ST and T wave changes associated with pericarditis include: (1) diffuse ST elevation (except for ST depression in aVR); (2) return of the ST segment to baseline with decreasing T wave amplitude; (3) T wave inversion; and (4) return of the ECG to normal. However, pericarditis may be focal (e.g., post-pericardiotomy) rather than diffuse, and result in regional rather than diffuse ST elevation. Also, classic ST and T wave changes are more likely to occur in purulent compared to idiopathic, rheumatic, or malignant pericarditis. Pericarditis does not typically affect P wave amplitude or contour, although P wave alternans may occur if pericardial effusion is present. While PR depression is common and often diffuse, it is typically ***elevated*** in lead aVR. Electrical alternans is present in a minority of patients with pericardial effusion. Likewise, pericardial effusion is present in less than 50% of patients with electrical alternans. Finally, in pericarditis, T wave inversion occurs ***after*** the ST segment returns to baseline, while in myocardial infarction, T wave inversion typically begins while the ST segment is still elevated. (Answer:

none)

— Quick Review 86 —

ST and/or T wave changes suggesting acute pericarditis	
• Classic evolutionary pattern consists of ____ stages	4
▸ Stage 1: Upwardly concave ST segment ____ in almost all leads	elevation
▸ Stage 2: ST junction (J point) returns to baseline and T wave amplitude begins to (increase/decrease)	decrease
▸ Stage 3: T waves (invert/remain upright)	invert
▸ Stage 4: ECG (does/does not) return to normal	does
• Other clues to acute pericarditis:	
▸ Sinus ____	tachycardia
▸ PR ____ early (PR elevation in aVR)	depression
▸ (High/low) voltage QRS	low
▸ Electrical alternans if pericardial ____ is present	effusion
Pericardial effusion	
• (High/low) voltage QRS	Low
• Electrical ____, especially if complicated by cardiac ____	alternans tamponade
• Other features of acute ____ may also be present	pericarditis

Don't Forget!

Age of myocardial infarction can be approximated from the ECG pattern:

- Acute MI: Abnormal Q waves, ST elevation (associated ST depression is sometimes present in noninfarct leads)
- Recent MI: Abnormal Q waves, isoelectric ST segments, ischemic (usually inverted) T waves
- Old MI: Abnormal Q waves, isoelectric ST segments, nonspecific or normal T waves

MI may be present without Q waves in:

- Anterior MI: May only see low anterior R wave forces with decreasing R wave progression in leads V_2-V_5
- Posterior MI: Dominant R wave and ST depression in leads V_1-V_3

RVH (item 10c), WPW (item 6h), and RBBB (item 7b) interfere with the ECG diagnosis of posterior MI

ECG 87. 83-year-old male with cardiomegaly and dyspnea on exertion:

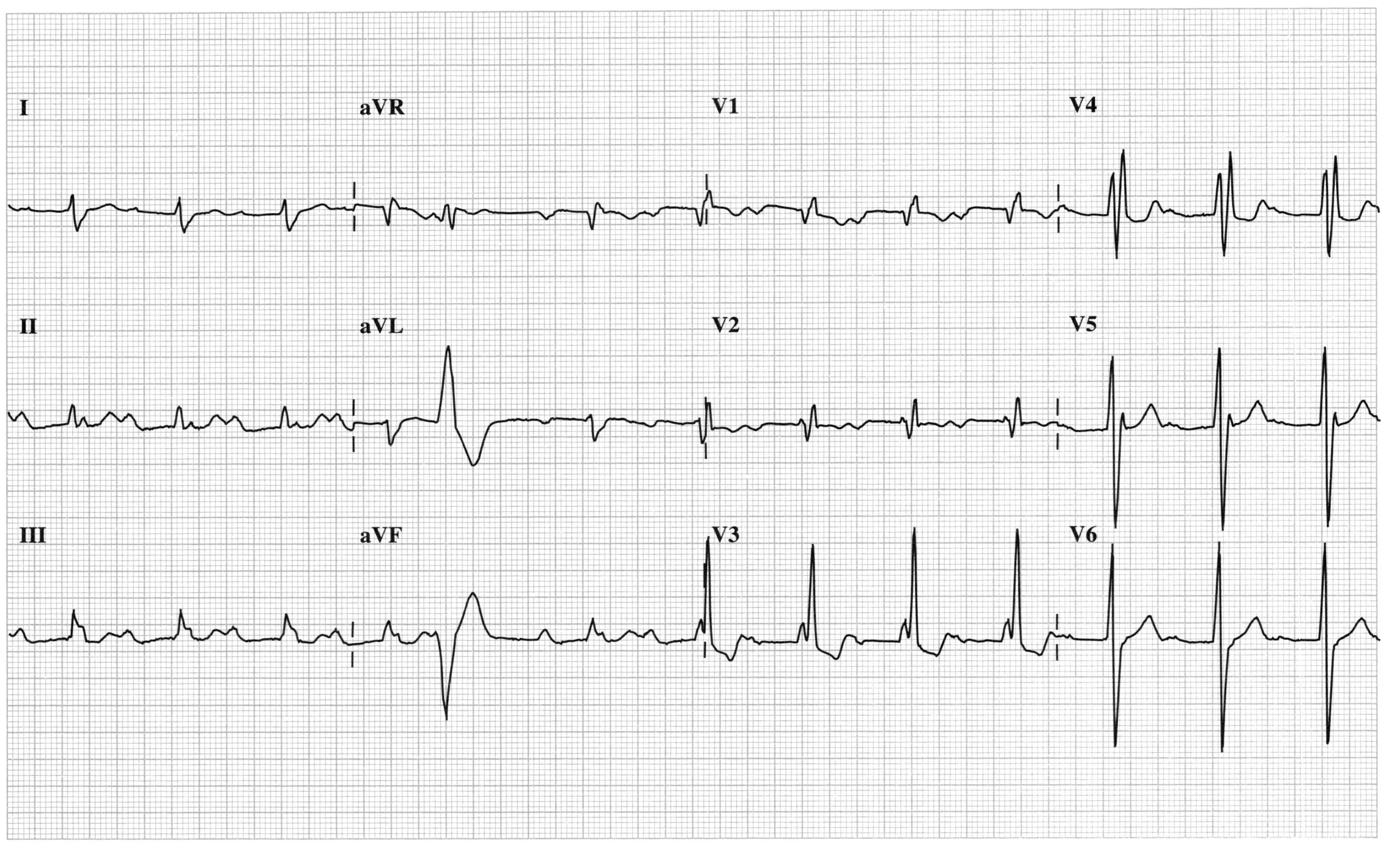

1. GENERAL FEATURES

☐ a. Normal ECG
☐ b. Borderline normal ECG or normal variant
☐ c. Incorrect electrode placement
☐ d. Artifact due to tremor

2. ATRIAL RHYTHMS

☐ a. Sinus rhythm
☐ b. Sinus arrhythmia
☐ c. Sinus bradycardia (< 60)
☐ d. Sinus tachycardia (> 100)
☐ e. Sinus pause or arrest
☐ f. Sinoatrial exit block
☐ g. Ecoptic atrial rhythm
☐ h. Wandering atrial pacemaker
☐ i. Atrial premature complexes, normally conducted
☐ j. Atrial premature complexes, nonconducted
☐ k. Atrial premature complexes with aberrant intraventricular conduction
☐ l. Atrial tachycardia (regular, sustained, 1:1 conduction)
☐ m. Atrial tachycardia, repetitive (short paroxysms)
☐ n. Atrial tachycardia, multifocal
☐ o. Atrial tachycardia with AV block
☐ p. Supraventricular tachycardia, unspecific
☐ q. Supraventricular tachycardia, paroxysmal
☐ r. Atrial flutter
☐ s. Atrial fibrillation
☐ t. Retrograde atrial activation

3. AV JUNCTIONAL RHYTHMS

☐ a. AV junctional premature complexes
☐ b. AV junctional escape complexes
☐ c. AV junctional rhythm, accelerated
☐ d. AV junctional rhythm

4. VENTRICULAR RHYTHMS

☐ a. Ventricular premature complex(es), uniform, fixed coupling
☐ b. Ventricular premature complex(es), uniform, nonfixed coupling
☐ c. Ventricular premature complexes(es), multiform
☐ d. Ventricular premature complexes, in pairs
☐ e. Ventricular parasystole
☐ f. Ventricular tachycardia (≥ 3 consecutive complexes)
☐ g. Accelerated idioventricular rhythm
☐ h. Ventricular escape complexes or rhythm
☐ i. Ventricular fibrillation

5. ATRIAL-VENTRICULAR INTERACTIONS IN ARRHYTHMIAS

☐ a. Fusion complexes
☐ b. Reciprocal (echo) complexes
☐ c. Ventricular capture complexes
☐ d. AV dissociation
☐ e. Ventriculophasic sinus arrhythmia

6. AV CONDUCTION ABNORMALITIES

☐ a. AV block, 1°
☐ b. AV block, 2° - Mobitz type I (Wenckebach)
☐ c. AV block, 2° - Mobitz type II
☐ d. AV block, 2:1
☐ e. AV block, 3°
☐ f. AV block, variable
☐ g. Short PR interval (with sinus rhythm and normal QRS duration)
☐ h. Wolff-Parkinson-White pattern

7. INTRAVENTRICULAR CONDUCTION DISTURBANCES

☐ a. RBBB, incomplete
☐ b. RBBB, complete
☐ c. Left anterior fascicular block
☐ d. Left posterior fascicular block
☐ e. LBBB, with ST-T wave suggestive of acute myocardial injury or infarction
☐ f. LBBB, complete
☐ g. LBBB, intermittent
☐ h. Intraventricular conduction disturbance, nonspecific
☐ i. Aberrant intraventricular conduction with supraventricular arrhythmia

8. P WAVE ABNORMALITIES

☐ a. Right atrial abnormality
☐ b. Left atrial abnormalities
☐ c. Nonspecific atrial abnormality

9. ABNORMALITIES OF QRS VOLTAGE OR AXIS

☐ a. Low voltage, limb leads only
☐ b. Low voltage, limb and precordial leads
☐ c. Left axis deviation (> - 30%)
☐ d. Right axis deviation (> + 100)
☐ e. Electrical alternans

10. VENTRICULAR HYPERTROPHY

☐ a. LVH by voltage only
☐ b. LVH by voltage and ST-T segment abnormalities
☐ c. RVH
☐ d. Combined ventricular hypertrophy

11. Q WAVE MYOCARDIAL INFARCTION

	Probably Acute or Recent	Probably Old or Age Indeterminate
Anterolateral	☐ a.	☐ g.
Anterior	☐ b.	☐ h.
Anteroseptal	☐ c.	☐ i.
Lateral/High lateral	☐ d.	☐ j.
Inferior	☐ e.	☐ k.
Posterior	☐ f.	☐ l.

☐ m. Probably ventricular aneurysm

12. ST, T, U, WAVE ABNORMALITIES

☐ a. Normal variant, early repolarization
☐ b. Normal variant, juvenile T waves
☐ c. Nonspecific ST and/or T wave abnormalities
☐ d. ST and/or T wave abnormalities suggesting myocardial ischemia
☐ e. ST and/or T wave abnormalities suggesting myocardial injury
☐ f. ST and/or T wave abnormalities suggesting acute pericarditis
☐ g. ST-T segment abnormalities secondary to intraventricular conduction disturbance or hypertrophy
☐ h. Post-extrasystolic T wave abnormality
☐ i. Isolated J point depression
☐ j. Peaked T waves
☐ k. Prolonged QT interval
☐ l. Prominent U waves

13. PACEMAKER FUNCTION AND RHYTHM

☐ a. Atrial or coronary sinus pacing
☐ b. Ventricular demand pacing
☐ c. AV sequential pacing
☐ d. Ventricular pacing, complete control
☐ e. Dual chamber, atrial sensing pacemaker
☐ f. Pacemaker malfunction, not constantly capturing (atrium or ventricle)
☐ g. Pacemaker malfunction, not constantly sensing (atrium or ventricle)
☐ h. Pacemaker malfunction, not firing
☐ i. Pacemaker malfunction, slowing

14. SUGGESTED OR PROBABLE CLINICAL DISORDERS

☐ a. Digitalis effect
☐ b. Digitalis toxicity
☐ c. Antiarrhythmic drug effect
☐ d. Antiarrhythmic drug toxicity
☐ e. Hyperkalemia
☐ f. Hypokalemia
☐ g. Hypercalcemia
☐ h. Hypocalcemia
☐ i. Atrial septal defect, secundum
☐ j. Atrial septal defect, primum
☐ k. Dextrocardia, mirror image
☐ l. Mitral valve disease
☐ m. Chronic lung disease
☐ n. Acute cor pulmonale, including pulmonary embolus
☐ o. Pericardial effusion
☐ p. Acute pericarditis
☐ q. Hypertrophic cardiomyopathy
☐ r. Coronary artery disease
☐ s. Central nervous system disorder
☐ t. Myxedema
☐ u. Hypothermia
☐ v. Sick sinus syndrome

ECG 87 was obtained in an 83-year-old male with cardiomegaly on chest x-ray and dyspnea on exertion. The ECG shows normal sinus rhythm with first-degree AV block and left atrial abnormality (arrowheads mark P waves in V_1). Also noted are right axis deviation due to left posterior fascicular block), a single ventricular premature complex (asterisk), and RBBB (arrows mark wide rSR' complexes in V_1 and V_2, and wide S waves in I, aVL, V_5, V_6) with associated ST-T abnormalities.

Codes:

2a	Sinus rhythm
4a	Ventricular premature complex(es), uniform, fixed coupling
6a	AV block, 1°
7b	RBBB, complete
7d	Left posterior fascicular block
8b	Left atrial abnormality
9d	Right axis deviation (> + 100°)
12g	ST-T segment abnormalities secondary to IVCD or hypertrophy

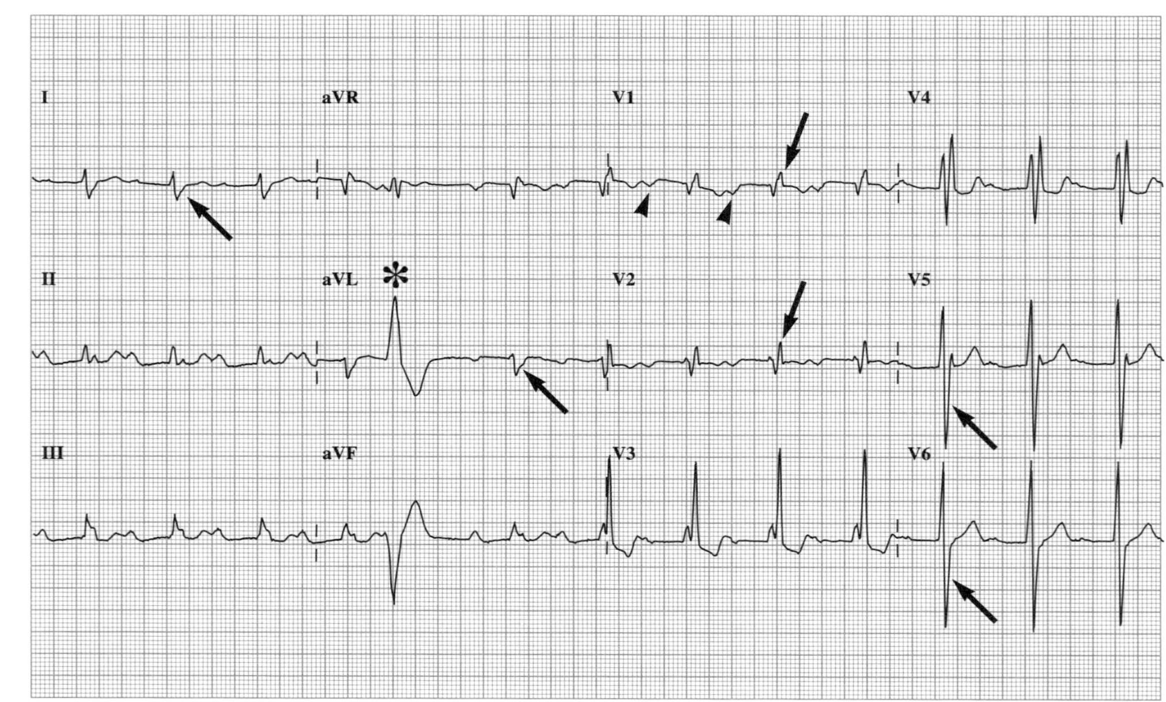

Questions: ECG 87

1. An rSr' pattern in leads V_1 and V_2 with a QRS duration < 0.09 seconds is most appropriately coded as:

   a. RBBB
   b. Incomplete RBBB
   c. Nonspecific intraventricular conduction disturbance
   d. Normal variant

2. Right axis deviation can be seen in:

   a. LVH
   b. Pulmonary embolism
   c. Obese individuals
   d. Thin individuals

Answers: ECG 87

1. A RBBB-like QRS pattern in leads V_1 and V_2 with a normal QRS duration is considered a normal variant finding. Incomplete RBBB should be coded when a typical RBBB pattern is present and the QRS duration is ≥ 0.09 but < 0.12 seconds; RBBB is coded when the QRS duration is ≥0.12 seconds. A nonspecific intraventricular conduction defect requires a QRS duration of ≥ 0.11 seconds that does not meet the morphological criteria for RBBB or LBBB. (Answer: d)

2. Right axis deviation is a common ECG finding and can be seen in the setting of acute pulmonary embolism, right ventricular hypertrophy, chronic obstructive pulmonary disease, and left posterior fascicular block. Right axis deviation may also be seen in thin individuals with a "vertical heart." In contrast, obese individuals are more likely to have a "horizontal heart" and tend to have leftward shift of the QRS axis. LVH is associated with a normal or leftward axis. (Answer: b, d)

— Quick Review 87 —

Ventricular premature complex(es), uniform, fixed coupling	
• A wide, notched or slurred ____ complex that is premature relative to the normal RR interval and is not preceded by a ____ wave	QRS P
• QRS duration is almost always > ____ seconds	0.12
• Initial direction of the QRS is often (similar to/different from) the QRS during sinus rhythm	different from
• Secondary ST & T wave changes in the (same/opposite) direction as the major deflection of the QRS (i.e., ST depression & T wave inversion in leads with a dominant _____wave; ST elevation and upright T wave in leads with a dominant _____ wave or ____ complex)	opposite R S QS
• Coupling interval is constant or varies by < ____ seconds	0.08
• Morphology of VPCs in any given lead is (the same/different)	the same
• Retrograde capture of atria may occur (true/false)	true
• A full ____ pause (PP interval containing the VPC is twice the normal PP interval) is usually evident	compensatory
Left posterior fascicular block	
• ____ axis deviation with a mean QRS axis between ____ and ____ degrees	right +100, +180
• ____ wave in lead I and ____ wave in lead III	s, q
• Normal or slightly prolonged QRS duration (true/false)	true
• No other cause for right axis deviation should be present (true/false)	true

Common Dilemmas in ECG Interpretation

Problem

With so many different criteria for the diagnosis of LVH, which should be used as the “gold-standard?”

Recommendation

The Cornell criteria (R wave in aVL + S wave in V_3 > than 24 mm in males and > 20 mm in females) is probably the most accurate of the voltage criteria. However, many ECGs meet voltage criteria in one area of the tracing but not in the others. Therefore, the best policy is know most or all of the various criteria used for the diagnosis of LVH. Remember to code item 10b (LVH with ST-T abnormalities) *and* item 12g (ST-T abnormalities secondary to IVCD or hypertrophy) when LVH with a “strain” pattern is present.

ECG 88. 78-year-old female with chest tightness three days ago:

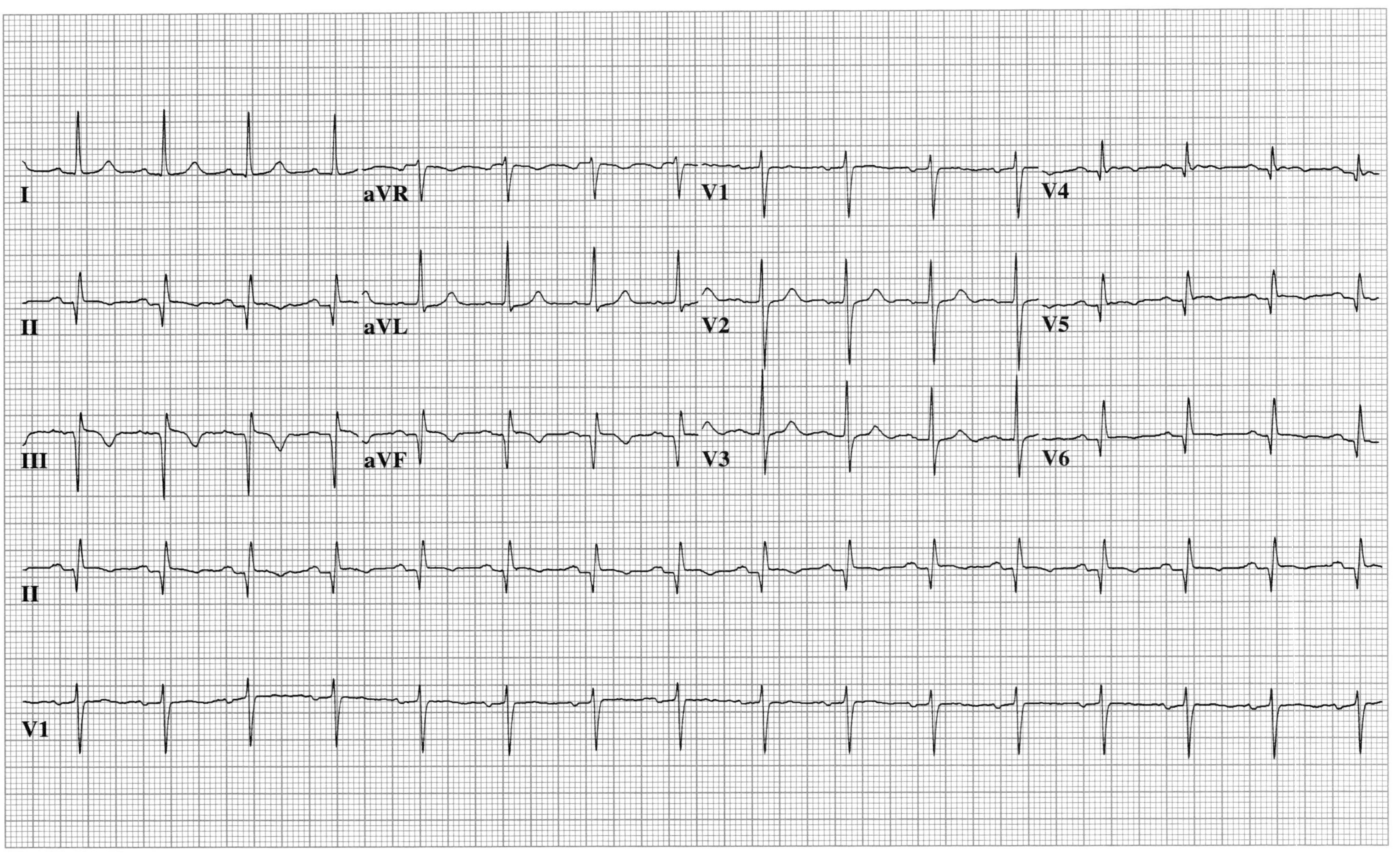

1. GENERAL FEATURES

- ☐ a. Normal ECG
- ☐ b. Borderline normal ECG or normal variant
- ☐ c. Incorrect electrode placement
- ☐ d. Artifact due to tremor

2. ATRIAL RHYTHMS

- ☐ a. Sinus rhythm
- ☐ b. Sinus arrhythmia
- ☐ c. Sinus bradycardia (< 60)
- ☐ d. Sinus tachycardia (> 100)
- ☐ e. Sinus pause or arrest
- ☐ f. Sinoatrial exit block
- ☐ g. Ecoptic atrial rhythm
- ☐ h. Wandering atrial pacemaker
- ☐ i. Atrial premature complexes, normally conducted
- ☐ j. Atrial premature complexes, nonconducted
- ☐ k. Atrial premature complexes with aberrant intraventricular conduction
- ☐ l. Atrial tachycardia (regular, sustained, 1:1 conduction)
- ☐ m. Atrial tachycardia, repetitive (short paroxysms)
- ☐ n. Atrial tachycardia, multifocal
- ☐ o. Atrial tachycardia with AV block
- ☐ p. Supraventricular tachycardia, unspecific
- ☐ q. Supraventricular tachycardia, paroxysmal
- ☐ r. Atrial flutter
- ☐ s. Atrial fibrillation
- ☐ t. Retrograde atrial activation

3. AV JUNCTIONAL RHYTHMS

- ☐ a. AV junctional premature complexes
- ☐ b. AV junctional escape complexes
- ☐ c. AV junctional rhythm, accelerated
- ☐ d. AV junctional rhythm

4. VENTRICULAR RHYTHMS

- ☐ a. Ventricular premature complex(es), uniform, fixed coupling
- ☐ b. Ventricular premature complex(es), uniform, nonfixed coupling
- ☐ c. Ventricular premature complexes(es), multiform
- ☐ d. Ventricular premature complexes, in pairs
- ☐ e. Ventricular parasystole
- ☐ f. Ventricular tachycardia (≥ 3 consecutive complexes)
- ☐ g. Accelerated idioventricular rhythm
- ☐ h. Ventricular escape complexes or rhythm
- ☐ i. Ventricular fibrillation

5. ATRIAL-VENTRICULAR INTERACTIONS IN ARRHYTHMIAS

- ☐ a. Fusion complexes
- ☐ b. Reciprocal (echo) complexes
- ☐ c. Ventricular capture complexes
- ☐ d. AV dissociation
- ☐ e. Ventriculophasic sinus arrhythmia

6. AV CONDUCTION ABNORMALITIES

- ☐ a. AV block, 1°
- ☐ b. AV block, 2° - Mobitz type I (Wenckebach)
- ☐ c. AV block, 2° - Mobitz type II
- ☐ d. AV block, 2:1
- ☐ e. AV block, 3°
- ☐ f. AV block, variable
- ☐ g. Short PR interval (with sinus rhythm and normal QRS duration)
- ☐ h. Wolff-Parkinson-White pattern

7. INTRAVENTRICULAR CONDUCTION DISTURBANCES

- ☐ a. RBBB, incomplete
- ☐ b. RBBB, complete
- ☐ c. Left anterior fascicular block
- ☐ d. Left posterior fascicular block
- ☐ e. LBBB, with ST-T wave suggestive of acute myocardial injury or infarction
- ☐ f. LBBB, complete
- ☐ g. LBBB, intermittent
- ☐ h. Intraventricular conduction disturbance, nonspecific
- ☐ i. Aberrant intraventricular conduction with supraventricular arrhythmia

8. P WAVE ABNORMALITIES

- ☐ a. Right atrial abnormality
- ☐ b. Left atrial abnormalities
- ☐ c. Nonspecific atrial abnormality

9. ABNORMALITIES OF QRS VOLTAGE OR AXIS

- ☐ a. Low voltage, limb leads only
- ☐ b. Low voltage, limb and precordial leads
- ☐ c. Left axis deviation (> - 30%)
- ☐ d. Right axis deviation (> + 100)
- ☐ e. Electrical alternans

10. VENTRICULAR HYPERTROPHY

- ☐ a. LVH by voltage only
- ☐ b. LVH by voltage and ST-T segment abnormalities
- ☐ c. RVH
- ☐ d. Combined ventricular hypertrophy

11. Q WAVE MYOCARDIAL INFARCTION

	Probably Acute or Recent	Probably Old or Age Indeterminate
Anterolateral	☐ a.	☐ g.
Anterior	☐ b.	☐ h.
Anteroseptal	☐ c.	☐ i.
Lateral/High lateral	☐ d.	☐ j.
Inferior	☐ e.	☐ k.
Posterior	☐ f.	☐ l.

☐ m. Probably ventricular aneurysm

12. ST, T, U, WAVE ABNORMALITIES

- ☐ a. Normal variant, early repolarization
- ☐ b. Normal variant, juvenile T waves
- ☐ c. Nonspecific ST and/or T wave abnormalities
- ☐ d. ST and/or T wave abnormalities suggesting myocardial ischemia
- ☐ e. ST and/or T wave abnormalities suggesting myocardial injury
- ☐ f. ST and/or T wave abnormalities suggesting acute pericarditis
- ☐ g. ST-T segment abnormalities secondary to intraventricular conduction disturbance or hypertrophy
- ☐ h. Post-extrasystolic T wave abnormality
- ☐ i. Isolated J point depression
- ☐ j. Peaked T waves
- ☐ k. Prolonged QT interval
- ☐ l. Prominent U waves

13. PACEMAKER FUNCTION AND RHYTHM

- ☐ a. Atrial or coronary sinus pacing
- ☐ b. Ventricular demand pacing
- ☐ c. AV sequential pacing
- ☐ d. Ventricular pacing, complete control
- ☐ e. Dual chamber, atrial sensing pacemaker
- ☐ f. Pacemaker malfunction, not constantly capturing (atrium or ventricle)
- ☐ g. Pacemaker malfunction, not constantly sensing (atrium or ventricle)
- ☐ h. Pacemaker malfunction, not firing
- ☐ i. Pacemaker malfunction, slowing

14. SUGGESTED OR PROBABLE CLINICAL DISORDERS

- ☐ a. Digitalis effect
- ☐ b. Digitalis toxicity
- ☐ c. Antiarrhythmic drug effect
- ☐ d. Antiarrhythmic drug toxicity
- ☐ e. Hyperkalemia
- ☐ f. Hypokalemia
- ☐ g. Hypercalcemia
- ☐ h. Hypocalcemia
- ☐ i. Atrial septal defect, secundum
- ☐ j. Atrial septal defect, primum
- ☐ k. Dextrocardia, mirror image
- ☐ l. Mitral valve disease
- ☐ m. Chronic lung disease
- ☐ n. Acute cor pulmonale, including pulmonary embolus
- ☐ o. Pericardial effusion
- ☐ p. Acute pericarditis
- ☐ q. Hypertrophic cardiomyopathy
- ☐ r. Coronary artery disease
- ☐ s. Central nervous system disorder
- ☐ t. Myxedema
- ☐ u. Hypothermia
- ☐ v. Sick sinus syndrome

ECG 88 was obtained in a 78-year-old asymptomatic female with chest tightness three days ago. The ECG shows a sinus rhythm with Q waves and ST-T changes to suggest recent inferior (arrows) and anterolateral myocardial infarctions (arrowheads). The ST-T changes are most appropriately coded as consistent with ischemia. Coronary artery disease should also be coded.

Codes:

2a	Sinus rhythm
11a	Anterolateral Q wave MI, probably acute or recent
11e	Inferior Q wave MI, probably acute or recent
12e	ST and/or T wave abnormalities suggesting myocardial injury
14r	Coronary artery disease

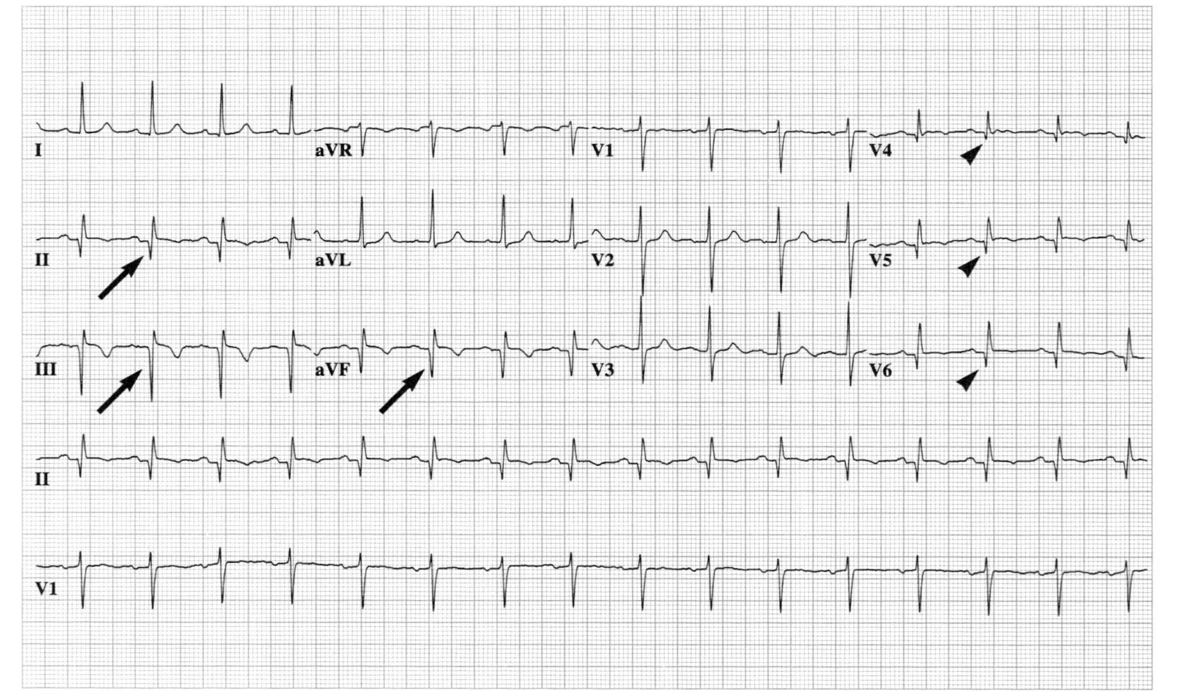

Questions: ECG 88

1. Which of the following statements about acute myocardial infarction are true?

   a. Abnormal Q waves always persist indefinitely
   b. T wave inversion begins while the ST segments are still elevated
   c. The presence of an abnormal Q wave signifies the presence of transmural infarction
   d. Acute myocardial infarction can occur without significant ST segment elevation or depression

Answers: ECG 88

1. Abnormal Q waves regress or disappear over months to years in up to 20% of patients with Q wave MI. Q wave MI, once considered the ECG hallmark of transmural MI, has clearly been shown to occur in subendocardial infarction as well. T wave inversion typically begins while the ST segments are still elevated (in contrast to pericarditis). Finally, acute infarction can occur without significant ST segment elevation or depression; up to 40% of patients with acute occlusion of the left circumflex coronary artery and 10-15% of patients with RCA or LAD occlusions may not have significant ECG changes. (Answer: b, d)

— Quick Review 88 —

Anterolateral MI, probably acute or recent	
• Abnormal Q waves (duration ≥ 0.03 seconds) and ST segment elevation in leads ____	V_4-V_6
Inferior MI, probably acute or recent	
• Abnormal Q waves and ST elevation in at least two of leads ____	II, III, aVF
• Associated ST depression is usually evident in leads I, aVL, V_1-V_3 (true/false)	true

ECG 89. 56-year-old female with breast cancer, shortness of breath, and weakness:

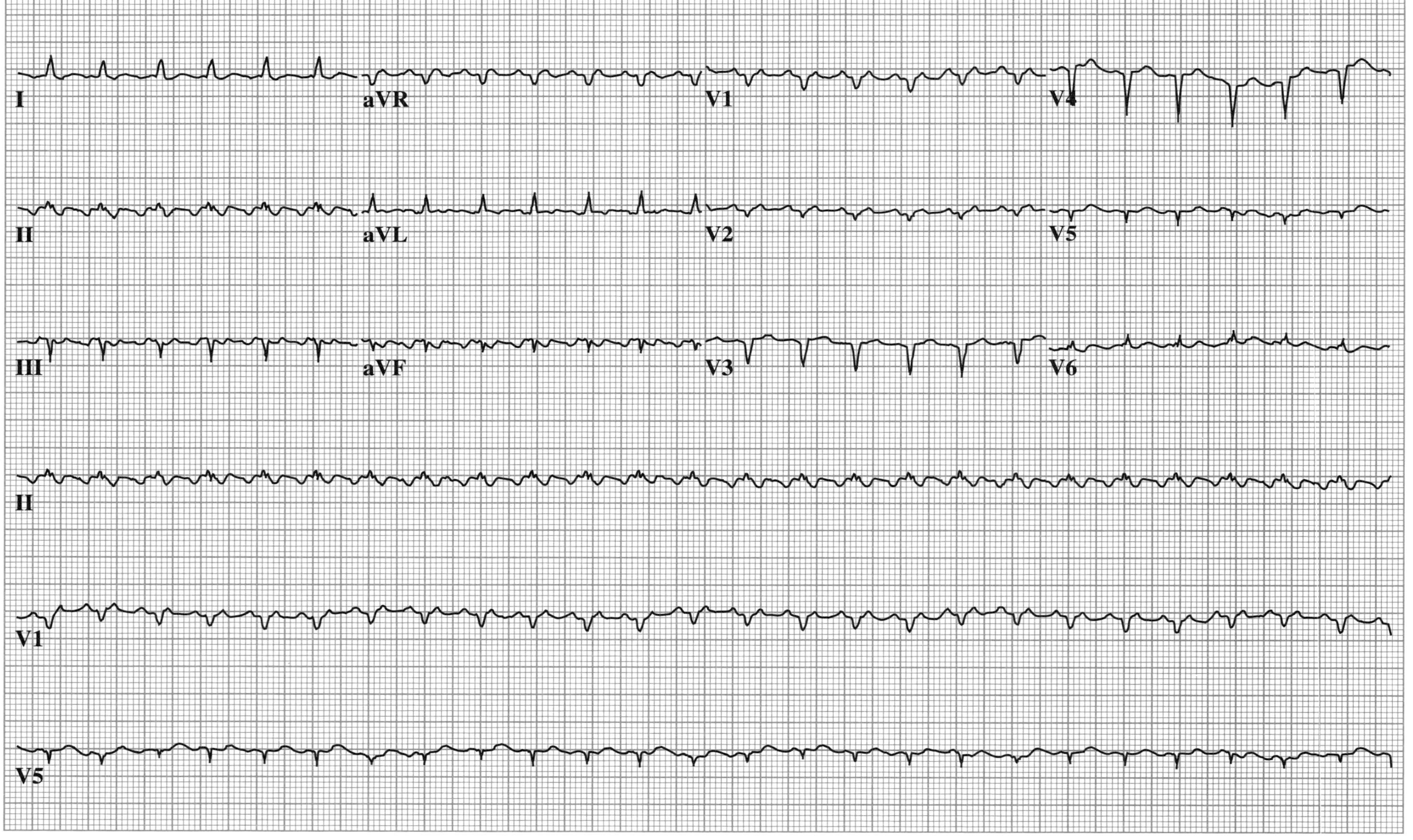

1. GENERAL FEATURES

- ☐ a. Normal ECG
- ☐ b. Borderline normal ECG or normal variant
- ☐ c. Incorrect electrode placement
- ☐ d. Artifact due to tremor

2. ATRIAL RHYTHMS

- ☐ a. Sinus rhythm
- ☐ b. Sinus arrhythmia
- ☐ c. Sinus bradycardia (< 60)
- ☐ d. Sinus tachycardia (> 100)
- ☐ e. Sinus pause or arrest
- ☐ f. Sinoatrial exit block
- ☐ g. Ecoptic atrial rhythm
- ☐ h. Wandering atrial pacemaker
- ☐ i. Atrial premature complexes, normally conducted
- ☐ j. Atrial premature complexes, nonconducted
- ☐ k. Atrial premature complexes with aberrant intraventricular conduction
- ☐ l. Atrial tachycardia (regular, sustained, 1:1 conduction)
- ☐ m. Atrial tachycardia, repetitive (short paroxysms)
- ☐ n. Atrial tachycardia, multifocal
- ☐ o. Atrial tachycardia with AV block
- ☐ p. Supraventricular tachycardia, unspecific
- ☐ q. Supraventricular tachycardia, paroxysmal
- ☐ r. Atrial flutter
- ☐ s. Atrial fibrillation
- ☐ t. Retrograde atrial activation

3. AV JUNCTIONAL RHYTHMS

- ☐ a. AV junctional premature complexes
- ☐ b. AV junctional escape complexes
- ☐ c. AV junctional rhythm, accelerated
- ☐ d. AV junctional rhythm

4. VENTRICULAR RHYTHMS

- ☐ a. Ventricular premature complex(es), uniform, fixed coupling
- ☐ b. Ventricular premature complex(es), uniform, nonfixed coupling
- ☐ c. Ventricular premature complexes(es), multiform
- ☐ d. Ventricular premature complexes, in pairs
- ☐ e. Ventricular parasystole
- ☐ f. Ventricular tachycardia (≥ 3 consecutive complexes)
- ☐ g. Accelerated idioventricular rhythm
- ☐ h. Ventricular escape complexes or rhythm
- ☐ i. Ventricular fibrillation

5. ATRIAL-VENTRICULAR INTERACTIONS IN ARRHYTHMIAS

- ☐ a. Fusion complexes
- ☐ b. Reciprocal (echo) complexes
- ☐ c. Ventricular capture complexes
- ☐ d. AV dissociation
- ☐ e. Ventriculophasic sinus arrhythmia

6. AV CONDUCTION ABNORMALITIES

- ☐ a. AV block, 1°
- ☐ b. AV block, 2° - Mobitz type I (Wenckebach)
- ☐ c. AV block, 2° - Mobitz type II
- ☐ d. AV block, 2:1
- ☐ e. AV block, 3°
- ☐ f. AV block, variable
- ☐ g. Short PR interval (with sinus rhythm and normal QRS duration)
- ☐ h. Wolff-Parkinson-White pattern

7. INTRAVENTRICULAR CONDUCTION DISTURBANCES

- ☐ a. RBBB, incomplete
- ☐ b. RBBB, complete
- ☐ c. Left anterior fascicular block
- ☐ d. Left posterior fascicular block
- ☐ e. LBBB, with ST-T wave suggestive of acute myocardial injury or infarction
- ☐ f. LBBB, complete
- ☐ g. LBBB, intermittent
- ☐ h. Intraventricular conduction disturbance, nonspecific
- ☐ i. Aberrant intraventricular conduction with supraventricular arrhythmia

8. P WAVE ABNORMALITIES

- ☐ a. Right atrial abnormality
- ☐ b. Left atrial abnormalities
- ☐ c. Nonspecific atrial abnormality

9. ABNORMALITIES OF QRS VOLTAGE OR AXIS

- ☐ a. Low voltage, limb leads only
- ☐ b. Low voltage, limb and precordial leads
- ☐ c. Left axis deviation (> - 30%)
- ☐ d. Right axis deviation (> + 100)
- ☐ e. Electrical alternans

10. VENTRICULAR HYPERTROPHY

- ☐ a. LVH by voltage only
- ☐ b. LVH by voltage and ST-T segment abnormalities
- ☐ c. RVH
- ☐ d. Combined ventricular hypertrophy

11. Q WAVE MYOCARDIAL INFARCTION

	Probably Acute or Recent	Probably Old or Age Indeterminate
Anterolateral	☐ a.	☐ g.
Anterior	☐ b.	☐ h.
Anteroseptal	☐ c.	☐ i.
Lateral/High lateral	☐ d.	☐ j.
Inferior	☐ e.	☐ k.
Posterior	☐ f.	☐ l.

☐ m. Probably ventricular aneurysm

12. ST, T, U, WAVE ABNORMALITIES

- ☐ a. Normal variant, early repolarization
- ☐ b. Normal variant, juvenile T waves
- ☐ c. Nonspecific ST and/or T wave abnormalities
- ☐ d. ST and/or T wave abnormalities suggesting myocardial ischemia
- ☐ e. ST and/or T wave abnormalities suggesting myocardial injury
- ☐ f. ST and/or T wave abnormalities suggesting acute pericarditis
- ☐ g. ST-T segment abnormalities secondary to intraventricular conduction disturbance or hypertrophy
- ☐ h. Post-extrasystolic T wave abnormality
- ☐ i. Isolated J point depression
- ☐ j. Peaked T waves
- ☐ k. Prolonged QT interval
- ☐ l. Prominent U waves

13. PACEMAKER FUNCTION AND RHYTHM

- ☐ a. Atrial or coronary sinus pacing
- ☐ b. Ventricular demand pacing
- ☐ c. AV sequential pacing
- ☐ d. Ventricular pacing, complete control
- ☐ e. Dual chamber, atrial sensing pacemaker
- ☐ f. Pacemaker malfunction, not constantly capturing (atrium or ventricle)
- ☐ g. Pacemaker malfunction, not constantly sensing (atrium or ventricle)
- ☐ h. Pacemaker malfunction, not firing
- ☐ i. Pacemaker malfunction, slowing

14. SUGGESTED OR PROBABLE CLINICAL DISORDERS

- ☐ a. Digitalis effect
- ☐ b. Digitalis toxicity
- ☐ c. Antiarrhythmic drug effect
- ☐ d. Antiarrhythmic drug toxicity
- ☐ e. Hyperkalemia
- ☐ f. Hypokalemia
- ☐ g. Hypercalcemia
- ☐ h. Hypocalcemia
- ☐ i. Atrial septal defect, secundum
- ☐ j. Atrial septal defect, primum
- ☐ k. Dextrocardia, mirror image
- ☐ l. Mitral valve disease
- ☐ m. Chronic lung disease
- ☐ n. Acute cor pulmonale, including pulmonary embolus
- ☐ o. Pericardial effusion
- ☐ p. Acute pericarditis
- ☐ q. Hypertrophic cardiomyopathy
- ☐ r. Coronary artery disease
- ☐ s. Central nervous system disorder
- ☐ t. Myxedema
- ☐ u. Hypothermia
- ☐ v. Sick sinus syndrome

ECG 89 was obtained in a 56-year-old female with breast cancer, shortness of breath, and weakness. The ECG shows atrial flutter with 2:1 AV block (2 flutter waves for every QRS complex); the flutter waves are inverted in lead II and upright in lead V_1, as is typically the case. Low voltage QRS is present in the limb and precordial leads. There is subtle evidence for electrical alternans, which is most noticeable in the rhythm strip (asterisk). These findings are consistent with pericardial effusion (which is probably malignant in this case). Q waves in leads V_1-V_4 (arrows) suggest old anteroseptal and anterior myocardial infarction. The Q waves in V_4-V_5 but not V_6 is insufficient for the diagnosis of anterolateral MI.

Codes:

2r	Atrial flutter
6d	AV block, 2:1
9b	Low voltage, limb and precordial leads
9e	Electrical alternans
11h	Anterior Q wave MI, probably old or age indeterminate
11i	Anteroseptal Q wave MI, probably old or age indeterminate
14o	Pericardial effusion
14r	Coronary artery disease

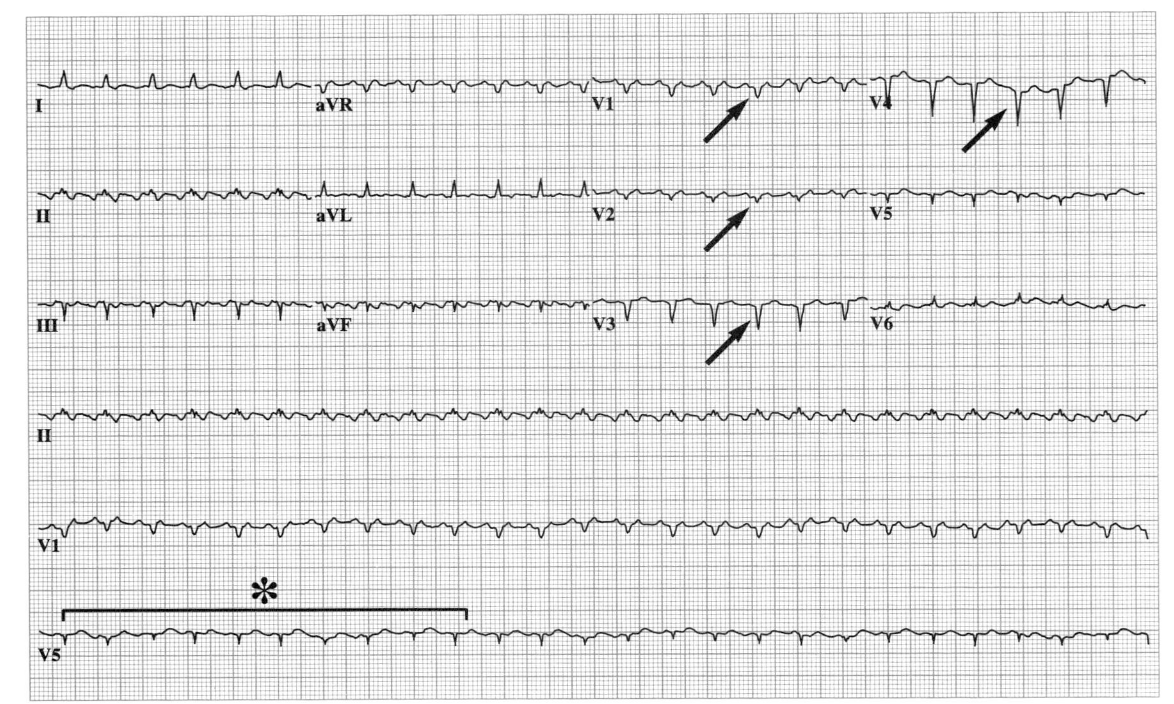

Questions: ECG 89

1. The diagnosis of low voltage in the limb leads requires a QRS amplitude less than ___ mm:

   a. 10
   b. 5
   c. 15
   d. 7

2. Atrial flutter with 2:1 block usually results in a ventricular rate of approximately ___ beats per minute:

   a. 150
   b. 100
   c. 300
   d. 180

3. ECG findings characteristic of pericardial effusion include:

   a. ST elevation
   b. Electrical alternans
   c. PR depression
   d. Low voltage QRS complexes

4. Anterior myocardial infarction is associated with pathologic Q waves in leads:

   a. V_4-V_6
   b. V_2-V_4
   c. V_1-V_3
   d. I, aVL

Answers: ECG 89

1. The diagnosis of low voltage in the limb leads requires a total QRS amplitude (maximal deflection of R + S wave) less than 5 mm. To diagnose low voltage in the precordial leads, the maximal QRS amplitude must be less than 10 mm in V_1-V_6. Clinical conditions associated with low voltage QRS complexes include pleural or pericardial effusion, restrictive or infiltrative cardiomyopathies, diffuse myocardial disease with multiple prior infarctions, and obesity. Emphysema (chronic lung disease) can result in electrical insulation of the heart and also cause low QRS complexes. (Answer: b)

2. In typical atrial flutter, flutter (or "F" waves) occur at a rate of 300 per minute. Therefore, atrial flutter with 2:1 block usually results in a ventricular rate of 150 per minute. Flutter waves are

sometimes difficult to recognize, and are usually best seen in the inferior leads (II, III, and aVF) and in lead V_1. The ventricular rhythm may be regular or irregular depending on whether AV nodal conduction is constant or variable. (Answer: a)

3. Low voltage QRS complexes and electrical alternans are consistent with (but not very sensitive or specific for) the diagnosis of pericardial effusion. ECG findings of acute pericarditis (PR depression, ST segment elevation) may or may not be present. (Answer: b, d)

4. It is important to identify leads with abnormal Q waves before localizing the area of infarction. Q waves in leads V_2 - V_4 should be coded as anterior myocardial infarction; if a Q wave is also present in lead V_1, anteroseptal myocardial infarction should be coded. (Answer: b)

— Quick Review 89 —

Atrial flutter	
• Rapid (regular/irregular) atrial undulations ("F" waves) at a rate of ____ per minute	regular 240-340
• Flutter rate may (increase/decrease) in the presence of Types IA, IC or III antiarrhythmic drugs	decrease
• Flutter waves in leads II, III, AVF are typically (inverted/upright) (with/without) an isoelectric baseline	inverted, without
• Flutter waves in lead V_1 are typically small (positive/negative) deflections (with/without) a distinct isoelectric baseline	positive, with
• QRS complex may be normal or aberrant (true/false)	true
• AV conduction ratio (ratio of flutter waves to QRS complexes) is usually (fixed/variable)	fixed
▸ Conduction ratios of 1:1 and 3:1 are (common/uncommon)	uncommon
▸ In untreated patients, AV block ≥ ____ suggests the coexistence of AV conduction disease	4:1
Pericardial effusion	
• (High/low) voltage QRS	Low
• Electrical ____, especially if complicated by cardiac ____	alternans tamponade
• Other features of acute ____ may also be present	pericarditis

Differential Diagnosis

INTRAVENTRICULAR CONDUCTION DISTURBANCE

(QRS duration $\geq$ 0.11 seconds in duration but QRS morphology does not meet criteria for LBBB (item 7f) or RBBB (item 7g), *or* abnormal notching of the QRS complex is present without prolongation)

- Antiarrhythmic drug toxicity (especially Type IA and IC agents) (item 14d)
- Hyperkalemia (item 14e)
- LVH (item 10a)
- Wolff-Parkinson-White (item 6h)
- Hypothermia (item 14u)
- Severe metabolic disturbances

ECG 90: Asymptomatic 67-year-old male:

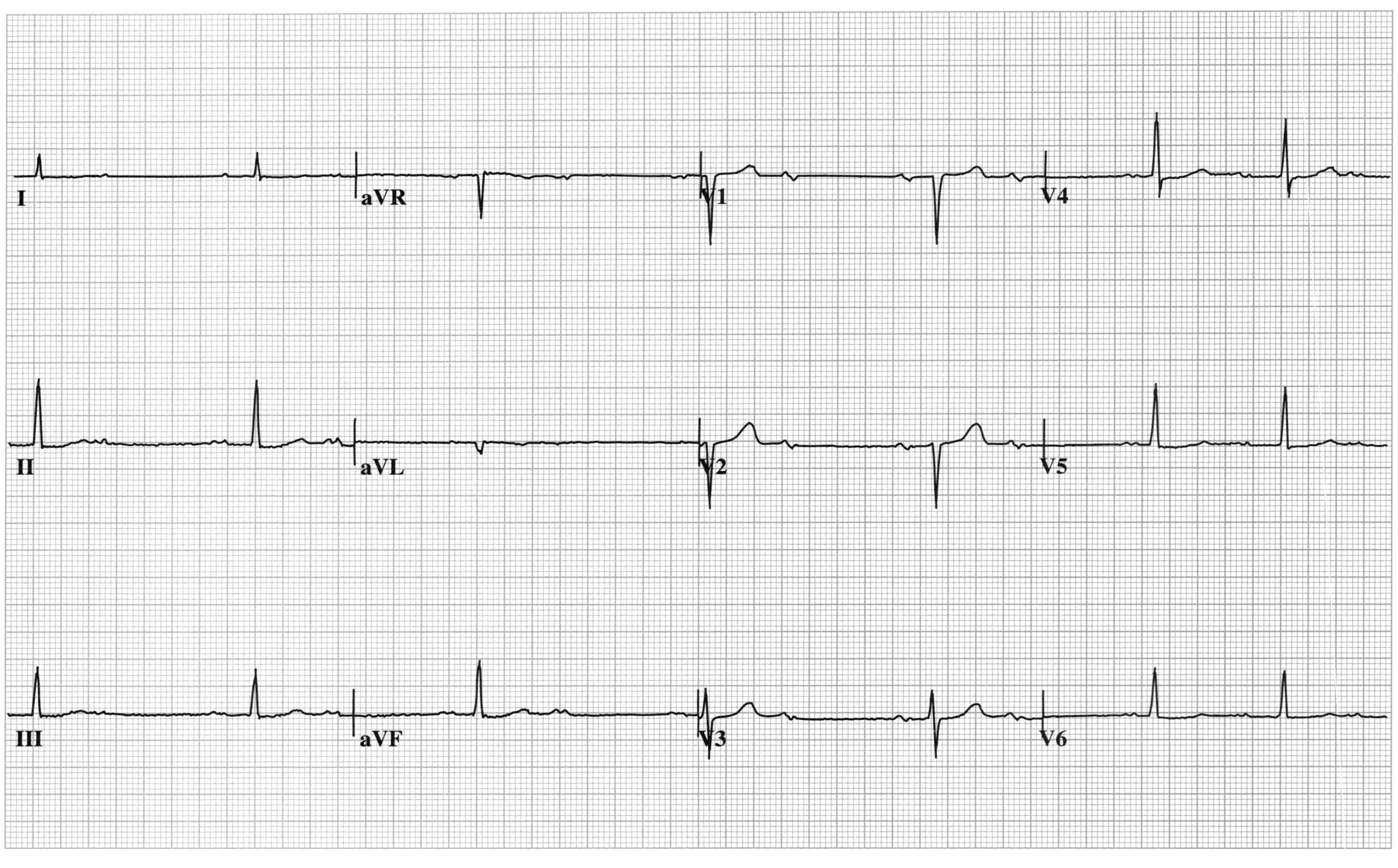

1. GENERAL FEATURES

☐ a. Normal ECG
☐ b. Borderline normal ECG or normal variant
☐ c. Incorrect electrode placement
☐ d. Artifact due to tremor

2. ATRIAL RHYTHMS

☐ a. Sinus rhythm
☐ b. Sinus arrhythmia
☐ c. Sinus bradycardia (< 60)
☐ d. Sinus tachycardia (> 100)
☐ e. Sinus pause or arrest
☐ f. Sinoatrial exit block
☐ g. Ecoptic atrial rhythm
☐ h. Wandering atrial pacemaker
☐ i. Atrial premature complexes, normally conducted
☐ j. Atrial premature complexes, nonconducted
☐ k. Atrial premature complexes with aberrant intraventricular conduction
☐ l. Atrial tachycardia (regular, sustained, 1:1 conduction)
☐ m. Atrial tachycardia, repetitive (short paroxysms)
☐ n. Atrial tachycardia, multifocal
☐ o. Atrial tachycardia with AV block
☐ p. Supraventricular tachycardia, unspecific
☐ q. Supraventricular tachycardia, paroxysmal
☐ r. Atrial flutter
☐ s. Atrial fibrillation
☐ t. Retrograde atrial activation

3. AV JUNCTIONAL RHYTHMS

☐ a. AV junctional premature complexes
☐ b. AV junctional escape complexes
☐ c. AV junctional rhythm, accelerated
☐ d. AV junctional rhythm

4. VENTRICULAR RHYTHMS

☐ a. Ventricular premature complex(es), uniform, fixed coupling
☐ b. Ventricular premature complex(es), uniform, nonfixed coupling
☐ c. Ventricular premature complexes(es), multiform
☐ d. Ventricular premature complexes, in pairs
☐ e. Ventricular parasystole
☐ f. Ventricular tachycardia (≥ 3 consecutive complexes)
☐ g. Accelerated idioventricular rhythm
☐ h. Ventricular escape complexes or rhythm
☐ i. Ventricular fibrillation

5. ATRIAL-VENTRICULAR INTERACTIONS IN ARRHYTHMIAS

☐ a. Fusion complexes
☐ b. Reciprocal (echo) complexes
☐ c. Ventricular capture complexes
☐ d. AV dissociation
☐ e. Ventriculophasic sinus arrhythmia

6. AV CONDUCTION ABNORMALITIES

☐ a. AV block, 1°
☐ b. AV block, 2° - Mobitz type I (Wenckebach)
☐ c. AV block, 2° - Mobitz type II
☐ d. AV block, 2:1
☐ e. AV block, 3°
☐ f. AV block, variable
☐ g. Short PR interval (with sinus rhythm and normal QRS duration)
☐ h. Wolff-Parkinson-White pattern

7. INTRAVENTRICULAR CONDUCTION DISTURBANCES

☐ a. RBBB, incomplete
☐ b. RBBB, complete
☐ c. Left anterior fascicular block
☐ d. Left posterior fascicular block
☐ e. LBBB, with ST-T wave suggestive of acute myocardial injury or infarction
☐ f. LBBB, complete
☐ g. LBBB, intermittent
☐ h. Intraventricular conduction disturbance, nonspecific
☐ i. Aberrant intraventricular conduction with supraventricular arrhythmia

8. P WAVE ABNORMALITIES

☐ a. Right atrial abnormality
☐ b. Left atrial abnormalities
☐ c. Nonspecific atrial abnormality

9. ABNORMALITIES OF QRS VOLTAGE OR AXIS

☐ a. Low voltage, limb leads only
☐ b. Low voltage, limb and precordial leads
☐ c. Left axis deviation (> - 30%)
☐ d. Right axis deviation (> + 100)
☐ e. Electrical alternans

10. VENTRICULAR HYPERTROPHY

☐ a. LVH by voltage only
☐ b. LVH by voltage and ST-T segment abnormalities
☐ c. RVH
☐ d. Combined ventricular hypertrophy

11. Q WAVE MYOCARDIAL INFARCTION

	Probably Acute or Recent	Probably Old or Age Indeterminate
Anterolateral	☐ a.	☐ g.
Anterior	☐ b.	☐ h.
Anteroseptal	☐ c.	☐ i.
Lateral/High lateral	☐ d.	☐ j.
Inferior	☐ e.	☐ k.
Posterior	☐ f.	☐ l.

☐ m. Probably ventricular aneurysm

12. ST, T, U, WAVE ABNORMALITIES

☐ a. Normal variant, early repolarization
☐ b. Normal variant, juvenile T waves
☐ c. Nonspecific ST and/or T wave abnormalities
☐ d. ST and/or T wave abnormalities suggesting myocardial ischemia
☐ e. ST and/or T wave abnormalities suggesting myocardial injury
☐ f. ST and/or T wave abnormalities suggesting acute pericarditis
☐ g. ST-T segment abnormalities secondary to intraventricular conduction disturbance or hypertrophy
☐ h. Post-extrasystolic T wave abnormality
☐ i. Isolated J point depression
☐ j. Peaked T waves
☐ k. Prolonged QT interval
☐ l. Prominent U waves

13. PACEMAKER FUNCTION AND RHYTHM

☐ a. Atrial or coronary sinus pacing
☐ b. Ventricular demand pacing
☐ c. AV sequential pacing
☐ d. Ventricular pacing, complete control
☐ e. Dual chamber, atrial sensing pacemaker
☐ f. Pacemaker malfunction, not constantly capturing (atrium or ventricle)
☐ g. Pacemaker malfunction, not constantly sensing (atrium or ventricle)
☐ h. Pacemaker malfunction, not firing
☐ i. Pacemaker malfunction, slowing

14. SUGGESTED OR PROBABLE CLINICAL DISORDERS

☐ a. Digitalis effect
☐ b. Digitalis toxicity
☐ c. Antiarrhythmic drug effect
☐ d. Antiarrhythmic drug toxicity
☐ e. Hyperkalemia
☐ f. Hypokalemia
☐ g. Hypercalcemia
☐ h. Hypocalcemia
☐ i. Atrial septal defect, secundum
☐ j. Atrial septal defect, primum
☐ k. Dextrocardia, mirror image
☐ l. Mitral valve disease
☐ m. Chronic lung disease
☐ n. Acute cor pulmonale, including pulmonary embolus
☐ o. Pericardial effusion
☐ p. Acute pericarditis
☐ q. Hypertrophic cardiomyopathy
☐ r. Coronary artery disease
☐ s. Central nervous system disorder
☐ t. Myxedema
☐ u. Hypothermia
☐ v. Sick sinus syndrome

ECG 90 was obtained in a 67-year-old asymptomatic male. The ECG shows a normal sinus rhythm at a rate of 72 bpm (arrows mark the P waves). The first two-thirds of the tracing show 2:1 AV block; the progressive prolongation of the PR interval in leads V_4 - V_6 supports the diagnosis of Mobitz type I (Wenkebach) second-degree AV block. Left atrial enlargement and nonspecific ST-T abnormalities are also present.

Codes:

2a	Sinus rhythm
6b	AV block, 2° - Mobitz type I (Wenckebach)
6d	AV block, 2:1
8b	Left atrial abnormality
12c	Nonspecific ST and/or T wave abnormalities

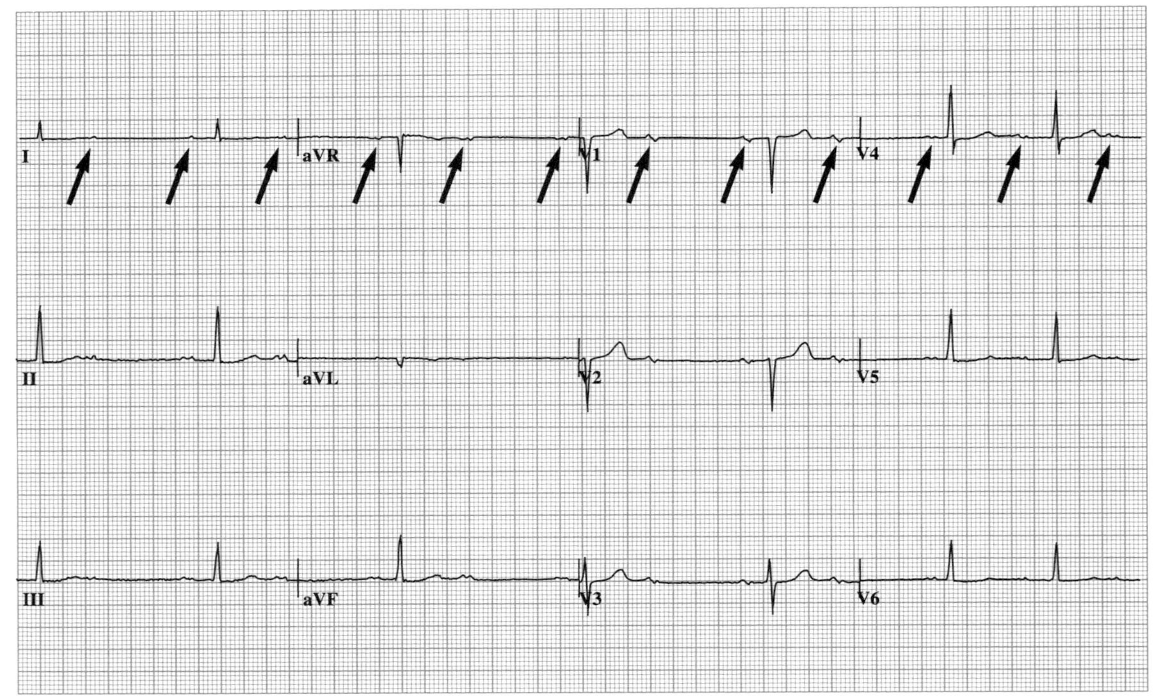

Questions: ECG 90

1. Manifestations of classic Wenckebach periodicity include:

   a. Constant PP interval
   b. Progressive lengthening of the PR interval and shortening of the RR interval until a P wave is blocked
   c RR interval containing the blocked P wave that is equal to 2 normal PP intervals.

2. Which of the findings in the setting of 2:1 block favor Mobitz Type I second-degree AV block over a Mobitz Type II mechanism:

   a. Narrow QRS complex
   b. Block worsens in response to atropine
   c. Block worsens in response to carotid sinus massage
   d. 2:1 block develops during inferior MI
   e. History of syncope

Answers: ECG 90

1. Manifestations of the Wenckebach phenomenon (Type I second-degree AV block) include a constant PP interval; progressive lengthening of the PR interval and shortening of the RR interval until a P wave is blocked; and an RR interval containing the blocked P wave that is ***shorter*** than 2 normal PP intervals. Classic Wenckbach phenomenon is often absent in Type I second-degree AV block due to the presence of sinus arrhythmia and/or changes in vagal tone. (Answer: a, b)

2. In the setting of 2:1 AV block, findings favoring a Mobitz Type I (Wenckebach) mechanism include a narrow QRS complex, improvement in AV block in response to maneuvers that increase heart rate and AV conduction (atropine, exercise), worsening in AV block in response to maneuvers that reduce heart rate and AV conduction (carotid sinus massage), the development of 2:1 block during inferior MI, and the presence of Type I on another part of the ECG. (Answer: a, c, d)

— Quick Review 90—

AV block, 2° - Mobitz Type I (Wenckebach)	
• Progressive prolongation of the ____ interval and shortening of the ____ interval until a P wave is blocked	PR RR
• RR interval containing the nonconducted P wave is (less than/equal to/greater than) the sum of two PP intervals	less than
• Results in ____ beating due to the presence of nonconducted P waves	group
Left atrial abnormality	
• Notched P wave with a duration ≥ ____ seconds in leads II, III or aVF, *or*	0.12
• Terminal negative portion of the P wave in lead V_1 ≥ 1 mm deep and ≥ ____ seconds in duration	0.04

— Comic Relief —

You're in the home stretch. Only 13 ECGs to go...

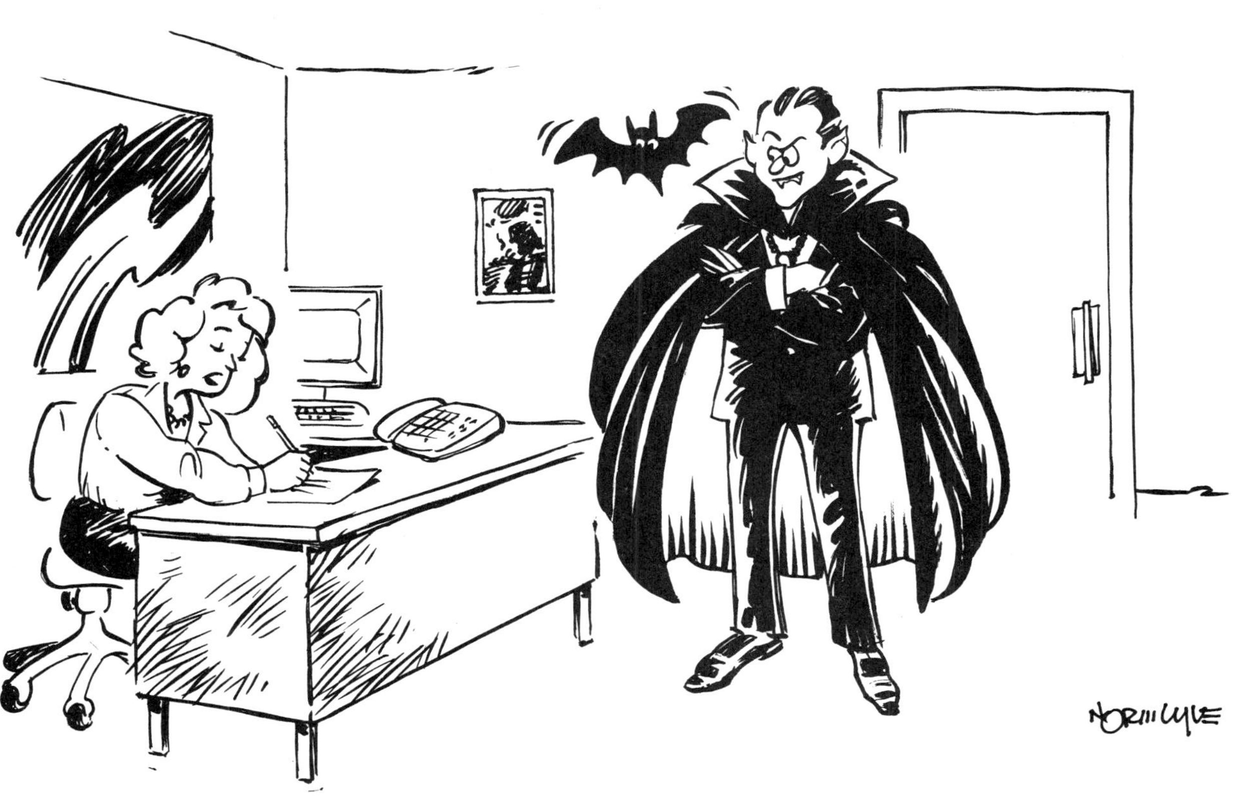

"And what experience have you had as a phlebotomist?"

...before you start all over again!

ECG 91. 73-year-old male with new onset neurological deficit:

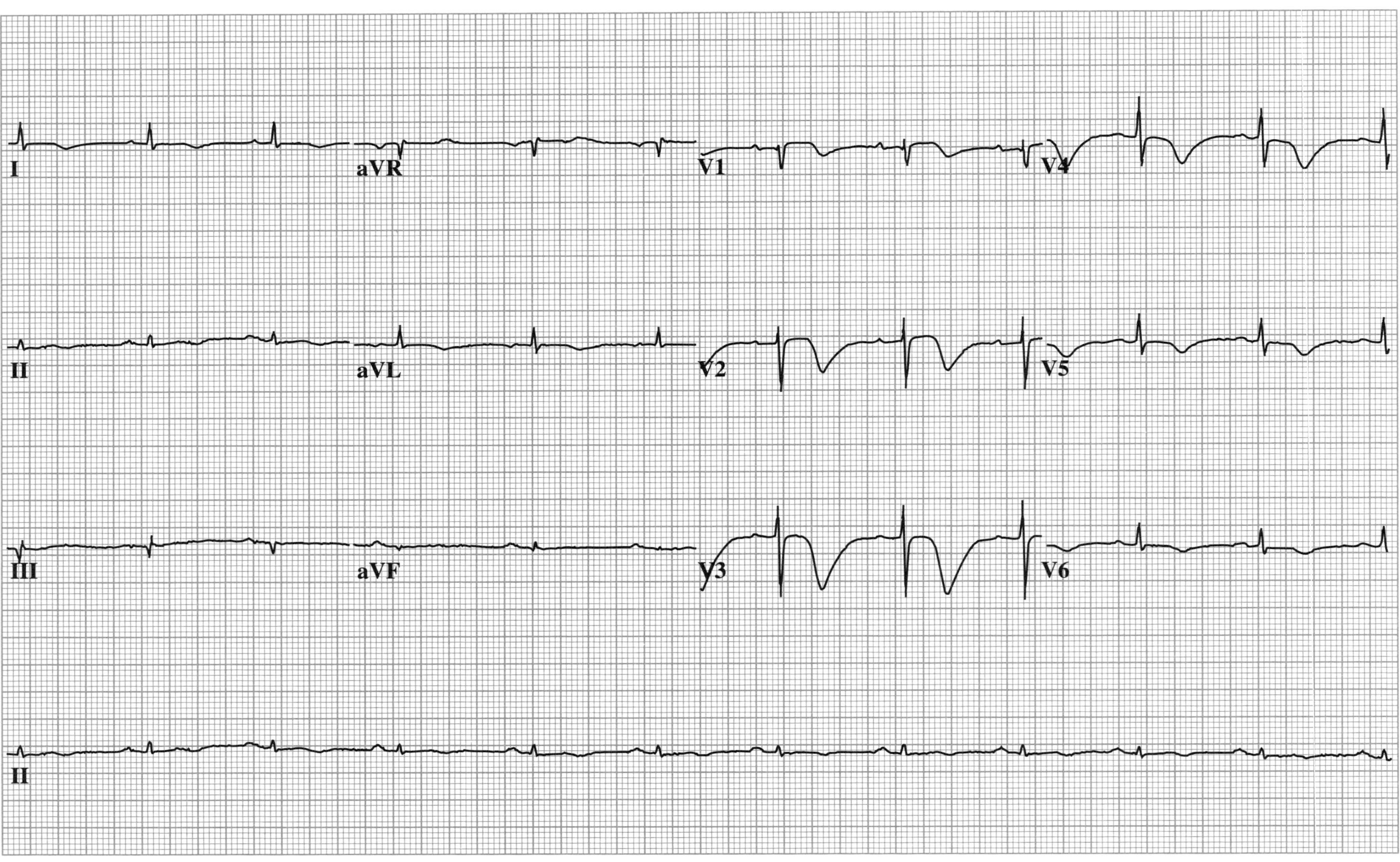

1. GENERAL FEATURES

☐ a. Normal ECG
☐ b. Borderline normal ECG or normal variant
☐ c. Incorrect electrode placement
☐ d. Artifact due to tremor

2. ATRIAL RHYTHMS

☐ a. Sinus rhythm
☐ b. Sinus arrhythmia
☐ c. Sinus bradycardia (< 60)
☐ d. Sinus tachycardia (> 100)
☐ e. Sinus pause or arrest
☐ f. Sinoatrial exit block
☐ g. Ecoptic atrial rhythm
☐ h. Wandering atrial pacemaker
☐ i. Atrial premature complexes, normally conducted
☐ j. Atrial premature complexes, nonconducted
☐ k. Atrial premature complexes with aberrant intraventricular conduction
☐ l. Atrial tachycardia (regular, sustained, 1:1 conduction)
☐ m. Atrial tachycardia, repetitive (short paroxysms)
☐ n. Atrial tachycardia, multifocal
☐ o. Atrial tachycardia with AV block
☐ p. Supraventricular tachycardia, unspecific
☐ q. Supraventricular tachycardia, paroxysmal
☐ r. Atrial flutter
☐ s. Atrial fibrillation
☐ t. Retrograde atrial activation

3. AV JUNCTIONAL RHYTHMS

☐ a. AV junctional premature complexes
☐ b. AV junctional escape complexes
☐ c. AV junctional rhythm, accelerated
☐ d. AV junctional rhythm

4. VENTRICULAR RHYTHMS

☐ a. Ventricular premature complex(es), uniform, fixed coupling
☐ b. Ventricular premature complex(es), uniform, nonfixed coupling
☐ c. Ventricular premature complexes(es), multiform
☐ d. Ventricular premature complexes, in pairs
☐ e. Ventricular parasystole
☐ f. Ventricular tachycardia (≥ 3 consecutive complexes)
☐ g. Accelerated idioventricular rhythm
☐ h. Ventricular escape complexes or rhythm
☐ i. Ventricular fibrillation

5. ATRIAL-VENTRICULAR INTERACTIONS IN ARRHYTHMIAS

☐ a. Fusion complexes
☐ b. Reciprocal (echo) complexes
☐ c. Ventricular capture complexes
☐ d. AV dissociation
☐ e. Ventriculophasic sinus arrhythmia

6. AV CONDUCTION ABNORMALITIES

☐ a. AV block, 1°
☐ b. AV block, 2° - Mobitz type I (Wenckebach)
☐ c. AV block, 2° - Mobitz type II
☐ d. AV block, 2:1
☐ e. AV block, 3°
☐ f. AV block, variable
☐ g. Short PR interval (with sinus rhythm and normal QRS duration)
☐ h. Wolff-Parkinson-White pattern

7. INTRAVENTRICULAR CONDUCTION DISTURBANCES

☐ a. RBBB, incomplete
☐ b. RBBB, complete
☐ c. Left anterior fascicular block
☐ d. Left posterior fascicular block
☐ e. LBBB, with ST-T wave suggestive of acute myocardial injury or infarction
☐ f. LBBB, complete
☐ g. LBBB, intermittent
☐ h. Intraventricular conduction disturbance, nonspecific
☐ i. Aberrant intraventricular conduction with supraventricular arrhythmia

8. P WAVE ABNORMALITIES

☐ a. Right atrial abnormality
☐ b. Left atrial abnormalities
☐ c. Nonspecific atrial abnormality

9. ABNORMALITIES OF QRS VOLTAGE OR AXIS

☐ a. Low voltage, limb leads only
☐ b. Low voltage, limb and precordial leads
☐ c. Left axis deviation (> - 30%)
☐ d. Right axis deviation (> + 100)
☐ e. Electrical alternans

10. VENTRICULAR HYPERTROPHY

☐ a. LVH by voltage only
☐ b. LVH by voltage and ST-T segment abnormalities
☐ c. RVH
☐ d. Combined ventricular hypertrophy

11. Q WAVE MYOCARDIAL INFARCTION

	Probably Acute or Recent	Probably Old or Age Indeterminate
Anterolateral	☐ a.	☐ g.
Anterior	☐ b.	☐ h.
Anteroseptal	☐ c.	☐ i.
Lateral/High lateral	☐ d.	☐ j.
Inferior	☐ e.	☐ k.
Posterior	☐ f.	☐ l.

☐ m. Probably ventricular aneurysm

12. ST, T, U, WAVE ABNORMALITIES

☐ a. Normal variant, early repolarization
☐ b. Normal variant, juvenile T waves
☐ c. Nonspecific ST and/or T wave abnormalities
☐ d. ST and/or T wave abnormalities suggesting myocardial ischemia
☐ e. ST and/or T wave abnormalities suggesting myocardial injury
☐ f. ST and/or T wave abnormalities suggesting acute pericarditis
☐ g. ST-T segment abnormalities secondary to intraventricular conduction disturbance or hypertrophy
☐ h. Post-extrasystolic T wave abnormality
☐ i. Isolated J point depression
☐ j. Peaked T waves
☐ k. Prolonged QT interval
☐ l. Prominent U waves

13. PACEMAKER FUNCTION AND RHYTHM

☐ a. Atrial or coronary sinus pacing
☐ b. Ventricular demand pacing
☐ c. AV sequential pacing
☐ d. Ventricular pacing, complete control
☐ e. Dual chamber, atrial sensing pacemaker
☐ f. Pacemaker malfunction, not constantly capturing (atrium or ventricle)
☐ g. Pacemaker malfunction, not constantly sensing (atrium or ventricle)
☐ h. Pacemaker malfunction, not firing
☐ i. Pacemaker malfunction, slowing

14. SUGGESTED OR PROBABLE CLINICAL DISORDERS

☐ a. Digitalis effect
☐ b. Digitalis toxicity
☐ c. Antiarrhythmic drug effect
☐ d. Antiarrhythmic drug toxicity
☐ e. Hyperkalemia
☐ f. Hypokalemia
☐ g. Hypercalcemia
☐ h. Hypocalcemia
☐ i. Atrial septal defect, secundum
☐ j. Atrial septal defect, primum
☐ k. Dextrocardia, mirror image
☐ l. Mitral valve disease
☐ m. Chronic lung disease
☐ n. Acute cor pulmonale, including pulmonary embolus
☐ o. Pericardial effusion
☐ p. Acute pericarditis
☐ q. Hypertrophic cardiomyopathy
☐ r. Coronary artery disease
☐ s. Central nervous system disorder
☐ t. Myxedema
☐ u. Hypothermia
☐ v. Sick sinus syndrome

ECG 91 was obtained in a 73-year-old male with an acute neurological deficit. The ECG shows sinus rhythm, low voltage in the limb leads, deep anterolateral T wave inversions (arrows), and a prolonged QT interval. Given the clinical presentation, the deeply inverted T waves and prolonged QT interval are likely to be due to the acute central nervous system disorder. Since myocardial ischemia may present with a similar ECG pattern, this diagnosis should be excluded.

Codes:

2a	Sinus rhythm
9a	Low voltage, limb leads only
12d	ST and/or T wave abnormality suggesting myocardial ischemia
12k	Prolonged QT interval
14s	Central nervous system disorder

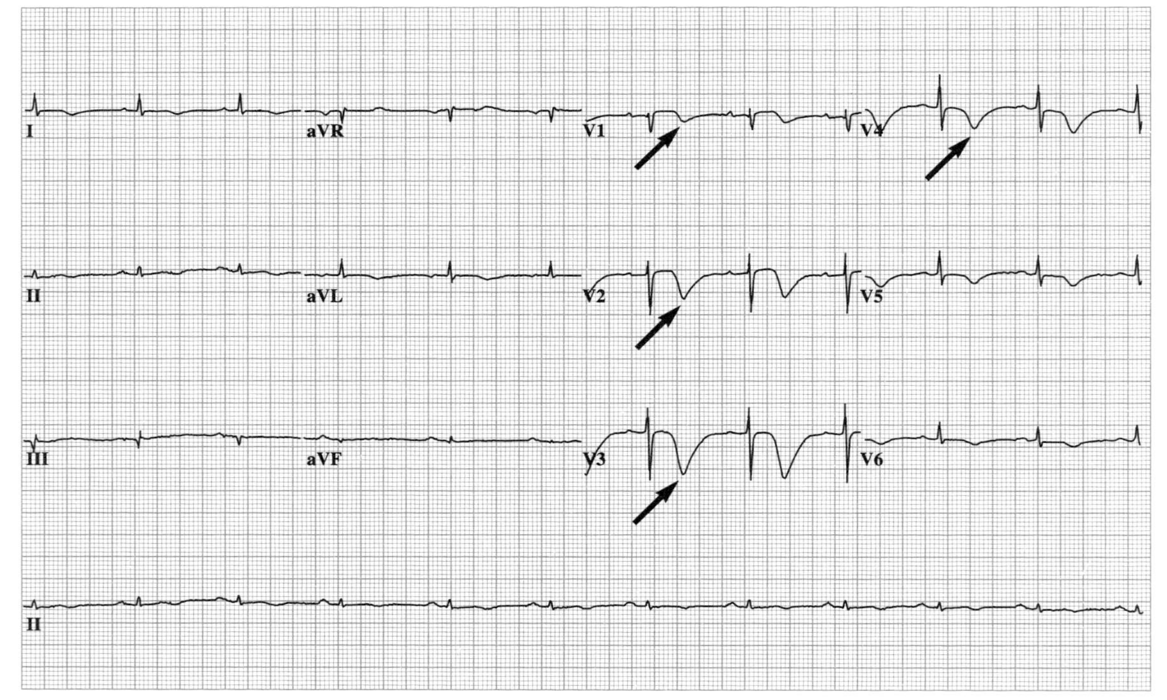

Questions: ECG 91

1. ECG features of acute central nervous system disorders such as cerebral or subarachnoid hemorrhage include:

   a. Large upright T waves in precordial leads
   b. Prolonged QT interval
   c. Deeply inverted T waves in precordial leads
   d. Increased QRS voltage
   e. Prominent U waves in precordial leads

2. Acute central nervous system disorders can cause ECG changes that mimic:

   a. Acute myocardial infarction
   b. Right ventricular hypertrophy
   c. Left ventricular hypertrophy
   d. Pericarditis
   e. Bifascicular block

Answers: ECG 91

1. Acute central nervous system disorders such as cerebral hemorrhage and subarachnoid hemorrhage can cause significant changes in the rhythm and QRS-ST-T complexes of the ECG. Classic changes usually occur in the precordial leads and include large upright or deeply inverted T waves, prolonged QT interval, and prominent U waves. Other changes can include T wave notching and loss of T wave amplitude; diffuse ST segment elevation (mimicking pericarditis or acute myocardial injury); abnormal Q waves (mimicking myocardial infarction); and abnormalities of cardiac rhythm including atrial fibrillation, ventricular tachycardia, sinus bradycardia, and sinus tachycardia. Increased QRS voltage is not a feature of acute CNS disorders. (Answer: All except d)

2. ECG changes associated with acute central nervous system disorders can mimic acute myocardial infarction (Q waves, large upright T waves), myocardial ischemia (deep T wave inversion), acute pericarditis (diffuse ST elevation), and drug effects (prolonged QT interval, prominent U waves). Ventricular hypertrophy and conduction abnormalities such as bifascicular block are not typically associated with acute central nervous system disorders. (Answer: a, d)

— Quick Review 91 —

Low voltage, limb leads only	
• Amplitude of the entire QRS complex (R+S) < ____ mm in all limb leads	5
Prolonged QT interval	
• Corrected QT interval (QTc) ≥ ____ seconds,	0.42-0.46
where QTc = QT interval divided by the square root of the preceding ____ interval	RR
• QT interval varies (directly/inversely) with heart rate	inversely
• The normal QT interval should be (less than/greater than) 50% of the RR interval	less than
Central nervous system disorder	
• "Classic changes" usually occur in the (limb/precordial) leads	precordial
▸ Large upright or deeply inverted ____ waves	T
▸ Prolonged ____ interval (often marked)	QT
▸ Prominent ____ waves	U
• Other changes:	
▸ ST segment changes:	
• Diffuse ST elevation mimicking acute ____	pericarditis
• Focal ST elevation mimicking ____	acute injury
• ST depression may also occur (true/false)	true
▸ Abnormal ____ waves mimicking MI	Q
▸ Almost any rhythm abnormality including sinus tachycardia or bradycardia, junctional rhythm, VPCs, ventricular tachycardia, etc. (true/false)	true

Differential Diagnosis

Group Beating

- Mobitz Type I second-degree AV block (item 6b)
- Blocked APCs (item 2j)
- Type II second-degree AV block (item 6c)
- Concealed His-bundle depolarizations

ECG 92. 79-year-old male complaining of chest and epigastric tightness:

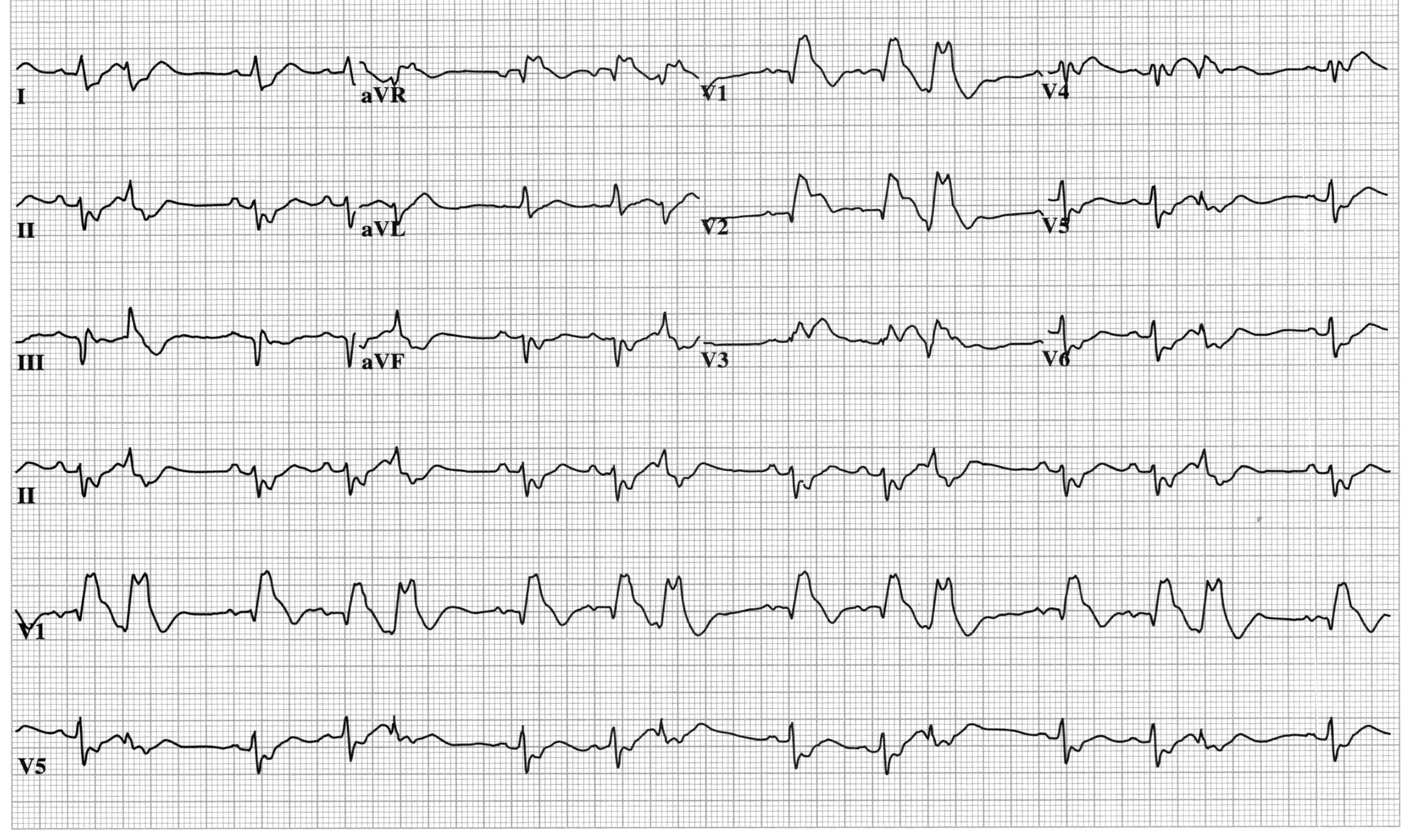

1. GENERAL FEATURES
☐ a. Normal ECG
☐ b. Borderline normal ECG or normal variant
☐ c. Incorrect electrode placement
☐ d. Artifact due to tremor

2. ATRIAL RHYTHMS
☐ a. Sinus rhythm
☐ b. Sinus arrhythmia
☐ c. Sinus bradycardia (< 60)
☐ d. Sinus tachycardia (> 100)
☐ e. Sinus pause or arrest
☐ f. Sinoatrial exit block
☐ g. Ecoptic atrial rhythm
☐ h. Wandering atrial pacemaker
☐ i. Atrial premature complexes, normally conducted
☐ j. Atrial premature complexes, nonconducted
☐ k. Atrial premature complexes with aberrant intraventricular conduction
☐ l. Atrial tachycardia (regular, sustained, 1:1 conduction)
☐ m. Atrial tachycardia, repetitive (short paroxysms)
☐ n. Atrial tachycardia, multifocal
☐ o. Atrial tachycardia with AV block
☐ p. Supraventricular tachycardia, unspecific
☐ q. Supraventricular tachycardia, paroxysmal
☐ r. Atrial flutter
☐ s. Atrial fibrillation
☐ t. Retrograde atrial activation

3. AV JUNCTIONAL RHYTHMS
☐ a. AV junctional premature complexes
☐ b. AV junctional escape complexes
☐ c. AV junctional rhythm, accelerated
☐ d. AV junctional rhythm

4. VENTRICULAR RHYTHMS
☐ a. Ventricular premature complex(es), uniform, fixed coupling
☐ b. Ventricular premature complex(es), uniform, nonfixed coupling
☐ c. Ventricular premature complexes(es), multiform
☐ d. Ventricular premature complexes, in pairs
☐ e. Ventricular parasystole
☐ f. Ventricular tachycardia (≥ 3 consecutive complexes)
☐ g. Accelerated idioventricular rhythm
☐ h. Ventricular escape complexes or rhythm
☐ i. Ventricular fibrillation

5. ATRIAL-VENTRICULAR INTERACTIONS IN ARRHYTHMIAS
☐ a. Fusion complexes
☐ b. Reciprocal (echo) complexes
☐ c. Ventricular capture complexes
☐ d. AV dissociation
☐ e. Ventriculophasic sinus arrhythmia

6. AV CONDUCTION ABNORMALITIES
☐ a. AV block, 1°
☐ b. AV block, 2° - Mobitz type I (Wenckebach)
☐ c. AV block, 2° - Mobitz type II
☐ d. AV block, 2:1
☐ e. AV block, 3°
☐ f. AV block, variable
☐ g. Short PR interval (with sinus rhythm and normal QRS duration)
☐ h. Wolff-Parkinson-White pattern

7. INTRAVENTRICULAR CONDUCTION DISTURBANCES
☐ a. RBBB, incomplete
☐ b. RBBB, complete
☐ c. Left anterior fascicular block
☐ d. Left posterior fascicular block
☐ e. LBBB, with ST-T wave suggestive of acute myocardial injury or infarction
☐ f. LBBB, complete
☐ g. LBBB, intermittent
☐ h. Intraventricular conduction disturbance, nonspecific
☐ i. Aberrant intraventricular conduction with supraventricular arrhythmia

8. P WAVE ABNORMALITIES
☐ a. Right atrial abnormality
☐ b. Left atrial abnormalities
☐ c. Nonspecific atrial abnormality

9. ABNORMALITIES OF QRS VOLTAGE OR AXIS
☐ a. Low voltage, limb leads only
☐ b. Low voltage, limb and precordial leads
☐ c. Left axis deviation (> - 30%)
☐ d. Right axis deviation (> + 100)
☐ e. Electrical alternans

10. VENTRICULAR HYPERTROPHY
☐ a. LVH by voltage only
☐ b. LVH by voltage and ST-T segment abnormalities
☐ c. RVH
☐ d. Combined ventricular hypertrophy

11. Q WAVE MYOCARDIAL INFARCTION

	Probably Acute or Recent	Probably Old or Age Indeterminate
Anterolateral	☐ a.	☐ g.
Anterior	☐ b.	☐ h.
Anteroseptal	☐ c.	☐ i.
Lateral/High lateral	☐ d.	☐ j.
Inferior	☐ e.	☐ k.
Posterior	☐ f.	☐ l.

☐ m. Probably ventricular aneurysm

12. ST, T, U, WAVE ABNORMALITIES
☐ a. Normal variant, early repolarization
☐ b. Normal variant, juvenile T waves
☐ c. Nonspecific ST and/or T wave abnormalities
☐ d. ST and/or T wave abnormalities suggesting myocardial ischemia
☐ e. ST and/or T wave abnormalities suggesting myocardial injury
☐ f. ST and/or T wave abnormalities suggesting acute pericarditis
☐ g. ST-T segment abnormalities secondary to intraventricular conduction disturbance or hypertrophy
☐ h. Post-extrasystolic T wave abnormality
☐ i. Isolated J point depression
☐ j. Peaked T waves
☐ k. Prolonged QT interval
☐ l. Prominent U waves

13. PACEMAKER FUNCTION AND RHYTHM
☐ a. Atrial or coronary sinus pacing
☐ b. Ventricular demand pacing
☐ c. AV sequential pacing
☐ d. Ventricular pacing, complete control
☐ e. Dual chamber, atrial sensing pacemaker
☐ f. Pacemaker malfunction, not constantly capturing (atrium or ventricle)
☐ g. Pacemaker malfunction, not constantly sensing (atrium or ventricle)
☐ h. Pacemaker malfunction, not firing
☐ i. Pacemaker malfunction, slowing

14. SUGGESTED OR PROBABLE CLINICAL DISORDERS
☐ a. Digitalis effect
☐ b. Digitalis toxicity
☐ c. Antiarrhythmic drug effect
☐ d. Antiarrhythmic drug toxicity
☐ e. Hyperkalemia
☐ f. Hypokalemia
☐ g. Hypercalcemia
☐ h. Hypocalcemia
☐ i. Atrial septal defect, secundum
☐ j. Atrial septal defect, primum
☐ k. Dextrocardia, mirror image
☐ l. Mitral valve disease
☐ m. Chronic lung disease
☐ n. Acute cor pulmonale, including pulmonary embolus
☐ o. Pericardial effusion
☐ p. Acute pericarditis
☐ q. Hypertrophic cardiomyopathy
☐ r. Coronary artery disease
☐ s. Central nervous system disorder
☐ t. Myxedema
☐ u. Hypothermia
☐ v. Sick sinus syndrome

ECG 92 was obtained in a 79-year-old male complaining of chest and epigastric tightness. The tracing shows a sinus rhythm (arrows mark sinus P waves) with frequent unifocal VPCs (asterisks), which appear in a trigeminal pattern and show fixed coupling and a compensatory pause. Left anterior fascicular block and left axis deviation are noted as well as RBBB. ST segment elevation is present in leads V_1-V_3 (arrowheads), consistent with acute anteroseptal myocardial injury. Since Q waves are present in V_1-V_2 but not V_3, acute anteroseptal MI should not be coded. The findings are also consistent with coronary artery disease.

Codes:

2a	Sinus rhythm
4a	Ventricular premature complex(es), uniform, fixed coupling
7b	RBBB, complete
7c	Left anterior fascicular block
9c	Left axis deviation (>-30°)
12e	ST and/or T wave abnormalities suggesting myocardial injury
14r	Coronary artery disease

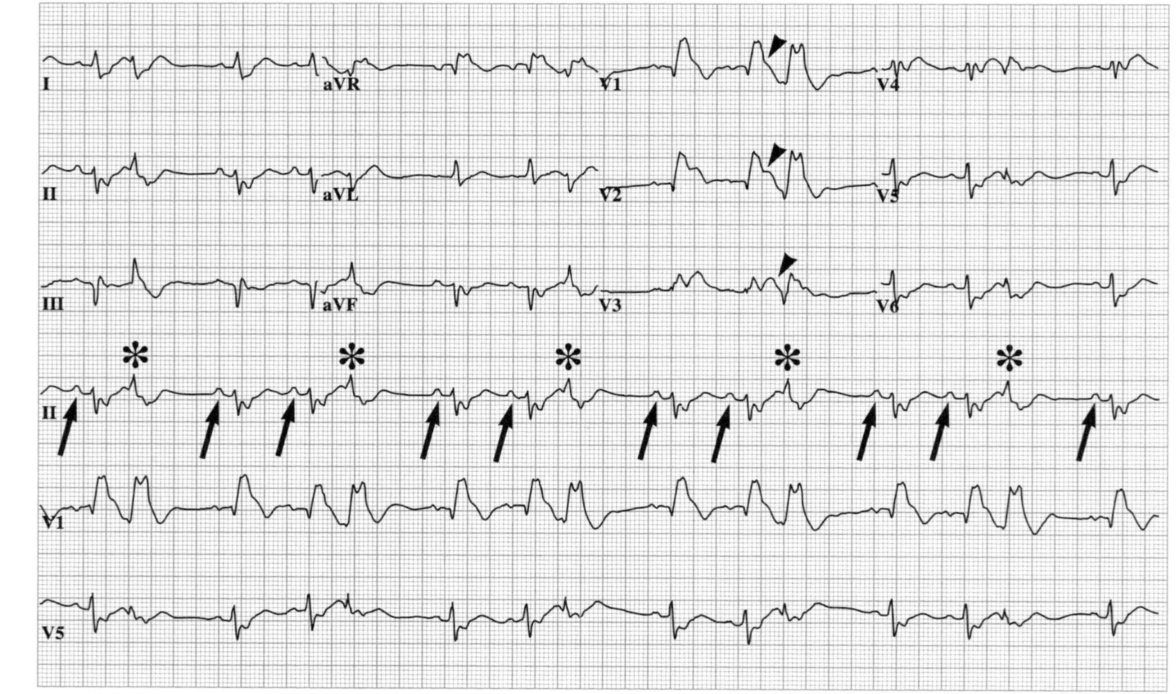

Questions: ECG 92

1. Which of the following statements about compensatory pauses are true?

   a. A full compensatory pause exists when the RR interval containing a ventricular premature complex (VPC) is twice the normal RR interval
   b. Compensatory pauses can occasionally follow supraventricular beats
   c. VPCs always demonstrate either a partial or full compensatory pause

2. Which of the following statements about ventricular premature complexes (VPCs) are true?

   a. Multifocal VPCs typically manifest a constant coupling interval
   b. VPCs always have a QRS duration > 0.12 seconds
   c. Uniform VPCs with nonfixed coupling should raise the suspicion of parasystole
   d. The QRS duration of a VPC may be shorter than the QRS of a sinus beat when bundle branch block is present
   e. VPCs with different morphology (multiform VPCs) can originate from the same ventricular focus

Answers: ECG 92

1. A full compensatory pause is present when the RR interval containing a VPC is two times the normal RR interval (unless sinus arrhythmia is also present). Interpolated VPCs are VPCs that are interposed between two consecutive sinus beats without disrupting the basic sinus rhythm; they result in neither a partial nor full compensatory pause. Compensatory pauses do not usually occur with supraventricular beats, but may on occasion follow low atrial or junctional beats. (Answer: a, b)

2. In general, unifocal ventricular premature complexes (VPC) demonstrate a constant coupling interval while multifocal VPCs do not. Multiform VPCs (VPCs with different morphologies) may be *multifocal or unifocal* in origin, and may therefore demonstrate nonfixed or fixed coupling. Uniform VPCs with nonfixed coupling should raise the suspicion of parasystole, in which an ectopic ventricular focus is protected from depolarization by an entrance block; this results in a varying coupling interval, RR intervals that are multiples of a basic inter-ectopic interval, and fusion beats. While typically associated with a wide and bizarre QRS, VPCs originating high in the interventricular septum may have a relatively normal QRS duration. VPCs frequently show a full compensatory pause, but this may be absent when an interpolated VPC occurs or ventriculoatrial conduction penetrates and resets the sinus node. Finally, when a VPC occurs just distal to the site of bundle branch block and near the interventricular septum, the QRS of the VPC may be narrower than the QRS of the bundle branch block. (Answer: c, d, e)

— Quick Review 92 —

Ventricular premature complex(es), uniform, fixed coupling	
• A wide, notched or slurred ____ complex that is premature relative to the normal RR interval and is not preceded by a ____ wave	QRS P
• QRS duration is almost always > ____ seconds	0.12
• Initial direction of the QRS is often (similar to/different from) the QRS during sinus rhythm	different from
• Secondary ST & T wave changes in the (same/opposite) direction as the major deflection of the QRS (i.e., ST depression & T wave inversion in leads with a dominant ____ wave; ST elevation and upright T wave in leads with a dominant ____ wave or ____ complex)	opposite R S QS
• Coupling interval is constant or varies by < ____ seconds	0.08
• Morphology of VPCs in any given lead is (the same/different)	the same
• Retrograde capture of atria may occur (true/false)	true
• A full ____ pause (PP interval containing the VPC is twice the normal PP interval) is usually evident	compensatory

— Quick Review 92 —

Left anterior fascicular block	
• ____ axis deviation with a mean QRS axis between ____ and ____ degrees	left -45, -90
• (qR/rS) complex in leads I and aVL	qR
• (qR/rS) complex in lead III	rS
• Normal or slightly prolonged QRS duration (true/false)	true
• No other cause for left axis deviation should be present (true/false)	true
• Poor R wave progression is (common/uncommon)	common
Anteroseptal MI, recent or acute	
• Abnormal Q or QS deflection and ST elevation in ____ (and sometimes V_4)	V_1-V_3
• The presence of a Q wave in lead ____ distinguishes anteroseptal from anterior infarction	V_1
ST and/or T wave changes suggesting myocardial injury	
• Acute ST segment (elevation/depression) with upward (convexity/concavity) in the leads representing the area of infarction	elevation convexity
• T waves invert (before/after) ST segments return to baseline	before
• Associated ST (elevation/depression) in the noninfarct leads is common	depression
• Acute ____ wall injury often has horizontal or downsloping ST segment depression with upright T waves in V_1-V_3, with or without a prominent R wave in these same leads	posterior

— POP QUIZ —

Make The Diagnosis

Instructions: Determine the clinical disorder that best corresponds to the ECG features listed below (see item 14 of score sheet for options)

ECG Features	Answer
• Sinus tachycardia and findings consistent with right ventricular pressure overload: ▸ Right atrial abnormality ▸ Inverted T waves in leads V_1-V_3 ▸ Right axis deviation ▸ S_1Q_3 or S_1Q_3 T_3 pattern ▸ Pseudoinfarct pattern in the inferior leads ▸ Incomplete or complete RBBB ▸ Supraventricular tachyarrhythmias are common • ECG abnormalities are often transient	Acute cor pulmonale, incl. pulmonary embolus
• Low voltage QRS • Electrical alternans and other features of acute pericarditis may be present	Pericardial effusion
• Right atrial abnormality is common • Majority have abnormal QRS complexes: ▸ Large amplitude QRS ▸ Large abnormal Q waves (can give pseudoinfarct pattern in inferior, lateral, and anterior precordial leads) ▸ Tall R wave with inverted T wave in V_1 simulating RVH ▸ Nonspecific ST and/or T wave abnormalities common ▸ Left axis deviation in 20%	Hypertrophic cardiomyopathy

ECG 93. 89-year-old male with dyspnea and confusion:

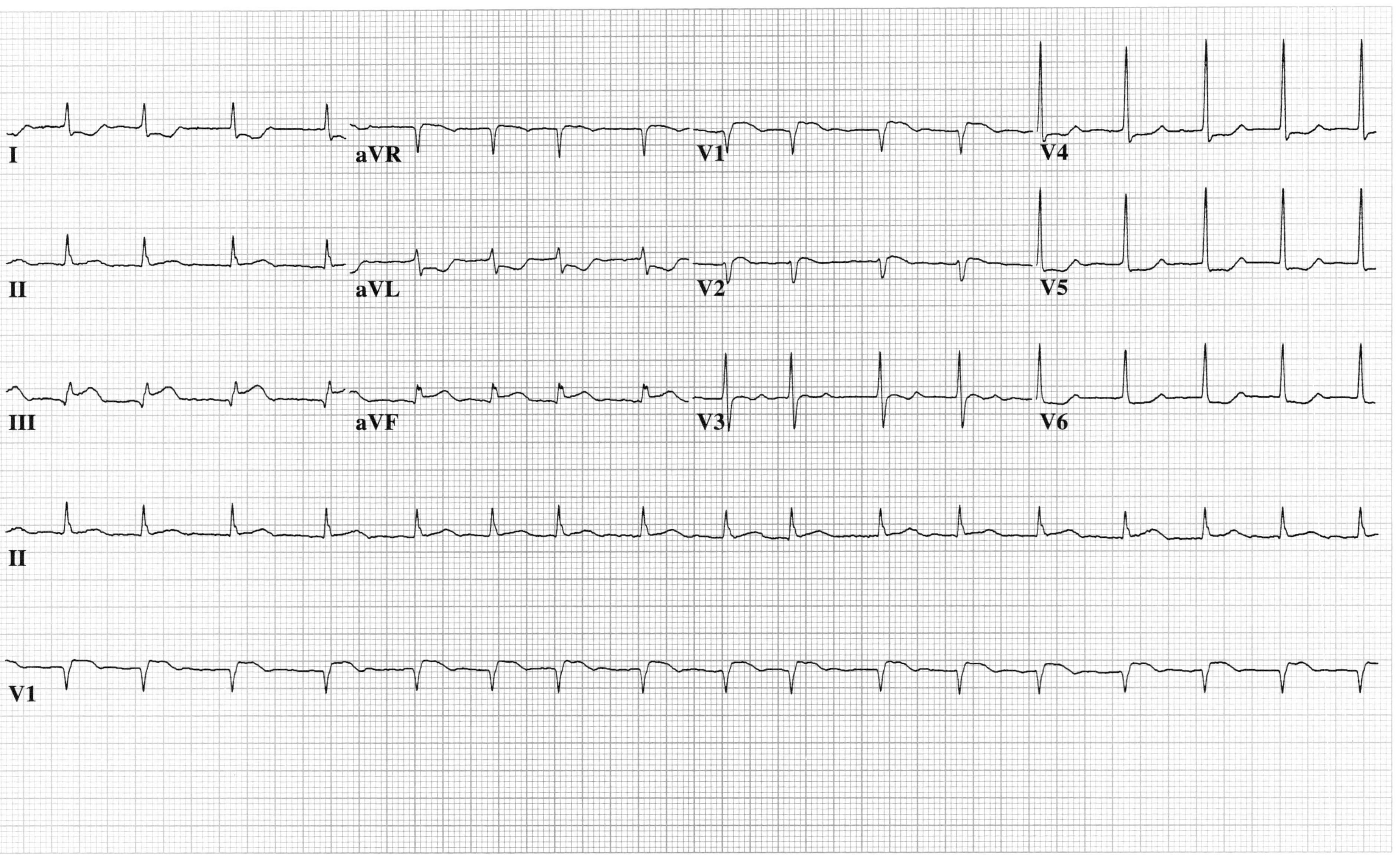

1. GENERAL FEATURES

- ☐ a. Normal ECG
- ☐ b. Borderline normal ECG or normal variant
- ☐ c. Incorrect electrode placement
- ☐ d. Artifact due to tremor

2. ATRIAL RHYTHMS

- ☐ a. Sinus rhythm
- ☐ b. Sinus arrhythmia
- ☐ c. Sinus bradycardia (< 60)
- ☐ d. Sinus tachycardia (> 100)
- ☐ e. Sinus pause or arrest
- ☐ f. Sinoatrial exit block
- ☐ g. Ecoptic atrial rhythm
- ☐ h. Wandering atrial pacemaker
- ☐ i. Atrial premature complexes, normally conducted
- ☐ j. Atrial premature complexes, nonconducted
- ☐ k. Atrial premature complexes with aberrant intraventricular conduction
- ☐ l. Atrial tachycardia (regular, sustained, 1:1 conduction)
- ☐ m. Atrial tachycardia, repetitive (short paroxysms)
- ☐ n. Atrial tachycardia, multifocal
- ☐ o. Atrial tachycardia with AV block
- ☐ p. Supraventricular tachycardia, unspecific
- ☐ q. Supraventricular tachycardia, paroxysmal
- ☐ r. Atrial flutter
- ☐ s. Atrial fibrillation
- ☐ t. Retrograde atrial activation

3. AV JUNCTIONAL RHYTHMS

- ☐ a. AV junctional premature complexes
- ☐ b. AV junctional escape complexes
- ☐ c. AV junctional rhythm, accelerated
- ☐ d. AV junctional rhythm

4. VENTRICULAR RHYTHMS

- ☐ a. Ventricular premature complex(es), uniform, fixed coupling
- ☐ b. Ventricular premature complex(es), uniform, nonfixed coupling
- ☐ c. Ventricular premature complexes(es), multiform
- ☐ d. Ventricular premature complexes, in pairs
- ☐ e. Ventricular parasystole
- ☐ f. Ventricular tachycardia (≥ 3 consecutive complexes)
- ☐ g. Accelerated idioventricular rhythm
- ☐ h. Ventricular escape complexes or rhythm
- ☐ i. Ventricular fibrillation

5. ATRIAL-VENTRICULAR INTERACTIONS IN ARRHYTHMIAS

- ☐ a. Fusion complexes
- ☐ b. Reciprocal (echo) complexes
- ☐ c. Ventricular capture complexes
- ☐ d. AV dissociation
- ☐ e. Ventriculophasic sinus arrhythmia

6. AV CONDUCTION ABNORMALITIES

- ☐ a. AV block, 1°
- ☐ b. AV block, 2° - Mobitz type I (Wenckebach)
- ☐ c. AV block, 2° - Mobitz type II
- ☐ d. AV block, 2:1
- ☐ e. AV block, 3°
- ☐ f. AV block, variable
- ☐ g. Short PR interval (with sinus rhythm and normal QRS duration)
- ☐ h. Wolff-Parkinson-White pattern

7. INTRAVENTRICULAR CONDUCTION DISTURBANCES

- ☐ a. RBBB, incomplete
- ☐ b. RBBB, complete
- ☐ c. Left anterior fascicular block
- ☐ d. Left posterior fascicular block
- ☐ e. LBBB, with ST-T wave suggestive of acute myocardial injury or infarction
- ☐ f. LBBB, complete
- ☐ g. LBBB, intermittent
- ☐ h. Intraventricular conduction disturbance, nonspecific
- ☐ i. Aberrant intraventricular conduction with supraventricular arrhythmia

8. P WAVE ABNORMALITIES

- ☐ a. Right atrial abnormality
- ☐ b. Left atrial abnormalities
- ☐ c. Nonspecific atrial abnormality

9. ABNORMALITIES OF QRS VOLTAGE OR AXIS

- ☐ a. Low voltage, limb leads only
- ☐ b. Low voltage, limb and precordial leads
- ☐ c. Left axis deviation (> - 30%)
- ☐ d. Right axis deviation (> + 100)
- ☐ e. Electrical alternans

10. VENTRICULAR HYPERTROPHY

- ☐ a. LVH by voltage only
- ☐ b. LVH by voltage and ST-T segment abnormalities
- ☐ c. RVH
- ☐ d. Combined ventricular hypertrophy

11. Q WAVE MYOCARDIAL INFARCTION

	Probably Acute or Recent	Probably Old or Age Indeterminate
Anterolateral	☐ a.	☐ g.
Anterior	☐ b.	☐ h.
Anteroseptal	☐ c.	☐ i.
Lateral/High lateral	☐ d.	☐ j.
Inferior	☐ e.	☐ k.
Posterior	☐ f.	☐ l.

- ☐ m. Probably ventricular aneurysm

12. ST, T, U, WAVE ABNORMALITIES

- ☐ a. Normal variant, early repolarization
- ☐ b. Normal variant, juvenile T waves
- ☐ c. Nonspecific ST and/or T wave abnormalities
- ☐ d. ST and/or T wave abnormalities suggesting myocardial ischemia
- ☐ e. ST and/or T wave abnormalities suggesting myocardial injury
- ☐ f. ST and/or T wave abnormalities suggesting acute pericarditis
- ☐ g. ST-T segment abnormalities secondary to intraventricular conduction disturbance or hypertrophy
- ☐ h. Post-extrasystolic T wave abnormality
- ☐ i. Isolated J point depression
- ☐ j. Peaked T waves
- ☐ k. Prolonged QT interval
- ☐ l. Prominent U waves

13. PACEMAKER FUNCTION AND RHYTHM

- ☐ a. Atrial or coronary sinus pacing
- ☐ b. Ventricular demand pacing
- ☐ c. AV sequential pacing
- ☐ d. Ventricular pacing, complete control
- ☐ e. Dual chamber, atrial sensing pacemaker
- ☐ f. Pacemaker malfunction, not constantly capturing (atrium or ventricle)
- ☐ g. Pacemaker malfunction, not constantly sensing (atrium or ventricle)
- ☐ h. Pacemaker malfunction, not firing
- ☐ i. Pacemaker malfunction, slowing

14. SUGGESTED OR PROBABLE CLINICAL DISORDERS

- ☐ a. Digitalis effect
- ☐ b. Digitalis toxicity
- ☐ c. Antiarrhythmic drug effect
- ☐ d. Antiarrhythmic drug toxicity
- ☐ e. Hyperkalemia
- ☐ f. Hypokalemia
- ☐ g. Hypercalcemia
- ☐ h. Hypocalcemia
- ☐ i. Atrial septal defect, secundum
- ☐ j. Atrial septal defect, primum
- ☐ k. Dextrocardia, mirror image
- ☐ l. Mitral valve disease
- ☐ m. Chronic lung disease
- ☐ n. Acute cor pulmonale, including pulmonary embolus
- ☐ o. Pericardial effusion
- ☐ p. Acute pericarditis
- ☐ q. Hypertrophic cardiomyopathy
- ☐ r. Coronary artery disease
- ☐ s. Central nervous system disorder
- ☐ t. Myxedema
- ☐ u. Hypothermia

ECG 93 was obtained in an 89-year-old male with dyspnea and confusion. The ECG shows atrial fibrillation with an early evolving inferior infarction. Because the inferior Q waves are not pathological as of yet, inferior myocardial injury should be coded (asterisks mark ST elevation in leads III and aVF) rather than Q wave infarction. Also evident is ST depression in leads I, aVL, V_5 and V_6 (arrows), consistent with lateral wall ischemia. The ST segment elevation in lead V_1 (arrowhead) may represent right ventricular infarction.

Codes:

2s	Atrial fibrillation
12d	ST and/or T wave abnormalities suggesting myocardial ischemia
12e	ST and/or T wave abnormalities suggesting myocardial injury
14r	Coronary artery disease

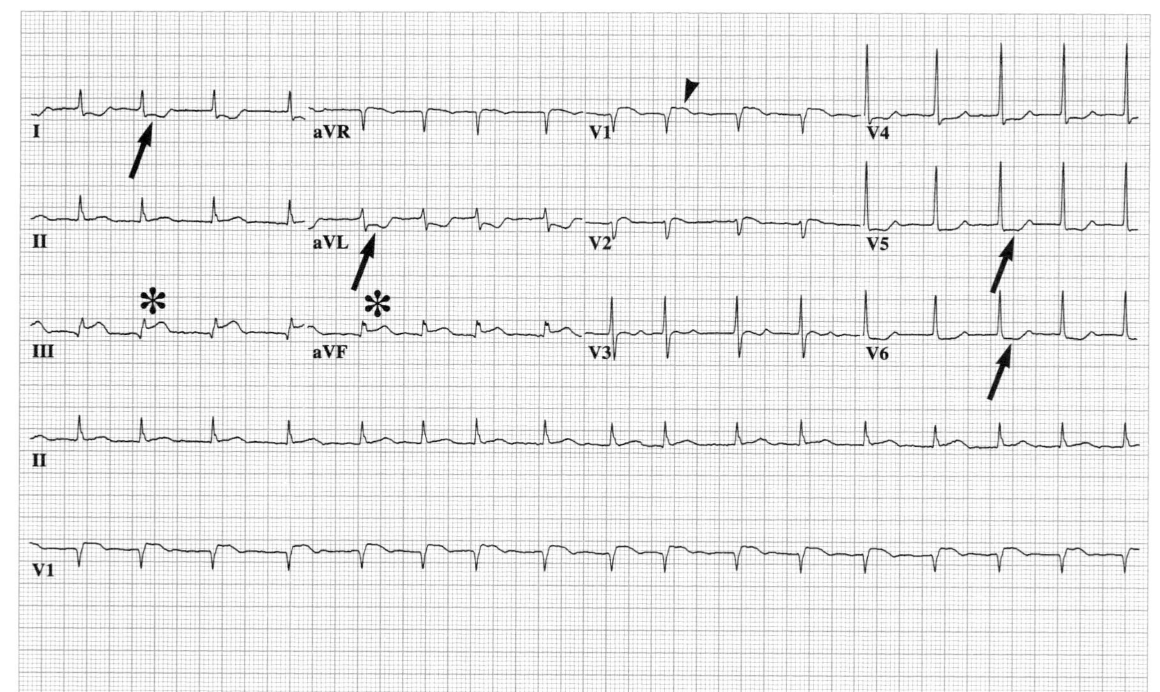

Questions: ECG 93

1. The diagnosis of an acute myocardial infarction requires:

   For non-posterior wall MI:
   a. Q waves alone
   b. ST elevation alone
   c. Q waves and ST elevation
   d. Q waves and ST depression

   For posterior wall MI:
   e. Q waves and ST elevation
   f. Dominant R waves in V_1 alone
   g. Dominant R wave and ST depression in V_1-V_3
   h. Dominant R wave and ST elevation in V_1-V_3

2. An irregularly irregular rhythm may be due to atrial fibrillation as well as:

   a. Multifocal atrial tachycardia
   b. Paroxysmal atrial tachycardia with variable AV block
   c. Monomorphic ventricular tachycardia

Answers: ECG 93

1. Two elements are generally required for the diagnosis of acute myocardial infarction. For non-posterior MIs (anterior, anteroseptal, anterolateral, high lateral, inferior), pathological Q waves and significant ST elevation should be present. For posterior MI, dominant R waves and significant ST segment depression in leads V_1-V_3 should be present. (Answer: c, g)

2. The differential diagnosis of an irregularly irregular rhythm includes multifocal atrial tachycardia, paroxysmal atrial tachycardia or atrial flutter with variable AV block, atrial fibrillation, and sinus or supraventricular rhythm with frequent APCs or VPCs. Ventricular tachycardia is generally a regular rhythm (but may be irregular). (Answer: a, b)

— Quick Review 93 —

Atrial fibrillation	
• ____ waves are absent	P
• Atrial activity is totally ____ and represented by fibrillatory (f) waves of varying amplitudes, duration and morphology	irregular
• Atrial activity is best seen in the ____ and ____ leads	right precordial, inferior
• Ventricular rhythm is (regularly/irregularly) irregular	irregularly
• ____ toxicity may result in regularization of the RR interval due to complete heart block with junctional tachycardia	Digitalis
• Ventricular rate is usually ____ per minute in the absence of drugs	100-180
▸ Think ____ if the ventricular rate is > 200 per minute and the QRS is > 0.12 seconds	Wolff-Parkinson-White

ECG 94. 79-year-old asymptomatic female:

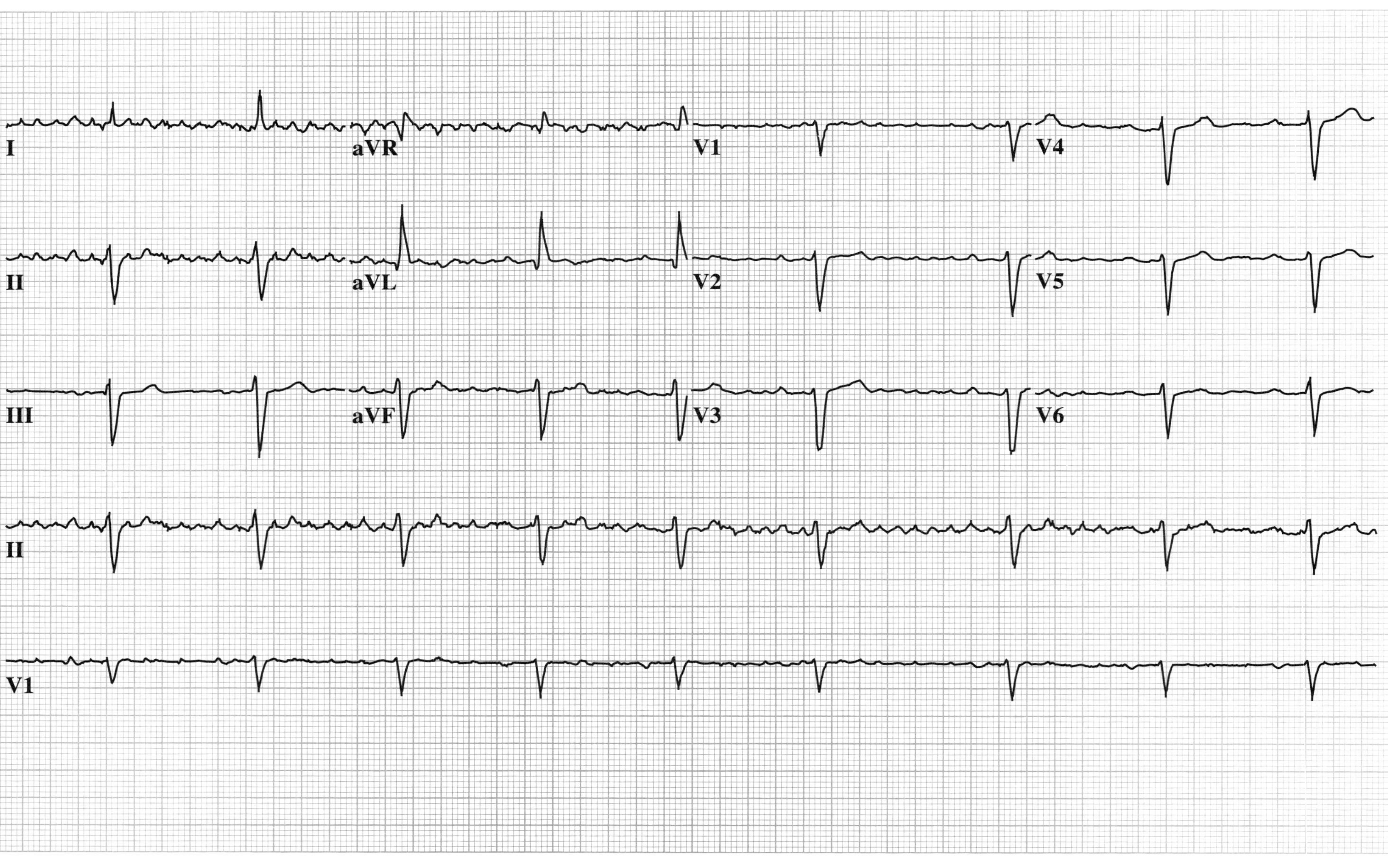

1. GENERAL FEATURES

- ☐ a. Normal ECG
- ☐ b. Borderline normal ECG or normal variant
- ☐ c. Incorrect electrode placement
- ☐ d. Artifact due to tremor

2. ATRIAL RHYTHMS

- ☐ a. Sinus rhythm
- ☐ b. Sinus arrhythmia
- ☐ c. Sinus bradycardia (< 60)
- ☐ d. Sinus tachycardia (> 100)
- ☐ e. Sinus pause or arrest
- ☐ f. Sinoatrial exit block
- ☐ g. Ecoptic atrial rhythm
- ☐ h. Wandering atrial pacemaker
- ☐ i. Atrial premature complexes, normally conducted
- ☐ j. Atrial premature complexes, nonconducted
- ☐ k. Atrial premature complexes with aberrant intraventricular conduction
- ☐ l. Atrial tachycardia (regular, sustained, 1:1 conduction)
- ☐ m. Atrial tachycardia, repetitive (short paroxysms)
- ☐ n. Atrial tachycardia, multifocal
- ☐ o. Atrial tachycardia with AV block
- ☐ p. Supraventricular tachycardia, unspecific
- ☐ q. Supraventricular tachycardia, paroxysmal
- ☐ r. Atrial flutter
- ☐ s. Atrial fibrillation
- ☐ t. Retrograde atrial activation

3. AV JUNCTIONAL RHYTHMS

- ☐ a. AV junctional premature complexes
- ☐ b. AV junctional escape complexes
- ☐ c. AV junctional rhythm, accelerated
- ☐ d. AV junctional rhythm

4. VENTRICULAR RHYTHMS

- ☐ a. Ventricular premature complex(es), uniform, fixed coupling
- ☐ b. Ventricular premature complex(es), uniform, nonfixed coupling
- ☐ c. Ventricular premature complexes(es), multiform
- ☐ d. Ventricular premature complexes, in pairs
- ☐ e. Ventricular parasystole
- ☐ f. Ventricular tachycardia (≥ 3 consecutive complexes)
- ☐ g. Accelerated idioventricular rhythm
- ☐ h. Ventricular escape complexes or rhythm
- ☐ i. Ventricular fibrillation

5. ATRIAL-VENTRICULAR INTERACTIONS IN ARRHYTHMIAS

- ☐ a. Fusion complexes
- ☐ b. Reciprocal (echo) complexes
- ☐ c. Ventricular capture complexes
- ☐ d. AV dissociation
- ☐ e. Ventriculophasic sinus arrhythmia

6. AV CONDUCTION ABNORMALITIES

- ☐ a. AV block, 1°
- ☐ b. AV block, 2° - Mobitz type I (Wenckebach)
- ☐ c. AV block, 2° - Mobitz type II
- ☐ d. AV block, 2:1
- ☐ e. AV block, 3°
- ☐ f. AV block, variable
- ☐ g. Short PR interval (with sinus rhythm and normal QRS duration)
- ☐ h. Wolff-Parkinson-White pattern

7. INTRAVENTRICULAR CONDUCTION DISTURBANCES

- ☐ a. RBBB, incomplete
- ☐ b. RBBB, complete
- ☐ c. Left anterior fascicular block
- ☐ d. Left posterior fascicular block
- ☐ e. LBBB, with ST-T wave suggestive of acute myocardial injury or infarction
- ☐ f. LBBB, complete
- ☐ g. LBBB, intermittent
- ☐ h. Intraventricular conduction disturbance, nonspecific
- ☐ i. Aberrant intraventricular conduction with supraventricular arrhythmia

8. P WAVE ABNORMALITIES

- ☐ a. Right atrial abnormality
- ☐ b. Left atrial abnormalities
- ☐ c. Nonspecific atrial abnormality

9. ABNORMALITIES OF QRS VOLTAGE OR AXIS

- ☐ a. Low voltage, limb leads only
- ☐ b. Low voltage, limb and precordial leads
- ☐ c. Left axis deviation (> - 30%)
- ☐ d. Right axis deviation (> + 100)
- ☐ e. Electrical alternans

10. VENTRICULAR HYPERTROPHY

- ☐ a. LVH by voltage only
- ☐ b. LVH by voltage and ST-T segment abnormalities
- ☐ c. RVH
- ☐ d. Combined ventricular hypertrophy

11. Q WAVE MYOCARDIAL INFARCTION

	Probably Acute or Recent	Probably Old or Age Indeterminate
Anterolateral	☐ a.	☐ g.
Anterior	☐ b.	☐ h.
Anteroseptal	☐ c.	☐ i.
Lateral/High lateral	☐ d.	☐ j.
Inferior	☐ e.	☐ k.
Posterior	☐ f.	☐ l.

- ☐ m. Probably ventricular aneurysm

12. ST, T, U, WAVE ABNORMALITIES

- ☐ a. Normal variant, early repolarization
- ☐ b. Normal variant, juvenile T waves
- ☐ c. Nonspecific ST and/or T wave abnormalities
- ☐ d. ST and/or T wave abnormalities suggesting myocardial ischemia
- ☐ e. ST and/or T wave abnormalities suggesting myocardial injury
- ☐ f. ST and/or T wave abnormalities suggesting acute pericarditis
- ☐ g. ST-T segment abnormalities secondary to intraventricular conduction disturbance or hypertrophy
- ☐ h. Post-extrasystolic T wave abnormality
- ☐ i. Isolated J point depression
- ☐ j. Peaked T waves
- ☐ k. Prolonged QT interval
- ☐ l. Prominent U waves

13. PACEMAKER FUNCTION AND RHYTHM

- ☐ a. Atrial or coronary sinus pacing
- ☐ b. Ventricular demand pacing
- ☐ c. AV sequential pacing
- ☐ d. Ventricular pacing, complete control
- ☐ e. Dual chamber, atrial sensing pacemaker
- ☐ f. Pacemaker malfunction, not constantly capturing (atrium or ventricle)
- ☐ g. Pacemaker malfunction, not constantly sensing (atrium or ventricle)
- ☐ h. Pacemaker malfunction, not firing
- ☐ i. Pacemaker malfunction, slowing

14. SUGGESTED OR PROBABLE CLINICAL DISORDERS

- ☐ a. Digitalis effect
- ☐ b. Digitalis toxicity
- ☐ c. Antiarrhythmic drug effect
- ☐ d. Antiarrhythmic drug toxicity
- ☐ e. Hyperkalemia
- ☐ f. Hypokalemia
- ☐ g. Hypercalcemia
- ☐ h. Hypocalcemia
- ☐ i. Atrial septal defect, secundum
- ☐ j. Atrial septal defect, primum
- ☐ k. Dextrocardia, mirror image
- ☐ l. Mitral valve disease
- ☐ m. Chronic lung disease
- ☐ n. Acute cor pulmonale, including pulmonary embolus
- ☐ o. Pericardial effusion
- ☐ p. Acute pericarditis
- ☐ q. Hypertrophic cardiomyopathy
- ☐ r. Coronary artery disease
- ☐ s. Central nervous system disorder
- ☐ t. Myxedema
- ☐ u. Hypothermia
- ☐ v. Sick sinus syndrome

ECG 94 was obtained in a 79-year-old asymptomatic female. The tracing, at first glance, appears to show atrial flutter. However, on closer inspection, sinus bradycardia is evident (arrows mark the P waves in leads III and V_4-V_6). The rapid undulation in baseline is therefore artifactual. Also evidence are first-degree AV block, sinus arrhythmia, left anterior fascicular block, and left axis deviation. The QRS measures 116 msec and thus exceeds the duration expected with left anterior fascicular block (0.08-0.10 msec); thus, nonspecific IVCD should also be coded.

Codes:

1d	Artifact due to tremor
2b	Sinus arrhythmia
2c	Sinus bradycardia < 60
6a	AV block, 1°
7c	Left anterior fascicular block
7h	IVCD, nonspecific type
9c	Left axis deviation (>-30°)

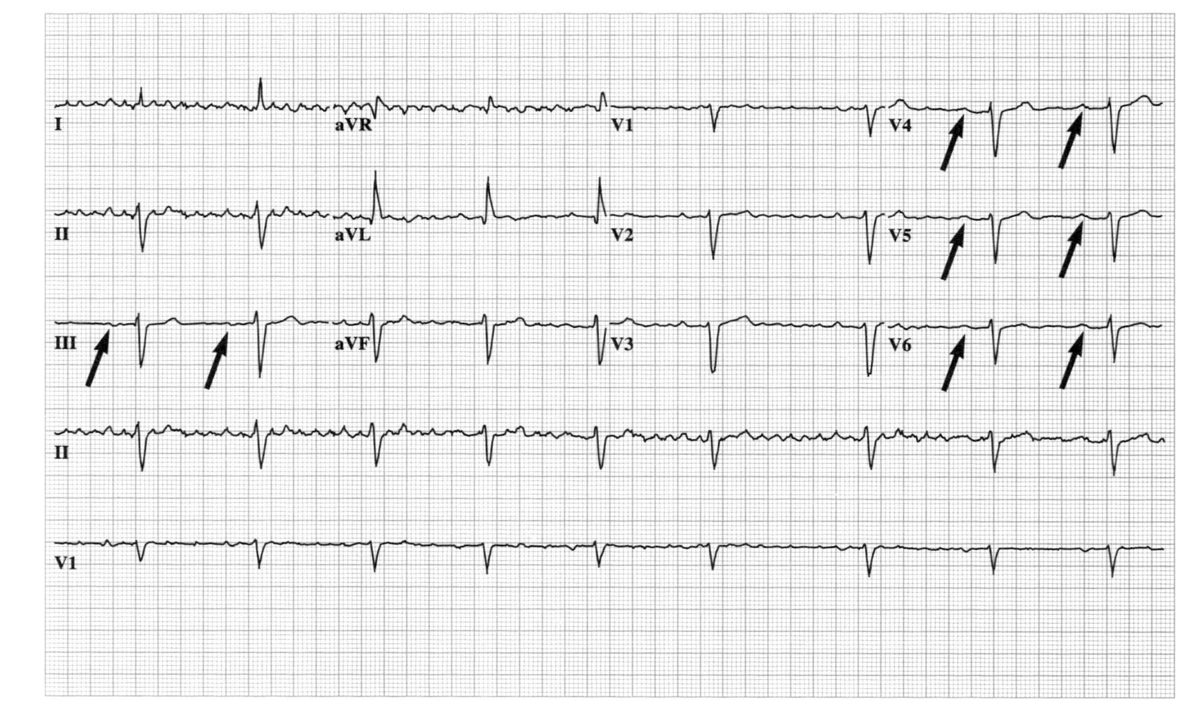

Questions: ECG 94

1. Causes of poor R wave progression include:

   a. Normal variant
   b. Anterior MI
   c. Cardiomyopathy
   d. Left ventricular hypertrophy
   e. Chronic obstructive pulmonary disease
   f. Left anterior fascicular block

Answers: ECG 94

1. Poor R wave progression (clockwise rotation of the precordial transition zone) is present when the precordial lead first manafesting comparable degrees of positive and negative deflection (R=S) is V_5 or V_6. Causes include anteroseptal or anterior MI, dilated or hypertrophic cardiomyopathy, LVH, RVH, COPD, cor pulmonale, WPW, and left anterior fascicular block. Up to 2% of normal individuals may also manifest this finding. (Answer: All)

— Quick Review 94 —

Artifact	
Commonly due to tremor	
• Parkinson's tremor simulates atrial ____ with a rate of ____ per second	flutter 4-6
• Physiologic tremor rate is ____ per second	7-9
• Tremor is most prominent in (limb/precordial) leads	limb
Sinus arrhythmia	
• (Sinus/nonsinus) P wave	Sinus
• Longest and shortest PP intervals vary by > ____ seconds or 10%	0.16
• Sinus arrhythmia differs from "ventriculophasic" sinus arrhythmia, the latter of which occurs in the setting of ____	heart block
Sinus bradycardia	
• Rate < ____ per minute	60
• If rate is < 40 per minute, think of 2:1 ____	sinoatrial exit block
AV block, 1°	
• PR interval ≥ ____ seconds	0.20

ECG 95. 51-year-old female with a history of orthopnea and paroxysmal nocturnal dyspnea:

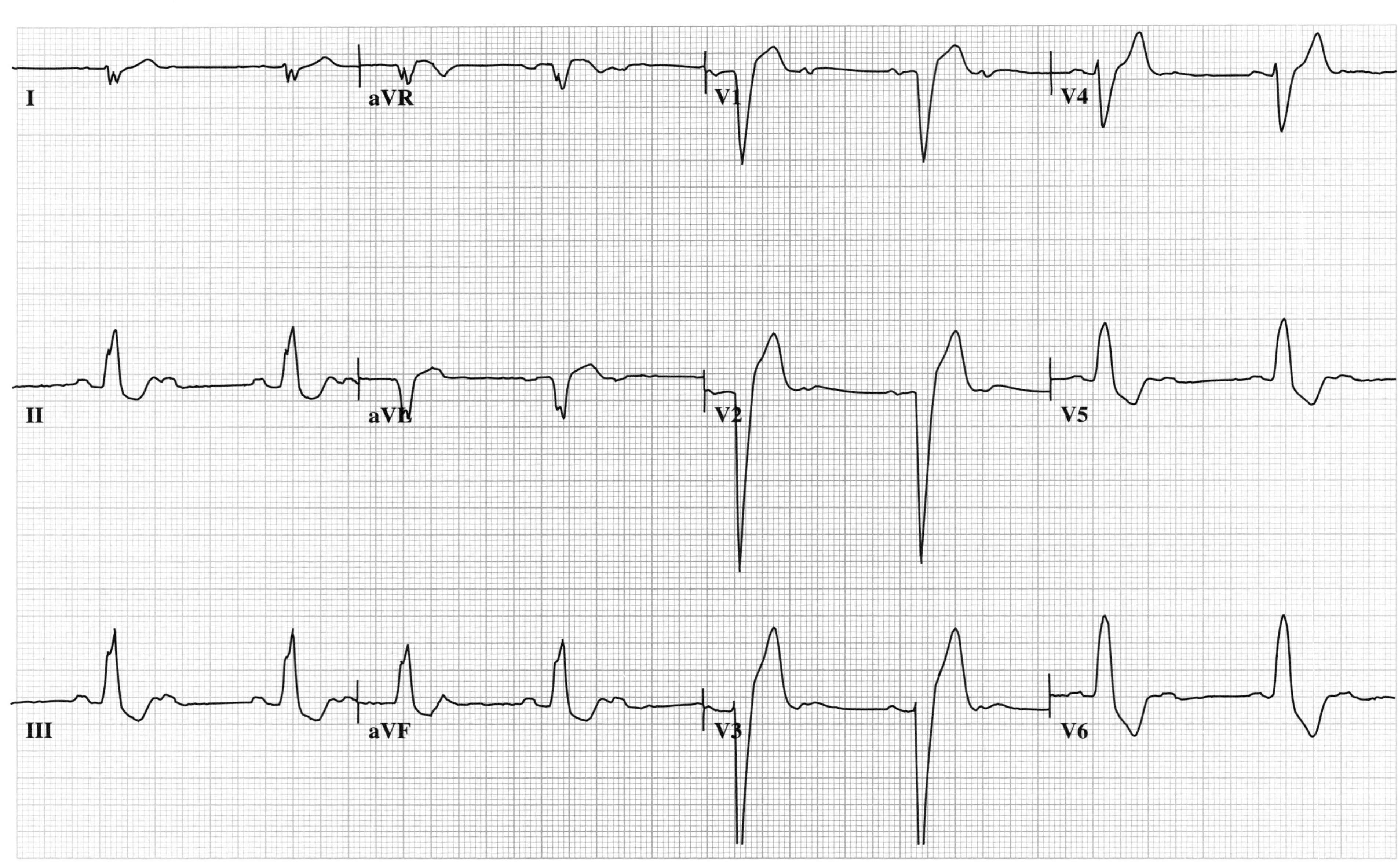

1. GENERAL FEATURES
- ☐ a. Normal ECG
- ☐ b. Borderline normal ECG or normal variant
- ☐ c. Incorrect electrode placement
- ☐ d. Artifact due to tremor

2. ATRIAL RHYTHMS
- ☐ a. Sinus rhythm
- ☐ b. Sinus arrhythmia
- ☐ c. Sinus bradycardia (< 60)
- ☐ d. Sinus tachycardia (> 100)
- ☐ e. Sinus pause or arrest
- ☐ f. Sinoatrial exit block
- ☐ g. Ecoptic atrial rhythm
- ☐ h. Wandering atrial pacemaker
- ☐ i. Atrial premature complexes, normally conducted
- ☐ j. Atrial premature complexes, nonconducted
- ☐ k. Atrial premature complexes with aberrant intraventricular conduction
- ☐ l. Atrial tachycardia (regular, sustained, 1:1 conduction)
- ☐ m. Atrial tachycardia, repetitive (short paroxysms)
- ☐ n. Atrial tachycardia, multifocal
- ☐ o. Atrial tachycardia with AV block
- ☐ p. Supraventricular tachycardia, unspecific
- ☐ q. Supraventricular tachycardia, paroxysmal
- ☐ r. Atrial flutter
- ☐ s. Atrial fibrillation
- ☐ t. Retrograde atrial activation

3. AV JUNCTIONAL RHYTHMS
- ☐ a. AV junctional premature complexes
- ☐ b. AV junctional escape complexes
- ☐ c. AV junctional rhythm, accelerated
- ☐ d. AV junctional rhythm

4. VENTRICULAR RHYTHMS
- ☐ a. Ventricular premature complex(es), uniform, fixed coupling
- ☐ b. Ventricular premature complex(es), uniform, nonfixed coupling
- ☐ c. Ventricular premature complexes(es), multiform
- ☐ d. Ventricular premature complexes, in pairs
- ☐ e. Ventricular parasystole
- ☐ f. Ventricular tachycardia (≥ 3 consecutive complexes)
- ☐ g. Accelerated idioventricular rhythm
- ☐ h. Ventricular escape complexes or rhythm
- ☐ i. Ventricular fibrillation

5. ATRIAL-VENTRICULAR INTERACTIONS IN ARRHYTHMIAS
- ☐ a. Fusion complexes
- ☐ b. Reciprocal (echo) complexes
- ☐ c. Ventricular capture complexes
- ☐ d. AV dissociation
- ☐ e. Ventriculophasic sinus arrhythmia

6. AV CONDUCTION ABNORMALITIES
- ☐ a. AV block, 1°
- ☐ b. AV block, 2° - Mobitz type I (Wenckebach)
- ☐ c. AV block, 2° - Mobitz type II
- ☐ d. AV block, 2:1
- ☐ e. AV block, 3°
- ☐ f. AV block, variable
- ☐ g. Short PR interval (with sinus rhythm and normal QRS duration)
- ☐ h. Wolff-Parkinson-White pattern

7. INTRAVENTRICULAR CONDUCTION DISTURBANCES
- ☐ a. RBBB, incomplete
- ☐ b. RBBB, complete
- ☐ c. Left anterior fascicular block
- ☐ d. Left posterior fascicular block
- ☐ e. LBBB, with ST-T wave suggestive of acute myocardial injury or infarction
- ☐ f. LBBB, complete
- ☐ g. LBBB, intermittent
- ☐ h. Intraventricular conduction disturbance, nonspecific
- ☐ i. Aberrant intraventricular conduction with supraventricular arrhythmia

8. P WAVE ABNORMALITIES
- ☐ a. Right atrial abnormality
- ☐ b. Left atrial abnormalities
- ☐ c. Nonspecific atrial abnormality

9. ABNORMALITIES OF QRS VOLTAGE OR AXIS
- ☐ a. Low voltage, limb leads only
- ☐ b. Low voltage, limb and precordial leads
- ☐ c. Left axis deviation (> - 30%)
- ☐ d. Right axis deviation (> + 100)
- ☐ e. Electrical alternans

10. VENTRICULAR HYPERTROPHY
- ☐ a. LVH by voltage only
- ☐ b. LVH by voltage and ST-T segment abnormalities
- ☐ c. RVH
- ☐ d. Combined ventricular hypertrophy

11. Q WAVE MYOCARDIAL INFARCTION

	Probably Acute or Recent	Probably Old or Age Indeterminate
Anterolateral	☐ a.	☐ g.
Anterior	☐ b.	☐ h.
Anteroseptal	☐ c.	☐ i.
Lateral/High lateral	☐ d.	☐ j.
Inferior	☐ e.	☐ k.
Posterior	☐ f.	☐ l.

☐ m. Probably ventricular aneurysm

12. ST, T, U, WAVE ABNORMALITIES
- ☐ a. Normal variant, early repolarization
- ☐ b. Normal variant, juvenile T waves
- ☐ c. Nonspecific ST and/or T wave abnormalities
- ☐ d. ST and/or T wave abnormalities suggesting myocardial ischemia
- ☐ e. ST and/or T wave abnormalities suggesting myocardial injury
- ☐ f. ST and/or T wave abnormalities suggesting acute pericarditis
- ☐ g. ST-T segment abnormalities secondary to intraventricular conduction disturbance or hypertrophy
- ☐ h. Post-extrasystolic T wave abnormality
- ☐ i. Isolated J point depression
- ☐ j. Peaked T waves
- ☐ k. Prolonged QT interval
- ☐ l. Prominent U waves

13. PACEMAKER FUNCTION AND RHYTHM
- ☐ a. Atrial or coronary sinus pacing
- ☐ b. Ventricular demand pacing
- ☐ c. AV sequential pacing
- ☐ d. Ventricular pacing, complete control
- ☐ e. Dual chamber, atrial sensing pacemaker
- ☐ f. Pacemaker malfunction, not constantly capturing (atrium or ventricle)
- ☐ g. Pacemaker malfunction, not constantly sensing (atrium or ventricle)
- ☐ h. Pacemaker malfunction, not firing
- ☐ i. Pacemaker malfunction, slowing

14. SUGGESTED OR PROBABLE CLINICAL DISORDERS
- ☐ a. Digitalis effect
- ☐ b. Digitalis toxicity
- ☐ c. Antiarrhythmic drug effect
- ☐ d. Antiarrhythmic drug toxicity
- ☐ e. Hyperkalemia
- ☐ f. Hypokalemia
- ☐ g. Hypercalcemia
- ☐ h. Hypocalcemia
- ☐ i. Atrial septal defect, secundum
- ☐ j. Atrial septal defect, primum
- ☐ k. Dextrocardia, mirror image
- ☐ l. Mitral valve disease
- ☐ m. Chronic lung disease
- ☐ n. Acute cor pulmonale, including pulmonary embolus
- ☐ o. Pericardial effusion
- ☐ p. Acute pericarditis
- ☐ q. Hypertrophic cardiomyopathy
- ☐ r. Coronary artery disease
- ☐ s. Central nervous system disorder
- ☐ t. Myxedema
- ☐ u. Hypothermia
- ☐ v. Sick sinus syndrome

ECG 95 was obtained in a 51-year-old female with a history of orthopnea and paroxysmal nocturnal dyspnea. The ECG shows sinus rhythm with predominantly 2:1 AV block (arrowheads mark P waves), LBBB with secondary ST-T changes, and right axis deviation. Upon close inspection, there is evidence for Mobitz Type I (Wenckebach) second-degree AV block (asterisk) — the third P wave conducts at a normal PR interval, the fourth P wave at a prolonged PR interval, and the fifth P wave (hidden in the T wave) is blocked. The Q waves and ST elevation in leads V_1 - V_3 are most likely due to LBBB rather than acute anteroseptal MI.

Codes:

2a	Sinus rhythm
6b	AV block, 2°- Mobitz type I (Wenckebach)
6d	AV block, 2:1
7f	LBBB, complete
9d	Right axis deviation (> + 100°)
12g	ST-T segment abnormalities secondary to IVCD or hypertrophy

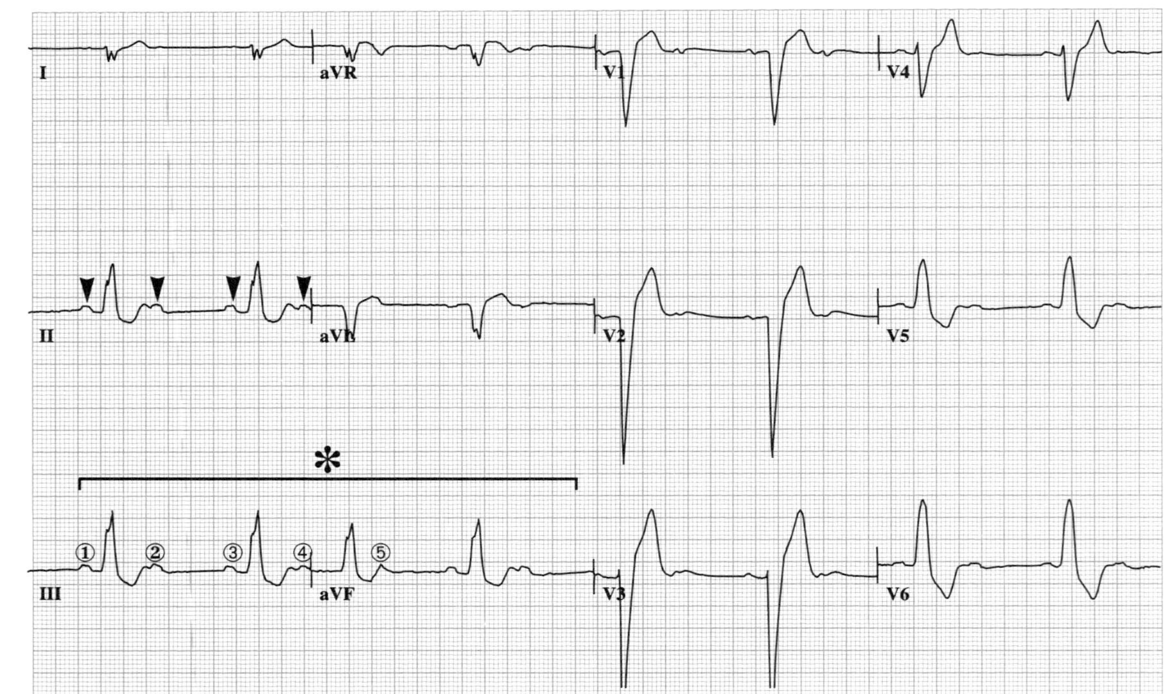

Questions: ECG 95

1. Right axis deviation is defined as a QRS axis rightward of:

   a. 70°
   b. 90°
   c. 100°
   d. 110°

2. The presence of a wide complex QRS in the setting of 2:1 AV block makes the etiology of the second-degree AV block more likely to be:

   a. Mobitz Type I
   b. Mobitz Type II

Answer: ECG 95

1. Right axis deviation is defined as a QRS axis between 100 and 254 degrees. (Answer: c)

2. It is often difficult to distinguish Mobitz I from Mobitz II second-degree AV block when 2:1 AV block is present throughout the tracing. If classic Mobitz I (Wenckebach) is present on another ECG or on monitoring strips, then 2:1 block is probably Mobitz I. On the other hand, if abnormal QRS conduction is present (e.g., LBBB or bifascicular block), Mobitz II is more likely. (Answer: b)

— Quick Review 95 —

AV block, 2° - Mobitz Type I (Wenckebach)	
• Progressive prolongation of the ____ interval and shortening of the ____ interval until a P wave is blocked	PR RR
• RR interval containing the nonconducted P wave is (less than/equal to/greater than) the sum of two PP intervals	less than
• Results in ____ beating due to the presence of nonconducted P waves	group
LBBB, complete	
• QRS duration ≥ ____ seconds	0.12
• Onset of intrinsicoid deflection in leads I, V_5, V_6 > ____ seconds	0.05
• Broad monophasic R waves in leads ____, which are usually notched or slurred	I, V_5, V_6
• Secondary ST & T wave changes in the (same/opposite) direction to the major QRS deflection	opposite
• ____ or ____ complex in the right precordial leads	rS or QS
• LBBB (does/does not) interfere with determination of QRS axis and the diagnoses of ventricular hypertrophy and acute MI	does

ECG 96. 76-year-old male with a permanent pacemaker:

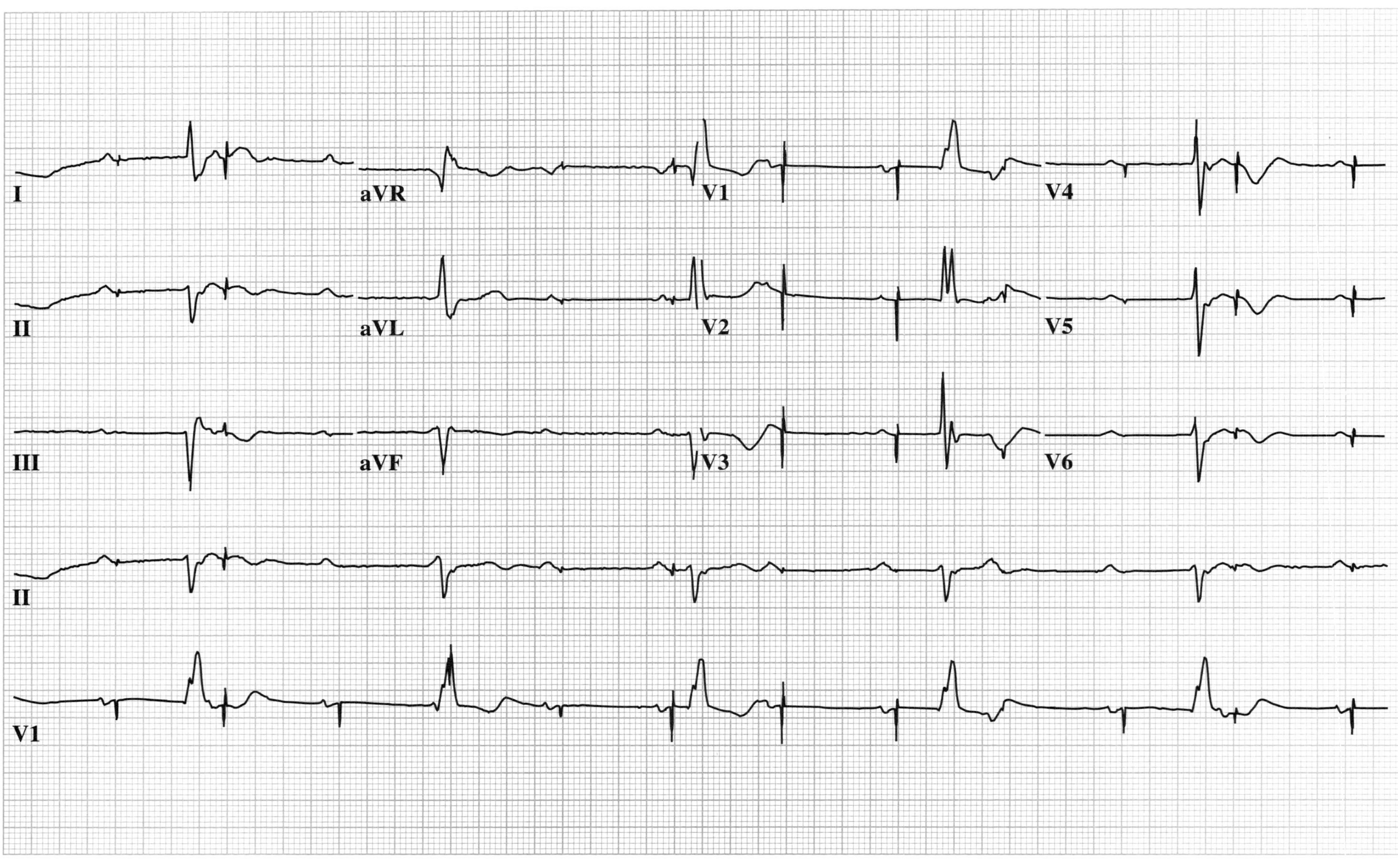

1. GENERAL FEATURES

☐ a. Normal ECG
☐ b. Borderline normal ECG or normal variant
☐ c. Incorrect electrode placement
☐ d. Artifact due to tremor

2. ATRIAL RHYTHMS

☐ a. Sinus rhythm
☐ b. Sinus arrhythmia
☐ c. Sinus bradycardia (< 60)
☐ d. Sinus tachycardia (> 100)
☐ e. Sinus pause or arrest
☐ f. Sinoatrial exit block
☐ g. Ecoptic atrial rhythm
☐ h. Wandering atrial pacemaker
☐ i. Atrial premature complexes, normally conducted
☐ j. Atrial premature complexes, nonconducted
☐ k. Atrial premature complexes with aberrant intraventricular conduction
☐ l. Atrial tachycardia (regular, sustained, 1:1 conduction)
☐ m. Atrial tachycardia, repetitive (short paroxysms)
☐ n. Atrial tachycardia, multifocal
☐ o. Atrial tachycardia with AV block
☐ p. Supraventricular tachycardia, unspecific
☐ q. Supraventricular tachycardia, paroxysmal
☐ r. Atrial flutter
☐ s. Atrial fibrillation
☐ t. Retrograde atrial activation

3. AV JUNCTIONAL RHYTHMS

☐ a. AV junctional premature complexes
☐ b. AV junctional escape complexes
☐ c. AV junctional rhythm, accelerated
☐ d. AV junctional rhythm

4. VENTRICULAR RHYTHMS

☐ a. Ventricular premature complex(es), uniform, fixed coupling
☐ b. Ventricular premature complex(es), uniform, nonfixed coupling
☐ c. Ventricular premature complexes(es), multiform
☐ d. Ventricular premature complexes, in pairs
☐ e. Ventricular parasystole
☐ f. Ventricular tachycardia (≥ 3 consecutive complexes)
☐ g. Accelerated idioventricular rhythm
☐ h. Ventricular escape complexes or rhythm
☐ i. Ventricular fibrillation

5. ATRIAL-VENTRICULAR INTERACTIONS IN ARRHYTHMIAS

☐ a. Fusion complexes
☐ b. Reciprocal (echo) complexes
☐ c. Ventricular capture complexes
☐ d. AV dissociation
☐ e. Ventriculophasic sinus arrhythmia

6. AV CONDUCTION ABNORMALITIES

☐ a. AV block, 1°
☐ b. AV block, 2° - Mobitz type I (Wenckebach)
☐ c. AV block, 2° - Mobitz type II
☐ d. AV block, 2:1
☐ e. AV block, 3°
☐ f. AV block, variable
☐ g. Short PR interval (with sinus rhythm and normal QRS duration)
☐ h. Wolff-Parkinson-White pattern

7. INTRAVENTRICULAR CONDUCTION DISTURBANCES

☐ a. RBBB, incomplete
☐ b. RBBB, complete
☐ c. Left anterior fascicular block
☐ d. Left posterior fascicular block
☐ e. LBBB, with ST-T wave suggestive of acute myocardial injury or infarction
☐ f. LBBB, complete
☐ g. LBBB, intermittent
☐ h. Intraventricular conduction disturbance, nonspecific
☐ i. Aberrant intraventricular conduction with supraventricular arrhythmia

8. P WAVE ABNORMALITIES

☐ a. Right atrial abnormality
☐ b. Left atrial abnormalities
☐ c. Nonspecific atrial abnormality

9. ABNORMALITIES OF QRS VOLTAGE OR AXIS

☐ a. Low voltage, limb leads only
☐ b. Low voltage, limb and precordial leads
☐ c. Left axis deviation (> - 30%)
☐ d. Right axis deviation (> + 100)
☐ e. Electrical alternans

10. VENTRICULAR HYPERTROPHY

☐ a. LVH by voltage only
☐ b. LVH by voltage and ST-T segment abnormalities
☐ c. RVH
☐ d. Combined ventricular hypertrophy

11. Q WAVE MYOCARDIAL INFARCTION

	Probably Acute or Recent	Probably Old or Age Indeterminate
Anterolateral	☐ a.	☐ g.
Anterior	☐ b.	☐ h.
Anteroseptal	☐ c.	☐ i.
Lateral/High lateral	☐ d.	☐ j.
Inferior	☐ e.	☐ k.
Posterior	☐ f.	☐ l.

☐ m. Probably ventricular aneurysm

12. ST, T, U, WAVE ABNORMALITIES

☐ a. Normal variant, early repolarization
☐ b. Normal variant, juvenile T waves
☐ c. Nonspecific ST and/or T wave abnormalities
☐ d. ST and/or T wave abnormalities suggesting myocardial ischemia
☐ e. ST and/or T wave abnormalities suggesting myocardial injury
☐ f. ST and/or T wave abnormalities suggesting acute pericarditis
☐ g. ST-T segment abnormalities secondary to intraventricular conduction disturbance or hypertrophy
☐ h. Post-extrasystolic T wave abnormality
☐ i. Isolated J point depression
☐ j. Peaked T waves
☐ k. Prolonged QT interval
☐ l. Prominent U waves

13. PACEMAKER FUNCTION AND RHYTHM

☐ a. Atrial or coronary sinus pacing
☐ b. Ventricular demand pacing
☐ c. AV sequential pacing
☐ d. Ventricular pacing, complete control
☐ e. Dual chamber, atrial sensing pacemaker
☐ f. Pacemaker malfunction, not constantly capturing (atrium or ventricle)
☐ g. Pacemaker malfunction, not constantly sensing (atrium or ventricle)
☐ h. Pacemaker malfunction, not firing
☐ i. Pacemaker malfunction, slowing

14. SUGGESTED OR PROBABLE CLINICAL DISORDERS

☐ a. Digitalis effect
☐ b. Digitalis toxicity
☐ c. Antiarrhythmic drug effect
☐ d. Antiarrhythmic drug toxicity
☐ e. Hyperkalemia
☐ f. Hypokalemia
☐ g. Hypercalcemia
☐ h. Hypocalcemia
☐ i. Atrial septal defect, secundum
☐ j. Atrial septal defect, primum
☐ k. Dextrocardia, mirror image
☐ l. Mitral valve disease
☐ m. Chronic lung disease
☐ n. Acute cor pulmonale, including pulmonary embolus
☐ o. Pericardial effusion
☐ p. Acute pericarditis
☐ q. Hypertrophic cardiomyopathy
☐ r. Coronary artery disease
☐ s. Central nervous system disorder
☐ t. Myxedema
☐ u. Hypothermia
☐ v. Sick sinus syndrome

ECG 96 was obtained in a 76-year-old male with a permanent pacemaker. The ECG shows an underlying sinus rhythm at approximately 70 beats/minute with complete heart block and a ventricular escape rhythm at 49 beats/minute. Nonspecific repolarization abnormalities are present (secondary to the conduction abnormality). A dual chamber atrial sensing pacemaker is apparent with failure to sense and capture appropriately; the failure to capture is obvious (arrow), while the failure to sense can be diagnosed from the second complex in the rhythm strip, which shows ventricular pacing very early after a native complex (arrowhead points to pacer spike superimposed on the QRS complex).

Codes:

2a	Sinus rhythm
4h	Ventricular escape complexes or rhythm
6e	AV block, 3°
12g	ST-T segment abnormalities secondary to IVCD or hypertrophy
13e	Dual chamber, atrial sensing pacemaker
13f	Pacemaker malfunction, not constantly capturing (atrium or ventricle)
13g	Pacemaker malfunction, not constantly sensing (atrium or ventricle)

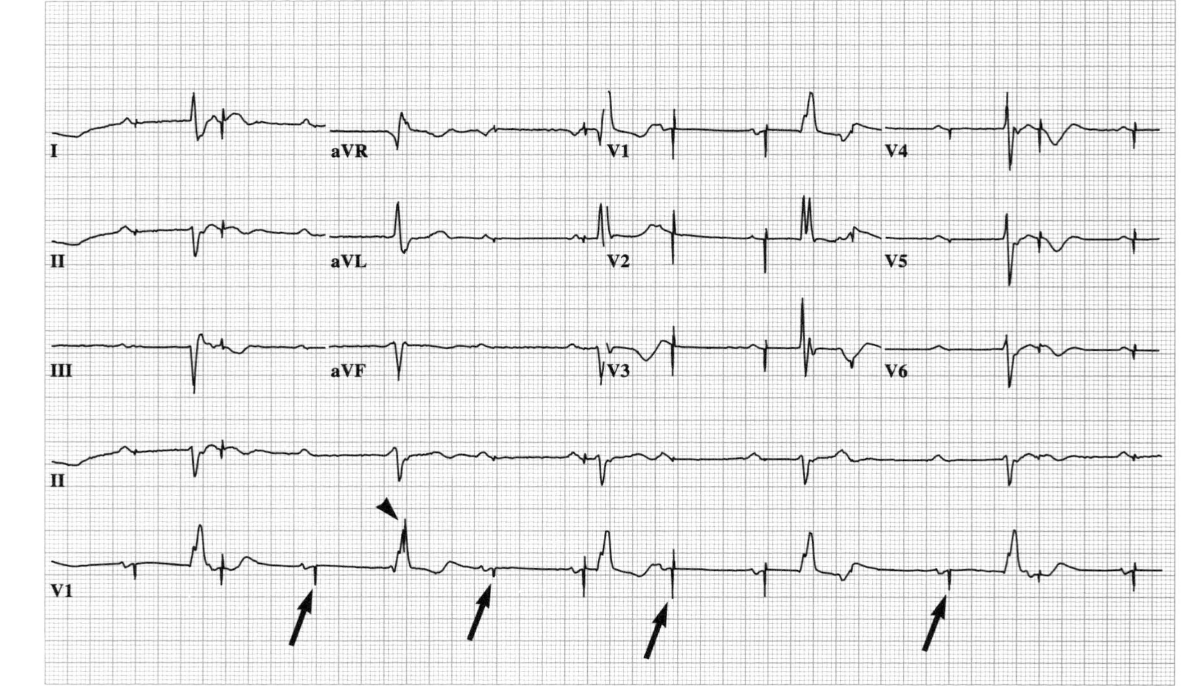

Questions: ECG 96

1. Disruption of the insulating sleeve (insulation fracture) can manifest as any of the following except:

   a. Battery depletion
   b. Oversensing
   c. Failure to capture
   d. Pacemaker-mediated tachycardia

Answers: ECG 96

1. Insulation sleeve fracture can result in oversensing, failure to capture, and/or early battery depletion. Pacemaker-mediated tachycardia is not a manifestation of insulation fracture. (Answer: d)

— Quick Review 96 —

Ventricular escape beats or rhythm	
• Ventricular rate of ____ per minute (can be ____ per minute)	30-40, 20-50
• QRS morphology is similar to ____	VPCs
• QRS complex occurs as a ____ phenomenon in response to decreased sinus impulse formation or conduction, or high-degree AV block	secondary
Dual chamber, atrial-sensing pacemaker	
• For atrial sensing, need to demonstrate inhibition of (atrial/ventricular) output and/or triggering of the (atrial/ventricular) stimulus in response to intrinsic atrial depolarization	atrial ventricular
• Includes____ and possibly VAT or VDD pacemakers	DDD
Pacemaker malfunction, not constantly capturing (atrium or ventricle)	
• Failure of pacemaker stimulus to be followed by a ____	depolarization
• Rule out "pseudo-malfunction" (i.e., pacer stimulus falls into the ____ period of ventricle)	refractory

— Quick Review 96 —

Pacemaker malfunction, not constantly sensing (atrium or ventricle)	
• Pacemakers in the inhibited mode: Pacemaker fails to be ____ by an appropriate intrinsic depolarization	inhibited
• Pacemakers in the triggered mode: Pacemaker fails to be ____ by an appropriate intrinsic depolarization	triggered
• Premature depolarizations may not be sensed if they fall within the programmed ____ period of the pacemaker, *or* have insufficient ____ at the sensing electrode site	refractory amplitude

Common Dilemmas in ECG Interpretation

Problem

Ischemic-looking ST segment elevation is present without pathological Q waves in a patient with chest pain. Should acute myocardial infarction be coded?

Recommendation

No. Convex upward ST segment elevation without pathological Q waves should be coded as 12e (ST and/or T abnormalities suggesting myocardial injury). Clinically, this usually represents the early stages of acute infarction or transient coronary spasm or occlusion. Nevertheless, in the absence of pathological Q waves (or pathological R waves in the case of posterior infarction), acute myocardial infarction should not be coded. Ischemic ST elevation alone, however, should prompt coding of 14r (coronary artery disease).

ECG 97. 66-year-old female smoker being evaluated for dyspnea:

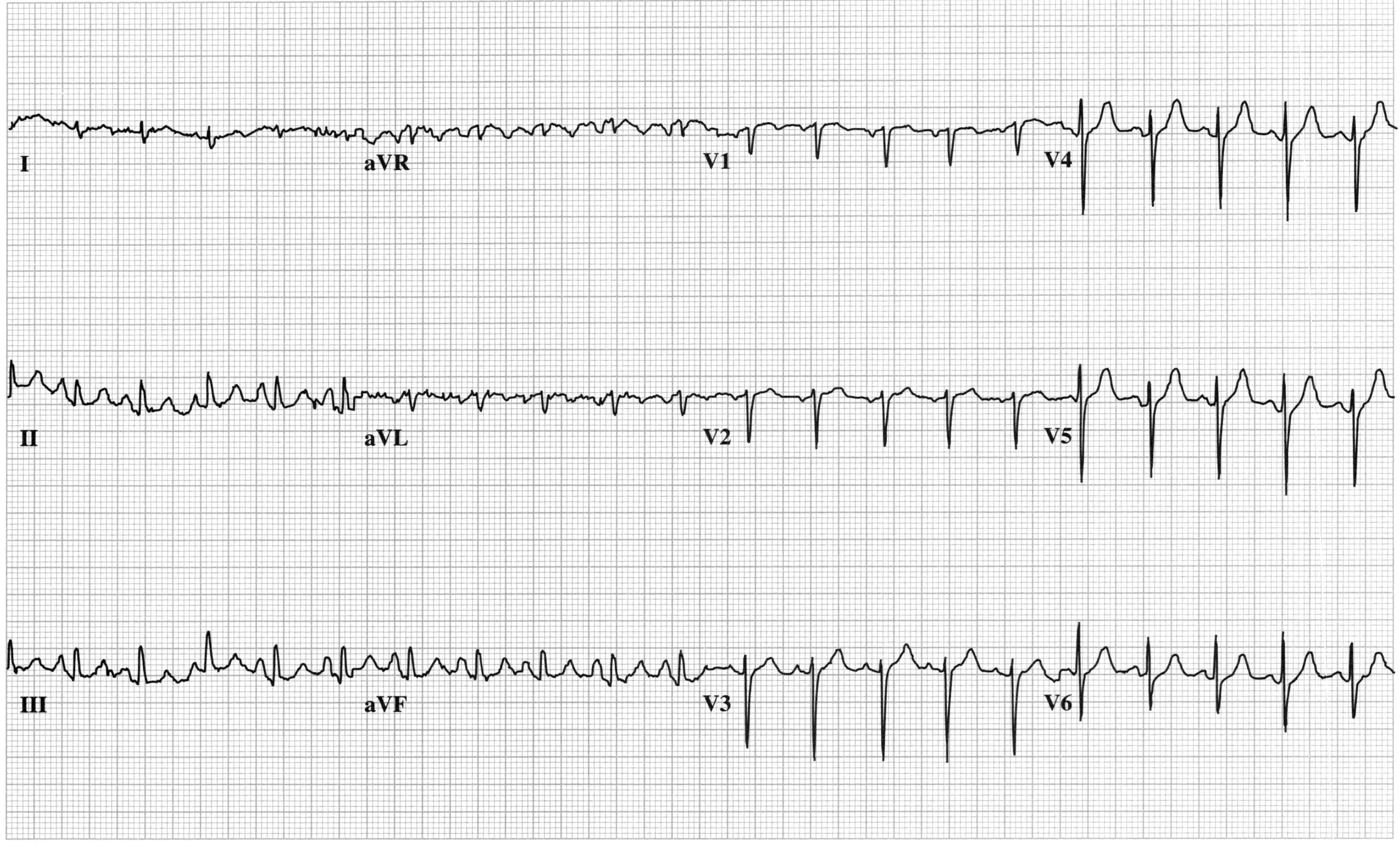

1. GENERAL FEATURES
- ☐ a. Normal ECG
- ☐ b. Borderline normal ECG or normal variant
- ☐ c. Incorrect electrode placement
- ☐ d. Artifact due to tremor

2. ATRIAL RHYTHMS
- ☐ a. Sinus rhythm
- ☐ b. Sinus arrhythmia
- ☐ c. Sinus bradycardia (< 60)
- ☐ d. Sinus tachycardia (> 100)
- ☐ e. Sinus pause or arrest
- ☐ f. Sinoatrial exit block
- ☐ g. Ecoptic atrial rhythm
- ☐ h. Wandering atrial pacemaker
- ☐ i. Atrial premature complexes, normally conducted
- ☐ j. Atrial premature complexes, nonconducted
- ☐ k. Atrial premature complexes with aberrant intraventricular conduction
- ☐ l. Atrial tachycardia (regular, sustained, 1:1 conduction)
- ☐ m. Atrial tachycardia, repetitive (short paroxysms)
- ☐ n. Atrial tachycardia, multifocal
- ☐ o. Atrial tachycardia with AV block
- ☐ p. Supraventricular tachycardia, unspecific
- ☐ q. Supraventricular tachycardia, paroxysmal
- ☐ r. Atrial flutter
- ☐ s. Atrial fibrillation
- ☐ t. Retrograde atrial activation

3. AV JUNCTIONAL RHYTHMS
- ☐ a. AV junctional premature complexes
- ☐ b. AV junctional escape complexes
- ☐ c. AV junctional rhythm, accelerated
- ☐ d. AV junctional rhythm

4. VENTRICULAR RHYTHMS
- ☐ a. Ventricular premature complex(es), uniform, fixed coupling
- ☐ b. Ventricular premature complex(es), uniform, nonfixed coupling
- ☐ c. Ventricular premature complexes(es), multiform
- ☐ d. Ventricular premature complexes, in pairs
- ☐ e. Ventricular parasystole
- ☐ f. Ventricular tachycardia (≥ 3 consecutive complexes)
- ☐ g. Accelerated idioventricular rhythm
- ☐ h. Ventricular escape complexes or rhythm
- ☐ i. Ventricular fibrillation

5. ATRIAL-VENTRICULAR INTERACTIONS IN ARRHYTHMIAS
- ☐ a. Fusion complexes
- ☐ b. Reciprocal (echo) complexes
- ☐ c. Ventricular capture complexes
- ☐ d. AV dissociation
- ☐ e. Ventriculophasic sinus arrhythmia

6. AV CONDUCTION ABNORMALITIES
- ☐ a. AV block, 1°
- ☐ b. AV block, 2° - Mobitz type I (Wenckebach)
- ☐ c. AV block, 2° - Mobitz type II
- ☐ d. AV block, 2:1
- ☐ e. AV block, 3°
- ☐ f. AV block, variable
- ☐ g. Short PR interval (with sinus rhythm and normal QRS duration)
- ☐ h. Wolff-Parkinson-White pattern

7. INTRAVENTRICULAR CONDUCTION DISTURBANCES
- ☐ a. RBBB, incomplete
- ☐ b. RBBB, complete
- ☐ c. Left anterior fascicular block
- ☐ d. Left posterior fascicular block
- ☐ e. LBBB, with ST-T wave suggestive of acute myocardial injury or infarction
- ☐ f. LBBB, complete
- ☐ g. LBBB, intermittent
- ☐ h. Intraventricular conduction disturbance, nonspecific
- ☐ i. Aberrant intraventricular conduction with supraventricular arrhythmia

8. P WAVE ABNORMALITIES
- ☐ a. Right atrial abnormality
- ☐ b. Left atrial abnormalities
- ☐ c. Nonspecific atrial abnormality

9. ABNORMALITIES OF QRS VOLTAGE OR AXIS
- ☐ a. Low voltage, limb leads only
- ☐ b. Low voltage, limb and precordial leads
- ☐ c. Left axis deviation (> - 30%)
- ☐ d. Right axis deviation (> + 100)
- ☐ e. Electrical alternans

10. VENTRICULAR HYPERTROPHY
- ☐ a. LVH by voltage only
- ☐ b. LVH by voltage and ST-T segment abnormalities
- ☐ c. RVH
- ☐ d. Combined ventricular hypertrophy

11. Q WAVE MYOCARDIAL INFARCTION

	Probably Acute or Recent	Probably Old or Age Indeterminate
Anterolateral	☐ a.	☐ g.
Anterior	☐ b.	☐ h.
Anteroseptal	☐ c.	☐ i.
Lateral/High lateral	☐ d.	☐ j.
Inferior	☐ e.	☐ k.
Posterior	☐ f.	☐ l.

☐ m. Probably ventricular aneurysm

12. ST, T, U, WAVE ABNORMALITIES
- ☐ a. Normal variant, early repolarization
- ☐ b. Normal variant, juvenile T waves
- ☐ c. Nonspecific ST and/or T wave abnormalities
- ☐ d. ST and/or T wave abnormalities suggesting myocardial ischemia
- ☐ e. ST and/or T wave abnormalities suggesting myocardial injury
- ☐ f. ST and/or T wave abnormalities suggesting acute pericarditis
- ☐ g. ST-T segment abnormalities secondary to intraventricular conduction disturbance or hypertrophy
- ☐ h. Post-extrasystolic T wave abnormality
- ☐ i. Isolated J point depression
- ☐ j. Peaked T waves
- ☐ k. Prolonged QT interval
- ☐ l. Prominent U waves

13. PACEMAKER FUNCTION AND RHYTHM
- ☐ a. Atrial or coronary sinus pacing
- ☐ b. Ventricular demand pacing
- ☐ c. AV sequential pacing
- ☐ d. Ventricular pacing, complete control
- ☐ e. Dual chamber, atrial sensing pacemaker
- ☐ f. Pacemaker malfunction, not constantly capturing (atrium or ventricle)
- ☐ g. Pacemaker malfunction, not constantly sensing (atrium or ventricle)
- ☐ h. Pacemaker malfunction, not firing
- ☐ i. Pacemaker malfunction, slowing

14. SUGGESTED OR PROBABLE CLINICAL DISORDERS
- ☐ a. Digitalis effect
- ☐ b. Digitalis toxicity
- ☐ c. Antiarrhythmic drug effect
- ☐ d. Antiarrhythmic drug toxicity
- ☐ e. Hyperkalemia
- ☐ f. Hypokalemia
- ☐ g. Hypercalcemia
- ☐ h. Hypocalcemia
- ☐ i. Atrial septal defect, secundum
- ☐ j. Atrial septal defect, primum
- ☐ k. Dextrocardia, mirror image
- ☐ l. Mitral valve disease
- ☐ m. Chronic lung disease
- ☐ n. Acute cor pulmonale, including pulmonary embolus
- ☐ o. Pericardial effusion
- ☐ p. Acute pericarditis
- ☐ q. Hypertrophic cardiomyopathy
- ☐ r. Coronary artery disease
- ☐ s. Central nervous system disorder
- ☐ t. Myxedema
- ☐ u. Hypothermia
- ☐ v. Sick sinus syndrome

ECG 97 was obtained in a 66-year-old female smoker being evaluated for dyspnea. The tracing shows sinus tachycardia at approximately 120 beats/minute. A rightward axis (at +97° it does not quite meet criteria for RAD), right atrial abnormality (arrow), relatively low voltage (not meeting criteria for coding of low voltage, however), and poor R wave progression are present. This constellation of findings is suggestive of chronic lung disease. The irregular baseline (best seen in lead I; asterisk) is consistent with tremor.

Codes:

1d	Artifact due to tremor
2d	Sinus tachycardia
8a	Right atrial abnormality
14m	Chronic lung disease

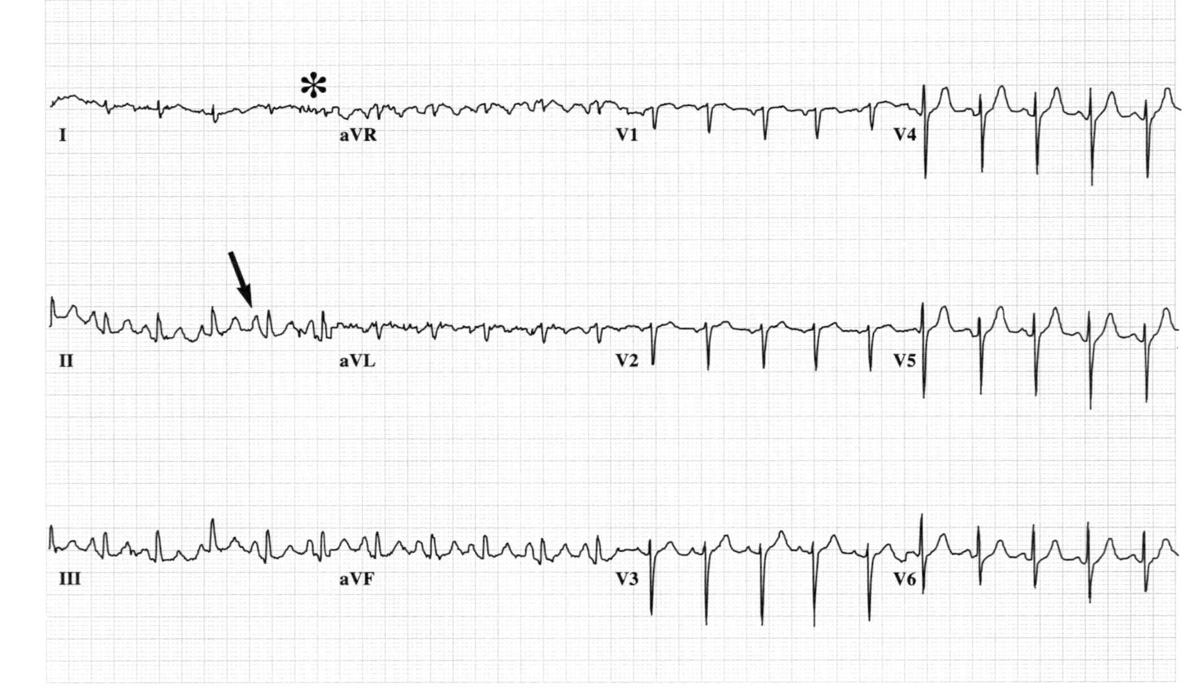

Questions: ECG 97

1. Typical ECG findings of chronic lung disease (COPD or emphysema) include:

   a. Inferior ST elevation
   b. Rightward and posterior shift of QRS axis
   c. Low QRS voltage
   d. Right atrial abnormality

2. Chronic lung disease can cause a pseudo-infarct pattern in leads:

   a. II, III, aVF
   b. V_4-V_6
   c. V_1-V_3
   d. I, aVL

3. Dysrhythmias associated with COPD include:

   a. Multifocal atrial tachycardia
   b. Sinus tachycardia
   c. Torsade de Pointes
   d. Atrial fibrillation

Answers: ECG 97

1. Chronic obstructive pulmonary disease typically causes changes in the 12-lead ECG. The QRS axis is often shifted to the right and posteriorly, (although not generally enough to meet criteria for right axis deviation). Low QRS voltage may be present since air (in the hyperexpanded lungs) is a poor electrical conductor. Right atrial abnormality (tall P waves in leads II, III, and aVF) are also often seen. ST segment elevation is not typically associated with chronic lung disease, but inferior ST segment depression can be a sign of right ventricular hypertrophy with strain. (Answer: b, c, d)

2. The posterior shift in mean QRS vector associated with chronic lung disease may result in low or absent R waves in the anterior precordial leads (V_1-V_3), mimicking anteroseptal MI. (Answer: c)

3. Transient supraventricular dysrhythmias commonly associated with COPD include multifocal atrial tachycardia, sinus tachycardia, atrial fibrillation, atrial flutter, and ectopic atrial tachycardia. Ventricular dysrhythmias, including torsade de pointes, are not typically seen with COPD. (Answer: All except c)

— Quick Review 97 —

Artifact	
Commonly due to tremor	
• Parkinson's tremor simulates atrial ____ with a rate	flutter
of ____ per second	4-6
• Physiologic tremor rate is ____ per second	7-9
• Tremor is most prominent in (limb/precordial) leads	limb
Sinus tachycardia (>100)	
• Rate > ____ per minute	100
• P wave amplitude often (increases/decreases) and	increases
PR interval often (increases/decreases) with increasing heart rate	shortens
Right atrial abnormality	
• Upright P wave > ____ mm in leads II, III and aVF	2.5
or > ____ mm in leads V_1 or V_2	1.5
• P wave axis ≥ ____ degrees	70
Chronic lung disease	
• (Right/left) ventricular hypertrophy	Right
• (Right/left) axis deviation	Right
• (Right/left) atrial abnormality	Right
• Shift of transitional zone (clockwise/counterclockwise)	counter-clockwise
• (High/low) voltage QRS	Low
• Pseudoinfarct pattern in the ____ leads	anteroseptal
• S waves in leads ____ (S_1 S_2 S_3 pattern)	I, II, and III
• May also see sinus tachycardia, junctional rhythm, various degrees of AV block, IVCD, and bundle branch block (true/false)	true

Don't Forget!

- Classic evolutionary ECG pattern of acute pericarditis consists of 4 stages (but is not always present):
  - Stage 1: Upwardly concave ST segment elevation in almost all leads except aVR; no reciprocal ST depression in other leads except aVR
  - Stage 2: ST junction (J point) returns to baseline and T wave amplitude begins to decrease
  - Stage 3: T waves invert
  - Stage 4: ECG returns to normal
- Digitalis toxicity can cause almost any type of cardiac dysrhythmia or conduction disturbance **except** bundle branch block.
- ECG findings in CNS disease can mimic those of:
  - Acute MI (item 11)
  - Acute pericarditis (item 14p)
  - Drug effect or toxicity (items 14c, d)

ECG 98. 90-year-old male with a remote myocardial infarction:

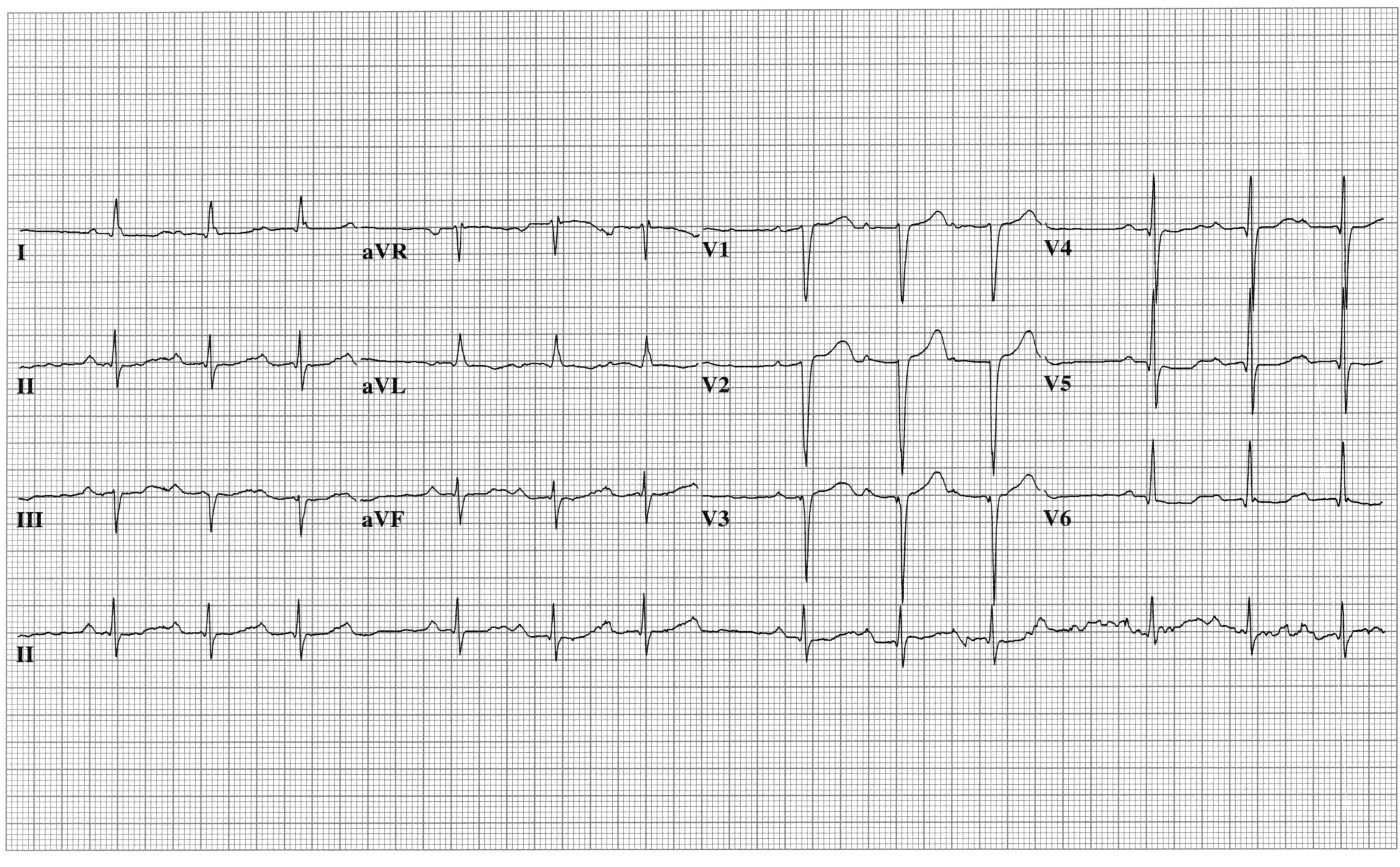

1. GENERAL FEATURES
- ☐ a. Normal ECG
- ☐ b. Borderline normal ECG or normal variant
- ☐ c. Incorrect electrode placement
- ☐ d. Artifact due to tremor

2. ATRIAL RHYTHMS
- ☐ a. Sinus rhythm
- ☐ b. Sinus arrhythmia
- ☐ c. Sinus bradycardia (< 60)
- ☐ d. Sinus tachycardia (> 100)
- ☐ e. Sinus pause or arrest
- ☐ f. Sinoatrial exit block
- ☐ g. Ecoptic atrial rhythm
- ☐ h. Wandering atrial pacemaker
- ☐ i. Atrial premature complexes, normally conducted
- ☐ j. Atrial premature complexes, nonconducted
- ☐ k. Atrial premature complexes with aberrant intraventricular conduction
- ☐ l. Atrial tachycardia (regular, sustained, 1:1 conduction)
- ☐ m. Atrial tachycardia, repetitive (short paroxysms)
- ☐ n. Atrial tachycardia, multifocal
- ☐ o. Atrial tachycardia with AV block
- ☐ p. Supraventricular tachycardia, unspecific
- ☐ q. Supraventricular tachycardia, paroxysmal
- ☐ r. Atrial flutter
- ☐ s. Atrial fibrillation
- ☐ t. Retrograde atrial activation

3. AV JUNCTIONAL RHYTHMS
- ☐ a. AV junctional premature complexes
- ☐ b. AV junctional escape complexes
- ☐ c. AV junctional rhythm, accelerated
- ☐ d. AV junctional rhythm

4. VENTRICULAR RHYTHMS
- ☐ a. Ventricular premature complex(es), uniform, fixed coupling
- ☐ b. Ventricular premature complex(es), uniform, nonfixed coupling
- ☐ c. Ventricular premature complexes(es), multiform
- ☐ d. Ventricular premature complexes, in pairs
- ☐ e. Ventricular parasystole
- ☐ f. Ventricular tachycardia (≥ 3 consecutive complexes)
- ☐ g. Accelerated idioventricular rhythm
- ☐ h. Ventricular escape complexes or rhythm
- ☐ i. Ventricular fibrillation

5. ATRIAL-VENTRICULAR INTERACTIONS IN ARRHYTHMIAS
- ☐ a. Fusion complexes
- ☐ b. Reciprocal (echo) complexes
- ☐ c. Ventricular capture complexes
- ☐ d. AV dissociation
- ☐ e. Ventriculophasic sinus arrhythmia

6. AV CONDUCTION ABNORMALITIES
- ☐ a. AV block, 1°
- ☐ b. AV block, 2° - Mobitz type I (Wenckebach)
- ☐ c. AV block, 2° - Mobitz type II
- ☐ d. AV block, 2:1
- ☐ e. AV block, 3°
- ☐ f. AV block, variable
- ☐ g. Short PR interval (with sinus rhythm and normal QRS duration)
- ☐ h. Wolff-Parkinson-White pattern

7. INTRAVENTRICULAR CONDUCTION DISTURBANCES
- ☐ a. RBBB, incomplete
- ☐ b. RBBB, complete
- ☐ c. Left anterior fascicular block
- ☐ d. Left posterior fascicular block
- ☐ e. LBBB, with ST-T wave suggestive of acute myocardial injury or infarction
- ☐ f. LBBB, complete
- ☐ g. LBBB, intermittent
- ☐ h. Intraventricular conduction disturbance, nonspecific
- ☐ i. Aberrant intraventricular conduction with supraventricular arrhythmia

8. P WAVE ABNORMALITIES
- ☐ a. Right atrial abnormality
- ☐ b. Left atrial abnormalities
- ☐ c. Nonspecific atrial abnormality

9. ABNORMALITIES OF QRS VOLTAGE OR AXIS
- ☐ a. Low voltage, limb leads only
- ☐ b. Low voltage, limb and precordial leads
- ☐ c. Left axis deviation (> - 30%)
- ☐ d. Right axis deviation (> + 100)
- ☐ e. Electrical alternans

10. VENTRICULAR HYPERTROPHY
- ☐ a. LVH by voltage only
- ☐ b. LVH by voltage and ST-T segment abnormalities
- ☐ c. RVH
- ☐ d. Combined ventricular hypertrophy

11. Q WAVE MYOCARDIAL INFARCTION

	Probably Acute or Recent	Probably Old or Age Indeterminate
Anterolateral	☐ a.	☐ g.
Anterior	☐ b.	☐ h.
Anteroseptal	☐ c.	☐ i.
Lateral/High lateral	☐ d.	☐ j.
Inferior	☐ e.	☐ k.
Posterior	☐ f.	☐ l.

☐ m. Probably ventricular aneurysm

12. ST, T, U, WAVE ABNORMALITIES
- ☐ a. Normal variant, early repolarization
- ☐ b. Normal variant, juvenile T waves
- ☐ c. Nonspecific ST and/or T wave abnormalities
- ☐ d. ST and/or T wave abnormalities suggesting myocardial ischemia
- ☐ e. ST and/or T wave abnormalities suggesting myocardial injury
- ☐ f. ST and/or T wave abnormalities suggesting acute pericarditis
- ☐ g. ST-T segment abnormalities secondary to intraventricular conduction disturbance or hypertrophy
- ☐ h. Post-extrasystolic T wave abnormality
- ☐ i. Isolated J point depression
- ☐ j. Peaked T waves
- ☐ k. Prolonged QT interval
- ☐ l. Prominent U waves

13. PACEMAKER FUNCTION AND RHYTHM
- ☐ a. Atrial or coronary sinus pacing
- ☐ b. Ventricular demand pacing
- ☐ c. AV sequential pacing
- ☐ d. Ventricular pacing, complete control
- ☐ e. Dual chamber, atrial sensing pacemaker
- ☐ f. Pacemaker malfunction, not constantly capturing (atrium or ventricle)
- ☐ g. Pacemaker malfunction, not constantly sensing (atrium or ventricle)
- ☐ h. Pacemaker malfunction, not firing
- ☐ i. Pacemaker malfunction, slowing

14. SUGGESTED OR PROBABLE CLINICAL DISORDERS
- ☐ a. Digitalis effect
- ☐ b. Digitalis toxicity
- ☐ c. Antiarrhythmic drug effect
- ☐ d. Antiarrhythmic drug toxicity
- ☐ e. Hyperkalemia
- ☐ f. Hypokalemia
- ☐ g. Hypercalcemia
- ☐ h. Hypocalcemia
- ☐ i. Atrial septal defect, secundum
- ☐ j. Atrial septal defect, primum
- ☐ k. Dextrocardia, mirror image
- ☐ l. Mitral valve disease
- ☐ m. Chronic lung disease
- ☐ n. Acute cor pulmonale, including pulmonary embolus
- ☐ o. Pericardial effusion
- ☐ p. Acute pericarditis
- ☐ q. Hypertrophic cardiomyopathy
- ☐ r. Coronary artery disease
- ☐ s. Central nervous system disorder
- ☐ t. Myxedema
- ☐ u. Hypothermia
- ☐ v. Sick sinus syndrome

ECG 98 was obtained in a 90-year-old male with a history of remote myocardial infarction. The ECG shows a sinus rhythm at 73 beats/minute. "Group beating" is noted (asterisks) consistent with Mobitz Type I (Wenckebach) second-degree AV block (PR lengthens and RR shortens between nonconducted P waves marked by arrows). Abnormal Q waves in leads V_2-V_6 suggest old or age indeterminate anterior and anterolateral myocardial infarctions. Nonspecific repolarization abnormalities and findings consistent with coronary artery disease are also noted.

Codes:

2a	Sinus rhythm
6b	AV block, 2° - Mobitz type I (Wenckebach)
11g	Anterolateral Q wave MI, probably old or age indeterminate
11h	Anterior Q wave MI, probably old or age indeterminate
12c	Nonspecific ST and/or T wave abnormalities
14r	Coronary artery disease

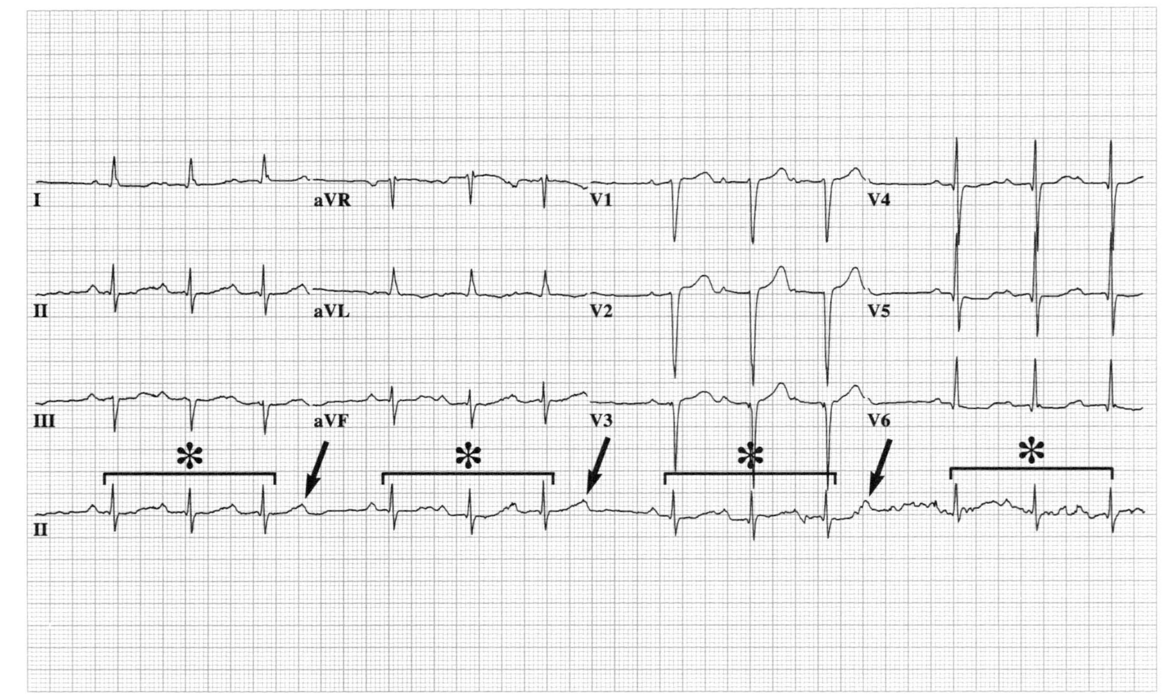

Questions: ECG 98

1. Which of the following statements about Mobitz Type I second-degree AV block are true?

   a. The QRS is usually narrow, and the level of block is usually at the AV node
   b. First-degree and third-degree AV block may coexist with Mobitz Type I block
   c. Progressive shortening of the RR interval is typical of Mobitz Type I, and is due to a decrease in the increment of the PR interval
   d. Progressive prolongation of the PR interval and shortening of the RR interval are not always present

2 In addition to Mobitz Type I block, causes of "group beating" include:

   a. Premature atrial contractions
   b. Type II second-degree AV block
   c. Type II sinoatrial exit block
   d. Concealed premature His-bundle depolarizations

3. What is the conduction ratio in the present tracing?

   a. 3:1
   b. 3:2
   c. 4:3
   d. 5:4

Answers: ECG 98

1. In second-degree AV block, there is intermittent failure of supraventricular beats to conduct to the ventricles. Mobitz Type I second-degree AV block (Wenckebach) is characterized by progressive prolongation of the PR interval and shortening the RR interval until a P wave is blocked; a constant PP interval; and an RR interval containing the nonconducted P wave that is shorter than the sum of two PP intervals. The progressive shortening of the RR interval is due to a decrease in the increment of PR interval prolongation. Type I block usually occurs at the level of the AV node, resulting in a narrow QRS complex. (In contrast, Type II second-degree AV block usually occurs within or below the bundle of His, and is associated with a wide QRS in 80% of cases.) Type I block may coexist with first-degree but not third-degree (complete) AV block. Classical Wenckebach periodicity (progressive prolongation of the PR

nterval and shortening of the RR interval up to the nonconducted P wave) is not always seen, especially when sinus arrhythmia is present. In Type I block with high conduction ratios, the PR interval of the beats immediately preceding the blocked P wave may be equal, suggesting Type II block. In these situations, it is best to compare the PR interval immediately before and after the blocked P wave; differences in the PR interval suggests Type I block, whereas a constant PR interval is evidence for Type II block. (Answer: a, c, d)

2. Type I second-degree AV block (Wenckebach) is often suspected by a pattern of "group beating." Other causes of group beating include blocked premature atrial contractions, Type II second-degree AV block, and concealed premature His depolarizations. Type II sinoatrial exit block may also result in group beating; however, this differs from the other causes listed in that the P-QRS ratio remains at 1:1. (Answer: All)

3. The conduction ratio is determined by the ratio of P waves to QRS complexes between pauses. In the present tracing, there are four P-waves and three QRS complexes between pauses, making the conduction ratio (P:QRS) is 4:3. Conduction ratio should not be confused with *conduction block*, which refers to the ratio of P waves to absent QRS complexes between pauses. In the present tracing, 4:1 AV conduction block is present. (Answer: c)

— Quick Review 98 —

AV block, 2° - Mobitz Type I (Wenckebach)	
• Progressive prolongation of the ____ interval and shortening of the ____ interval until a P wave is blocked	PR RR
• RR interval containing the nonconducted P wave is (less than/equal to/greater than) the sum of two PP intervals	less than
• Results in ____ beating due to the presence of nonconducted P waves	group

Differential Diagnosis

Fusion Complexes

(Simultaneous activation of the ventricle from two sources, resulting in a QRS complex intermediate in morphology between the QRS complexes of each source)

- Ventricular premature complexes (item 4a-d)
- Ventricular tachycardia (item 4f)
- Ventricular parasystole (item 4e)
- Accelerated idioventricular rhythm (item 4g)
- Wolff-Parkinson-White Syndrome (item 6h)
- Paced rhythm

ECG 99. 70-year-old male hospitalized with recent severe neck and left shoulder pain:

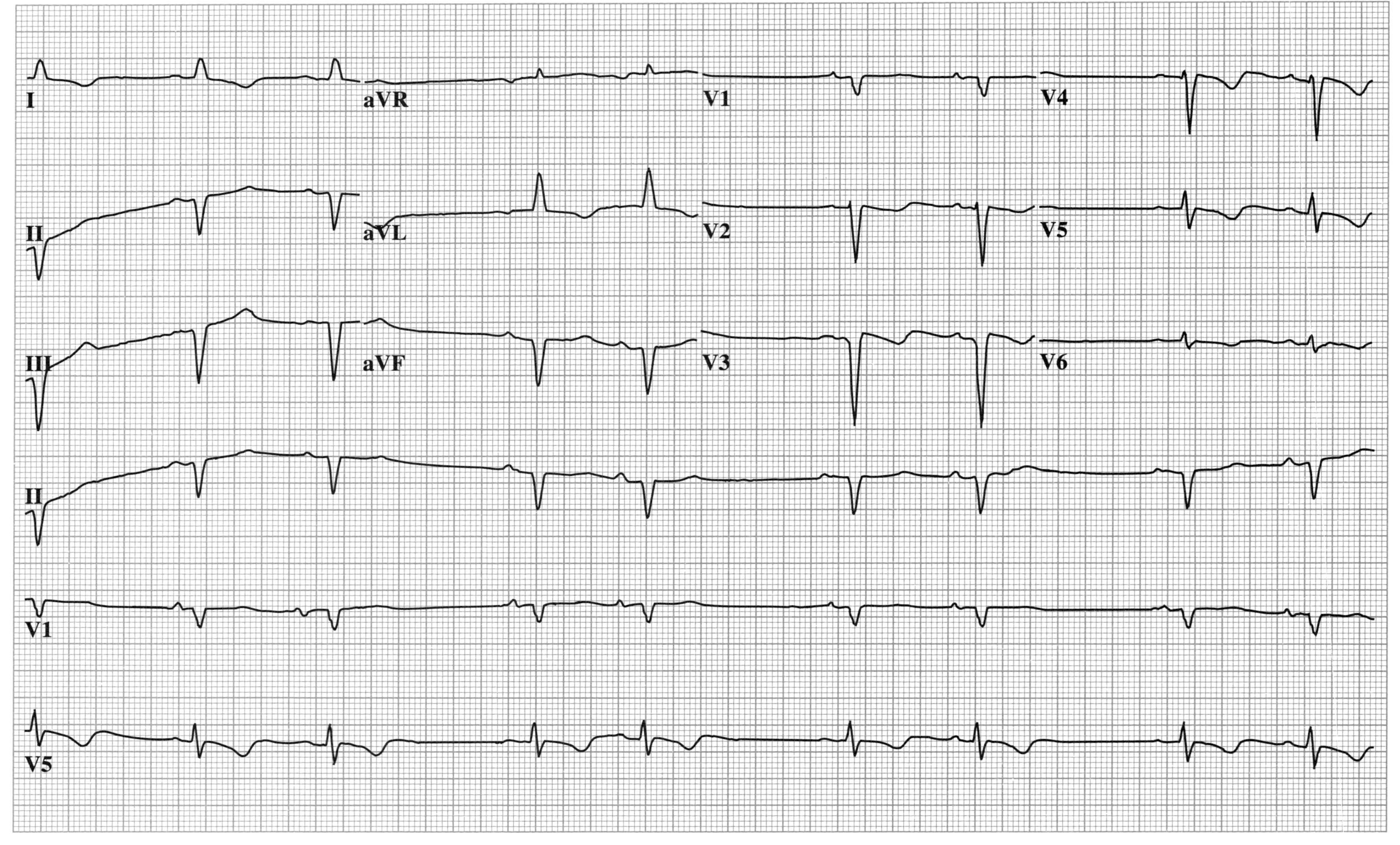

1. GENERAL FEATURES

- ☐ a. Normal ECG
- ☐ b. Borderline normal ECG or normal variant
- ☐ c. Incorrect electrode placement
- ☐ d. Artifact due to tremor

2. ATRIAL RHYTHMS

- ☐ a. Sinus rhythm
- ☐ b. Sinus arrhythmia
- ☐ c. Sinus bradycardia (< 60)
- ☐ d. Sinus tachycardia (> 100)
- ☐ e. Sinus pause or arrest
- ☐ f. Sinoatrial exit block
- ☐ g. Ecoptic atrial rhythm
- ☐ h. Wandering atrial pacemaker
- ☐ i. Atrial premature complexes, normally conducted
- ☐ j. Atrial premature complexes, nonconducted
- ☐ k. Atrial premature complexes with aberrant intraventricular conduction
- ☐ l. Atrial tachycardia (regular, sustained, 1:1 conduction)
- ☐ m. Atrial tachycardia, repetitive (short paroxysms)
- ☐ n. Atrial tachycardia, multifocal
- ☐ o. Atrial tachycardia with AV block
- ☐ p. Supraventricular tachycardia, unspecific
- ☐ q. Supraventricular tachycardia, paroxysmal
- ☐ r. Atrial flutter
- ☐ s. Atrial fibrillation
- ☐ t. Retrograde atrial activation

3. AV JUNCTIONAL RHYTHMS

- ☐ a. AV junctional premature complexes
- ☐ b. AV junctional escape complexes
- ☐ c. AV junctional rhythm, accelerated
- ☐ d. AV junctional rhythm

4. VENTRICULAR RHYTHMS

- ☐ a. Ventricular premature complex(es), uniform, fixed coupling
- ☐ b. Ventricular premature complex(es), uniform, nonfixed coupling
- ☐ c. Ventricular premature complexes(es), multiform
- ☐ d. Ventricular premature complexes, in pairs
- ☐ e. Ventricular parasystole
- ☐ f. Ventricular tachycardia ($\geq$ 3 consecutive complexes)
- ☐ g. Accelerated idioventricular rhythm
- ☐ h. Ventricular escape complexes or rhythm
- ☐ i. Ventricular fibrillation

5. ATRIAL-VENTRICULAR INTERACTIONS IN ARRHYTHMIAS

- ☐ a. Fusion complexes
- ☐ b. Reciprocal (echo) complexes
- ☐ c. Ventricular capture complexes
- ☐ d. AV dissociation
- ☐ e. Ventriculophasic sinus arrhythmia

6. AV CONDUCTION ABNORMALITIES

- ☐ a. AV block, 1°
- ☐ b. AV block, 2° - Mobitz type I (Wenckebach)
- ☐ c. AV block, 2° - Mobitz type II
- ☐ d. AV block, 2:1
- ☐ e. AV block, 3°
- ☐ f. AV block, variable
- ☐ g. Short PR interval (with sinus rhythm and normal QRS duration)
- ☐ h. Wolff-Parkinson-White pattern

7. INTRAVENTRICULAR CONDUCTION DISTURBANCES

- ☐ a. RBBB, incomplete
- ☐ b. RBBB, complete
- ☐ c. Left anterior fascicular block
- ☐ d. Left posterior fascicular block
- ☐ e. LBBB, with ST-T wave suggestive of acute myocardial injury or infarction
- ☐ f. LBBB, complete
- ☐ g. LBBB, intermittent
- ☐ h. Intraventricular conduction disturbance, nonspecific
- ☐ i. Aberrant intraventricular conduction with supraventricular arrhythmia

8. P WAVE ABNORMALITIES

- ☐ a. Right atrial abnormality
- ☐ b. Left atrial abnormalities
- ☐ c. Nonspecific atrial abnormality

9. ABNORMALITIES OF QRS VOLTAGE OR AXIS

- ☐ a. Low voltage, limb leads only
- ☐ b. Low voltage, limb and precordial leads
- ☐ c. Left axis deviation (> - 30%)
- ☐ d. Right axis deviation (> + 100)
- ☐ e. Electrical alternans

10. VENTRICULAR HYPERTROPHY

- ☐ a. LVH by voltage only
- ☐ b. LVH by voltage and ST-T segment abnormalities
- ☐ c. RVH
- ☐ d. Combined ventricular hypertrophy

11. Q WAVE MYOCARDIAL INFARCTION

	Probably Acute or Recent	Probably Old or Age Indeterminate
Anterolateral	☐ a.	☐ g.
Anterior	☐ b.	☐ h.
Anteroseptal	☐ c.	☐ i.
Lateral/High lateral	☐ d.	☐ j.
Inferior	☐ e.	☐ k.
Posterior	☐ f.	☐ l.

- ☐ m. Probably ventricular aneurysm

12. ST, T, U, WAVE ABNORMALITIES

- ☐ a. Normal variant, early repolarization
- ☐ b. Normal variant, juvenile T waves
- ☐ c. Nonspecific ST and/or T wave abnormalities
- ☐ d. ST and/or T wave abnormalities suggesting myocardial ischemia
- ☐ e. ST and/or T wave abnormalities suggesting myocardial injury
- ☐ f. ST and/or T wave abnormalities suggesting acute pericarditis
- ☐ g. ST-T segment abnormalities secondary to intraventricular conduction disturbance or hypertrophy
- ☐ h. Post-extrasystolic T wave abnormality
- ☐ i. Isolated J point depression
- ☐ j. Peaked T waves
- ☐ k. Prolonged QT interval
- ☐ l. Prominent U waves

13. PACEMAKER FUNCTION AND RHYTHM

- ☐ a. Atrial or coronary sinus pacing
- ☐ b. Ventricular demand pacing
- ☐ c. AV sequential pacing
- ☐ d. Ventricular pacing, complete control
- ☐ e. Dual chamber, atrial sensing pacemaker
- ☐ f. Pacemaker malfunction, not constantly capturing (atrium or ventricle)
- ☐ g. Pacemaker malfunction, not constantly sensing (atrium or ventricle)
- ☐ h. Pacemaker malfunction, not firing
- ☐ i. Pacemaker malfunction, slowing

14. SUGGESTED OR PROBABLE CLINICAL DISORDERS

- ☐ a. Digitalis effect
- ☐ b. Digitalis toxicity
- ☐ c. Antiarrhythmic drug effect
- ☐ d. Antiarrhythmic drug toxicity
- ☐ e. Hyperkalemia
- ☐ f. Hypokalemia
- ☐ g. Hypercalcemia
- ☐ h. Hypocalcemia
- ☐ i. Atrial septal defect, secundum
- ☐ j. Atrial septal defect, primum
- ☐ k. Dextrocardia, mirror image
- ☐ l. Mitral valve disease
- ☐ m. Chronic lung disease
- ☐ n. Acute cor pulmonale, including pulmonary embolus
- ☐ o. Pericardial effusion
- ☐ p. Acute pericarditis
- ☐ q. Hypertrophic cardiomyopathy
- ☐ r. Coronary artery disease
- ☐ s. Central nervous system disorder
- ☐ t. Myxedema
- ☐ u. Hypothermia

ECG 99 was obtained in a 70-year-old male hospitalized with recent severe neck and left shoulder pain. The ECG shows an atrial bradycardia with multiple P wave morphologies (asterisk) suggestive of wandering atrial pacemaker. A probably old or age indeterminate inferior infarction is noted (arrowheads) with a probably recent anterior myocardial infarction. The downsloping ST segments and T wave inversions in the precordial leads are consistent with ischemia (arrows). The QRS measures 116 msec in duration, yielding a diagnosis of nonspecific IVCD. These findings are suggestive of coronary artery disease and sick sinus syndrome. Although the axis is leftward, left anterior fascicular block should not be diagnosed in the presence of other conditions that can cause left axis deviation, such as inferior myocardial infarction.

Codes:

2h	Wandering atrial pacemaker
7h	IVCD, nonspecific type
9c	Left axis deviation (> -30°)
11b	Anterior Q wave MI, probably acute or recent
11k	Inferior Q wave MI, probably old or age indeterminate
12d	ST and/or T wave abnormalities suggesting myocardial ischemia
14r	Coronary artery disease
14v	Sick sinus syndrome

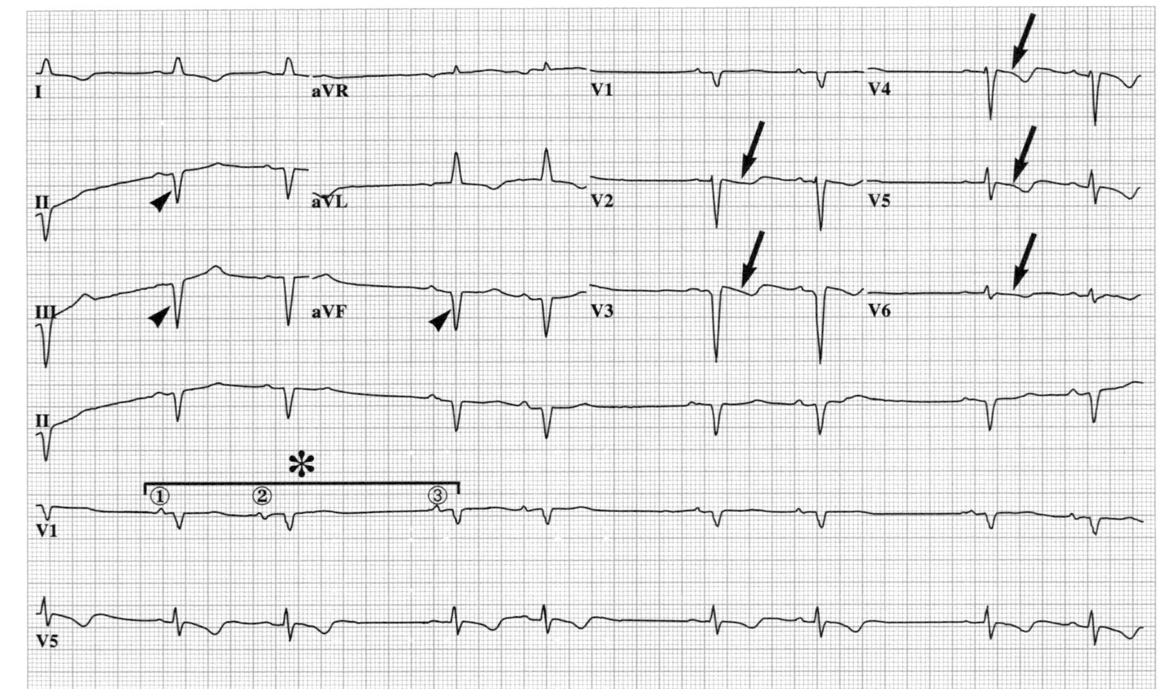

Questions: ECG 99

1. The diagnosis of wandering atrial pacemaker requires the presence of ___ or more P wave morphologies:

   a. 2
   b. 3
   c. 4

2. The heart rate with wandering atrial pacemaker is:

   a. < 100 BPM
   b. ≥ 100 BPM

Answers: ECG 99

1. Wandering atrial pacemaker is a supraventricular rhythm characterized by the presence of 3 or more P wave morphologies and varying PR, RR, and RP intervals. (Answer: b)

2. The heart rate with wandering atrial pacemaker is less than 100 beats per minute. If 3 or more P wave morphologies are present but the heart rate exceeds 100 BPM, the arrhythmia should be classified as multifocal atrial tachycardia. (Answer: a)

— Quick Review 99 —

Wandering atrial pacemaker	
• Rate < ____ per minute	100
• P waves with ≥ ____ morphologies	3
• PR, RR, and RP intervals (are constant/vary)	vary
• May be confused with sinus rhythm with multifocal APCs, or atrial fibrillation/flutter with a moderate ventricular response, but:	
▸ Unlike sinus rhythm with multifocal APCs, wandering atrial pacemaker (does/does not) manifest a dominant P wave morphology	does not
▸ Unlike atrial fibrillation/flutter, wandering atrial pacemaker has a distinct ____ baseline	isoelectric
• P waves may be blocked or conducted with a narrow or aberrant QRS complex (true/false)	true
Sick sinus syndrome	
• Marked sinus ____	bradycardia
• ____ arrest or ____ exit block	Sinus, sinoatrial
• Bradycardia alternating with ____	tachycardia
• Atrial fibrillation with ____ ventricular response preceded or followed by sinus bradycardia, sinus arrest, or sinoatrial exit block	slow
• Prolonged sinus node ____ time after atrial premature complex or atrial tachyarrhythmias	recovery
• AV junctional ____ rhythm	escape
• Additional conduction system disease is often present, including AV block, IVCD, and/or bundle branch block (true/false)	true

ECG 100. 67-year-old asymptomatic male:

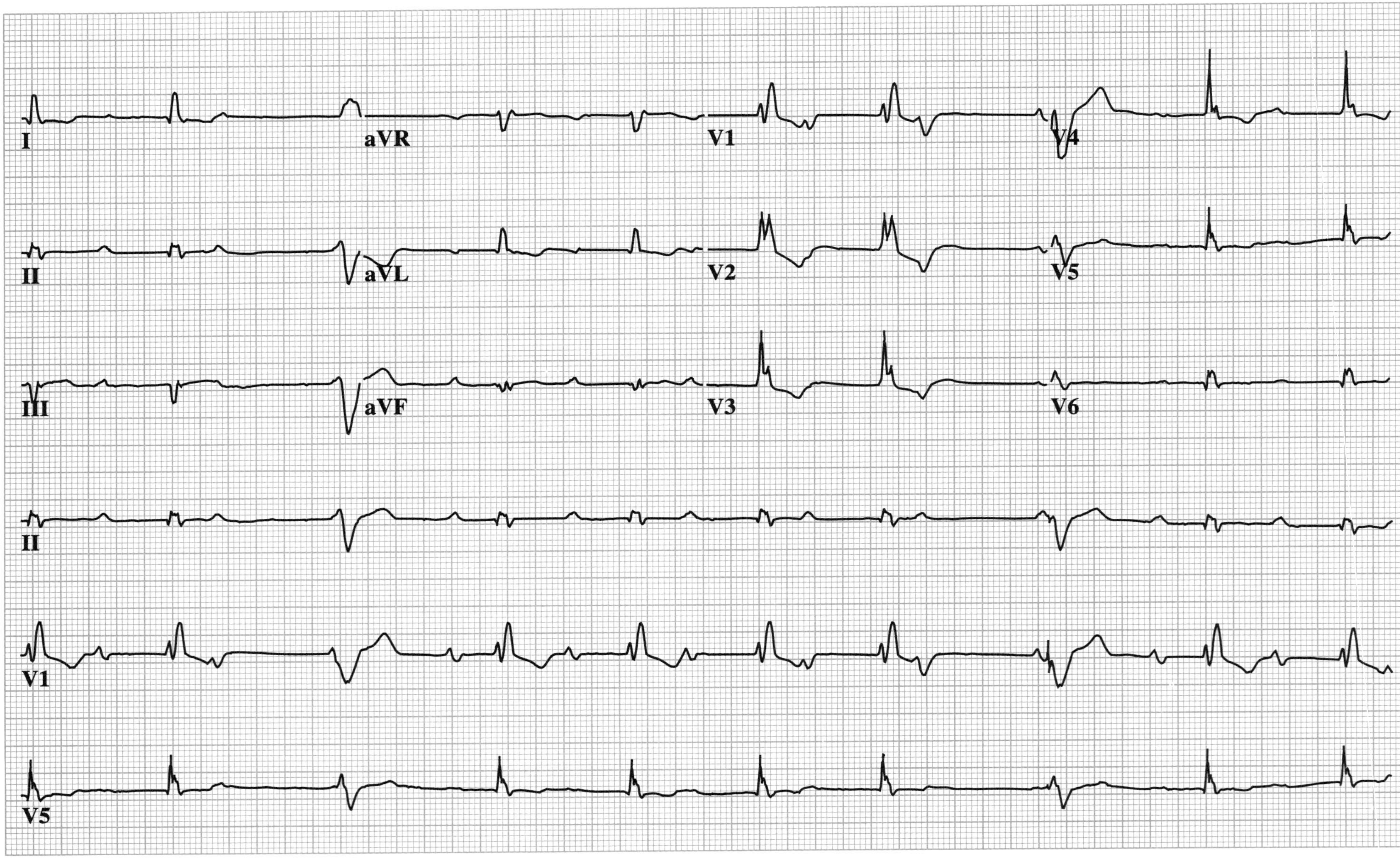

1. GENERAL FEATURES
- ☐ a. Normal ECG
- ☐ b. Borderline normal ECG or normal variant
- ☐ c. Incorrect electrode placement
- ☐ d. Artifact due to tremor

2. ATRIAL RHYTHMS
- ☐ a. Sinus rhythm
- ☐ b. Sinus arrhythmia
- ☐ c. Sinus bradycardia (< 60)
- ☐ d. Sinus tachycardia (> 100)
- ☐ e. Sinus pause or arrest
- ☐ f. Sinoatrial exit block
- ☐ g. Ecoptic atrial rhythm
- ☐ h. Wandering atrial pacemaker
- ☐ i. Atrial premature complexes, normally conducted
- ☐ j. Atrial premature complexes, nonconducted
- ☐ k. Atrial premature complexes with aberrant intraventricular conduction
- ☐ l. Atrial tachycardia (regular, sustained, 1:1 conduction)
- ☐ m. Atrial tachycardia, repetitive (short paroxysms)
- ☐ n. Atrial tachycardia, multifocal
- ☐ o. Atrial tachycardia with AV block
- ☐ p. Supraventricular tachycardia, unspecific
- ☐ q. Supraventricular tachycardia, paroxysmal
- ☐ r. Atrial flutter
- ☐ s. Atrial fibrillation
- ☐ t. Retrograde atrial activation

3. AV JUNCTIONAL RHYTHMS
- ☐ a. AV junctional premature complexes
- ☐ b. AV junctional escape complexes
- ☐ c. AV junctional rhythm, accelerated
- ☐ d. AV junctional rhythm

4. VENTRICULAR RHYTHMS
- ☐ a. Ventricular premature complex(es), uniform, fixed coupling
- ☐ b. Ventricular premature complex(es), uniform, nonfixed coupling
- ☐ c. Ventricular premature complexes(es), multiform
- ☐ d. Ventricular premature complexes, in pairs
- ☐ e. Ventricular parasystole
- ☐ f. Ventricular tachycardia (≥ 3 consecutive complexes)
- ☐ g. Accelerated idioventricular rhythm
- ☐ h. Ventricular escape complexes or rhythm
- ☐ i. Ventricular fibrillation

5. ATRIAL-VENTRICULAR INTERACTIONS IN ARRHYTHMIAS
- ☐ a. Fusion complexes
- ☐ b. Reciprocal (echo) complexes
- ☐ c. Ventricular capture complexes
- ☐ d. AV dissociation
- ☐ e. Ventriculophasic sinus arrhythmia

6. AV CONDUCTION ABNORMALITIES
- ☐ a. AV block, 1°
- ☐ b. AV block, 2° - Mobitz type I (Wenckebach)
- ☐ c. AV block, 2° - Mobitz type II
- ☐ d. AV block, 2:1
- ☐ e. AV block, 3°
- ☐ f. AV block, variable
- ☐ g. Short PR interval (with sinus rhythm and normal QRS duration)
- ☐ h. Wolff-Parkinson-White pattern

7. INTRAVENTRICULAR CONDUCTION DISTURBANCES
- ☐ a. RBBB, incomplete
- ☐ b. RBBB, complete
- ☐ c. Left anterior fascicular block
- ☐ d. Left posterior fascicular block
- ☐ e. LBBB, with ST-T wave suggestive of acute myocardial injury or infarction
- ☐ f. LBBB, complete
- ☐ g. LBBB, intermittent
- ☐ h. Intraventricular conduction disturbance, nonspecific
- ☐ i. Aberrant intraventricular conduction with supraventricular arrhythmia

8. P WAVE ABNORMALITIES
- ☐ a. Right atrial abnormality
- ☐ b. Left atrial abnormalities
- ☐ c. Nonspecific atrial abnormality

9. ABNORMALITIES OF QRS VOLTAGE OR AXIS
- ☐ a. Low voltage, limb leads only
- ☐ b. Low voltage, limb and precordial leads
- ☐ c. Left axis deviation (> - 30%)
- ☐ d. Right axis deviation (> + 100)
- ☐ e. Electrical alternans

10. VENTRICULAR HYPERTROPHY
- ☐ a. LVH by voltage only
- ☐ b. LVH by voltage and ST-T segment abnormalities
- ☐ c. RVH
- ☐ d. Combined ventricular hypertrophy

11. Q WAVE MYOCARDIAL INFARCTION

	Probably Acute or Recent	Probably Old or Age Indeterminate
Anterolateral	☐ a.	☐ g.
Anterior	☐ b.	☐ h.
Anteroseptal	☐ c.	☐ i.
Lateral/High lateral	☐ d.	☐ j.
Inferior	☐ e.	☐ k.
Posterior	☐ f.	☐ l.

- ☐ m. Probably ventricular aneurysm

12. ST, T, U, WAVE ABNORMALITIES
- ☐ a. Normal variant, early repolarization
- ☐ b. Normal variant, juvenile T waves
- ☐ c. Nonspecific ST and/or T wave abnormalities
- ☐ d. ST and/or T wave abnormalities suggesting myocardial ischemia
- ☐ e. ST and/or T wave abnormalities suggesting myocardial injury
- ☐ f. ST and/or T wave abnormalities suggesting acute pericarditis
- ☐ g. ST-T segment abnormalities secondary to intraventricular conduction disturbance or hypertrophy
- ☐ h. Post-extrasystolic T wave abnormality
- ☐ i. Isolated J point depression
- ☐ j. Peaked T waves
- ☐ k. Prolonged QT interval
- ☐ l. Prominent U waves

13. PACEMAKER FUNCTION AND RHYTHM
- ☐ a. Atrial or coronary sinus pacing
- ☐ b. Ventricular demand pacing
- ☐ c. AV sequential pacing
- ☐ d. Ventricular pacing, complete control
- ☐ e. Dual chamber, atrial sensing pacemaker
- ☐ f. Pacemaker malfunction, not constantly capturing (atrium or ventricle)
- ☐ g. Pacemaker malfunction, not constantly sensing (atrium or ventricle)
- ☐ h. Pacemaker malfunction, not firing
- ☐ i. Pacemaker malfunction, slowing

14. SUGGESTED OR PROBABLE CLINICAL DISORDERS
- ☐ a. Digitalis effect
- ☐ b. Digitalis toxicity
- ☐ c. Antiarrhythmic drug effect
- ☐ d. Antiarrhythmic drug toxicity
- ☐ e. Hyperkalemia
- ☐ f. Hypokalemia
- ☐ g. Hypercalcemia
- ☐ h. Hypocalcemia
- ☐ i. Atrial septal defect, secundum
- ☐ j. Atrial septal defect, primum
- ☐ k. Dextrocardia, mirror image
- ☐ l. Mitral valve disease
- ☐ m. Chronic lung disease
- ☐ n. Acute cor pulmonale, including pulmonary embolus
- ☐ o. Pericardial effusion
- ☐ p. Acute pericarditis
- ☐ q. Hypertrophic cardiomyopathy
- ☐ r. Coronary artery disease
- ☐ s. Central nervous system disorder
- ☐ t. Myxedema
- ☐ u. Hypothermia

ECG 100 was obtained in a 67-year-old asymptomatic male. The ECG shows sinus rhythm with both first-degree and second-degree AV block. The second-degree AV block is Mobitz Type I (Wenckebach), as indicated by progressive prolongation of the PR interval between nonconducted P waves (asterisks). RBBB with secondary ST-T changes is also present. Appropriate ventricular demand pacing is noted (arrowhead). The third QRS on the rhythm strip (arrow) is a paced complex (note similarity in morphology between the third and eight beats); pacer spikes may not be consistently recorded by the ECG due to sampling rate.

Codes:

2a	Sinus rhythm
6a	AV block, 1°
6b	AV block, 2° - Mobitz type I (Wenckebach)
7b	RBBB, complete
12g	ST-T segment abnormalities secondary to IVCD or hypertrophy

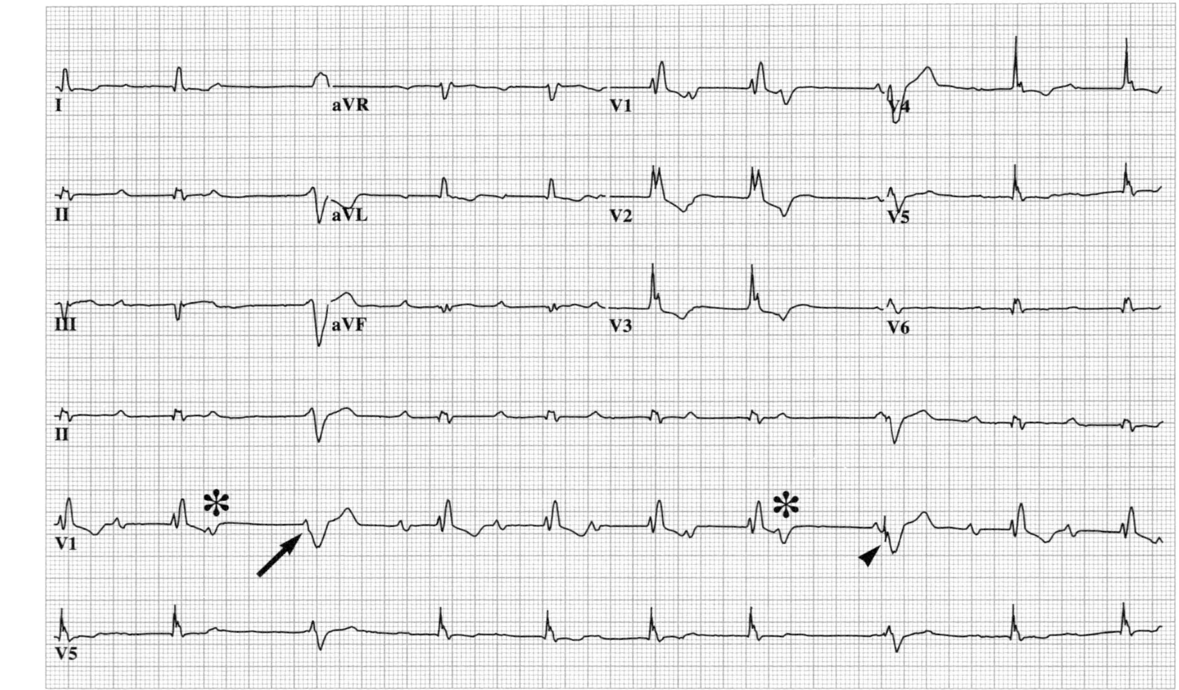

Questions: ECG 100

1. The typical rate of a ventricular escape rhythm is ___ BPM:

   a. 10-30
   b. 30-40
   c. 40-60
   d. > 60

2. With VVI pacing, the escape interval from the last QRS to the ventricular spike should be constant:

   a. True
   b. False

Answers: ECG 100

1. The typical rate of a ventricular escape rhythm is 30-40 beats/minute, but can vary between 20-50 beats/minute. The QRS complexes are wide (usually > 0.14 seconds) and have ST-T changes in a direction opposite to the major deflection of the QRS. (Answer: b)

2. With VVI pacing, the ventricle is the only chamber sensed and paced. When a native ventricular complex is sensed, the output of the ventricular pacemaker is inhibited. The escape interval is programmed and should be constant relative to native QRS complexes originating from the same focus. Minor variation in the escape interval can be seen when native QRS complexes originate from different locations in the ventricle. (Answer: a)

— Quick Review 100 —

Ventricular escape beats or rhythm	
• Ventricular rate of ____ per minute (can be ____ per minute)	30-40, 20-50
• QRS morphology is similar to ____	VPCs
• QRS complex occurs as a ____ phenomenon in response to decreased sinus impulse formation or conduction, or high-degree AV block	secondary
RBBB, complete	
• QRS duration ≥ ____ seconds	0.12
• Secondary R wave (R') in lead ____ is usually (shorter/taller) than the initial R wave	V_1 taller
• Onset of intrinsicoid deflection in leads V_1 and V_2 > ____ seconds	0.05
• ST segment (depression/elevation) and (upright/inverted) T wave in V_1, V_2	depression inverted
• Wide slurred S wave in leads ____	I, V_5, V_6
• QRS axis is usually (normal/leftward/rightward)	normal
• RBBB (does/does not) interfere with the ECG diagnosis of ventricular hypertrophy or Q wave MI	does not
Ventricular demand pacing	
• Pacemaker stimulus followed by a QRS complex that has (the same/different) morphology compared to the intrinsic QRS	different
• Must demonstrate ____ of pacemaker output in response to intrinsic QRS	inhibition

ECG 101. 61-year-old asymptomatic female:

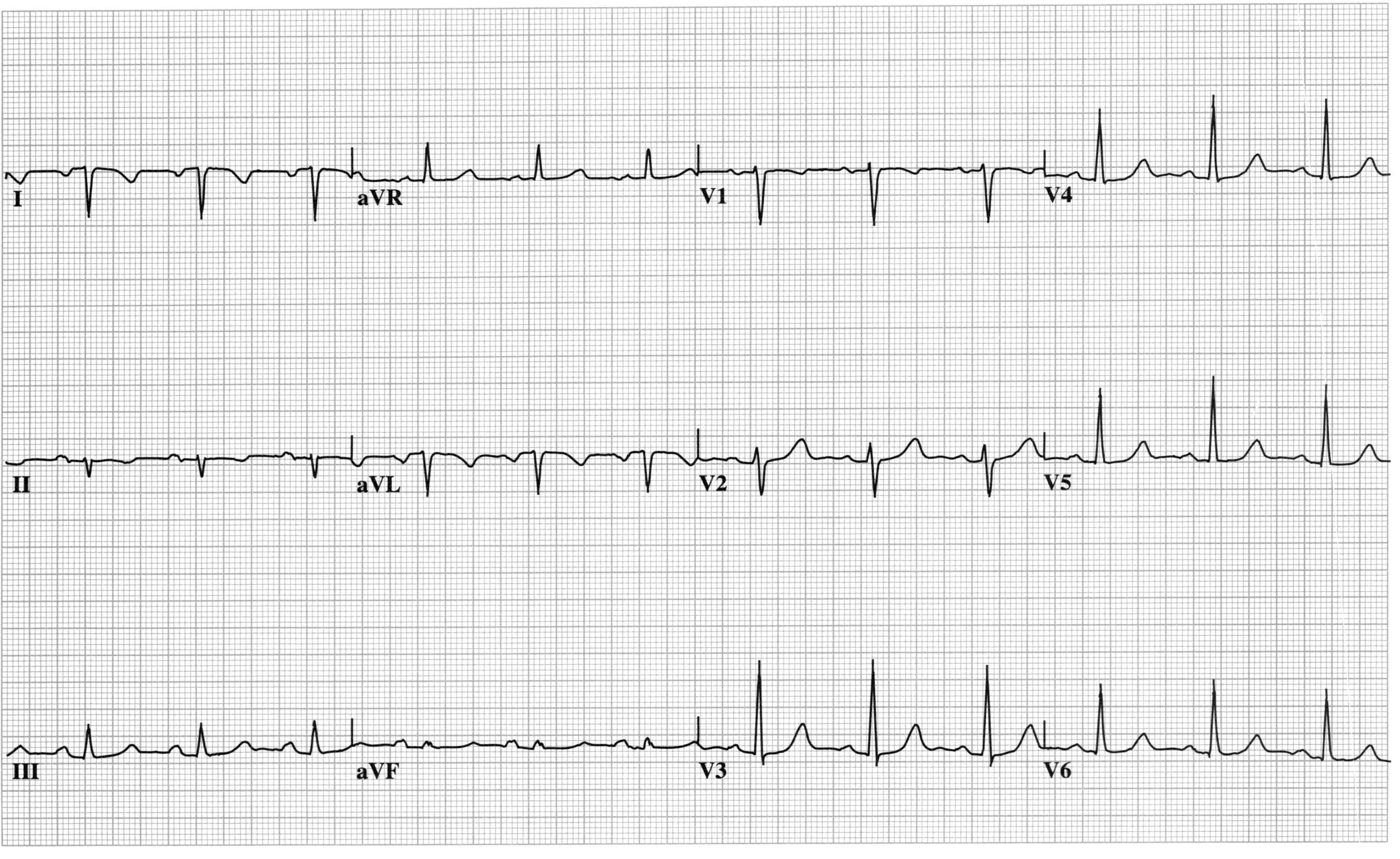

1. GENERAL FEATURES

- ☐ a. Normal ECG
- ☐ b. Borderline normal ECG or normal variant
- ☐ c. Incorrect electrode placement
- ☐ d. Artifact due to tremor

2. ATRIAL RHYTHMS

- ☐ a. Sinus rhythm
- ☐ b. Sinus arrhythmia
- ☐ c. Sinus bradycardia (< 60)
- ☐ d. Sinus tachycardia (> 100)
- ☐ e. Sinus pause or arrest
- ☐ f. Sinoatrial exit block
- ☐ g. Ecoptic atrial rhythm
- ☐ h. Wandering atrial pacemaker
- ☐ i. Atrial premature complexes, normally conducted
- ☐ j. Atrial premature complexes, nonconducted
- ☐ k. Atrial premature complexes with aberrant intraventricular conduction
- ☐ l. Atrial tachycardia (regular, sustained, 1:1 conduction)
- ☐ m. Atrial tachycardia, repetitive (short paroxysms)
- ☐ n. Atrial tachycardia, multifocal
- ☐ o. Atrial tachycardia with AV block
- ☐ p. Supraventricular tachycardia, unspecific
- ☐ q. Supraventricular tachycardia, paroxysmal
- ☐ r. Atrial flutter
- ☐ s. Atrial fibrillation
- ☐ t. Retrograde atrial activation

3. AV JUNCTIONAL RHYTHMS

- ☐ a. AV junctional premature complexes
- ☐ b. AV junctional escape complexes
- ☐ c. AV junctional rhythm, accelerated
- ☐ d. AV junctional rhythm

4. VENTRICULAR RHYTHMS

- ☐ a. Ventricular premature complex(es), uniform, fixed coupling
- ☐ b. Ventricular premature complex(es), uniform, nonfixed coupling
- ☐ c. Ventricular premature complexes(es), multiform
- ☐ d. Ventricular premature complexes, in pairs
- ☐ e. Ventricular parasystole
- ☐ f. Ventricular tachycardia (≥ 3 consecutive complexes)
- ☐ g. Accelerated idioventricular rhythm
- ☐ h. Ventricular escape complexes or rhythm
- ☐ i. Ventricular fibrillation

5. ATRIAL-VENTRICULAR INTERACTIONS IN ARRHYTHMIAS

- ☐ a. Fusion complexes
- ☐ b. Reciprocal (echo) complexes
- ☐ c. Ventricular capture complexes
- ☐ d. AV dissociation
- ☐ e. Ventriculophasic sinus arrhythmia

6. AV CONDUCTION ABNORMALITIES

- ☐ a. AV block, 1°
- ☐ b. AV block, 2° - Mobitz type I (Wenckebach)
- ☐ c. AV block, 2° - Mobitz type II
- ☐ d. AV block, 2:1
- ☐ e. AV block, 3°
- ☐ f. AV block, variable
- ☐ g. Short PR interval (with sinus rhythm and normal QRS duration)
- ☐ h. Wolff-Parkinson-White pattern

7. INTRAVENTRICULAR CONDUCTION DISTURBANCES

- ☐ a. RBBB, incomplete
- ☐ b. RBBB, complete
- ☐ c. Left anterior fascicular block
- ☐ d. Left posterior fascicular block
- ☐ e. LBBB, with ST-T wave suggestive of acute myocardial injury or infarction
- ☐ f. LBBB, complete
- ☐ g. LBBB, intermittent
- ☐ h. Intraventricular conduction disturbance, nonspecific
- ☐ i. Aberrant intraventricular conduction with supraventricular arrhythmia

8. P WAVE ABNORMALITIES

- ☐ a. Right atrial abnormality
- ☐ b. Left atrial abnormalities
- ☐ c. Nonspecific atrial abnormality

9. ABNORMALITIES OF QRS VOLTAGE OR AXIS

- ☐ a. Low voltage, limb leads only
- ☐ b. Low voltage, limb and precordial leads
- ☐ c. Left axis deviation (> - 30%)
- ☐ d. Right axis deviation (> + 100)
- ☐ e. Electrical alternans

10. VENTRICULAR HYPERTROPHY

- ☐ a. LVH by voltage only
- ☐ b. LVH by voltage and ST-T segment abnormalities
- ☐ c. RVH
- ☐ d. Combined ventricular hypertrophy

11. Q WAVE MYOCARDIAL INFARCTION

	Probably Acute or Recent	Probably Old or Age Indeterminate
Anterolateral	☐ a.	☐ g.
Anterior	☐ b.	☐ h.
Anteroseptal	☐ c.	☐ i.
Lateral/High lateral	☐ d.	☐ j.
Inferior	☐ e.	☐ k.
Posterior	☐ f.	☐ l.

- ☐ m. Probably ventricular aneurysm

12. ST, T, U, WAVE ABNORMALITIES

- ☐ a. Normal variant, early repolarization
- ☐ b. Normal variant, juvenile T waves
- ☐ c. Nonspecific ST and/or T wave abnormalities
- ☐ d. ST and/or T wave abnormalities suggesting myocardial ischemia
- ☐ e. ST and/or T wave abnormalities suggesting myocardial injury
- ☐ f. ST and/or T wave abnormalities suggesting acute pericarditis
- ☐ g. ST-T segment abnormalities secondary to intraventricular conduction disturbance or hypertrophy
- ☐ h. Post-extrasystolic T wave abnormality
- ☐ i. Isolated J point depression
- ☐ j. Peaked T waves
- ☐ k. Prolonged QT interval
- ☐ l. Prominent U waves

13. PACEMAKER FUNCTION AND RHYTHM

- ☐ a. Atrial or coronary sinus pacing
- ☐ b. Ventricular demand pacing
- ☐ c. AV sequential pacing
- ☐ d. Ventricular pacing, complete control
- ☐ e. Dual chamber, atrial sensing pacemaker
- ☐ f. Pacemaker malfunction, not constantly capturing (atrium or ventricle)
- ☐ g. Pacemaker malfunction, not constantly sensing (atrium or ventricle)
- ☐ h. Pacemaker malfunction, not firing
- ☐ i. Pacemaker malfunction, slowing

14. SUGGESTED OR PROBABLE CLINICAL DISORDERS

- ☐ a. Digitalis effect
- ☐ b. Digitalis toxicity
- ☐ c. Antiarrhythmic drug effect
- ☐ d. Antiarrhythmic drug toxicity
- ☐ e. Hyperkalemia
- ☐ f. Hypokalemia
- ☐ g. Hypercalcemia
- ☐ h. Hypocalcemia
- ☐ i. Atrial septal defect, secundum
- ☐ j. Atrial septal defect, primum
- ☐ k. Dextrocardia, mirror image
- ☐ l. Mitral valve disease
- ☐ m. Chronic lung disease
- ☐ n. Acute cor pulmonale, including pulmonary embolus
- ☐ o. Pericardial effusion
- ☐ p. Acute pericarditis
- ☐ q. Hypertrophic cardiomyopathy
- ☐ r. Coronary artery disease
- ☐ s. Central nervous system disorder
- ☐ t. Myxedema
- ☐ u. Hypothermia

ECG 101 was obtained in a 61-year-old asymptomatic female. The P, QRS, and T waves are all inverted in leads I and aVL (asterisks) and upright in aVR. These findings are characteristic of incorrect limb lead electrode placement. The normal R wave progression in the precordial leads helps distinguish limb lead reversal from dextrocardia, the latter of which manifests reverse R wave progression. The axis is difficult to determine due to incorrect electrode placement and labeling. First-degree AV block is also present.

Codes:

1c	Incorrect electrode placement
2a	Sinus rhythm
6a	AV block, 1°

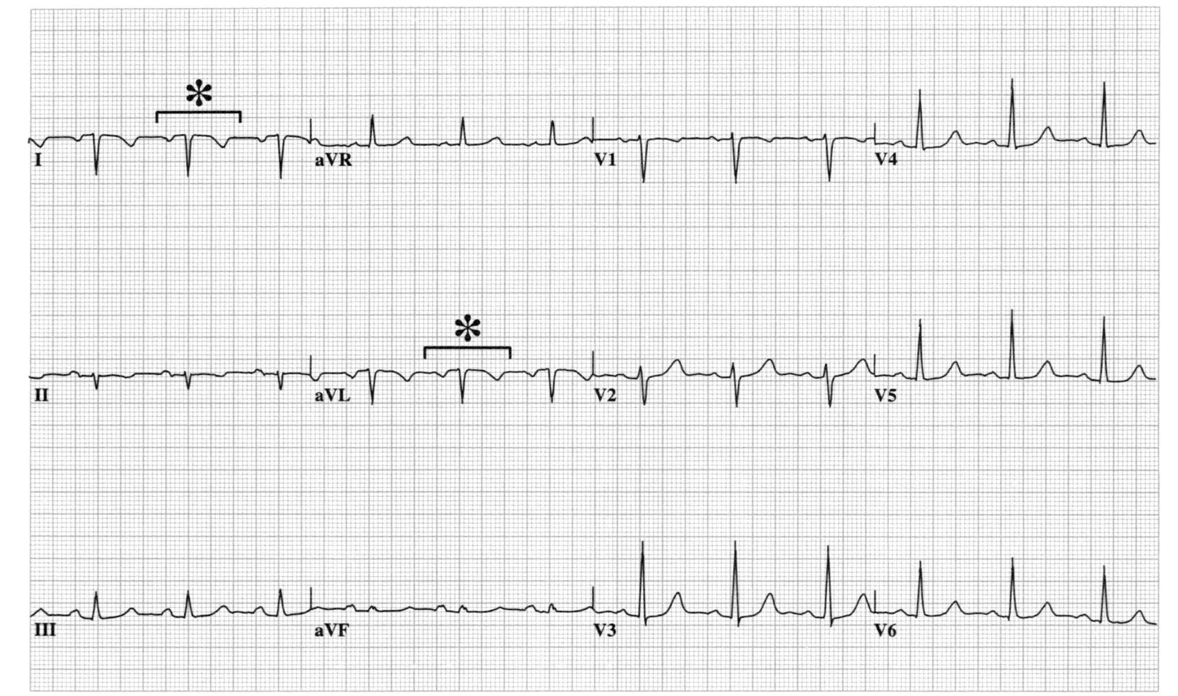

Questions: ECG 101

1. Incorrect placement of limb lead electrodes results in a "mirror-image" of the normal P-QRS-T in leads ____ and _____:

   a. I and aVL
   b. I and II
   c. II and III
   d. aVL and aVR

2. Limb lead reversal is associated with reverse R wave progression in leads V_1-V_6:

   a. True
   b. False

Answers: ECG 101

1. Incorrect placement of the limb lead electrodes results in inversion of the P-QRS-T in leads I and aVL. This gives the mistaken impression of right axis deviation, and may be confused with mirror-image dextrocardia. (Answer: a)

2. Dextrocardia and limb lead electrode reversal result in right axis deviation of the P, QRS, and T waves. Dextrocardia is associated with reverse R wave progression in leads V_1-V_6, while limb lead reversal shows normal R wave progression in these leads . (Answer: b)

— Quick Review 101 —	
Incorrect electrode placement	
Limb lead reversal (reversal of right and left arm leads)	
• Resultant ECG mimics dextrocardia with ____ of	inversion
the P-QRS-T in leads ____ and aVL	I
• To distinguish between these conditions, look at precordial leads: dextrocardia shows (reverse/normal) R wave progression, while limb	reverse
lead reversal shows (reverse/normal) R wave progression.	normal
Precordial lead reversal: Unexplained decrease in ____ voltage in two consecutive leads (e.g., V_1, V_2) with a return to normal progression in the following leads	R wave

ECG 102: 88-year-old male with an irregular pulse:

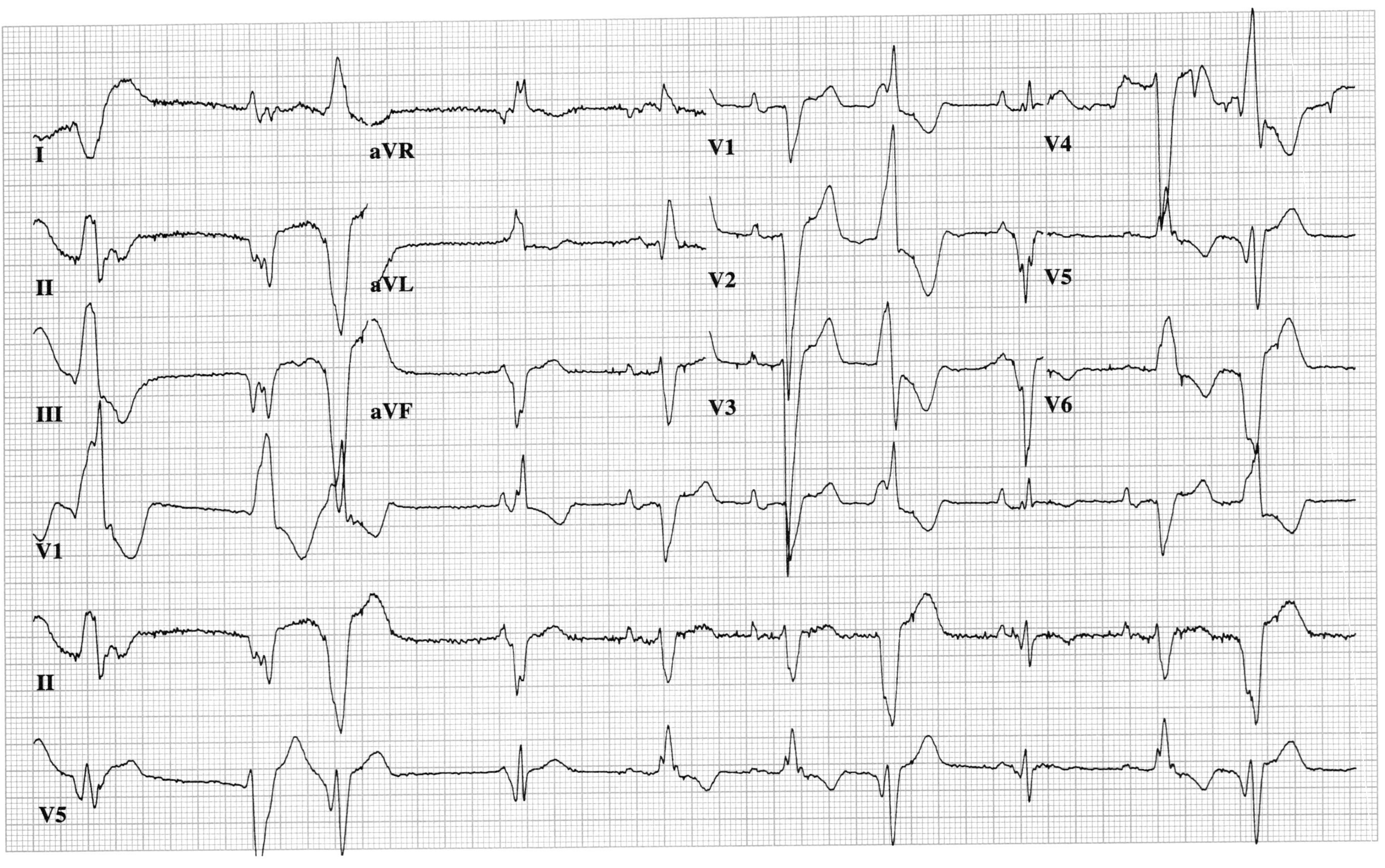

1. GENERAL FEATURES

☐ a. Normal ECG
☐ b. Borderline normal ECG or normal variant
☐ c. Incorrect electrode placement
☐ d. Artifact due to tremor

2. ATRIAL RHYTHMS

☐ a. Sinus rhythm
☐ b. Sinus arrhythmia
☐ c. Sinus bradycardia (< 60)
☐ d. Sinus tachycardia (> 100)
☐ e. Sinus pause or arrest
☐ f. Sinoatrial exit block
☐ g. Ecoptic atrial rhythm
☐ h. Wandering atrial pacemaker
☐ i. Atrial premature complexes, normally conducted
☐ j. Atrial premature complexes, nonconducted
☐ k. Atrial premature complexes with aberrant intraventricular conduction
☐ l. Atrial tachycardia (regular, sustained, 1:1 conduction)
☐ m. Atrial tachycardia, repetitive (short paroxysms)
☐ n. Atrial tachycardia, multifocal
☐ o. Atrial tachycardia with AV block
☐ p. Supraventricular tachycardia, unspecific
☐ q. Supraventricular tachycardia, paroxysmal
☐ r. Atrial flutter
☐ s. Atrial fibrillation
☐ t. Retrograde atrial activation

3. AV JUNCTIONAL RHYTHMS

☐ a. AV junctional premature complexes
☐ b. AV junctional escape complexes
☐ c. AV junctional rhythm, accelerated
☐ d. AV junctional rhythm

4. VENTRICULAR RHYTHMS

☐ a. Ventricular premature complex(es), uniform, fixed coupling
☐ b. Ventricular premature complex(es), uniform, nonfixed coupling
☐ c. Ventricular premature complexes(es), multiform
☐ d. Ventricular premature complexes, in pairs
☐ e. Ventricular parasystole
☐ f. Ventricular tachycardia (≥ 3 consecutive complexes)
☐ g. Accelerated idioventricular rhythm
☐ h. Ventricular escape complexes or rhythm
☐ i. Ventricular fibrillation

5. ATRIAL-VENTRICULAR INTERACTIONS IN ARRHYTHMIAS

☐ a. Fusion complexes
☐ b. Reciprocal (echo) complexes
☐ c. Ventricular capture complexes
☐ d. AV dissociation
☐ e. Ventriculophasic sinus arrhythmia

6. AV CONDUCTION ABNORMALITIES

☐ a. AV block, 1°
☐ b. AV block, 2° - Mobitz type I (Wenckebach)
☐ c. AV block, 2° - Mobitz type II
☐ d. AV block, 2:1
☐ e. AV block, 3°
☐ f. AV block, variable
☐ g. Short PR interval (with sinus rhythm and normal QRS duration)
☐ h. Wolff-Parkinson-White pattern

7. INTRAVENTRICULAR CONDUCTION DISTURBANCES

☐ a. RBBB, incomplete
☐ b. RBBB, complete
☐ c. Left anterior fascicular block
☐ d. Left posterior fascicular block
☐ e. LBBB, with ST-T wave suggestive of acute myocardial injury or infarction
☐ f. LBBB, complete
☐ g. LBBB, intermittent
☐ h. Intraventricular conduction disturbance, nonspecific
☐ i. Aberrant intraventricular conduction with supraventricular arrhythmia

8. P WAVE ABNORMALITIES

☐ a. Right atrial abnormality
☐ b. Left atrial abnormalities
☐ c. Nonspecific atrial abnormality

9. ABNORMALITIES OF QRS VOLTAGE OR AXIS

☐ a. Low voltage, limb leads only
☐ b. Low voltage, limb and precordial leads
☐ c. Left axis deviation (> - 30%)
☐ d. Right axis deviation (> + 100)
☐ e. Electrical alternans

10. VENTRICULAR HYPERTROPHY

☐ a. LVH by voltage only
☐ b. LVH by voltage and ST-T segment abnormalities
☐ c. RVH
☐ d. Combined ventricular hypertrophy

11. Q WAVE MYOCARDIAL INFARCTION

	Probably Acute or Recent	Probably Old or Age Indeterminate
Anterolateral	☐ a.	☐ g.
Anterior	☐ b.	☐ h.
Anteroseptal	☐ c.	☐ i.
Lateral/High lateral	☐ d.	☐ j.
Inferior	☐ e.	☐ k.
Posterior	☐ f.	☐ l.

☐ m. Probably ventricular aneurysm

12. ST, T, U, WAVE ABNORMALITIES

☐ a. Normal variant, early repolarization
☐ b. Normal variant, juvenile T waves
☐ c. Nonspecific ST and/or T wave abnormalities
☐ d. ST and/or T wave abnormalities suggesting myocardial ischemia
☐ e. ST and/or T wave abnormalities suggesting myocardial injury
☐ f. ST and/or T wave abnormalities suggesting acute pericarditis
☐ g. ST-T segment abnormalities secondary to intraventricular conduction disturbance or hypertrophy
☐ h. Post-extrasystolic T wave abnormality
☐ i. Isolated J point depression
☐ j. Peaked T waves
☐ k. Prolonged QT interval
☐ l. Prominent U waves

13. PACEMAKER FUNCTION AND RHYTHM

☐ a. Atrial or coronary sinus pacing
☐ b. Ventricular demand pacing
☐ c. AV sequential pacing
☐ d. Ventricular pacing, complete control
☐ e. Dual chamber, atrial sensing pacemaker
☐ f. Pacemaker malfunction, not constantly capturing (atrium or ventricle)
☐ g. Pacemaker malfunction, not constantly sensing (atrium or ventricle)
☐ h. Pacemaker malfunction, not firing
☐ i. Pacemaker malfunction, slowing

14. SUGGESTED OR PROBABLE CLINICAL DISORDERS

☐ a. Digitalis effect
☐ b. Digitalis toxicity
☐ c. Antiarrhythmic drug effect
☐ d. Antiarrhythmic drug toxicity
☐ e. Hyperkalemia
☐ f. Hypokalemia
☐ g. Hypercalcemia
☐ h. Hypocalcemia
☐ i. Atrial septal defect, secundum
☐ j. Atrial septal defect, primum
☐ k. Dextrocardia, mirror image
☐ l. Mitral valve disease
☐ m. Chronic lung disease
☐ n. Acute cor pulmonale, including pulmonary embolus
☐ o. Pericardial effusion
☐ p. Acute pericarditis
☐ q. Hypertrophic cardiomyopathy
☐ r. Coronary artery disease
☐ s. Central nervous system disorder
☐ t. Myxedema
☐ u. Hypothermia

ECG 102 was obtained in an 88-year-old male with an irregular pulse. This complex ECG shows sinus rhythm at a rate of 65 per minute (asterisk marks the sinus interval), first-degree AV block, right atrial enlargement (arrowheads), and left bundle branch block with secondary ST-T repolarization abnormalities. Also noted is ventricular parasystole, diagnosed by the presence of ventricular premature complexes (VPC) without fixed coupling to the previous normal QRS complex, fusion complexes (FUS), and VPC-to-VPC intervals that bear a mathematical relationship (2X, 3X, etc.) to each other. The key to interpreting this ECG is to recognize that the interval between VPC 2 and VPC 3, and the interval between the fusion beat (FUS) and VPC 2 are the same and equal to twice the interval between VPC 1 and the fusion beat (i.e., the parasystolic interval; double asterisk). With this relationship determined, it is then possible to set your calipers on the parasystolic interval and march forward from VPC 1 to the fusion beat (FUS), and then to a point during the ST segment of beat 5 when the ventricle is refractory (REF) and will not conduct the parasystolic impulse, and then to VPC 2, and then to a point during the ST segment of beat 8 when the ventricle is again refractory, and then to VPC 3. You can also march back from VPC 1 to a point on the ST segment of beat 1 when the ventricle is refractory. The second wide QRS complex represents a ventricular escape beat. The beat following VPC 2 is preceeded by a normal P wave with a PR interval that is shorter than the other sinus beats and a QRS morphology that differs from the other beats — this represents a fusion complex from a sinus beat and a VPC originating from a focus other than the parasystolic focus.

Codes:	2a	Sinus rhythm	6a	AV block, 1°
	4e	Ventricular parasystole	7f	LBBB, complete
	4h	Ventricular escape complexes	8a	Right atrial abnormality
	5a	Fusion complexes	12g	ST-T segment abnormalities secondary to IVCD or hypertrophy

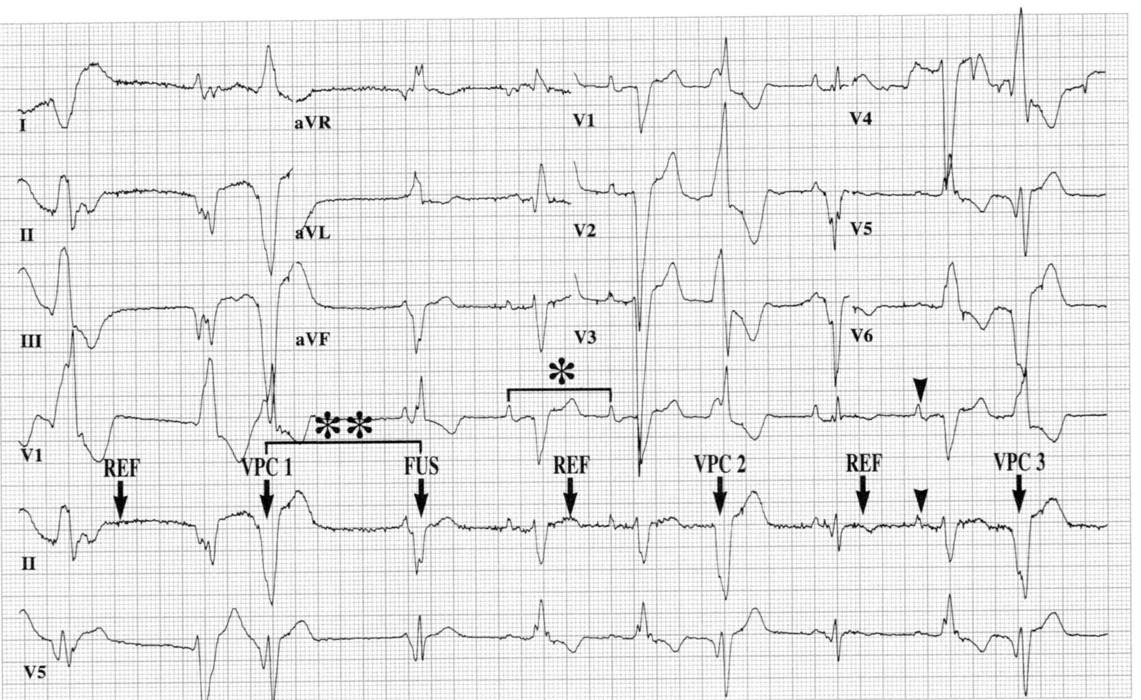

Questions: ECG 102

1. Ventricular parasystole is due to:

   a. Local reentry coupled to the prior sinus beat
   b. Automatic focus with entrance block

2. ECG features consistent with ventricular parasystole include:

   a. Varying relationship of the VPC to the preceding sinus beat
   b. Constant relationship of the VPC to the preceding sinus beat
   c. Interectopic intervals are a multiple of a constant shortest interval
   d. Fusion beats
   e. Capture beats

Answers: ECG 102

1. Ventricular parasystole is due to an automatic focus in the ventricle that is isolated from (i.e., cannot be depolarized by) the normal sinus impulse due to entrance block into the focus. The ventricular focus fires at a regular cycle length and results in a VPC that bears no constant relationship to the previous sinus beat (i.e., nonfixed coupling). In contrast to ventricular parasystole, uniform VPC's due to local reentry initiated by prior sinus activation of the ventricle show fixed coupling. (Answer: b)

2. Ventricular parasystole is due to presence of an automatic and independent focus and has a varying relationship (nonfixed coupling) to the preceding sinus beat. Since the parasystolic focus fires at a regular rate and inscribes a QRS complex whenever the ventricles are not refractory, all interectopic intervals are a multiple of a constant shortest interval. Fusion complexes may be present, resulting from simultaneous activation of the ventricles by atrial and parasystolic impulses. Capture beats do not occur with ventricular parasystole. (Answer: a, c, d)

— Quick Review 102 —

Ventricular parasystole	
• Ventricular ectopic beats occur at a rate of ____ per minute (can range from ____ per minute)	30-50 20-400
• VPCs show (fixed/nonfixed) coupling	nonfixed
• Fusion complexes are required for the diagnosis (true/false)	false
• All interectopic intervals are a ____ of the shortest interectopic interval	multiple
• Ventricular parasystole is due to the presence of an ectopic ventricular focus that activates the ventricles ____ of the basic sinus or supraventricular rhythm, and is protected from depolarization by an (entrance/exit) block	independent entrance
• Think of parasystole when you see ventricular complexes with ____ coupling and ____ beats	nonfixed, fusion
Fusion complexes	
• Due to simultaneous activation of the ventricle from ____ sources, resulting in a QRS complex that is ____ in morphology between each source	2 intermediate

— POP QUIZ —

Find The Mistake

Instructions: Identify the incorrect ECG feature(s) for each of the ECG diagnoses listed below

ECG Features	Answer

CNS disorder
• "Classic changes" usually occur in the limb leads
  ▸ Large upright or deeply inverted T waves
  ▸ Prolonged QT interval (often marked)
  ▸ Prominent U waves
• Other changes:
  ▸ ST segment mimicking acute pericarditis or injury
  ▸ ST depression may also occur
  ▸ Abnormal Q waves mimicking MI
  ▸ Almost any rhythm abnormality including sinus tachycardia or bradycardia, junctional rhythm, VPCs, ventricular tachycardia, etc.
	"Classic changes" usually occur in the precordial (not limb) leads

Myxedema • Low QRS voltage in all leads • Sinus bradycardia • Peaked T waves • PR interval may be prolonged • Frequently associated with pericardial effusion • Electrical alternans may occur	T waves are flattened or inverted (not peaked)
Hypothermia • Sinus bradycardia • PR, QRS, and QT prolonged • Osborne ("J") wave: late upright terminal deflection of QRS complex • Atrial fibrillation in 50-60%	All are correct!

ECG 103. 40-year-old male runner with palpitations:

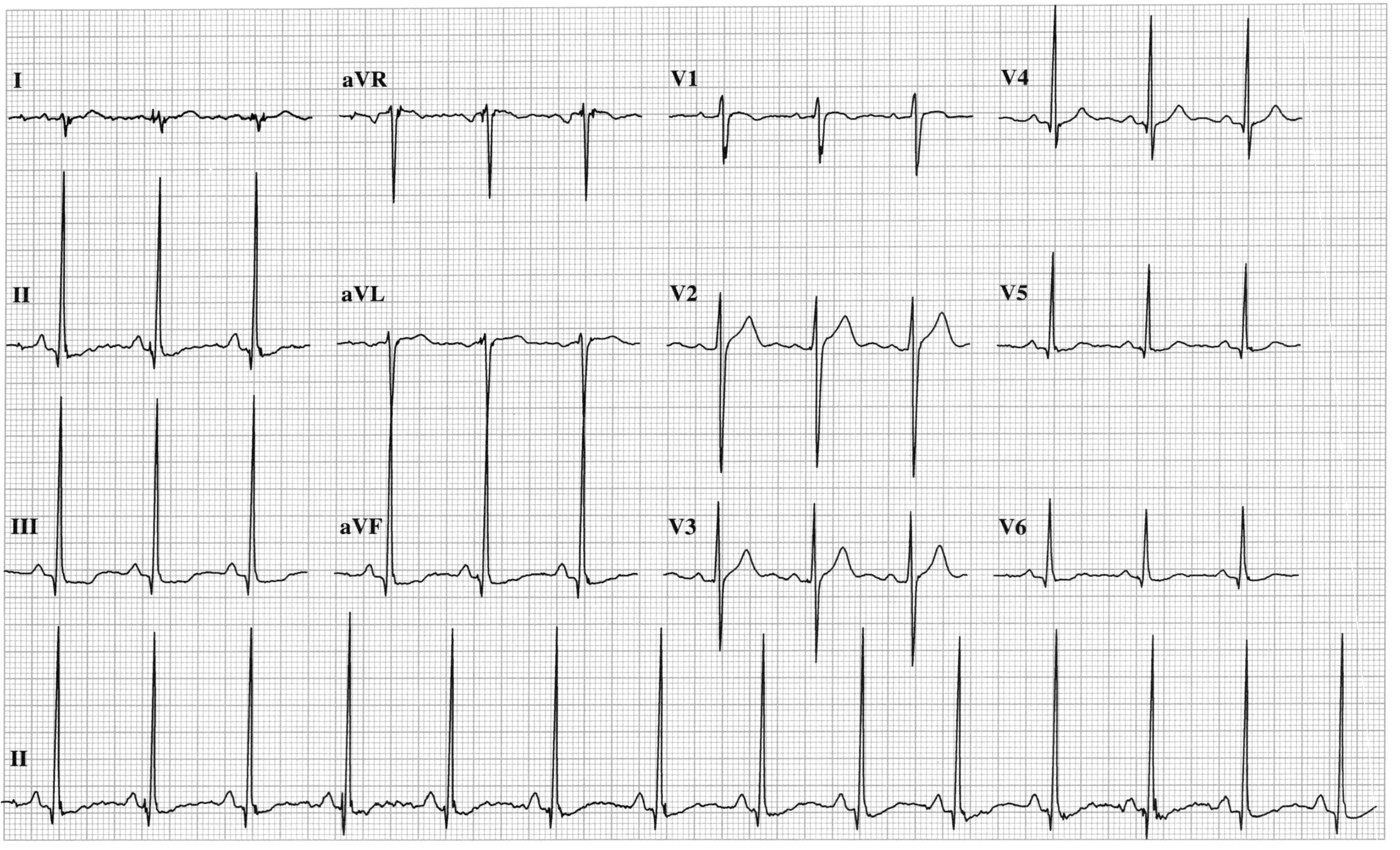

1. GENERAL FEATURES
- ☐ a. Normal ECG
- ☐ b. Borderline normal ECG or normal variant
- ☐ c. Incorrect electrode placement
- ☐ d. Artifact due to tremor

2. ATRIAL RHYTHMS
- ☐ a. Sinus rhythm
- ☐ b. Sinus arrhythmia
- ☐ c. Sinus bradycardia (< 60)
- ☐ d. Sinus tachycardia (> 100)
- ☐ e. Sinus pause or arrest
- ☐ f. Sinoatrial exit block
- ☐ g. Ecoptic atrial rhythm
- ☐ h. Wandering atrial pacemaker
- ☐ i. Atrial premature complexes, normally conducted
- ☐ j. Atrial premature complexes, nonconducted
- ☐ k. Atrial premature complexes with aberrant intraventricular conduction
- ☐ l. Atrial tachycardia (regular, sustained, 1:1 conduction)
- ☐ m. Atrial tachycardia, repetitive (short paroxysms)
- ☐ n. Atrial tachycardia, multifocal
- ☐ o. Atrial tachycardia with AV block
- ☐ p. Supraventricular tachycardia, unspecific
- ☐ q. Supraventricular tachycardia, paroxysmal
- ☐ r. Atrial flutter
- ☐ s. Atrial fibrillation
- ☐ t. Retrograde atrial activation

3. AV JUNCTIONAL RHYTHMS
- ☐ a. AV junctional premature complexes
- ☐ b. AV junctional escape complexes
- ☐ c. AV junctional rhythm, accelerated
- ☐ d. AV junctional rhythm

4. VENTRICULAR RHYTHMS
- ☐ a. Ventricular premature complex(es), uniform, fixed coupling
- ☐ b. Ventricular premature complex(es), uniform, nonfixed coupling
- ☐ c. Ventricular premature complexes(es), multiform
- ☐ d. Ventricular premature complexes, in pairs
- ☐ e. Ventricular parasystole
- ☐ f. Ventricular tachycardia (≥ 3 consecutive complexes)
- ☐ g. Accelerated idioventricular rhythm
- ☐ h. Ventricular escape complexes or rhythm
- ☐ i. Ventricular fibrillation

5. ATRIAL-VENTRICULAR INTERACTIONS IN ARRHYTHMIAS
- ☐ a. Fusion complexes
- ☐ b. Reciprocal (echo) complexes
- ☐ c. Ventricular capture complexes
- ☐ d. AV dissociation
- ☐ e. Ventriculophasic sinus arrhythmia

6. AV CONDUCTION ABNORMALITIES
- ☐ a. AV block, 1°
- ☐ b. AV block, 2° - Mobitz type I (Wenckebach)
- ☐ c. AV block, 2° - Mobitz type II
- ☐ d. AV block, 2:1
- ☐ e. AV block, 3°
- ☐ f. AV block, variable
- ☐ g. Short PR interval (with sinus rhythm and normal QRS duration)
- ☐ h. Wolff-Parkinson-White pattern

7. INTRAVENTRICULAR CONDUCTION DISTURBANCES
- ☐ a. RBBB, incomplete
- ☐ b. RBBB, complete
- ☐ c. Left anterior fascicular block
- ☐ d. Left posterior fascicular block
- ☐ e. LBBB, with ST-T wave suggestive of acute myocardial injury or infarction
- ☐ f. LBBB, complete
- ☐ g. LBBB, intermittent
- ☐ h. Intraventricular conduction disturbance, nonspecific
- ☐ i. Aberrant intraventricular conduction with supraventricular arrhythmia

8. P WAVE ABNORMALITIES
- ☐ a. Right atrial abnormality
- ☐ b. Left atrial abnormalities
- ☐ c. Nonspecific atrial abnormality

9. ABNORMALITIES OF QRS VOLTAGE OR AXIS
- ☐ a. Low voltage, limb leads only
- ☐ b. Low voltage, limb and precordial leads
- ☐ c. Left axis deviation (> - 30%)
- ☐ d. Right axis deviation (> + 100)
- ☐ e. Electrical alternans

10. VENTRICULAR HYPERTROPHY
- ☐ a. LVH by voltage only
- ☐ b. LVH by voltage and ST-T segment abnormalities
- ☐ c. RVH
- ☐ d. Combined ventricular hypertrophy

11. Q WAVE MYOCARDIAL INFARCTION

	Probably Acute or Recent	Probably Old or Age Indeterminate
Anterolateral	☐ a.	☐ g.
Anterior	☐ b.	☐ h.
Anteroseptal	☐ c.	☐ i.
Lateral/High lateral	☐ d.	☐ j.
Inferior	☐ e.	☐ k.
Posterior	☐ f.	☐ l.

- ☐ m. Probably ventricular aneurysm

12. ST, T, U, WAVE ABNORMALITIES
- ☐ a. Normal variant, early repolarization
- ☐ b. Normal variant, juvenile T waves
- ☐ c. Nonspecific ST and/or T wave abnormalities
- ☐ d. ST and/or T wave abnormalities suggesting myocardial ischemia
- ☐ e. ST and/or T wave abnormalities suggesting myocardial injury
- ☐ f. ST and/or T wave abnormalities suggesting acute pericarditis
- ☐ g. ST-T segment abnormalities secondary to intraventricular conduction disturbance or hypertrophy
- ☐ h. Post-extrasystolic T wave abnormality
- ☐ i. Isolated J point depression
- ☐ j. Peaked T waves
- ☐ k. Prolonged QT interval
- ☐ l. Prominent U waves

13. PACEMAKER FUNCTION AND RHYTHM
- ☐ a. Atrial or coronary sinus pacing
- ☐ b. Ventricular demand pacing
- ☐ c. AV sequential pacing
- ☐ d. Ventricular pacing, complete control
- ☐ e. Dual chamber, atrial sensing pacemaker
- ☐ f. Pacemaker malfunction, not constantly capturing (atrium or ventricle)
- ☐ g. Pacemaker malfunction, not constantly sensing (atrium or ventricle)
- ☐ h. Pacemaker malfunction, not firing
- ☐ i. Pacemaker malfunction, slowing

14. SUGGESTED OR PROBABLE CLINICAL DISORDERS
- ☐ a. Digitalis effect
- ☐ b. Digitalis toxicity
- ☐ c. Antiarrhythmic drug effect
- ☐ d. Antiarrhythmic drug toxicity
- ☐ e. Hyperkalemia
- ☐ f. Hypokalemia
- ☐ g. Hypercalcemia
- ☐ h. Hypocalcemia
- ☐ i. Atrial septal defect, secundum
- ☐ j. Atrial septal defect, primum
- ☐ k. Dextrocardia, mirror image
- ☐ l. Mitral valve disease
- ☐ m. Chronic lung disease
- ☐ n. Acute cor pulmonale, including pulmonary embolus
- ☐ o. Pericardial effusion
- ☐ p. Acute pericarditis
- ☐ q. Hypertrophic cardiomyopathy
- ☐ r. Coronary artery disease
- ☐ s. Central nervous system disorder
- ☐ t. Myxedema
- ☐ u. Hypothermia

ECG 103 was obtained from a 40-year-old male runner with palpitations. The ECG shows normal sinus rhythm at a rate of 77 bpm. LVH with secondary repolarization abnormality is present (S wave in aVR ≥ 15 mm; R wave in aVF > 21 mm). The axis is shifted rightward but is < 100° (so right axis deviation should not be coded). Likewise, the P wave in lead II, Q waves in leads II, III, and aVF, and U waves in leads V_2 and V_3 do not meet criteria for right atrial abnormality, Q-wave MI, or prominent U waves. This ECG was obtained from Mark Freed, MD, one of the editors of this book and a very active runner. The rightward axis, large P wave in lead II, and prominent inferior voltage are consistent with a vertical heart, thin body habitus, and "physiologic hypertrophy," not uncommon in well-trained athletes. The palpitations were due to the combination of coffee, chocolate, and lack of sleep — all related to finishing this book on time!

Codes:

2a	Sinus rhythm
10b	LVH by both voltage and ST-T wave abnormalities

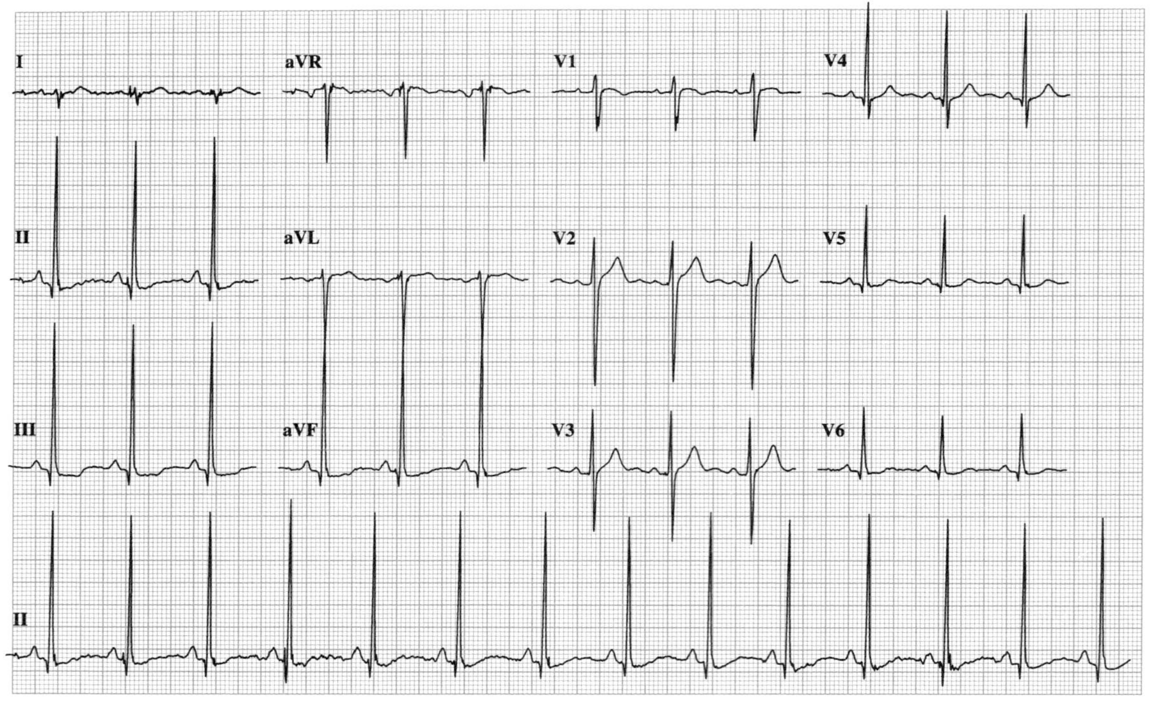

Questions: ECG 103

1. Causes of right axis deviation include:

   a. RVH
   b. COPD
   c. Horizontal heart
   d. Left posterior fascicular block
   e. Dextrocardia
   f. Ostium primum ASD
   g. Reversal of right and left arm leads

2. Factors/conditions that reduce the specificity (i.e., increase the rate of false-positives) for the diagnosis of LVH by voltage criteria include:

   a. Obesity
   b. Thin body habitus
   c. Severe COPD
   d. Pericardial or plural effusion
   e. Coronary artery disease
   f. Pneumothorax
   g. Sarcoidosis or amyloidosis of the heart
   h. Severe RVH
   i. Left anterior fascicular block

Answers: ECG 103

1. Causes of right axis deviation include RVH, vertical heart, COPD, pulmonary embolus, left posterior fascicular block, lateral wall MI, dextrocardia, reversal of right and left arm leads, and ostium secundum ASD. Horizontal hearts and ostium primum ASDs are associated with a leftward shift of the mean QRS axis. (Answer: a, b, d, e, g)

2. Thin body habitus and the presence of left anterior fascicular block may increase QRS amplitude and reduce the specificity for the diagnosis of LVH by voltage criteria. In contrast, conditions that decrease QRS amplitude and reduce the sensitivity (i.e., increase the rate of false-negatives) for the diagnosis of LVH by voltage criteria include conditions that increase the amount of body tissue (obesity), air (COPD, pneumothorax), fluid (pericardial or plural effusion), or fibrous tissue (coronary artery disease, sarcoid or amyloid of the heart) between the myocardium and ECG electrodes. Severe RVH can also underestimate the ECG diagnosis of LVH by cancelling prominent QRS forces from the thickened LV. (Answer: b, i)

— Quick Review 103 —	
Right axis deviation • Mean QRS axis between ____ and ____ degrees	101, 254

— Section II —

General Features of Major ECG Diagnoses

1. GENERAL FEATURES

1a. Normal ECG

- No abnormalities of rate, rhythm, or axis
- Normal amplitude, duration, and configuration of the P-QRS-T:

P Wave		
	Duration:	0.08 - 0.11 seconds
	Axis:	0 - 75^0
	Morphology:	Upright in I, II; upright or inverted in aVF; inverted or biphasic in III, aVL, V_1, V_2; small notching may be present
	Amplitude:	Limb leads: < 2.5 mm; V_1: positive deflection < 1.5 mm and negative deflection < 1 mm
PR Interval		
	Duration:	0.12 - 0.20 seconds
	PR segment:	Usually isoelectric; may be displaced in a direction opposite to the P wave; elevation usually < 0.5 mm; depression usually < 0.8 mm
QRS Complex		
	Duration:	0.06 - 0.10 seconds
	Axis:	-30^0 to 105^0
	*Transition zone**	V_2 - V_4
	Q wave:	Small Q waves (duration < 0.04 seconds and amplitude < 2 mm) are common in most leads except aVR, V_1 and V_2
	*OID***	Right precordial leads < 0.035 seconds; left precordial leads < 0.045 seconds
ST Segment:		Usually isoelectric; may vary from 0.5 mm below to 1 mm above baseline in limb leads; up to 3 mm concave upward elevation in precordial leads may be seen (early repolarization, item 12a)
T Wave:	*Morphology:*	Upright in I, II, V_3-V_6; inverted in aVR, V_1; may be upright, flat or biphasic in III, aVL, aVF, V_1,V_2; T wave inversion may be present in V_1-V_3 in healthy young adults (juvenile T waves, item 12b)
	Amplitude:	Usually < 6 mmm in limb leads and ≤ 10 mm in precordial leads
QT Interval:		Corrected QT 0.30 - 0.46 seconds; varies inversely with heart rate
U Wave:	*Morphology:*	Upright in all leads except aVR
	Amplitude:	5-25% the height of the T wave (usually < 1.5 mm)

* Precordial leads with equal positive and negative deflection

** Onset of intrinsicoid deflection: beginning of QRS to peak of R wave

1b. Borderline normal ECG or normal variant

- Early repolarization (item 12a)
- Juvenile T waves (item 12b)
- S wave in leads I, II, and III (S_1 S_2 S_3 pattern)

  Note: Present in up to 20% of healthy adults.
- RSR' or rSr' in lead V_1 with:
  - QRS duration <0.10 seconds and <7 mm in height, *and*
  - r' amplitude smaller than r or S waves

  Note: Seen in 2% of normals.

  Note: Can also be seen in pathological states:
  - RVH
  - Posterior MI
  - Skeletal deformities (pectus excavation, straight back syndrome)
  - High electrode placement of V_1 (in 3rd intercostal space instead of 4th)

1c. Incorrect electrode placement

Most commonly:

- Limb lead reversal (reversal of right and left arm leads)
  - Resultant ECG mimics dextrocardia with inversion of the P-QRS-T in leads I and aVL

  Note: To distinguish between these conditions, look at precordial leads: dextrocardia shows reverse R wave progression, while limb lead reversal shows normal R wave progression.
- Precordial lead reversal
  - Typically manifests as an unexplained decrease in R wave voltage in two consecutive leads (e.g., V_1, V_2) with a return to normal R wave progression on the following leads

1d. Artifact

- Commonly due to tremor
  - Parkinson's tremor simulates atrial flutter with a rate of ~ 300 per minute (4-6 per second)
  - Physiologic tremor rate is 500 per minute (7-9 per second)

  - Most prominent in limb leads
- Other common artifacts
  - AC electrical interference
  - Skeletal muscle fasciculations

2. ATRIAL RHYTHMS

2a. Sinus rhythm

- Normal P wave axis and morphology (item 1a)
- Atrial rate is 60-100 per minute and regular (PP interval varies by < 0.16 seconds or 10%

2b. Sinus arrhythmla

- Normal P wave morphology and axis (item 1a)
- Gradual phasic change in PP interval (may sometimes be abrupt)
- Longest and shortest PP intervals vary by >0.16 seconds or 10%

Note: Sinus arrhythmia differs from "ventriculophasic" sinus arrhythmia, the latter of which occurs in the setting of partial or complete heart block (item 5e).

2c. Sinus bradycardia (<60)

- Normal P wave axis and morphology (item 1a)
- Rate <60 per minute

Note: If the atrial rate is < 40 per minute, think of 2:1 sinoatrial exit block (item 2f)

2d. Sinus tachycardia (>100)

- Normal P wave axis and morphology (item 1a)
- Rate >100 per minute

Note: P wave amplitude often increases and PR interval often shortens with increasing heart rate (e.g., during exercise)

2e. Sinus pause or arrest

- PP interval (pause) greater than 1.6-2.0 seconds

- Sinus rhythm resumes at a PP interval that is not a multiple of the basic sinus PP interval

  Note: If sinus rhythm resumes at a multiple of the basic PP, consider sinoatrial exit block (item 2f).

Note: Sinus pause/arrest is due to transient failure of impulse formation at the SA node

Note: Sinus pauses must be differentiated from:

- ▸ Sinus arrhythmia (item 2b): Phasic, gradual change in PP interval
- ▸ Second-degree sinoatrial exit block, Mobitz I (Wenckebach) (item 2f): Progressive shortening of PP interval until a P wave fails to appear
- ▸ Second-degree sinoatrial exit block, Mobitz II (item 2f): Resumption of sinus rhythm at a PP interval that is a multiple (e.g., 2x, 3x, etc.) of the basic sinus rhythm
- ▸ Third-degree sinoatrial exit block (item 2f): Complete failure of sinoatrial conduction; cannot be differentiated from complete sinus arrest on surface ECG
- ▸ Abrupt change in autonomic tone
- ▸ "Pseudo" sinus pause due to nonconducted APCs (item 2j): P wave appears to be absent but is actually buried in the T wave — look for subtle deformity of the T wave just preceding the pause to detect nonconducted atrial premature complexes

2f. Sinoatrial (SA) exit block

- First-degree: Conduction of sinus impulses to the atrium is delayed, but 1:1 response is maintained; not detectable on surface ECG
- Second-degree: Some sinus impulses fail to capture the atria (i.e., intermittent absence of a P wave)
  - ▸ Type I (Mobitz I):
    - P wave morphology and axis consistent with a sinus node origin
    - "Group beating" with:

      (1) Shortening of the PP interval leading up to pause

      (2) Constant PR interval

      (3) PP pause less than twice the normal PP interval
  - ▸ Type II (Mobitz II)
    - Constant PP interval followed by a pause that is a multiple (e.g., 2x, 3x,

etc.) of the normal PP interval

Note: The pause may be slightly less than twice the normal PP interval but is usually within 0.10 seconds.

- Third-degree: Complete failure of sinoatrial conduction; cannot be differentiated from complete sinus arrest (item 2e)

2g. Ectopic atrial rhythm

- P wave axis or morphology different from sinus node (item 1a)
- Rate <100 per minute
- PR interval >0.11 seconds

Note: Inverted P waves in II, III, aVF suggest either an AV junctional rhythm with retrograde atrial activation or a low atrial rhythm. To distinguish between these mechanisms, measure the PR interval:

  - PR > 0.11 seconds suggests a low atrial rhythm
  - PR ≤ 0.11 seconds suggests an AV junctional rhythm

2h. Wandering atrial pacemaker

- P waves with ≥ 3 morphologies
- Rate <100 per minute
- Varying PR, RR, and RP intervals

Note: May be confused with:

  - Sinus rhythm with multifocal APCs: Sinus rhythm with multifocal APCs demonstrates one dominant atrial pacemaker (i.e., the sinus node); in wandering atrial pacemaker, *no* dominant atrial pacemaker (i.e., no dominant P wave morphology) is present.
  - Atrial fibrillation/flutter with a moderate ventricular response: In atrial fib/flutter, there is lack of an isoelectric baseline; in wandering atrial pacemaker, a distinct isoelectric baseline is present.

Note: P waves may be blocked (i.e., not followed by a QRS complex), or may be conducted with a narrow or aberrant QRS complex.

2i. Atrial premature complexes, normally conducted

- P wave that is abnormal in configuration and premature relative to the normal PP interval

- QRS complex is similar in morphology to the QRS complex present during sinus rhythm

Note: The PR interval may be normal, increased, or decreased.

Note: The post-extrasystolic pause is usually *noncompensatory* (i.e., premature P to subsequent P wave interval is less than two PP intervals). However, an interpolated APC or a full compensatory may be evident when sinoatrial (SA) entrance block is present and the SA node is not reset.

2j. Atrial premature complexes, nonconducted

- Premature P wave with abnormal morphology not followed by a QRS-T complex

Note: The sinus node is usually reset, resulting in a noncompensatory pause (item 2i)

Note: P waves are often hidden in the preceding T wave — when you see an RR pause, look for a deformed T wave immediately preceding the pause to identify the presence of a nonconducted atrial premature beat.

2k. Atrial premature complexes with aberrant intraventricular conduction

- P wave occurs very early relative to the normal PP interval (also see item 2i)
- QRS morphology is most often RBBB pattern, but can be LBBB or variable

2l. Atrial tachycardia (regular, sustained, 1:1 conduction)

- P wave axis or morphology different from sinus node (item 1a)
- Three or more beats in succession at an atrial rate of 100-180 per minute (may be up to 240 per minute)
- Regular rhythm (constant RR interval), except for a warm-up period in the automatic type
- QRS complex follows each P wave
- QRS morphology usually resembles QRS during sinus rhythm, but may be wide and bizarre if aberrant
- PR interval may be within normal limits or prolonged
- Nonspecific ST-T changes (item 12c) may occur

2m. Atrial tachycardia, repetitive (short paroxysm)

- Recurring short runs of atrial tachycardia (item 2l) interrupted by normal sinus rhythm

2n. Atrial tachycardia, multifocal (chaotic atrial tachycardia)

- Atrial rate >100 per minute
- P waves with ≥ 3 morphologies
- Varying PR, RR and RP intervals

Note: Multifocal atrial tachycardia may be confused with:

- Sinus tachycardia with multifocal APCs, which demonstrates one dominant atrial pacemaker (i.e., the sinus node). In contrast, in multifocal atrial tachycardia, *no* dominant atrial pacemaker (i.e., no dominant P wave morphology) is present.
- Atrial fibrillation/flutter, in which there is lack of an isoelectric baseline. In contrast, multifocal atrial tachycardia demonstrates a distinct isoelectric baseline and P waves.

Note: P waves may be blocked (i.e., not followed by a QRS complex), or may be conducted with a narrow or aberrant QRS complex.

2o. Atrial tachycardia with AV block

- P wave axis or morphology different from sinus node (item 1a)
- Atrial rate of 150-240 per minute (may be as low as 100 per minute)
- Isoelectric intervals between P waves in all leads
- Second- or third-degree AV block
- Atrial rhythm is regular (but may see ventriculophasic arrhythmia [item 5e])

Note: May be secondary to digoxin toxicity (item 14b).

Note: May be confused with atrial flutter. Atrial tachycardia with AV block has a distinct isoelectric baseline between P waves, whereas atrial flutter does not (except in lead V_1).

2p. Supraventricular tachycardia, unspecified

- Regular rhythm
- Rate >100 per minute
- P waves not easily identified
- QRS complex is usually narrow (but occasionally aberrant)

Note: If rate is 150 per minute, atrial flutter with 2:1 block may be present.

2q. Supraventricular tachycardia (paroxysmal)

- Onset and termination of SVT (item 2p) is sudden
- SVT is episodic and does not persist throughout the entire tracing
- May see retrograde atrial activation (item 2t)

2r. Atrial flutter

- Rapid regular atrial undulations (flutter or "F" waves) at 240-340 per minute

  Note: Flutter rate may be faster in children, and slower in the presence of antiarrhythmic drugs (Type IA, IC, III) and massively dilated atria.
- Typical atrial flutter morphology usually present:
  - Leads II, III, AVF: Inverted F waves without an isoelectric baseline ("picket-fence" or "sawtooth" appearance)
  - Lead V_1: Small positive deflections with a distinct isoelectric baseline
- QRS complex may be normal or aberrant
- Rate and regularity of QRS complexes depend on the AV conduction sequence
  - AV conduction ratio (ratio of flutter waves to QRS complexes) is usually fixed (e.g., 2:1, 4:1), but may vary.

    Note: Conduction ratios of 1:1 and 3:1 are uncommon. In untreated patients, ≥ 4:1 block suggests the coexistence of AV conduction disease.
  - Complete heart block with a junctional or ventricular escape rhythm may be present.

Note: Think digitalis toxicity when complete heart block with junctional tachycardia is present.

Note: Flutter waves can deform QRS, ST and/or T to mimic intraventricular conduction delay and/or myocardial ischemia.

2s. Atrial fibrillation

- P waves absent
- Atrial activity is totally irregular and represented by fibrillatory (f) waves of varying amplitude, duration and morphology, causing random oscillation of the baseline

  Note: Atrial activity is best seen in the V_1, V_2 and the inferior leads (II, III, aVF).

- Ventricular rhythm is irregularly irregular

  Note: If the RR interval is regular, third-degree AV block (item 6e) is present.

  Note: Digoxin toxicity may result in regularization of the QRS due to complete heart block with junctional tachycardia.

- Ventricular rate is usually 100-180 per minute in the absence of drugs

  Note: If the rate without AV blocking drugs is less than 100 beats per minute, AV conduction system disease is likely to be present.

  Note: Think Wolff-Parkinson-White (item 6h) if the ventricular rate is >200 per minute and the QRS is > 0.12 seconds.

Note: Conditions mimicking atrial fibrillation include:

- Multifocal atrial tachycardia (item 2n)
- Paroxysmal atrial tachycardia with block (item 2o)
- Atrial flutter (item 2r)

2t. Retrograde atrial activation

- Inverted P waves in leads II, III and aVF

Note: Look for retrograde P waves after ventricular premature complexes and other junctional, ventricular, or low ectopic atrial rhythms.

3. AV JUNCTIONAL RHYTHMS

3a. AV junctional premature complexes

- Premature QRS complex (relative to the basic RR interval), which may be narrow or aberrant
- Inverted P waves in leads II, III, aVF (item 2t) and upright P waves in leads I and aVL is commonly seen

  Note: The atrium may occasionally be activated by the sinus node, resulting in a normal sinus P wave. This occurs when retrograde block exists between the AV junctional focus and the atrium.

  Note: The P wave may precede the QRS by ≤ 0.11 seconds (retrograde atrial activation, item 2t), may be buried in the QRS (and not visualized), or may follow the QRS complex.

Note: A constant coupling interval and noncompensatory pause are usually present.

3b. AV junctional escape complexes

- Rate is typically 40-60 per minute
- Atrial mechanism may be sinus rhythm, paroxysmal atrial tachycardia, atrial flutter, or atrial fibrillation
- QRS morphology is similar to the sinus or supraventricular impulse

<u>Note:</u> QRS complex occurs as a secondary phenomenon in response to decreased sinus impulse formation or conduction, high-degree AV block, or after the pause following termination of atrial tachycardia, atrial flutter, or atrial fibrillation.

3c. AV junctional rhythm, accelerated

- Regular QRS rhythm at rate >60 per minute
- P wave may proceed, be buried in, or follow the QRS complex
- QRS is usually narrow but may be wide if aberrant or preexisting IVCD
- Relationship between atrial and ventricular rates may vary:
  - If retrograde block is present, the atria remain in sinus rhythm and ***AV dissociation*** will be present
  - If retrograde atrial activation (item 2t) occurs, a constant QRS-P interval is usually present (occasionally there is 2:1 VA conduction)

<u>Note:</u> Think digitalis toxicity (item 14b) if atrial fibrillation or flutter with a regular RR is seen — this often represents complete heart block with accelerated junctional rhythm.

3d. AV junctional rhythm (rate $\leq$60/minute)

- P wave and QRS complex as described in item 3a
- RR interval of escape rhythm is usually constant (< 0.04 seconds variation)
- May have isorhythmic AV dissociation (item 5d)

4. VENTRICULAR RHYTHMS

4a. Ventricular premature complex(es), uniform, fixed coupling

Requires <u>all</u> of the following:

- A wide, notched or slurred QRS complex that is:
  - Premature relative to the normal RR interval, *and*
  - Not preceded by a P wave

  <u>Note:</u> QRS is almost always > 0.12 seconds.

Note: Initial direction of the QRS is often different from the QRS during sinus rhythm.

- Secondary ST & T wave changes in a direction opposite to the major deflection of the QRS (i.e., ST depression & T wave inversion in leads with a dominant R wave; ST elevation and upright T wave in leads with a dominant S wave or QS complex)
- Coupling interval (relation of VPCs to the preceding QRS) is constant (or varies by < 0.08 seconds)
- Morphology of VPCs in any given lead is the same (i.e., uniform)

Note: Retrograde capture of atria may occur (item 2t)

Note: A full compensatory pause (PP interval containing the VPC is twice the normal PP interval) is usually evident, and requires undisturbed sinus depolarization due to:

- ▸ Ventriculoatrial (VA) conduction block
- ▸ Sinoatrial (SA) entrance block if atrial capture occurs
- ▸ SA node discharge prior to arrival of retrograde wavefront

4b. Ventricular premature complexes, nonfixed coupling

- Relationship of VPCs to preceding QRS (coupling interval) is variable
- See item 4a for QRS morphology

4c. Ventricular premature complex(es), multiform

- VPCs with ≥ 2 morphologies

Note: Although multiform VPCs are usually multifocal in origin (i.e., originate from more than one ventricular focus), a single ventricular focus can produce VPCs of varying morphology.

4d. Ventricular premature complexes, in pairs (two consecutive)

- Two consecutive ventricular premature complexes (items 4a, c) of not necessarily the same morphology

4e. Ventricular parasystole

- Ventricular ectopic beats (VEB) occur at a rate of 30-50 per minute (but may range from 20-400 per minute, depending upon the degree of exit block and the refractoriness of the ventricle)
- Resultant ventricular premature complexes (VPC) vary in relationship to the preceding sinus or supraventricular beats (i.e., nonfixed coupling)

- VPCs typically manifest the same morphology (which resembles a VPC, item 4a) unless fusion occurs (item 5a)

  Note: Fusion complexes are commonly seen but are not required for the diagnosis.

  Note: When the ectopic ventricular focus originates on the same side as a bundle branch block, the resulting fusion complex can be narrow.

- All interectopic intervals are a multiple (2x, 3x, etc.) of the shortest interectopic interval present

Note: Ventricular parasystole is due to the presence of an ectopic ventricular focus that activates the ventricles independent of the basic sinus or supraventricular rhythm, and is protected from depolarization by an entrance block.

Note: Think of parasystole when you see ventricular premature complexes with nonfixed coupling and fusion beats.

4f. Ventricular tachycardia (≥ 3 consecutive beats)

- Rapid succession of three or more premature ventricular beats (item 4a) at a rate > 100 per minute
- RR interval is usually regular but may be irregular
- Abrupt onset and termination of arrhythmia is evident
- AV dissociation (item 5d) is common
- On occasion, retrograde atrial activation (item 2t) and capture occur

  Note: Look for ventricular capture complexes (item 5c) and fusion beats (item 5a) as markers for VT.

Note: In the setting of a wide QRS tachycardia, certain findings may help distinguish ventricular tachycardia from supraventricular tachycardia with aberrancy (Table 1).

4g. Accelerated idioventricular rhythm

- Regular or slightly irregular ventricular rhythm
- Rate of 60-110 per minute
- QRS morphology similar to VPCs (item 4a)
- AV dissociation is often present (item 5d)
- Ventricular capture complexes (item 5c) and fusion beats (item 5a) are common

Table 1. Origin of Wide QRS Tachycardia

	FAVORS VT	FAVORS SVT WITH ABERRANCY
QRS morphology	Similar to VPCs	Similar to sinus rhythm or aberrantly conducted APCs
Tachycardia initiated by	VPCs	APCs
AV dissociation[1]	Yes	No
Capture[2] or fusion beats[3]	Yes	No
QRS duration when QRS is narrow during sinus rhythm	> 0.14 sec. if RBBB morphology; > 0.16 sec. if LBBB morphology	
QRS deflection in precordial leads	All positive or negative (concordance)	Some positive and some negative (discordance)
Axis	Left or northwest	---
RSR' in V_1	R wave taller than R'	R' taller than R wave

1. *See item 5d*
2. *See item 5c*
3. *See item 5a*
4. *When the ventricular focus originates high in interventricular septum near the normal conduction system, ventricular tachycardia may have a relatively narrow QRS complex*

4h. Ventricular escape beats or rhythm

- Regular or slightly irregular ventricular rhythm
- Rate of 30-40 per minute (can be 20-50 per min)
- QRS morphology similar to VPCs (item 4a)

Note: QRS complex occurs as a secondary phenomenon in response to decreased sinus impulse formation or conduction, high-degree AV block, or after the pause following termination of atrial tachycardia, atrial flutter, or atrial fibrillation.

4i. Ventricular fibrillation

- An extremely rapid and irregular ventricular rhythm demonstrating:
  - Chaotic and irregular deflections of varying amplitude and contour, *and*
  - Absence of distinct P waves, QRS complexes, or T waves

5. ATRIOVENTRICULAR INTERACTIONS

5a. Fusion complexes

- Simultaneous activation of the ventricle from two sources, resulting in a QRS complex intermediate in morphology between the QRS complexes of each source

Note: Fusion complexes may be seen with:

  - Ventricular premature complexes (item 4a-d)
  - Ventricular tachycardia (item 4f)
  - Ventricular parasystole (item 4e)
  - Accelerated idioventricular rhythm (item 4g)
  - Wolff-Parkinson-White Syndrome (item 6h)
  - Paced rhythm

5b. Reciprocal (echo) complexes

- An impulse activates a chamber (atria or ventricle), returns to site of origin, and reactivates the same chamber again
- A form of nonsustained reentry

5c. Ventricular capture complexes

- Occurs when an atrial impulse is conducted to and stimulates the ventricles during ventricular tachycardia. The "captured" ventricle results in a:
  - Fusion complex (item 5a), *or*
  - QRS complex similar to that during sinus rhythm

Note: The presence of a ventricular capture complex in the setting of a wide QRS tachycardia strongly suggests the diagnosis of ventricular tachycardia.

5d. AV dissociation

- Atrial and ventricular rhythms are independent of each other, *and the*
- Ventricular rate is *equal to or faster* than the atrial rate

Note: AV dissociation is always a secondary phenomenon resulting from some other disturbance of cardiac rhythm. Examples include:

- ▸ Slowing of the atrial rate (sinus bradycardia, sinus arrest, sinoatrial exit block) below the intrinsic rate of a subsidiary AV junctional or ventricular pacemaker, *or*
- ▸ Acceleration of a subsidiary pacemaker (e.g., junctional or ventricular tachycardia) to a rate faster then the normal sinus rate.

5e. Ventriculophasic sinus arrhythmia

- PP interval containing a QRS complex is less than the PP interval without a QRS complex

Note: Occurs in 30-50% of patients with partial or complex AV block.

6. AV CONDUCTION ABNORMALITIES

6a. AV block, 1°

- PR interval ≥0.20 seconds (usually 0.21-0.40 seconds but may be as long as 0.80 seconds)
- Each P wave is followed by a QRS complex

6b. AV block, 2° - Mobitz Type I (Wenckebach)

- Progressive prolongation of the PR interval and shortening of the RR interval until a P wave is blocked, *and the*
- RR interval containing the nonconducted P wave is less than two PP intervals

Note: Classical Wenckebach periodicity may not always be evident, especially when sinus arrhythmia is present or an abrupt change in autonomic tone occurs.

Note: Mobitz Type I results in "group" or "pattern beating" due to the presence of nonconducted P waves. Other causes of group beating include:

- ▸ Blocked APCs (item 2j)
- ▸ Type II second-degree AV block (item 6c)
- ▸ Concealed His-bundle depolarizations

6c. AV block, 2° - Mobitz Type II

- Regular sinus or atrial rhythm (item 2g) with intermittent nonconducted P waves and no evidence for atrial prematurity, *and*
- PR interval in the conducted beats is constant, *and*
- RR interval containing the nonconducted P wave is equal to two PP intervals

Note: 2:1 AV block can be Mobitz Type I or II. Features suggesting (but not proving) one mechanism over another are listed in Table 2.

Table 2. Features Suggesting the Mechanism of 2:1 AV Block

	Mobitz Type I	Mobitz Type II
QRS duration	Narrow	Wide
Response to maneuvers that increase heart rate & AV conduction (e.g., atropine, exercise)	Block improves	Block worsens
Response to maneuvers that reduce heart rate & AV conduction (e.g., carotid sinus massage)	Block worsens	Block improves
Develops during acute MI	Inferior MI	Anterior MI
Other	Mobitz I on another part of ECG	History of syncope

6d. AV block, 2:1

- Regular sinus or atrial rhythm with two P waves for each QRS complex (i.e., every other P wave is nonconducted)

Note: Can be Mobitz Type I or II second-degree AV block (see Table 2).

6e. AV block, 3°

- Atrial and ventricular rhythms are independent of each other
- Atrial rate is usually faster than ventricular rate
- Ventricular rhythm is maintained by a junctional or idioventricular escape rhythm or a ventricular pacemaker

Note: Ventriculophasic sinus arrhythmia (item 5a) may be present in 30-50%.

Note: Complete heart block may present with an atrial rate slower than the ventricular escape rate. This is identified by the presence of nonconducted P waves when the AV node and ventricle are not refractory.

6f. AV block, variable

- Varying degrees of AV block (1°, 2°, 3°)

  Note: Consider this diagnosis in atrial flutter with variable intervals between flutter waves and R waves after ruling out third-degree AV block

6g. Short PR interval (with sinus rhythm and normal QRS duration)

- Normal P wave axis and morphology (item 1a)
- PR interval <0.12 seconds
- No delta wave (QRS <0.11 seconds)
- No sinus rhythm with AV dissociation

6h. Wolff-Parkinson-White pattern

- Normal P wave axis and morphology (item 1a)
- PR interval <0.12 seconds (rarely >0.12 seconds)
- Initial slurring of QRS (delta wave) resulting in an abnormally wide QRS (>0.10 seconds)
- Secondary ST-T wave changes (opposite in direction to main deflection of QRS)

Note: PJ interval (beginning of P wave to end of QRS complex) is constant and ≤ 0.26 seconds

Note: Think WPW when atrial fibrillation or flutter is associated with a QRS that varies in width (generally wide) and has a rate >200 per minute

7. INTRAVENTRICULAR CONDUCTION DISTURBANCES

7a. RBBB, incomplete

- RBBB morphology (rSR' in V_1; item 7b) with a QRS duration between 0.09 and less than 0.12 seconds

Note: Other causes of RSR' pattern < 0.12 seconds in lead V_1 include:

- Normal variant (present in ~ 2% of healthy adults) (item 1b)
- Right ventricular hypertrophy (item 10c)

- Posterior wall MI (item 11l)
- Incorrect lead placement (electrode for lead V_1 placed in 3rd instead of 4th intercostal space) (item 1c)
- Skeletal deformities (e.g., pectus excavatum)

7b. RBBB, complete

- Prolonged QRS duration (≥ 0.12 seconds)
- Secondary R wave (R') in leads V_1 and V_2 (rsR' or rSR') with R' usually taller than the initial R wave
- Delayed onset of intrinsicoid deflection (beginning of QRS to peak of R wave > 0.05 seconds) in V_1 and V_2
- Secondary ST & T-wave changes (downsloping ST segment, T-wave inversion) in leads V_1 and V_2 (item 12g)
- Wide slurred S wave in leads I, V_5, and V_6

Note: In RBBB, mean QRS axis is determined by the initial unblocked 0.06-0.08 seconds of QRS, and should be normal unless left anterior fascicular block (item 7c) or left posterior fascicular block (item 7d) is present.

Note: RBBB does not interfere with the ECG diagnosis of ventricular hypertrophy or Q-wave MI.

7c. Left anterior fascicular block

- Left axis deviation with mean QRS axis between -45° and -90° (item 9c)
- qR complex (or an R wave) in leads I and aVL
- rS complex in lead III
- Normal or slightly prolonged QRS duration (0.08-0.10 seconds)
- No other factors responsible for left axis deviation:
    - LVH (items 10a, b)
    - Inferior wall MI (items 11e, k)
    - Emphysema (chronic lung disease) (item 14m)
    - Left bundle branch block (item 7f)
    - Ostium primum atrial septal defect (item 14j)
    - Severe hyperkalemia (item 14f)

Note: LAFB may result in a false-positive diagnosis of LVH based on voltage criteria using leads I or aVL.

Note: Poor R-wave progression is common.

Note: Left anterior fascicular block can mask the presence of inferior wall MI.

7d. Left posterior fascicular block

- Right axis deviation with mean QRS axis between +100° and +180° (item 9d)
- S_1 Q_3 pattern (deep S wave in lead I; Q wave in lead III sometimes seen)
- Normal or slightly prolonged QRS duration (0.08-0.10 seconds)
- No other factors responsible for right axis deviation:
  - RVH (item 10c)
  - Vertical heart
  - Emphysema (chronic lung disease) (item 14m)
  - Pulmonary embolism (item 14n)
  - Lateral wall MI (items 10d, j)
  - Dextrocardia (item 14k)
  - Lead reversal (item 1c)
  - Wolff-Parkinson-White (item 6h)

Note: Left posterior fascicular block can mask the presence of lateral wall MI.

7e. LBBB, with ST-T waves suggestive of acute myocardial injury or infarction

- Fulfills criteria for LBBB (item 7f) (also valid for LBBB due to artificial pacemaker)
- Three criteria with independent value for diagnosing acute myocardial injury in setting of LBBB (in descending order of significance):
  - ST elevation ≥ 1 mm concordant to (same direction as) the major deflection of the QRS
  - ST depression ≥ 1 mm in V_1, V_2, or V_3
  - ST elevation ≥ 5mm discordant with (opposite direction to) the major deflection of the QRS

7f. LBBB, complete

- Prolonged QRS duration (≥ 0.12 seconds)
- Delayed onset of intrinsicoid deflection in leads I, V_5, V_6 (i.e., beginning of QRS to peak of R wave > 0.05 seconds)
- Broad monophasic R waves in leads I, V_5, V_6 that are usually notched or slurred

- Secondary ST & T wave changes opposite in direction to the major QRS deflection (i.e., ST depression & T wave inversion in leads I, V_5, V_6; ST elevation & upright T wave in leads V_1 and V_2)
- rS or QS complex in right precordial leads

Note: Left axis deviation may be present (item 9c).

Note: LBBB interferes with determination of QRS axis and the ECG diagnoses of ventricular hypertrophy and acute MI.

7g. LBBB, intermittent

- See item 7f for features of LBBB

Note: More commonly seen at high rates (tachycardia-dependent) but may be bradycardia-dependent as well.

7h. Intraventricular conduction disturbance, nonspecific type

- QRS ≥ 0.11 seconds in duration but morphology does not meet criteria for LBBB (item 7f) or RBBB (item 7g), *or* abnormal QRS notching without prolongation

Note: IVCD may be seen with:

- Antiarrhythmic drug toxicity (especially Type IA and IC agents) (item 14d)
- Hyperkalemia (item 14e)
- LVH (item 10a)
- Wolff-Parkinson-White (item 6h)
- Hypothermia (item 14u)
- Severe metabolic disturbances

7i. Aberrant intraventricular conduction with supraventricular arrhythmia

Note: See item 4f for criteria to distinguish between SVT with aberrancy vs. VT.

8. P WAVE ABNORMALITIES

8a. Right atrial abnormality

- Upright P wave:
  - >2.5 mm in leads II, III, and aVF (P-pulmonale), *or*
  - >1.5 mm in leads V_1 or V_2
- P wave axis shifted rightward (i.e., axis ≥ 70°)

Note: In up to 30% of cases, P pulmonale may actually represent left atrial enlargement. Suspect this possibility when left atrial abnormality (item 8b) is present in lead V_1.

8b. Left atrial abnormality

- Notched P wave with a duration ≥0.12 seconds in leads II, III or aVF (P-mitrale), *or*
- Terminal negative portion of the P wave in lead V_1 ≥ 1 mm deep and ≥ 0.04 seconds in duration (i.e., one small box deep and one small box wide)

Bi-atrial enlargement is suggested by any of the following:

- Large biphasic P wave in V_1 ≥ 0.04 seconds with:
  - An initial positive amplitude > 1.5 mm, *and*
  - A terminal negative amplitude ≥ 1 mm
- Tall peaked P waves (>1.5 mm) in the right precordial leads (V_1-V_3) and wide notched P waves in the left precordial leads (V_5-V_6)
- P wave amplitude ≥2.5 mm in the limb leads with a duration ≥0.12 seconds

8c. Nonspecific atrial abnormality

- Abnormal P wave morphology not fulfilling criteria for right (item 8a) or left atrial abnormality (item 8b)

9. ABNORMALITIES OF QRS VOLTAGE OR AXIS

9a. Low voltage, limb leads only

- Amplitude of the entire QRS complex (R+S) < 5 mm in all limb leads

Note: See item 9b for causes.

9b. Low voltage, limb and precordial leads

- Amplitude of the entire QRS complex (R+S) < 10 mm in each precordial lead, *and*
- Amplitude of R+S < 5 mm in all limb leads

Note: Causes include:

- Chronic lung disease (item 14m)
- Pericardial effusion (item 14o)
- Myxedema (item 14t)
- Obesity
- Pleural effusion

- Restrictive or infiltrative cardiomyopathies
- Diffuse coronary disease

9c. Left axis deviation (>-30°).

- Mean QRS axis between -30° and -106°

Note: Causes include:

- Left anterior fascicular block (if axis > -45°, item 7c)
- Inferior wall MI (item 11e, k)
- LBBB (item 7f)
- LVH (items 10 a, b)
- Ostium primum ASD (item 14j)
- COPD (item 14m)
- Hyperkalemia (item 14e)

9d. Right axis deviation (>+100°)

- Mean QRS axis between 101° and 254°
- Pure right axis deviation (left posterior fascicular block) should have an S wave in lead I and a Q wave in lead III (S_1 Q_3 pattern)

Note: Causes include:

- RVH (item 10c)
- Vertical heart
- Chronic obstructive pulmonary disease (item 14m)
- Pulmonary embolus (item 14n)
- Left posterior fascicular block (item 7d)
- Lateral wall myocardial infarction (items 11d, j)
- Dextrocardia (item 14k)
- Lead reversal (item 1c)
- Ostium secundum ASD (item 14i)

9e. Electrical alternans

- Alternation in the amplitude and/or direction of P, QRS, and/or T waves

Note: Causes include:

- Pericardial effusion (item 14o). (If electrical alternans involves the P, QRS, and T ["total alternans"], effusion with tamponade is often present. Yet, only 12% of patients with pericardial effusions have electrical alternans.)

- Severe left ventricular failure
- Hypertension
- Coronary artery disease
- Rheumatic heart disease
- Supraventricular or ventricular tachycardia
- Deep respirations

10. VENTRICULAR HYPERTROPHY

10a. Left ventricular hypertrophy by voltage only

- **Cornell Criteria** (most accurate) R wave in aVL + S wave in V_3
  - >24 mm in males
  - >20 mm in females
- **Other commonly used voltage-based criteria**
  - Precordial leads (one or more)
    (1) R wave in V_5 or V_6 + S wave in V_1
      - > 35 mm if age > 30 years
      - > 40 mm if age 20-30 years
      - > 60 mm if age 16-19 years

    (2) Maximum R wave + S wave in precordial leads > 45 mm
    (3) R wave in V_5 > 26 mm
    (4) R wave in V_6 > 20 mm
  - Limb leads (one or more)
    (1) R wave in lead I + S wave in lead II ≥ 26 mm
    (2) R wave in lead I ≥ 14 mm
    (3) S wave in aVR ≥ 15 mm
    (4) R wave in aVL ≥ 12 mm (a highly specific finding)
    (5) R wave in aVF ≥ 21 mm

- **Non-voltage related criteria for LVH** (often seen with or without prominent voltage and ST-T changes in patients with LVH)

- Left atrial abnormality (item 8b)
- Left axis deviation (item 9c)
- Nonspecific intraventricular conduction delay (item 7h)
- Delayed onset of intrinsicoid deflection (beginning of QRS to peak of R wave > 0.05 seconds)
- Small or absent R waves in V_1-V_3 (low anterior forces)
- Absent Q waves in leads I, V_5, V_6
- Abnormal Q waves in leads II, III, aVF (due to left axis deviation)
- Prominent U waves (item 12l)
- R wave in $V_6 > V_5$, provided there are dominant R waves in these leads

10b. Left ventricular hypertrophy by both voltage and ST-T segment abnormalities

- Voltage criteria for LVH (item 10a)
- ST-T segment abnormalities (one or more):
  - ST segment and T wave deviation opposite in direction to the major deflection of QRS
  - ST segment depression in leads I, aVL, III, aVF, and/or V_4-V_6
  - Subtle ST elevation (< 1-2 mm) in leads V_1-V_3
  - Inverted T waves in leads I, aVL, V_4-V_6
  - Prominent or inverted U waves

10c. Right ventricular hypertrophy

- Right axis deviation with mean QRS axis $\geq +100°$
- Dominant R wave
  - R/S ratio in V_1 or V_{3R} >1, *or* R/S ration in V_5 or $V_6 \leq 1$
  - R wave in $V_1 \geq 7$mm
  - R wave in V_1 + S wave in V_5 or V_6 >10.5 mm
  - rSR' in V_1 with R' >10 mm
  - qR complex in V_1
- Secondary ST-T changes (downsloping ST depression, T-wave inversion) in right precordial leads
- Right atrial abnormality (item 8a)
- Onset of intrinsicoid deflection in V_1 between 0.035 and 0.055 seconds

Note: For ECG features of RVH in the setting of chronic lung disease, see item 14m.

Note: Conditions that may present with right axis deviation and/or a dominant R wave and possibly mimic RVH include:

- Posterior or inferoposterolateral wall MI (item 11f)
- Right bundle branch block (item 7b)
- Wolff-Parkinson-White syndrome (type A) (item 6h)
- Dextroposition
- Left posterior fascicular block (item 7d)
- Normal variant (especially in children)

10d. Combined ventricular hypertrophy

Suggested by any of the following:

- ECG meets one or more diagnostic criteria for both isolated LVH (item 10a, b) and RVH (item 10c)
- Precordial leads show LVH but QRS axis is >90°
- LVH *plus:*
    - R wave > Q wave in aVR, *and*
    - S wave > R wave in V_5, *and*
    - T wave inversion in V_1
- Large amplitude, equiphasic (R=S) complexes in V_3 and V_4 (Kutz-Wachtel phenomenon)
- Right atrial abnormality (item 8a) with LVH pattern (item 10a, b) in precordial leads

11. Q-WAVE MYOCARDIAL INFARCTION

General considerations:

- Age of infarct can be approximated from ECG pattern:
    - Probably acute or recent
        - Acute MI: Abnormal Q waves, ST elevation (associated ST depression is sometimes present in noninfarct leads)
        - Recent MI: Abnormal Q waves, isoelectric ST segments, ischemic (usually inverted) T waves
    - Probably old or age indeterminate

- Old MI: Abnormal Q waves, isoelectric ST segments, nonspecific or normal T waves

Note: Exception: MI may be present without Q waves in:

- Anterior MI: May only see low anterior R wave forces with decreasing R wave progression in leads V_2-V_5
- Posterior MI: Dominant R wave and ST depression in leads V_1-V_3

- Myocardial infarction vs. injury vs. ischemia:
  - Infarction: Abnormal Q waves; ST segment elevation or depression; T waves inverted, normal, or upright & symmetrically peaked
  - Injury: ST segment elevation; Q waves absent
  - Ischemia: ST segment depression: T waves usually inverted; Q waves absent

  Note: Exception: MI may be present without Q waves in:

  - Anterior MI: May only see low anterior R wave forces with decreasing R wave progression in leads V_2-V_5
  - Posterior MI: Dominant R wave and ST depression in leads V_1-V_3
- Abnormal Q waves
  - Duration ≥ 0.03 seconds for most leads
  - Duration ≥ 0.04 seconds in leads III, aVL, aVF, and V_1
- Significant ST elevation
  - ≥ 1-2 mm in two or more contiguous leads
  - Usually with upwardly convex configuration
  - Can persist 48 hours to 4 weeks after MI

  Note: Persistent ST elevation beyond 4 weeks suggests the presence of a ventricular aneurysm (item 11m)
- T wave inversions may persist indefinitely
- Conditions causing "pseudoinfarcts" (ECG pattern mimics myocardial infarction):
  - Wolff-Parkinson-White (item 6h)
  - Hypertrophic cardiomyopathy (item 14q)
  - LVH (items 10a, b)
  - RVH (item 10c)
  - Left anterior fascicular block (item 7c)
  - Chronic lung disease (item 14m)
  - Amyloid heart (or other infiltrative diseases)

- Cardiomyopathy
- Chest deformity (e.g., pectus excavatum)
- Pulmonary embolism (item 14n)
- Myocarditis
- Myocardial tumors
- Hyperkalemia (item 14g)
- Pneumothorax
- Lead reversal (item 1c)
- Corrected transposition
- Dextrocardia (item 14k)

- Diagnosis of Q wave MI in the presence of bundle branch block
  - RBBB: Does not interfere with the diagnosis of Q wave MI; Q wave criteria apply for all infarctions
  - LBBB: Difficult to diagnose any infarct in the presence of LBBB. However, acute injury is sometimes apparent (item 7e)

11a. Anterolateral infarction, recent or probably acute

- Abnormal Q waves (duration $\geq$ 0.03 seconds) in leads V_4-V_6, *accompanied by*
- ST segment elevation

11b. Anterior infarction, recent or probably acute

- rS in V_1, *followed by*
- QS or QR complexes (Q wave duration $\geq$ 0.03 seconds) and ST segment elevation in two of leads V_2-V_4, *or*
- Decreasing R wave amplitude from V_2-V_5

11c. Anteroseptal infarction, recent or probably acute

- Abnormal Q or QS deflection in V_1-V_3 and sometimes V_4 (Q wave duration $\geq$ 0.04 seconds in V_1 and $\geq$ 0.03 seconds in V_2-V_4), *accompanied by*
- ST segment elevation

Note: Some electrocardiographers read anteroseptal infarction when abnormal Q waves are present in V_1-V_2 but not in V_3 or any other leads.

Note: The presence of a Q wave in V_1 distinguishes anteroseptal from anterior infarction.

11d - 11k

11d. Lateral or high lateral infarction, recent or probably acute

- Abnormal Q wave in lead I (duration ≥ 0.03 seconds) and aVL (duration ≥ 0.04 seconds), *accompanied by*
- ST segment elevation

Note: An isolated Q wave in aVL does not qualify as a lateral MI.

11e. Inferior (diaphragmatic) infarct, recent or probably acute

- Abnormal Q waves in at least two of leads II, III, aVF (Q wave duration ≥ 0.03 seconds in lead II and ≥ 0.04 seconds in leads III and aVF), *accompanied by*
- ST segment elevation

Note: Associated ST depression is usually evident in leads I, aVL, V_1-V_3.

11f. Posterior infarct, recent or probably acute

- Initial R wave ≥0.04 seconds in V_1 and V_2 with:
  - R wave ≥ S wave, *and*
  - ST segment depression (usually ≥ 2 mm) with upright T waves

Note: Posterior MI is usually seen in the setting of acute inferior MI.

Note: RVH (item 10c), WPW (item 6h), and RBBB (item 7b) interfere with the ECG diagnosis of posterior MI.

11g. Anterolateral infarction, age indeterminate or probably old

- See item 11a, no ST segment elevation

11h. Anterior infarction, age indeterminate or probably old

- See item 11b, no ST segment elevation

11i. Anteroseptal infarction, age indeterminate or probably old

- See item 11c, no ST segment elevation

11j. Lateral or high lateral infarction, age indeterminate or probably old

- See item 11d, no ST segment elevation

11k. Inferior (diaphragmatic) infarct, age indeterminate or probably old

- See item 11e, no ST segment elevation

11l. Posterior infarct, age indeterminate or probably old

- See item 11f , no ST segment depression characteristic of acute posterior injury

11m. Probable ventricular aneurysm

- ST segment elevation ≥ 1 mm persisting 4 or more weeks after acute MI in leads with abnormal Q waves

12. ST, T, U WAVE ABNORMALITIES

12a. Normal variant, early repolarization

Suggested by the following:

- Elevated take-off of ST segment at the junction between the QRS and ST segment (J junction)
- Concave upward ST elevation ending with a symmetrical upright T wave (often of large amplitude)
- Distinct notch or slur on downstroke of R wave
- Most commonly involves leads V_2-V_5; sometimes seen in leads II, III, and aVF
- No reciprocal ST segment depression

Note: Some degree of ST elevation is present in the majority of young healthy individuals, especially in the precordial leads.

12b. Normal variant, juvenile T waves

Suggested by the following:

- Persistently negative T waves (usually not symmetrical or deep) in leads V_1-V_3 in normal adults
- T waves still upright I, II, V_5, V_6

Note: Most frequently seen in young healthy females.

12c. Nonspecific ST and/or T wave abnormalities

- Slight (< 1mm) ST depression or elevation, *and/or*
- T wave flat or slightly inverted

Note: T wave is usually ≥ 10% the height of the R wave

Note: Can be seen in:

  - Organic heart disease

- Drugs (e.g., quinidine)
- Electrolyte disorders (e.g., hypokalemia, item 14f)
- Hyperventilation
- Hypothyroidism (item 14t)
- Stress
- Pancreatitis
- Pericarditis (item 14p)
- CNS disorders (item 14s)
- LVH (item 10b)
- RVH (item 10c)
- Bundle branch block (items 7a, f)
- Healthy adults (normal variant) (item 1b)

12d. ST and/or T wave abnormalities suggesting myocardial ischemia

- Ischemic T wave changes
  - Biphasic T waves with or without ST depression
  - Symmetrical or deeply inverted T waves

Note: QT interval is usually prolonged.

Note: Reciprocal T wave changes may be evident (e.g., tall upright T waves in inferior leads with deeply inverted T waves in anterior leads).

Note: Prominent U waves (upright or inverted) (item 12l) are often present.

Note: Tall upright T waves may also be seen in:

  - Normal healthy adults (item 1b)
  - Hyperkalemia (item 14e)
  - Early MI
  - LVH (item 10b)
  - CNS disorders (item 14s)
  - Anemia

- Ischemic ST segment changes
  - Horizontal or downsloping ST segments with or without T wave inversion

12e. ST and/or T wave changes suggesting myocardial injury

- Acute ST segment elevation with upward convexity in the leads representing the area of infarction
- ST & T wave changes evolve: T waves invert before ST segments return to baseline
- Associated ST depression in the noninfarct leads is common
- Acute posterior wall injury often has horizontal or downsloping ST segment depression with upright T-waves in V_1-V_3, with or without a prominent R wave in these same leads

Note: ST & T wave changes suggesting myocardial injury can also be seen in:

- ▸ Post-tachycardia sinus beats (T wave inversion) (item 12h)
- ▸ Apical hypertrophic cardiomyopathy (item 14q)
- ▸ Central nervous system disease (item 14s)

12f. ST and/or T wave changes suggesting acute pericarditis

- Classic evolutionary pattern consists of 4 stages (but is not always present):
  - ▸ Stage 1: Upwardly concave ST segment elevation in almost all leads except aVR; no reciprocal ST depression in other leads except aVR
  - ▸ Stage 2: ST junction (J point) returns to baseline and T wave amplitude begins to decrease
  - ▸ Stage 3: T waves invert
  - ▸ Stage 4: ECG returns to normal
- Other clues to acute pericarditis:
  - ▸ Sinus tachycardia
  - ▸ PR depression early (PR elevation in aVR)
  - ▸ Low voltage QRS (item 8b)
  - ▸ Electrical alternans (item 9e) if pericardial effusion (item 14o)

12g. ST and/or T wave changes secondary to intraventricular conduction disturbance or hypertrophy

- *LVH:* ST segment and T wave displacement opposite to the major QRS deflection:
  - ▸ ST depression (upwardly concave) & T wave inversion when the QRS is mainly positive (leads I, V_5, V_6)

- Subtle ST elevation and upright T waves when the QRS is mainly negative (leads V_1, V_2)

- ***RVH:*** ST segment depression and T wave inversion in leads V_1-V_3 and sometimes in leads II, III, aVF
- ***LBBB:*** ST segment and T wave displacement opposite to the major QRS deflection
- ***RBBB:*** Uncomplicated RBBB has little ST displacement. T wave vector is opposite to the terminal slurred portion of QRS (upright in leads I, V_5, V_6; inverted in leads V_1,V_2)

12h. Post-extrasystolic T wave abnormality

- Any alternation in contour, amplitude and/or direction of the T wave in the sinus beat(s) following an ectopic beat or beats

12i. Isolated J point depression

- ST segment depression ≥ 1 mm at the junction of the QRS and ST segment (J-point) lasting ≥ 0.08 seconds

Note: Most frequently seen during exercise testing.

12j. Peaked T waves

- T wave > 6 mm in limb leads, *or*
- T wave > 10 mm in precordial leads

Note: Causes of peaked T waves include:

- Acute MI (item 12e)
- Normal variant (item 1b); most common in mid-precordial leads
- Hyperkalemia (item 14e): QT normal
- Intracranial bleeding (item 14s): prolonged QT (item 12k); prominent U waves (item 12l)
- LVH (item 10b)
- LBBB (item 7f)

12k. Prolonged QT interval

- Corrected QT interval (QTc) ≥ 0.42-0.46 seconds, *where*

  QTc = QT interval divided by the square root of the preceding RR interval

  Note: Be sure to measure the QT interval in a lead with a large T wave and distinct termination.

  Note: QT interval varies inversely with heart rate.
- Easier methods to determine QT interval:

- Use 0.40 seconds as the normal QT interval for a heart rate of 70. For every 10 BPM change in heart rate above (or below) 70, subtract (or add) 0.02 seconds. (Measured value should be within ±0.07 seconds of the calculated normal.) Example: For a HR of 100 BPM, the calculated "normal" QT interval = 0.34 ± .07 seconds [(3 x 0.02 seconds) - 0.040 seconds]. For a HR of 50 BPM, the calculated "normal" QT interval = 0.44 ± .07 seconds [(2 x 0.02 seconds + 0.40 seconds].
- The normal QT interval should be less than 50% of the RR interval

Note: Conditions associated with a prolonged QT interval include:

Acquired

- Drugs (quinidine, procainamide, disopyramide, amiodarone, sotalol, phenothiazine, tricyclics, lithium) (item 14c, d)
- Hypomagnesemia
- Hypocalcemia (item 14h)
- Marked bradyarrhythmias
- Intracranial hemorrhage (item 14s)
- Myocarditis
- Mitral valve prolapse
- Hypothyroidism (item 14t)
- Hypothermia (item 14u)
- Liquid protein diets

Congenital

- Romano-Ward syndrome (normal hearing)
- Jervell and Lange-Nielson syndrome (deafness)

12l. Prominent U waves

- Amplitude ≥ 1.5 mm

  Note: The U wave is normally 5-25% the height of the T wave, and is largest in leads V_2 and V_3

  Note: Causes include:

  - Hypokalemia (item 14f)
  - Bradyarrhythmias
  - Hypothermia (item 14u)
  - LVH (item 10b)
  - Organic heart disease
  - Drugs (digitalis, quinidine, amiodarone, isoproterenol) (items 14a, c)

13. PACEMAKER FUNCTION AND RHYTHM

13a. Atrial or coronary sinus pacing

- Pacemaker stimulus followed by an atrial depolarization

13b. Ventricular demand pacing

- Pacemaker stimulus followed by a QRS complex of different morphology than intrinsic QRS
- Must demonstrate <u>inhibition</u> of pacemaker output in response to intrinsic QRS

13c. AV sequential pacing

- Atrial followed by ventricular pacing
- Could be DVI, DDD, DDI, or DOO pacing mode

13d. Ventricular pacing, fixed rate (asynchronous)

- Ventricular pacing with no demonstrable output inhibition by intrinsic QRS complexes

13e. Dual chamber, atrial-sensing pacemaker

- For atrial sensing, need to demonstrate inhibition of atrial output and/or triggering of ventricular stimulus in response to intrinsic atrial depolarization
- DDD and possibly VAT or VDD

13f. Pacemaker malfunction, not constantly capturing (atrium or ventricle)

- Failure of pacemaker stimulus to be followed by depolarization

<u>Note:</u> Rule out "pseudo-malfunction" (i.e., pacer stimulus falls into refractory period of ventricle)

13g. Pacemaker malfunction, not constantly sensing (atrium or ventricle)

- Pacemakers in Inhibited Mode: Failure of pacemaker to be inhibited by an appropriate intrinsic depolarization
- Pacemakers in Triggered Mode: Failure of pacemaker to be triggered by an appropriate intrinsic depolarization

<u>Note:</u> Watch for "pseudo-malfunction" (i.e., pacer stimulus falls into refractory period of ventricle)

<u>Note:</u> Premature depolarizations may not be sensed if they:

- Fall within the programmed refractory period of the pacemaker
- Have insufficient amplitude at the sensing electrode site

Note: Any stimulus falling within the QRS complex probably does not represent sensing malfunction (commonly seen with right ventricular electrodes in RBBB).

13h. Pacemaker malfunction, not firing

- Failure of appropriate pacemaker output

13i. Pacemaker malfunction, slowing

- Increase in stimulus intervals over the programmed intervals

Note: Usually an indicator of battery end of life

Note: Often noted first during magnet application

14. SUGGESTED OR PROBABLE CLINICAL DISORDERS

14a. Digitalis effect

- Sagging ST segment depression with upward concavity
- T wave flat, inverted, or biphasic
- QT interval shortened
- U wave amplitude increased
- PR interval lengthened

Note: ST changes are difficult to interpret in the setting of LVH, RVH, or bundle branch block. However, if typical sagging ST segments are present and the QT interval is shortened, consider digitalis effect.

14b. Digitalis toxicity

- Digitalis toxicity can cause almost any type of cardiac dysrhythmia or conduction disturbance **except bundle branch block**. Typical abnormalities include:
  - Paroxysmal atrial tachycardia with block (item 2o)
  - Atrial fibrillation with complete heart block (regular RR intervals)
  - Second or third-degree AV block (items 6b, c, e)
  - Complete heart block (item 6e) with accelerated junctional rhythm (item 3c) or accelerated idioventricular rhythm (items 4g)
  - Supraventricular tachycardia with alternating bundle branch block

14c. Antiarrhythmic drug effect

Suggested by the following:

- Prolonged QT interval (item 12k)
- Prominent U waves (one of the earliest findings) (item 12l)

- Nonspecific ST and/or T wave changes (item 12c)
- Decrease in atrial flutter rate

14d. Antiarrhythmic drug toxicity

Suggested by the following:

- Prolonged QT (item 12k)
- Ventricular arrhythmias including "Torsade de Pointes" (paroxysms of irregular ventricular tachyarrhythmia at a rate of 200-250 BPM with sinusoidal cycles of changing QRS amplitude and polarity in the setting of a prolonged QT interval)
- Wide QRS complex
- Various degrees of AV block
- Marked sinus bradycardia (item 2c), sinus arrest (item 2e), or SA block (item 2f)

14e. Hyperkalemia

- K^+ = 5.5 - 6.5 mEq/L
  - Tall, peaked, narrow based T waves
  - QT interval shortening
  - Reversible left anterior fascicular block (item 7c) or left posterior fascicular block (item 7d)
- K^+ = 6.5 - 7.5 mEq/L
  - First-degree AV block (item 6a)
  - Flattening and widening of the P wave
  - ST segment depression
  - QRS widening
- K^+ > 7.5 mEq/L
  - Disappearance of P waves, which may be caused by:
    - Sinus arrest (item 2e), *or*
    - "Sinoventricular conduction" (sinus impulses conducted to the ventricles via specialized atrial fibers *without* atrial depolarization)
  - LBBB (item 7f), RBBB (item 7b), or markedly widened and diffuse intraventricular conduction delay (item 7h) resembling a sine wave pattern
  - Arrhythmias and conduction disturbances including VT (item 4f), VF (item 4i), idioventricular rhythm, asystole

14f. Hypokalemia

Suggested by the following:

- Prominent U waves (item 12l)
- ST segment depression
- Flattened T waves
- Increased amplitude and duration of the P wave
- Prolonged QT sometimes seen
- Arrhythmias and conduction disturbances, including paroxysmal atrial tachycardia with block (item 2o), first-degree AV block (item 6a), Type I second-degree AV block (item 6b), AV dissociation (item 5d), VPCs (item 4a), ventricular tachycardia (item 4f), and ventricular fibrillation (item 4i).

  Note: These may be digitalis related.

14g. Hypercalcemia

- QTc shortening
- May see PR prolongation

  Note: Little if any effect on P, QRS, or T wave.

14h. Hypocalcemia

- Prolonged QTc (item 12k) (earliest and most common finding)

  Note: Due to ST segment prolongation, which occurs without changing the duration of the T wave; only hypothermia and hypocalcemia do this.
- Occasional flattening, peaking, or inversion of T waves

14i. Atrial septal defect, secundum

Suggested by the following:

- Typical RSR' or rSR' complex in V_1 with a QRS duration < 0.11 seconds
- Incomplete RBBB
- Right axis deviation (item 9d) ± right ventricular hypertrophy (item 10c)
- Right atrial abnormality (item 8a) in ~ 30%
- First-degree AV block (item 6a) in < 20%

Note: Secundum ASDs represent 70% of all ASDs, and are due to deficient tissue in the region of the fossa ovalis.

14j. Atrial septal defect, primum

Suggested by the following:

- RSR' complex in V_1
- Left axis deviation (in contrast to right axis deviation in secundum ASD)
- First-degree AV block (item 6a) in 15-40%

- Advanced cases have biventricular hypertrophy (item 10d)

Note: Primum ASDs represent 15% of all ASDs, and are due to deficient tissue in the lower portion of the septum. These ASDs are usually large, may be accompanied by anomalous pulmonary venous drainage, and are associated with a cleft anterior mitral valve leaflet, mitral regurgitation, and Down's syndrome.

14k. Dextrocardia, mirror image

Suggested by the following:

- P-QRS-T in leads I and aVL are inverted or "upside down"
- Decreasing R wave amplitude from leads V_1-V_6

Note: Dextrocardia and lead reversal (item 1c) can both produce an upside down P-QRS-T in leads I and aVL. To distinguish between these conditions, look at the R wave pattern in V_1 - V_6:

  - Reverse R wave progression suggests dextrocardia
  - Normal R wave progression suggests lead reversal

14l. Mitral valve disease

- Mitral stenosis
  - Combination of right ventricular hypertrophy (item 10c) and left atrial abnormality (item 8b) is suggestive
- Mitral valve prolapse
  - Flattened or inverted T waves in leads II, III and aVF (and sometimes in right precordial leads) ± ST segment depression, which is sometimes present in the left precordial leads
  - Prominent U waves (item 12l)
  - Prolonged QT interval (item 12k)

14m. Chronic lung disease

Suggested by any of the following:

- Right ventricular hypertrophy (item 10c)
- Right axis deviation (item 9d)
- Right atrial abnormality (item 8a)
- Shift of transitional zone clockwise (poor R wave progression)
- Low voltage QRS (items 9a, b)
- Pseudo-anteroseptal infarct pattern (low anterior forces)
- S waves in leads I, II, and III (S_1 S_2 S_3 pattern)
- May also see sinus tachycardia (item 2d), junctional rhythm (item 3d), various degrees of AV block, IVCD (item 7h), and bundle branch block

Note: Right ventricular hypertrophy in the setting of chronic lung disease is suggested by:

- Rightward shift of QRS
- T wave inversion in V_1, V_2
- ST depression in leads II, III, aVF
- Transient RBBB
- RSR' or QR complex in V_1

14n. Acute cor pulmonale including pulmonary embolus

- Sinus tachycardia (most common) (item 2d)
- Findings consistent with right ventricular pressure overload:
  - Right atrial abnormality (item 8a)
  - Inverted T waves in V_1-V_3
  - Right axis deviation (item 9d)
  - S_1Q_3 or $S_1Q_3T_3$ pattern
  - Pseudoinfarct pattern in inferior leads
  - Incomplete or complete RBBB
  - Various supraventricular tachyarrhythmias

Note: ECG abnormalities are often *transient*

14o. Pericardial effusion

Suggested by either of the following:

- Low voltage QRS (item 9a, b)
- Electrical alternans (item 9e)
- Other features of acute pericarditis (item 12f)

14p. Acute pericarditis

- Refer to item 12f for criteria

14q. Hypertrophic cardiomyopathy

- Left atrial abnormality (item 8b) is common; right atrial abnormality (item 8a) on occasion
- Majority have abnormal QRS
  - Large amplitude QRS
  - Large abnormal Q waves (can give pseudoinfarct pattern in inferior, lateral, and anterior precordial leads)
  - Tall R wave with inverted T wave in V_1 simulating RVH
  - Nonspecific ST and/or T wave abnormalities are common (item 12c)

- ST and/or T wave changes secondary to ventricular hypertrophy or conduction abnormalities (item 12g)
- Apical variant of hypertrophic cardiomyopathy has deep T wave inversions in V_4-V_6
- Left axis deviation (item 9c) in 20%

14r. Coronary artery disease

- Use only when definitive evidence of myocardial injury or infarction is present

14s. Central nervous system disorder

- "Classic changes" usually in precordial leads
    - Large upright or deeply inverted T waves
    - Prolonged QT interval (often marked) (item 12k)
    - Prominent U waves (item 12l)
- Other changes:
    - T wave notching with loss of amplitude
    - ST segment changes:
        - Diffuse ST elevation mimicking acute pericarditis, *or*
        - Focal ST elevation mimicking acute myocardial injury, *or*
        - ST depression
    - Abnormal Q waves mimicking MI
    - Almost any rhythm abnormality (sinus tachycardia or bradycardia, junctional rhythm, VPCs, ventricular tachycardia, etc.)

<u>Note:</u> ECG findings in CNS disease can mimic those of:

- Acute MI (item 11)
- Acute pericarditis (item 14p)
- Drug effect or toxicity (items 14c, d)

14t. Myxedema

- Low QRS voltage in all leads (item 9b)
- Sinus bradycardia (item 2c)
- T wave flattened or inverted
- PR interval may be prolonged (item 6a)
- Frequently associated with pericardial effusion (item 14o)
- Electrical alternans (item 9e) may occur

14u. Hypothermia

- Sinus bradycardia (item 2a)
- PR, QRS, and QT prolonged (items 2a, 12k)
- Osborne ("J") wave: late upright terminal deflection of QRS complex ("camel hump" sign); amplitude increases as temperature declines
- Atrial fibrillation (item 2s) in 50-60%
- Other arrhythmias include AV junctional rhythm (item 3d), ventricular tachycardia (item 4f), ventricular fibrillation (item 4i)

14v. Sick sinus syndrome

One or more of the following:

- Marked sinus bradycardia (item 2c)
- Sinus arrest (item 2e) or sinoatrial exit block (item 2f)
- Bradycardia alternating with tachycardia
- Atrial fibrillation with slow ventricular response preceded or followed by sinus bradycardia, sinus arrest, or sinoatrial exit block
- Prolonged sinus node recovery time after atrial premature complex or atrial tachyarrhythmias
- AV junctional escape rhythm
- Additional conduction system disease is often present, including AV block (items 6a-f), IVCD (item 7h), and/or bundle branch block

* * * * *

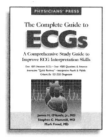

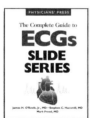

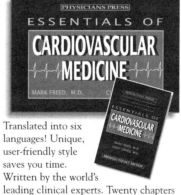

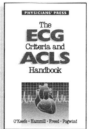

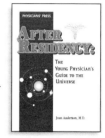

Interventional Cardiology

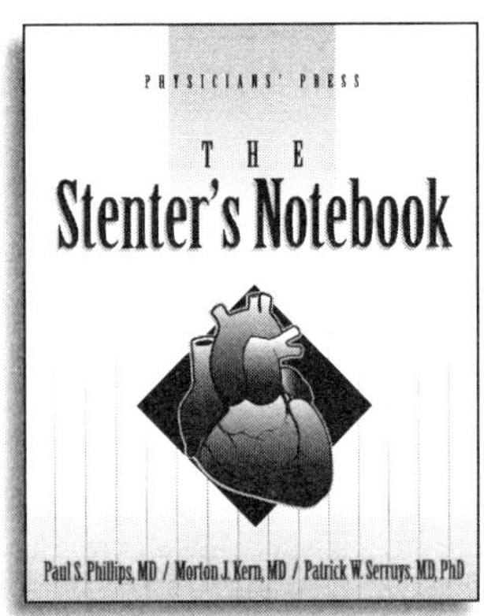

The Stenter's Notebook

Paul Phillips, MD
Morton Kern, MD
Patrick Serruys, MD, PhD

Case studies, equipment selection, simple and advanced stenting techniques, adjunctive imaging and pharmacotherapy, and management of complications. Includes a stent design compendium covering more than twenty stents.

210 pages; 71/2" x 9"
all figures in color

$59.95

The Stenter's Notebook SLIDE SERIES

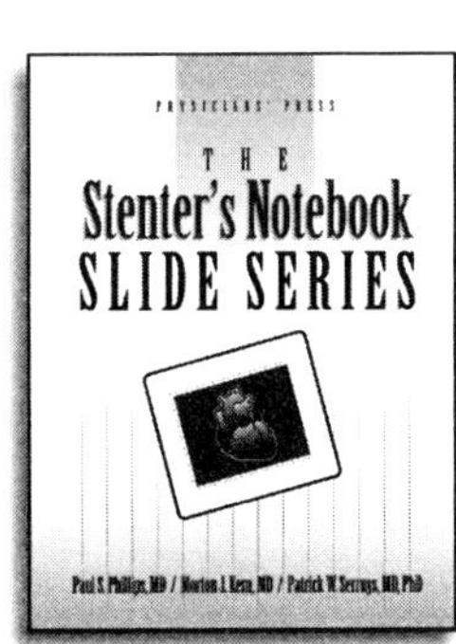

25 slide companion to *The Stenter's Notebook* in 3-ring binder with jackets and paper reference copies.

$49.95

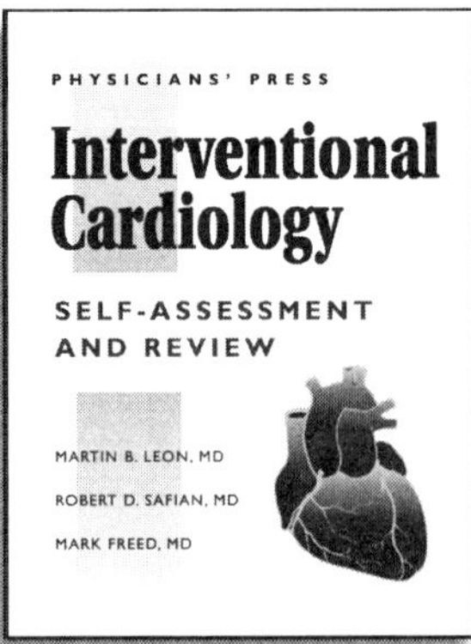

Interventional Cardiology Self-Assessment and Review

Martin B. Leon, MD
Robert D. Safian, MD
Mark Freed, MD

Start Preparing for Interventional Boards Today!

More than 500 questions and answers (with literature references) on simple and complex angioplasty; acute ischemic syndromes; lesion morphology and location; intraprocedural complications; adjunctive pharmacotherapy, imaging and hemodynamic support; valvuloplasty; and more.

500 pages; 9" x 12" **$45**

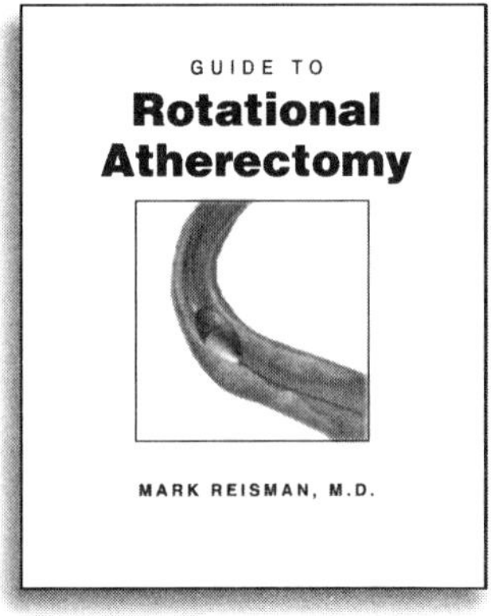

Guide to Rotational Atherectomy

by Mark Reisman, MD

A lesion-specific approach to Rotational Atherectomy. Case studies, equipment selection, simple and advanced Rotablator techniques, adjunctive imaging and pharmacotherapy, and management of complications.

350 pages; 71/2" x 9";
all figures in color

$59.95

with CD-ROM **$69.95**

TOUGH CALLS In Interventional Cardiology

Robert D. Safian, MD, and Mark Freed, MD

Unique instructional atlas contains over 200 interventional cases (with angiographic images), followed by detailed management recommendations from 40 leading experts representing 10 countries.

USA experts include: *Spencer King III, MD; William O'Neill, MD, Gary Roubin, MD, PhD; Marty Leon, MD; Eric Topol, MD; Donald Baim, MD; Richard Schatz*, MD and many more.

International experts include:
Antonio Columbo, MD (Italy); Nicolaus Reifert, MD (Germany); Patrick Serruys, MD, PhD (The Netherlands); Masakiyo Nobuyoshi, MD (Japan); Ulrich Sigwart, MD (England); Bernhard Meier, MD (Switzerland) and more.

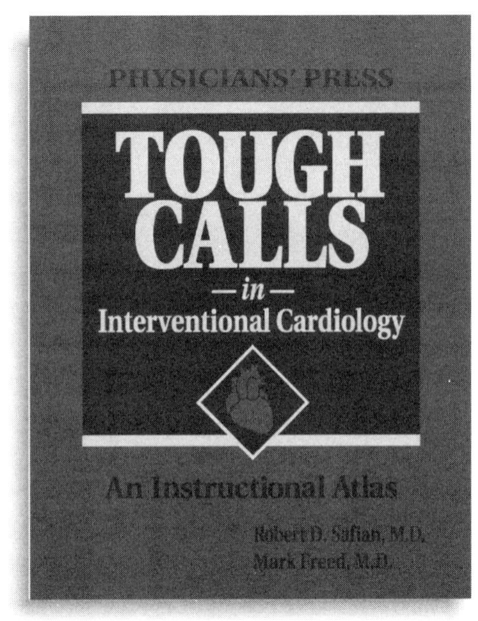

200 CASES IN ALL!

"The most unique and practical reference in the field! An outstanding way to receive multiple 'second opinions' about difficult cases and controversial issues."

Cindy Grines, MD

NOW IN SOFTCOVER!

700 pages; 9" x 12";

$69.95

The Device Guide – 2nd Edition

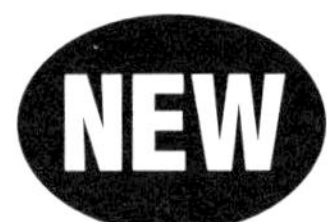

Robert D. Safian, MD, and Mark Freed, MD

OVER 500 PAGES! Labcoat pocket-sized reference offers step-by-step instruction, lesion-specific techniques, and troubleshooting for:

More Than 20 Stents • Atherectomy, Thrombectomy and Excimer Laser • Intravascular Ultrasound • Doppler FloWire, Pressure Wire, Guard Wire, Vascular Closure Devices • Intra-Aortic Balloon Pump • CPS

"An outstanding and completley unique publication that will certainly add greatly to patient care."

Martin Leon, MD

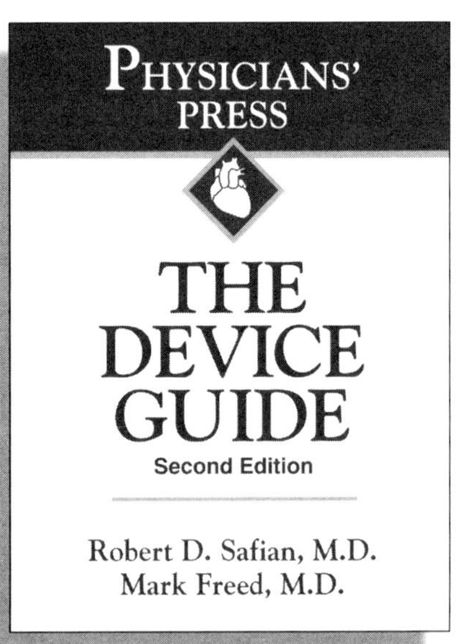

560 pages; 5" x 7";
Softcover; Fits Labcoat Pocket

$39.95

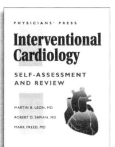

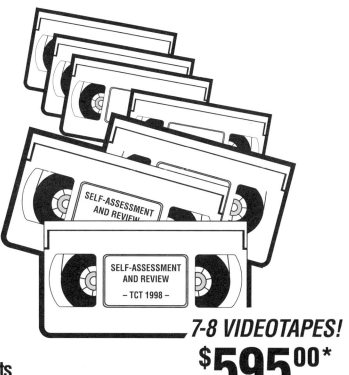

ORDERING INFORMATION

ELECTROCARDIOGRAPHY

ITEM	DESCRIPTION	PRICE (US Dollars)	
1	The Complete Guide to ECGs	$ 49.95	
2	The Complete Guide to ECGs Slide Set (100 slides)	69.95	
3	The ECG Criteria and ACLS Handbook	12.95	
3b	The Complete Guide to ECGs & Slide Set (Items 1 & 2)	104.95	**SAVE $15**

INTERVENTIONAL CARDIOLOGY

ITEM	DESCRIPTION	PRICE (US Dollars)	
4	The New Manual of Interventional Cardiology	84.95	
5	The New Manual of Interventional Cardiology Slide Series *(650 slides; 3-ring binder; protective slide jackets; paper copy of slides*	595.00	**SAVE $150**
6	Tough Calls in Interventional Cardiology – Soft Cover	69.95	
7	**The Device Guide-2nd Edition** *(All Sales Final*)*	**39.95***	
8	Guide to Rotational Atherectomy (with CD-ROM)	69.95	
9	Interventional Cardiology: Self-Assessment & Review	45.00	
10	The Stenter's Notebook	39.95	
11	The Stenter's Notebook Slide Series	49.95	
12	**NEW – Interventional Cardiology– Self-Assessment and Review** **2-day Minicourse from TCT X** (Washington D.C., Oct. '98) 40 lectures with self-assessment questions throughout on 12 hours of Super VHS tape. Includes testing sheets, and item #9 above ***Visit our website (www.physicianspress.com) for description, pricing and availablity for the following videotape series from TCT X:*** Stent Series; Unstable Ischemic Syndromes/Pharmacotherapy Series; Peripheral & Visceral Intervention Series	Entire Set: $ 595.00 Day 1 or Day 2 Tape: $ 350.00	

INTERVENTIONAL DISCOUNT PACKAGES

ITEM	DESCRIPTION	PRICE (US Dollars)	
13	Interventional Package I: Items 4, 6, & 7	164.95	**SAVE $30**
14	Interventional Package II: Items 4, 5, 6, & 7	749.95	**SAVE $120**
15	Interventional Package III: Items 4-11	1469.55	**SAVE $350**

OTHER TITLES

ITEM	DESCRIPTION	PRICE (US Dollars)
16	Essentials of Cardiovascular Medicine - unabridged	29.95
17	Essentials of Cardiovascular Medicine - abridged	12.95
18	Cardiovascular Disease in African-Americans (70 pg. monograph)	6.95
19	After Residency: The Young Physician's Guide to the Universe	9.95
20	The Magic of Children: A Celebration of Life, Love & Happiness	12.95
	***VISIT OUR WEB SITE (www.physicianspress.com) FOR INFORMATION, PRICING AND AVAILABLITY FOR THE FOLLOWING TITLES:** Essentials of Cardiovascular Medicine (2nd Edition); Quick Guide to Peripheral Vascular Stenting; Quick Guide to Emergency Medicine; Arrhythmia Essentials; The Complete Guide to Nuclear Cardiology; The Heart Failure Book; Antibiotic Essentials; Essentials of Infectious Diseases; Drug Essentials & Differential Diagnosis; The Psychiatrist's Little Book of Wisdom; Beyond Training: Mastering the Art of Contemporary Medicine; The Health Information Organizer	

FAX/MAIL ORDER FORM

TITLE	QUANTITY	TOTAL COST (US Dollars)

Sales Tax ____________
(Michigan residents add 6%; Canadian residents add 7% GST)

Shipping ____________
(Compute shipping charge based on chart below)

TOTAL (U.S. DOLLARS) $ ____________

4 Ways to Order:

By Phone:
(USA) (800) 642-5494
(Outside USA) (248) 616-3023

By Fax:
Fax order page to:
(248) 616-3003

By Mail: *Mail to:*
Physicians' Press
620 Cherry Street
Royal Oak, MI
USA 48073

By Internet:
www.physicianspress.com

TOTAL PURCHASE	USA	OUTSIDE USA*		
	UPS Ground; arrives 3–7 days	**US Postal Surface** Arrives 6–8 weeks	**US Postal Air** Arrives 10-14 Days	**Express Air** UPS, FEDEX, DHL arrives 2-5 Days
$1–35	Add $4	Add $10	Add $20	Add $30
$36–90	Add $7	Add $15	Add $30	Add $60
$91–150	Add $12	Add $20	Add $40	Add $75
$151–400	Add $14	Add $25	Add $50	Add $90
$401–750	Add $16	Add $30	Add $60	Add $120
$751–1000	Add $20	Add $35	Add $70	Add $150
$1000 +	Add $30	Add $50	Add $80	Add $180

** If shipping charges exceed those listed in the chart, you will be contacted for approval prior to shipment.*

For shipping outside USA, check one:
☐ Express Air ☐ US Postal Air ☐ US Postal Surface

☐ Check Enclosed *(US Dollars from US Bank)* ☐ Bill Me ☐ Credit Card: ☐ Visa ☐ MasterCard ☐ AMEX

☐ 3-Payment Plan:
Orders over $300, bill my credit card each month for 3 consecutive months.

Name: *(Please Print)* ____________________

Address: ____________________

____

Card No.: ____________________ Exp. Date: __________

Signature: ____________________ e-mail __________

Telephone *(important)*: ____________ FAX *(important)*: ____________

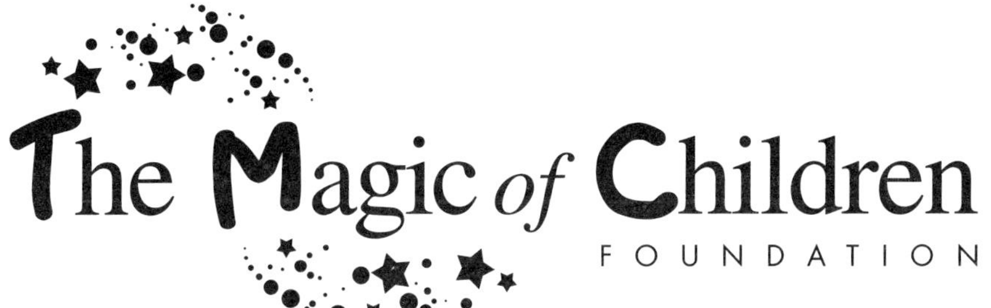

Planting the seeds for lifelong health and well-being

Dear Colleagues:

To help young people with the many challenges that confront them, we have established *The Magic of Children Foundation,* a new non-profit organization dedicated to promoting the physical, emotional, and social well-being of children.

Our flagship program, *Adopt-a-Doc™/ Adopt-a-Nurse™*, offers kindergartners through second-graders basic information about health, safety, and personal power. Doctors, nurses and other health care professionals will choose or be matched with a classroom that "adopts" them for the school year. Through monthly visits to the classroom, the doctors and nurses will present a highly acclaimed and tested health and safety curriculum of nine modules, each consisting of a presentation, experiential activities, and worksheet exercises.

By reaching children at an impressionable stage of life and by developing personal, trusting relationships with the volunteer doctors and nurses, the program seeks to instill children with positive health habits, personal safety skills, and the ability to resist peer pressure and manage their emotions in healthy, constructive ways. Other goals of the program include creating a meaningful and worthwhile opportunity for those who volunteer in the classrooms and developing relationships between schools, families and the medical community. Partial proceeds from all Physicians' Press titles go to *The Magic of Children Foundation.*

To learn more about *The Magic of Children Foundation* and the *Adopt-a-Doc™/Adopt-a-Nurse™* Program, you can either send us e-mail through our web site at: www.magicofchildren.org

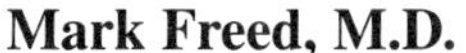

or write us at: The Magic of Children Foundation, 620 Cherry Street, Royal Oak, Michigan 48073.

Warmest regards and best wishes,

Mark Freed, M.D.
President and Editor-in-Chief
Physicians' Press
Founder and Chairman
The Magic of Children Foundation

THE MAGIC OF CHILDREN

Tell me a secret about Grandpa.

"He can take his hair off his head and spin it on his finger."

Charlene, age 5.

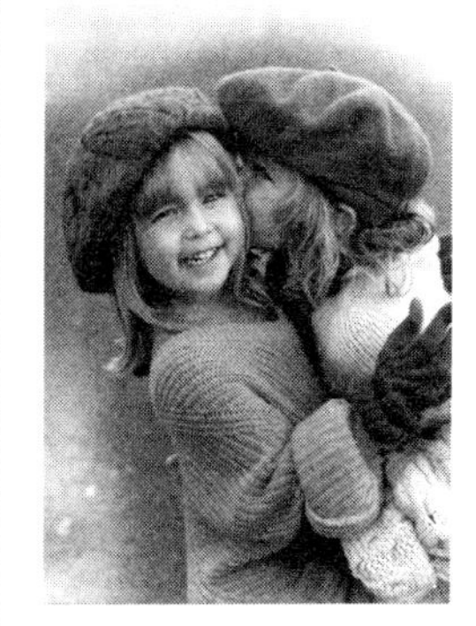

"A truly magical book of love and feelings that all families will want to share."

JACK CANFIELD, CO-AUTHOR
Chicken Soup for the Soul Series

Bring The Magic of Children Into the Lives of Those You Care About Most!

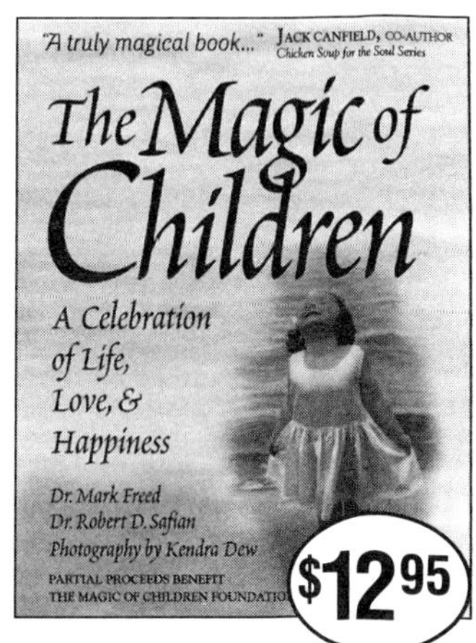

The Magic of Children by Drs. Mark Freed and Robert Safian is a warm and original collection of quotations and photographs that will tickle your funnybone and tug at your heartstrings as children share their thoughts and secrets about moms, dads, grandparents, brothers and sisters, and love and marriage. The authors also share touching and inspirational stories of hope and compassion drawn from their experiences as physicians.

Hardcover w/dust jacket; 6" x 7"; 160 pp.

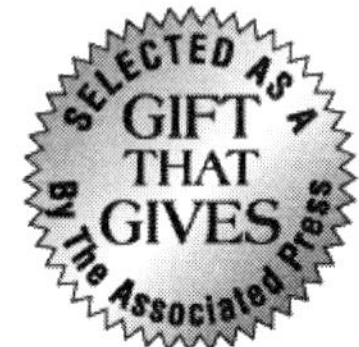

Partial Proceeds Benefit The Magic of Children Foundation

Available at Bookstores Everywhere (or call 1-800-642-5494, fax 248-616-3003 or visit www.magicofchildren.com)